Chronic Illness in Children

GEORGIA TRAVIS

Chronic Illness in Children

ITS IMPACT ON CHILD AND FAMILY

Stanford University Press
STANFORD, CALIFORNIA
1976

Stanford University Press
Stanford, California
© 1976 by the Board of Trustees of the
Leland Stanford Junior University
Printed in the United States of America
ISBN 0-8047-0893-2
LC 75-185

Preface

This book was written to provide social work practitioners and students with information about the psychosocial implications of various chronic illnesses in children. To know the practical problems facing family and child, the emotional burdens, and the effect of the illness on family relationships, the worker needs a framework of medical information. The medical data must be selected for their meaning to the patient group; they must be presented in lay terms and related to fundamentals of child development and family service. I had not been able to find a reference work meeting these requirements that I could recommend to students and workers, and I tried therefore to gather the necessary information and write the book myself.

It was a long task. Although I had worked many years in hospitals and community agencies, my experience could serve merely as a screen for the relevance of data, an amalgam to hold the information together, and a basis for synthesis. My contribution became largely that of a conduit for the experience and ideas of others. I am responsible, however, for the conclusions drawn.

Conviction about the importance of greater sensitivity to the problems of chronically ill children and their families, and a desire to share the ways they had found to ease burdens, prompted a multitude of persons to respond to my requests for information. Numerous California hospitals and community agencies opened their group meetings to me, gave individual staff members time to talk about their experiences, in some instances shared case records, arranged home visits, prepared the way for parents or foster parents to describe their experiences, and permitted me to observe children's activities. Librarians were equally generous in making possible the extensive bibliographic search.

Space prohibits my thanking more than those who contributed most substantially to this book. Those whose contributions of technical information have been used directly are credited in the body of the text. The names of many whose ideas are reported are given in footnotes as well as in the Notes section at the back of the book. The medical advisers are listed on pp. xv–xvi. These physicians gave hours of their time and thoughtful attention, gratis, in order that the purpose of the book might be fulfilled. Without them, a book based on medical information could not have been written. My gratitude is boundless. Other physicians deserve credit, too. Those who gave with unusual generosity over a period of time were Vincent Marenkovitch, M.D., former Director of the Pediatric Allergy Service of the Children's Hospital at Stanford; Oliver Nichols, M.D., former Chief of the Myelodysplasia Clinic, Orthopedic Hospital, Los Angeles; Gary E. Gathman, M.D., Associate Chief, Pediatric Cardiology, Department of Pediatrics of the Santa Clara Valley Medical Center; John H. Mazur, M.D., former Chief of the Cardiac Service at the Mercy Hospital in San Diego; and Bernice B. Widrow, M.D., former Medical Director of the Artificial Kidney Unit, El Camino Hospital, Mountain View, California.

I owe a particular debt to the staff of four institutions. Ruth Cox Brunings, Director of Social Work at Rancho Los Amigos Hospital in Downey, and the former Medical Director there, Vernon L. Nickel, M.D., gave me access to the current experiences and ideas of the staff and patients of their large rehabilitation hospital over a period of many months. Dr. David Kaplan, Director of Social Work, and Rose Grobstein, Chief Pediatric Social Worker, at the Stanford University Medical Center, not only shared with me much of their professional wisdom but gave me entrée to Stanford's pediatric staff and meetings. Harry Jennison, M.D., Medical Director of the Children's Hospital at Stanford; Miriam Pachacki, former Director of Social Work there; and Gerald Rubin, who followed in that position, afforded me a similar opportunity. Catherine Wilson, former Medical Social Worker at the Mercy Hospital in San Diego, arranged for me to volunteer at the Guadalupe Clinic, where I could observe and interview. Thanks to Henry Milton and Patricia Klein, former Director and teacher, respectively, of the Education Department of the San Diego Zoo, I was able to observe and interact with the handicapped children who took part in a special educational program there. Linda Tavazi, Director of Social Work at the Santa Clara Valley Medical Center, has given me access to her staff's experience. I want also to convey special thanks to Rosalie Friedman, Medical Social Worker at the Children's Hospital in Los Angeles; Betty Gitlin and Charles Hurt of the Social Service Department at the Orthopedic Hospital in Los Angeles; and Cecilia Mikkleson and Carol Levin, Clinical Social Workers at the University of California Medical Center in

PREFACE

San Francisco. Many other social workers, nurses, dieticians, and therapists at various institutions have contributed their valuable experiences to this book as well.

Kazuyoshi Ide, Public Health Social Work Consultant, California State Department of Health, and the medical, nursing, and social work staff of the Crippled Children's Services of Santa Clara County, gave me valuable information. The departments of public welfare and public health of San Diego, San Mateo, and Santa Clara counties, California, were very generous. I should like to thank especially Frederick B. Gillette, Director, Santa Clara County Department of Social Services, and his supervisors and staff in child welfare, adoptions, training, and medical care; and Frances M. Morrow, Program Deputy, Health Care Social Services, and Beatrice R. Moore, supervisor, Chope Community Hospital, San Mateo County Department of Public Health and Welfare.

Charles R. Hall, Associate Regional Commissioner for Community Services, San Francisco Regional Office of the Department of Health, Education, and Welfare; and Boyd M. Swartz, Program Officer, District Office and Professional Groups, provided information regarding Social Security and Public Social Service programs. The specialists who helped me understand the complexities of revenue-sharing and the current trends in public welfare are Elizabeth B. MacLatchie, consultant for Technical Assistance and Planning Associates, Ltd., Chicago; and Professor Jack Stumpf of the San Diego State University School of Social Work. To these persons, and to other colleagues, friends, and students who gave me stimulation and knowledge, I am most grateful. Among my former colleagues I am particularly indebted to Ernest and Irmgard Witte, whose lives inspire others to strive toward dedication and scholarship; and to Virginia Clary, whose judgment I value and who read the manuscript and made suggestions about my presentation of basic theory and practice in social work.

Leona Miu, Patient Services Coordinator of the Muscular Dystrophy Association of the Bay Area, contributed enormously to my understanding of the implications of muscular dystrophy. Jean Vavasseau and Aaron Smith, of the Los Angeles Sickle Cell Center and the Midpeninsula Sickle Cell Foundation, respectively, helped me to understand this disease and its meaning. Among other private health agencies who were especially helpful were the American Lung Association of San Diego and Imperial counties, which conducted a special program for asthmatic children and their parents; the Artificial Kidney Club of the South Bay Area; the American Heart Association; and the Northern California Diabetes Association and its branch in the Santa Clara Valley.

The parents and children who took part in these and similar organizations, and all those who recounted often painful and highly personal experiences in order that others might benefit, provided uniquely valuable insights. To them I offer my highest regard and deepest thanks.

Of the special education teachers and administrators who permitted me to observe children's classes and recreational activities and to learn about school programs, I am in special debt to Marjorie Abbott and Gail Rosenberry, Principal and Vice-Principal of the Chandler Tripp School of Santa Clara County.

Though this book doubtless has a Western bias, parochialism fortunately is unnecessary in a computerized age. Paul Hanson, skilled computer librarian at Stanford Lane Library, Stanford Medical Center, helped me to gain access to the storehouse of bibliographic data generated by "Medline," the Remote-Access Retrieval Service of the National Library of Medicine. The patient service of Eldora Pollex and Edna Graun, Santa Clara Valley Medical Center librarians, and that of the librarians of the San Diego and San Jose State Universities, have also been especially appreciated.

The research could not have been performed without preliminary grant no. MH 17213-01 from the National Institute of Mental Health in 1969–70, and financial assistance later from the Lois and Samuel Silberman Foundation. I am very grateful for the financial assistance, and even more for the faith and encouragement of the Silbermans and their consultant, Dr. Harold Lewis, Dean of the Hunter College School of Social Work, who read the entire manuscript and galley proof. C. M. Binger, M.D., a children's psychiatrist with expert knowledge of the emotional consequence of chronic illness, also read the galley proof, and to him too I am most grateful. And I must thank the Institute of Medical Research of Santa Clara Valley for administrative assistance.

To Miriam Pachacki, who contributed her special knowledge of psychotherapy with families of asthmatic children, and to Doris Harvey, who wrote a section beyond my competence (that on genetic transmission), I am indebted for their faith, knowledge, and friendship. And finally, participating in the transition of a manuscript to a book has been a pleasant and interesting experience thanks to William W. Carver, Executive Editor, and Elizabeth Spurr, Associate Editor, of Stanford University Press.

None of the contributors can be blamed for the biases that will become apparent to the reader. Something that appears to be a bias, but is not, is the use of "she" for worker and "he" for child. The usage is a grammatical convenience, to avoid pronoun confusion in referring to both worker and child in the same sentence. A real bias is the belief that behavior is formed in early life, is motivated by need, and must later manifest the effects of deprivation and trauma during the formative years. I am also biased in the direction of children's rights to health and security, a concept that sounds innocuous but involves hard decisions when it is followed to the end.

"Understanding comes only with information. One cannot completely understand a complicated problem in human relationships on the basis of common sense. It becomes the responsibility of all of us to provide a basis of understanding to our patients and students, and to their friends and relatives."* The physician who said this might have added: "—and to the social workers and others who strive to help."

* Robert Solow, M.D., "The Emotional and Social Aspects of Muscular Dystrophy," paper presented at a Symposium on Muscular Dystrophy for Special Education Personnel, September 25, 1971, Muscular Dystrophy Association of America, Los Angeles.

Contents

Medical Advisers   xv

1. *Introduction*   1

   Underlying assumptions, 1. Size and distribution of the problem, 4. Organization and use of the book, 7.

2. *A Conceptual Foundation for Work with Handicapped Children*   10

   Basic premises about human life, 11. Basic premises in child development, 21. The significance of experience, 36.

3. *The Experience of Chronic Illness in Childhood*   42

   Effects of the character of the illness on family and child, 43. Effects of the family's size, structure, and relationships, 49. Effects of age and disruption of basic childhood tasks, 57. Effects of the child's reaction to the stress of illness, 64. Effects of hospitalization, 70.

4. *Community Resources*   75

   Medical care, 76. Financial aid, 81. Public social services, 84. Homemaker services, 88. Day care, 89. Foster home care, 91. Adoption, 98. Collaboration with members of the health team, 104.

5. *The Unborn Child and the Mother*   119

   High-risk mothers: demography and definition, 120. Psychosocial risk factors, 122. Medical risk factors, 135. Prevention or termination of pregnancy, 144. Prevention of genetic disease, 152. Normal needs during pregnancy, 157. Psychological needs, or the foundation for maternal care, 160.

6. *Asthma*   164

   THE MEDICAL REALITIES, 165. What is an allergy? 165. Nature and symptoms of asthma, 166. Cause of attacks, 168. Psychological origins, 168. Treatment, 171. Outlook, 174.

PSYCHOSOCIAL IMPLICATIONS, 174. Family adjustment, 175. Quality of medical care, 176. Dietary and housekeeping problems, 177. Moving, 180. Pets, 181. Financial problems, 182. Foster care, 183. School-age problems, 183. The child's personality, 187.

Severe, emotionally triggered asthma, 189. Psychodynamics, 189. The parent-child relationship, 191. The treatment approach, 192.

7. *Chronic Kidney Diseases*   195

THE MEDICAL REALITIES, 196. The kidneys and their function, 196. Tests of kidney function, 197. Recurrent urinary tract infections, 198. Malformations or congenital anomalies, 199. Glomerulonephritis, 200. Nephrosis or nephrotic syndrome, 201. Chronic renal failure, 203. Complications, 203. Diet, 205. Dialysis, 206. Transplantation, 208.

PSYCHOSOCIAL IMPLICATIONS, 211. The young child, 211. Latency and early adolescence, 215. Dialysis and transplantation, 218. Post-transplant adjustment, 229. Family reactions to dialysis and transplant, 230.

8. *Congenital Heart Disease*   233

THE MEDICAL REALITIES, 233. Defects and their damage, 234. Symptoms and diagnosis, 235. Surgical treatment, 237. The surgical risk, 239. Medical management, 241. Common defects and the outlook for treatment, 242.

PSYCHOSOCIAL IMPLICATIONS, 247. Financial problems, 248. Transportation, 249. The working mother, 250. Family adjustment, 252. Discipline, 257. The effects of long-term disability, 259. The surgical experience, 260. Growth retardation, 262. Sibling relationships, 263. School adjustment and social relationships, 263. The multihandicapped child, 265.

9. *Cystic Fibrosis*   269

THE MEDICAL REALITIES, 270. Nature and symptoms, 270. Treatment, 272. Outlook, 274.

PSYCHOSOCIAL IMPLICATIONS, 275. Family adjustment, 275. Financial problems, 277. Housing, 278. Household assistance and foster care, 279. The parents' anxiety, 280. The child's anxiety, 281. Special problems of adolescents, 282.

10. *Head Injury*   287

THE MEDICAL REALITIES, 288. The brain and its functions, 288. Nature and course of recovery, 289. Aftereffects, 291.

PSYCHOSOCIAL IMPLICATIONS, 292. The early stage, 293. The later stage, 295. Special problems of adolescents, 296. Development of needed resources, 298.

11. *Hemophilia*   300

THE MEDICAL REALITIES, 301. Pattern of inheritance, 301. Course of the disease, 301. Treatment, 302. Dental care, 304.

CONTENTS

PSYCHOSOCIAL IMPLICATIONS, 304. Family problems, 305. The child's adjustment, 312. The worker's role in the community, 318. Special problems in adoption, 318.

12. *Juvenile Rheumatoid Arthritis* — 320

THE MEDICAL REALITIES, 321. Onset and symptoms, 321. Course and prognosis, 322. Complications, 323. Treatment, 324.

PSYCHOSOCIAL IMPLICATIONS, 327. Family adjustment, 327. Financial problems, 329. Housing and transportation, 330. Problems with treatment, 331. Pain, 335. Limitation of activity, 337. School attendance problems, 340. Personality, 341.

13. *Juvenile Diabetes* — 343

THE MEDICAL REALITIES, 344. Onset, symptoms, and course, 344. Treatment goals, 346. Insulin injections, 347. Testing urine, 349. Nutrition, 350. Insulin reaction and coma, 351. Long-term complications, 353.

PSYCHOSOCIAL IMPLICATIONS, 354. Financial problems, 355. Medical care, 357. The child's adjustment, 358. Family adjustment, 361. Managing away from home, 363. Marriage, sex, and pregnancy, 365. Resources for diabetic children, 366.

14. *Leukemia* — 367

THE MEDICAL REALITIES, 367. The disease, its cause and distribution, 367. Course and outlook, 368. The pains and limitations of treatment, 370.

PSYCHOSOCIAL IMPLICATIONS, 373. The family and the medical team, 374. The crisis of diagnosis, 377. The phenomenon of denial, 380. Informing the child, 381. Financial problems, 384. The family and the first remission, 385. Sibling relationships, 387. Adjustments and anxieties of the child, 388. School, 392. The family and the early terminal stage, 394. The dying child, 399.

15. *Muscular Dystrophy: Duchenne's Form* — 403

THE MEDICAL REALITIES, 404. Cause and hereditary pattern, 404. Symptoms, diagnosis, and course, 405. Treatment, 406. Mental status, 409.

PSYCHOSOCIAL IMPLICATIONS, 410. The family, 411. The physical burden, 413. Transportation, 416. Finances, 417. Coping with the fatality of the disease, 418. Effects on the child, 420.

16. *Sickle Cell Anemia* — 432

THE MEDICAL REALITIES, 433. Sickle cell disease, 433. Significance of sickle cell trait, 434. Pattern of inheritance, 435. Symptoms, course, and outlook, 435. Treatment, 437.

PSYCHOSOCIAL IMPLICATIONS, 438. Stigma and lack of information, 438. Financial problems, 439. Housing and diet, 440. Medical care, 442. Hospitalization, 444. Family adjustment, 445. School, 448. Effect on personality, 449. Implications for marriage and childbearing, 451. Foster care and adoption, 453. Sources of information, 454.

17. *Spina Bifida: Myelomeningocele Form*   455

    THE MEDICAL REALITIES, 456. Symptoms, 456. Outlook, 458. Treatment, 460. Management of bladder and bowel incontinence, 462. Coordination of treatment, 465.

    PSYCHOSOCIAL IMPLICATIONS, 465. Family adjustment, 466. Financial problems, 470. Incontinence, 471. Diet, 473. School, 474. Adolescence, 475. Out-of-home care, 477.

18. *Spinal Cord Injury*   481

    THE MEDICAL REALITIES, 481. The spinal cord, 482. Treatment, 483. Complications, 485. Bladder control, 486. Bowel control, 489. Sexual problems of the paraplegic youth, 491.

    PSYCHOSOCIAL IMPLICATIONS, 491. The person and his grief, 491. Family adjustment, 493. Financial problems, 494. Recreation, 495. Vocational preparation, 496.

Notes   499

Index   541

Medical Advisers

The following specialists, all in California, guided the author in understanding the medical realities that underlie the meaning and impact of a disease for both family and child, and generously edited the synthesis of medical content to assure accuracy.

5. *The Unborn Child and the Mother.* Bernice Giansiracusa, M.D., Director of Public Health; and former Chief, Maternal and Child Health, Santa Clara County Health Department, San Jose

Material on prevention of genetic disease by Howard M. Cann, M.D., Associate Professor of Pediatrics, Stanford University School of Medicine

6. *Asthma.* Minoru Yamate, M.D., Clinical Associate Professor of Pediatrics, Stanford University Medical Center; and Consultant, Pediatrics Allergy, Children's Hospital at Stanford

7. *Chronic Kidney Diseases.* Donald E. Potter, M.D., Assistant Professor of Pediatrics, University of California School of Medicine, San Francisco; and Director, Pediatric Dialysis Unit, University of California Medical Center, San Francisco

8. *Congenital Heart Disease.* Paul R. Lurie, M.D., Professor of Pediatrics, University of Southern California School of Medicine; and Head, Division of Cardiology, Children's Hospital, Los Angeles

9. *Cystic Fibrosis.* Birt Harvey, M.D., Associate Clinical Professor of Pediatrics, Stanford University School of Medicine; and former Chief, Pulmonary Disease Service, Children's Hospital at Stanford

10. *Head Injury.* Joyce Brink, M.D., Associate Clinical Professor of Pediatrics, University of Southern California School of Medicine; and Chief, Pediatric Service, Rancho Los Amigos Hospital, Downey

11. *Hemophilia.* T. John Gribble, M.D., Senior Attending Physician and Clinical Associate Professor of Pediatrics, Division of Hematology, Stanford University School of Medicine; and Chief, Hemophilia Service, Children's Hospital at Stanford (see also 14 and 16, below)

12. *Juvenile Rheumatoid Arthritis.* John J. Miller III, M.D., Ph.D., Chief, Rheumatic Disease Service, Children's Hospital at Stanford

13. *Juvenile Diabetes.* Robert O. Christiansen, M.D., Assistant Professor of Pediatrics and Human Development, Stanford University School of Medicine; and Director, Pediatric Metabolic Service, Stanford University Medical Center

14. *Leukemia.* T. John Gribble (see under 11, above)

15. *Muscular Dystrophy: Duchenne's Form.* Hans J. Zwang, M.D., Director, Muscular Dystrophy Clinic, Herrick Memorial Hospital, Berkeley

16. *Sickle Cell Anemia.* T. John Gribble (see under 11, above)

17. *Spina Bifida: Myelomeningocele Form.* Luigi Luzzatti, M.D., Professor of Pediatrics, Stanford University School of Medicine; and Director, Birth Defects Center, Stanford University Medical Center

18. *Spinal Cord Injury.* E. Shannon Stauffer, M.D., Associate Clinical Professor of Surgery (Orthopedics), University of Southern California School of Medicine; and Chief, Spinal Injuries Service, Rancho Los Amigos Hospital, Downey

Material on severe, emotionally triggered asthma by Miriam Pachacki, A.C.S.W., Clinical Social Worker, Director of Fair Oaks Mental Health Center, Sunnyvale, Santa Clara County Mental Health

Material on prevention of genetic disease by Doris Harvey, Research Assistant, Palo Alto

Chronic Illness in Children

CHAPTER ONE

Introduction

THIS BOOK views the child with long-term illness as a biopsychosocial being who functions as a whole in a changing matrix of relationships and events to which he responds and upon which he acts. The task is elusive, because of the constancy of change. A chronic illness grows better or worse; the increasing age of the child places his illness in a different developmental framework; the parents bend, straighten, or collapse under the stress of the child's illness and other events and relationships; siblings and friends, schools and neighborhoods change. "The picture of an arrow snapped in flight, frozen forever against the sky, conveys nothing of this great moment in the arrow's existence."[1] Within the limitations of the endeavor, the book examines some of the more prevalent long-term illnesses and conditions of childhood, and attempts to describe what these illnesses mean for children and their families. Throughout, the book emphasizes the crucial role of the social component in both adaptation and rehabilitation.

UNDERLYING ASSUMPTIONS

Several theses underlie my approach. The first is that the chronically ill child spends most of his life in the community, not in a hospital, and thereby comes under the purview of all who work with families and children. Physicians come rarely to the home. Modern hospital practice limits stays to an absolute minimum. Long-term convalescent institutions for children are nearing extinction under the burden of staggering medical costs. Money for the child's food, lodging, medicine, transportation, and supervision comes from the parents or community agencies. The administration of medication, preparation of special diet, transportation to the doctor, supervision of schoolwork, and often the performance of physical therapy are provided not by hospital staff but by mother, teacher, baby-sitter, day-care operator, or foster mother.

The chronically ill child, then, is not the concern of doctors and nurses alone. He is the concern of social workers, teachers, psychologists, educational counselors, recreational workers, eligibility clerks, day-care personnel, foster parents, adoptive parents, public and private health agency personnel, clergy, and all of the others who will be working with him or his family in one way or another through the long course of his illness.

My second thesis was well framed by Selma Fraiberg,[2] who in a speech given at the 1973 graduation ceremonies of the Smith College School of Social Work remarked that "those qualities we call 'human'—the capacity for enduring love and the exercise of conscience—are not given in human biology; they are the achievement of the earliest human partnership between a child and his parents." War had taught us, she reminded her audience, that life-threatening events were not as destructive to children's minds and emotions as separation from their parents. But of course "it is not only in times of war that children are deprived of mothering and family nurture." She described the permanent impairments in capacity to love, learn, judge, and abide by the tenets of the human community that occur in persons who knew shifting and uncertain partnerships in the formative period of personality.

Like war, chronic illness and ugly defects are often shattering events, especially because they separate infants and young children from their parents, both physically and emotionally. Enabling the parents to love and sustain the child is an obligation of those who would prevent later psychic distortions. The force of the relationship is brought home to us with particular clarity by the research that documents Mrs. Fraiberg's statements. In summarizing various research projects, Bloom reports the consistent finding that "variation in the environment has greatest quantitative effect on a characteristic at its most rapid period of change and least effect on the characteristic during the least rapid period of change."[3] Infancy and early childhood are the periods of most rapid change. In other words, early childhood is the time when trauma can be most severe and *also the time when we can be of greatest help*.

The third underlying assumption has to do with the nature of service. The book addresses itself primarily to an understanding of the problems that chronic illness creates, not to the art of helping. No one writer's philosophy or method could apply to all who strive to help chronically ill children and their families. Agencies have a great variety of functions. In addition, social work and related counseling fields are sprouting a myriad of approaches, as the human services struggle to find means of helping that suit the change and turmoil in society. Nevertheless, no reference work written by a social worker for practitioners in the human services can avoid some interjection of appropriate ways of response to problems discussed. My assumptions are based on a philosophy of practice that combines services with counseling, or "middle range" practice, the objectives of which

Hollis defines as "to enable change to occur in the individual(s) or in the situation or both."⁴ It further assumes that there is a great deal of what is sometimes called "brokerage" and coordination involved, and action in behalf of persons who are unable to perform all needed tasks for themselves. The only exception to middle-range practice is a section contributed by an expert on psychotherapy with families of children with severe, emotionally triggered asthma.

A fourth premise is that chronic illness is not an entity but an umbrella. Each illness is unique, and thus has a different impact on the child and his family. Arthritis means something different than asthma; leukemia does not have the same implications as diabetes. It follows that the psychosocial constellations differ because each facet of a system acts on the other facets, or, to use Erikson's seemingly abstruse but actually succinct statement, "An item in one process gains relevance by giving significance to and receiving significance from items in the other."⁵

To make this explicit, an understanding of the medical problem is essential to effective social service. Why? Because one cannot assess mental health without knowing whether sleeplessness, pain, fear, death, debt, or physical burden exist; one cannot assess financial need without knowing the cost of drugs, hospitalization, transportation, diet, and the way the breadwinner is affected. The specifics of a given illness and resources for treatment in many cases determine whether the child will live. The symptoms and manner of treatment determine the extent of trauma he will be required to incorporate into his personality and, to some extent, when. The characteristics of the child's illness determine whether he has the sensory and motor opportunities to learn, to know the enrichment of communication, to compete with his peers, to play his accustomed social role. They determine whether he can meet life vigorously or only in a debilitated fashion; whether he is free to explore and express his desires, or chained to pain or bed or chair or house.

The limitations imposed by a child's long-term illness and the requirements of getting well or making maximum adjustment greatly affect the plans of the entire family. The budget, housing, transportation, educational plans, need for supplemental resources, relatives' involvement, amount of free energy available to child and parents, and the feasibility of goals are influenced by the sick child's needs and physical abilities.

One cannot help a marriage, counsel a youth, determine a foster or adoptive home placement, guide toward rehabilitation, or sustain or console without knowing the role changes, family burdens, and distortions that long-term illness in one family member creates.

The final premise can be stated briefly. Chronic illness is the nation's number one health problem. Billions are spent on medical care and rehabilitation. Acute illness requiring miracle drugs or surgery depends for cure primarily on the physician. Chronic illness depends for maximum recovery on the patient and his family. Chronic illness needs good medical guidance, to be sure, but the dietary restriction, activity limitation, and life readjustment so often essential are performed not by the doctor but by the patient and his family. Many can make these adjustments alone, without help. Many others cannot. The contribution of social welfare is not only incalculable, it is essential.

SIZE AND DISTRIBUTION OF THE PROBLEM

How big is the problem? No one knows how many chronically ill children there are in the United States. Definitions vary, and surveys have serious weaknesses. Comparisons are not valid because of differences in definition. Some studies are of limited populations, and their findings may not apply nationally. Figures on specific conditions quoted with fundraising in mind may enlarge the boundaries of the probable numbers of persons affected. Some studies discuss "incidence," or new cases in a given period; others, "prevalence," or the accumulation of all cases in the population at one time. Rough estimates therefore are the most to be hoped for.

A few things *are* known. One is that the youngest and oldest are weakest, and thus at greatest risk of disease. Because of the vulnerability of the very young, many infants with potential long-term illness die. Nonetheless the rate of chronic conditions among children increases with age—for the development, diagnosis, and accumulation of many chronic conditions in the population take time. The largest number is in the group aged 10–16.[6]

The National Health Survey, a continuous survey based on household interviews, is the best source of information, and for the year 1966–67 it reported that 23 percent of children under 17 years of age had one or more chronic conditions.[7]

The National Health Survey provided physical examinations for a probability sample of children 6–11 years of age in 1963–65 and of youths 12–17 years of age in 1966–70. The findings showed that *one child in eight and one youth in five* had "one or more *significant* cardiovascular, neurological, musculoskeletal, or other physical abnormalities."[8]

Despite the serious nature of these findings, a chronic condition or significant abnormality may not disable or seriously handicap. According to the American Public Health Association, "A child is considered to be handicapped if he cannot within limits play, learn, work, or do things other children his age can do; if he is hindered in achieving his full physical, mental, and social potentialities."[9]

In a study of 18-year-old youths rejected by Selective Service in 1965, 15 percent were rejected because of chronic handicapping conditions. It was estimated that a third of these conditions could have been prevented or corrected if found before the young men had reached age nine, and almost two-thirds if found before age 15. Between 20 and 40 percent of children in low-income families suffer from one or more chronic conditions, of which only 40 percent were said to be under treatment, in an analysis presented in August 1974 by the Department of Health, Education, and Welfare in connection with a description of the Medicaid Early Diagnosis and Periodic Screening program for children.[10]

Handicap or abnormality is not synonymous with chronic illness. A child with a severe mental or neurological handicap may be well physically. Thus, in defining chronic illness, we must combine the long-term aspect of the chronic "condition" with the functional disability of the "handicap," and add the concept of disease, an active process.

Mattsson, who has studied the problem widely, uses the following definition: "Long-term or chronic illness refers to a disorder with a protracted course which can be progressive and fatal, or associated with a relatively normal life span despite impaired physical and mental functioning. Such a disease frequently shows periods of acute exacerbations requiring intensive medical attention."[11]

Some gauge of the size of the problem does stem from activity limitation. About 1.4 million children in the United States under 17 years of age have "activity limitation," and more than 2 million handicapped children require care.[12]

Many of the children with chronic conditions severe enough to limit activity have birth defects or congenital malformations. One reliable study reports an incidence of 7 percent of congenital malformations in a group of 6,000 children followed until one year of age.[13] Only one-half had been discovered at birth; how many more birth defects might show up later was not predicted, nor how many of those with malformations would live to be over a year old. Another report states that "of the viable infants born, between 4 percent and 7 percent have moderately serious birth defects." This same report states that the Secretary of the Department of Health, Education, and Welfare reported to the President in 1963 on the health of schoolchildren, saying, "By educational standards, it is usually estimated that about 12 percent of the children of school age are in need of special education because of handicapping conditions."[14] This of course vastly overstates the number of chronically ill because it includes the developmentally handicapped. Mattsson states that if only serious chronic illness of primarily physical origin is considered, surveys show that 7 to 10 percent of all children are afflicted.[15]

Limited population surveys shed some light on the problem to the extent that they can project to wider populations. An Erie County (New York) survey used medical and school records and those of public agencies, and concerned itself primarily with chronic illnesses, such as cystic fibrosis, muscular dystrophy, nephrosis, and arthritis. The study analyzed every known hospitalized case of seven chronic diseases from 1946 to 1961. Diabetes had the highest rate among hospitalized White children, 57.2 per 100,000 children under 16, and sickle cell anemia by far the highest prevalence rate for Black children, 190 per 100,000. (Asthma, the leading cause of school absence among children and the most prevalent chronic disease, was not included in the analysis.[16] The National Health Survey reported one in ten children as having a chronic allergic condition.[17])

Another in-depth study of a small population estimated that 162 children per 1,000 had chronic disabling conditions, including speech and hearing defects.[18] National Health Survey information taken from household interviews about the prevalence of heart disease shows that six children under 17 years of age per 1,000 persons have congenital heart defects, with a larger proportion among preschool than schoolchildren.[19]

General statistics are not only inadequate; they can be misleading. A larger number of children with chronic conditions are reported in household surveys by higher-income household respondents. The more affluent mothers have opportunities to take their children to physicians for diagnosis early and are more concerned with preventive care. One gross misinterpretation results from statistics that poor children under 15 spend fewer days at restricted activity than those from more affluent families, and that they also spend fewer days in bed.[20] This does not mean that "Children in well-to-do families experienced many more acute conditions than the children in low-income families," as one sociologist reports (the word "experienced" to mean psychological as well as physical experience); instead, it very likely shows that mothers at work, preoccupied with problems of poverty, or uneducated in preventive care, are less apt to see that their children maintain activity restriction or to report them ill when they have colds, flu, or other self-limiting health problems. The actual number of school-loss days owing to illness is inversely related to income (6.2 days per year for children in families with income under $3,000 vs. 4.6 days for children from families with $15,000 or more income).[21]

The poor are underrepresented in some specialty centers, such as those for hemophilia and renal dialysis and those in some mental-retardation agencies, despite the lack of any known genetic reasons, and are underrepresented as well in centers for cystic fibrosis, where a genetic disposition for Caucasians does exist. Many of these children who attend specialty clinics or who concern pediatricians or hospital staffs are children of working parents who maintain moderate standards of living.

However, the death rate for babies of low-income Black families is nearly double that for White infants; obvious serious impairments such as paralysis and blindness are reported more frequently by the poor than by the more affluent; hospitalization is less frequent for poor children but their stays are longer; and the lack of comprehensive effective care for poor children is so widely documented that Ellen Winston, then U.S. Commissioner of Welfare, said in 1965, "The health status of needy children remains a national disgrace."[22]

Too many variables exist to permit accurate analysis of children's conditions by socioeconomic class. However, the general trends are all in the same direction. In summarizing the results of the physical examinations performed as part of the National Health Survey, the report stated, "A significant relationship was evident between family income and the health of these children and youths. The proportion found abnormal on examination decreased consistently as family income level increased."[23] In a speech before the National Health Forum, Commissioner Howard Newman said, "In certain areas, a child in a poor family has only half the chance of those with higher incomes to live to his or her first birthday. . . . Poor children have three times more heart disease, six times more hearing defects, five times more mental illnesses than the more affluent."[24] And we know that by the time of adulthood, a direct relationship exists between income, health, and life expectancy.[25]

ORGANIZATION AND USE OF THE BOOK

Chapters 2, 3, and 4 deal with the subject of chronic illness as a whole. Chapter 2 discusses the concepts of human life and child development that are implicit in the later discussions of the chronically ill child. This is done not only to prepare the reader for the philosophy he may expect in the text but to anchor firmly the idea that a sick child is, first of all, a child and a child in a family. The third chapter is a synthesis of the medical conditions and practical considerations taken up in the later chapters; it seeks to identify the shared and the different psychosocial meanings and problems of various disease entities, and to discuss some of the recurring problems. Chapter 4 explores the major social provisions that may be available to relieve stress in the families of chronically ill children.

Chapter 5, on prevention, focuses on the child between conception and birth—or, in other words, on the mother. It is oriented particularly to the needs of workers or students concerned with pregnant teenage girls, or with families in which the mother is pregnant. This chapter includes a special section prepared by a social worker with the help of a geneticist, as well as a brief summary of genetic transmission and the diagnosis of transmissible disorders.

Eleven of the final 13 chapters deal with representative chronic disease conditions, two with the residual problems of common accidents. This portion, the heart of the book, is long but not comprehensive. One might ask about the omissions. It has seemed useful to concentrate on the active, changing, physical diseases, because their psychosocial meaning has not been presented elsewhere as fully as has that of the static handicaps, such as cerebral palsy, blindness, and mental retardation. The seemingly curious inclusion of two accidents in a book about the problems of childhood disease is due to their relative newness and the paucity of information about their psychosocial implications. Spinal cord injury replaces poliomyelitis as a major cause of paraplegia and quadriplegia, with the added tragedy of incontinence. Head injury is of special interest; the problems differ from those of children with brain damage from birth, because of the sudden, radical, and permanent change in the lives of the affected children and their families.

The opening or summary chapters may be used by teachers or in-service training supervisors who are preparing their students or workers to approach the problem of children's chronic illness in general. Chapter 3, on the experience of illness, is especially important as a background for single chapters on the problems created by specific diseases. However, a busy student or worker, particularly one grounded in the basic materials, can open the book to one of the later chapters about a particular problem and find much of the information that she will need in understanding what the child and family may be going through; she will find clues to the significance of remarks or behaviors that may need to be pursued. She need not read the other chapters, since each is designed to stand virtually alone. Some topics are necessarily treated at several different points in the volume. The Contents pages and the Index should enable the reader to locate all of the contexts of a given topic, and the Notes section provides suggestions for further reading.

A recurrent subject touched upon in different guises is that of bioethics, or the philosophy of life and death. In Chapter 5, on prevention, amniocentesis and abortion are discussed, as are contraception and sterilization. The prolongation of life—the obverse of these topics—is discussed at length in the kidney disease chapter, through the account of dialysis and transplantation. Whether the family should be given the right to permit a child to die, and at what age a child should be able to make his own decision about time of death, are mentioned in connection with dialysis and with the treatment of leukemia. Passive euthanasia, or withholding surgery that may save or prolong life, most closely approaches the most controversial of all subjects, active euthanasia, which enters into the consideration of children with multiple birth defects, like those occurring in rubella syndrome and spina bifida.

The issue of bioethics is most often raised in connection with aging, suicide, and intractable pain in adults, but one cannot think long and carefully about chronic illness in children without encountering the problem. The reader should expect to find himself disagreeing, perhaps strongly, with the way I have treated certain topics. In this difficult and emotional area I am of course no more an authority than the reader; each person has his own ideas about the right to life and the right to death. The more experience one accumulates with painful, miserable lives, the more one wonders about quality of life as opposed to length of life; many who work in hospitals and watch children suffer are concerned most deeply about quality.

The "God-squads" that are more and more coming into being should include human services workers who know or are involved with the family. A substantial literature has accumulated on bioethics. Those who wish to read about the subject may want to look at Daniel C. Maguire's *Death by Choice* (Garden City, N.Y.: Doubleday, 1974), Edward Shil, *Life or Death* (Seattle: University of Washington Press, 1968), and the Quaker presentation of the issues involved, *Who Shall Live?* (American Friends Service Committee; New York: Hill and Wang, 1970).

The writer's personal bias is toward prevention. This bias stands out in several contexts, such as in the discussion of the mating of two persons with known recessive genes for the same disease, or of increasing the size of a family where the mother is a demonstrated carrier of sex-linked genetic disease. Where most social workers would opt for complete personal freedom of the parents in mating, I interject the unborn child's right to avoid a miserable life. Needless to say, this does not imply approval of compulsion—the forcing of the worker's own religion, politics, or philosophy of eugenics on a client—but neither does it mean that the worker has no religious belief, political preference, or philosophical values. I propose conferences of all who are concerned with the child when decisions must be made about life or death, in order that the personal biases of the different members will be balanced one against the other, and in order that the pooling of knowledge will yield the greatest wisdom.

CHAPTER TWO

A Conceptual Foundation for Work with Handicapped Children

HANDICAPPED CHILDREN share the characteristics of other children; and all children share the characteristics of the human species. The social implications of the diseases or disabilities of children therefore rest upon broad assumptions about the nature of people, and especially about how children develop. Theories differ, however, and they are multitudinous. Only a few can be offered here.

Personal predilections influence selection. The theories to be presented spring from the writer's view of man as a biopsychosocial organism who is in constant interaction with his environment. A further winnowing of the range of concepts occurs in response to their relevance in understanding and helping sick children and their families. For example, the concept of experience has been selected because the book is about the ways children and families experience the child's chronic illness; the concept of stress, because illness is stress.

Unfortunately, each of the concepts presented is the subject of volumes, and adherents of different approaches have outlined their theses in separate vocabularies; practicality prevents presenting them as their various purists would demand. Fortunately, the concepts used are generally familiar. The admittedly superficial summaries in this chapter are buttressed with references, so that those interested may turn to the sources themselves. The material presented seeks merely to lay out for the reader the general ideas involved and to select certain elements that seem especially to impinge on work with sick or handicapped children.

Six concepts are presented that apply to all human life. These are the importance of preventing disability, the psychosomatic or unitary approach to individuals, the social systems concept, the determinants of stress, the concept and nature of crisis, and dependence as opposed to independence. Selected ideas about child development, drawn from psychodynamic and learning theory, follow. A final discussion draws together general factors determining the effects of experience on the individual—the experience of receiving help, as well as the experiences that accompany illness.

BASIC PREMISES ABOUT HUMAN LIFE

Childhood as a Period of Prevention

When nature substituted socialization for jaws and claws as a means of man's survival, she provided him with a long childhood. Man needs a long time to learn the skills he will require, having no in-dwelling weapons but the potential of a large brain pan. The family thus became a necessary corollary to long childhood, providing protection during the long learning period and forging, through its interrelationships, an individual capable of loving and helping others and contributing his share to his society.

Nature further improved the learning opportunity of childhood by making it a time when impressions sink deep. The younger and more helpless the child, the more imperative that he learn quickly, if he is to survive. Research confirms that at no other time does man learn so much so fast, for at no other time is he so open to imprint. The earliest time of life and the other times of rapid growth are the periods when man is most vulnerable to experience.[1]

This vulnerability of the young to experience, known proverbially in terms of "as the twig is bent,"[2] means that the bruised twig becomes the warped tree. Human services workers are concerned, therefore, with the prevention of unnecessary pain or limitations of movement, intelligence, or sensory experience. We are concerned to prevent the actuality and derivatives of terror, insecurity, and perception of parents as untrustworthy and of grown-ups as pain-inducers. We are concerned that parents and siblings should not be taxed beyond their capacities by the physical burdens or grotesqueries of an abnormal or ill family member. We are concerned, in short, that no one should suffer unnecessary physical or mental misery. Positively speaking, the central interest of social work is helping to "develop the capacity and the opportunity to lead personally satisfying and socially useful lives."[3] Social workers and other helping persons, therefore, are concerned with preventing illness or handicap and minimizing the effects of what cannot be prevented.

In practice, this concern sometimes shrinks into the background. Except for some child welfare and child guidance workers, most community agency staff relate primarily to the parents or foster parents. The marital discord, lack of funds, imminent eviction, incarceration, desertion, depression, psychosis, or other problems that bring parents to the agency tend to absorb the worker's attention. The baby with earache presents himself not as a person with *otitis media* who can be prevented from developing into a deaf person, but as a crying distraction for whom the worker is vaguely sorry and whose trip to clinic will require extra carfare and a delay for the parents from the main business at hand.

Are social workers callous and shortsighted? No, merely human. Concentrating on several things at once, especially when one of them may be an emergency, is difficult. And prevention is not dramatic. Further, children do not verbalize well, they are incapable of abstractions, they are in the shadow of the parents and in the background of the interview. They do not stand out as the adults of tomorrow whose lives are being shaped today.

In addition, the sick or handicapped child may seem to be the province of some other profession—that of the nurse or physician or hospital. Communication with members of other professional and health agencies itself may raise barriers. Not only does a real problem exist sometimes in working with other professions, but the worker may be uncomfortable in the presence of illness or handicap.

Thus, despite ready agreement on the importance of childhood, implementation of preventive measures requires conscious major effort. The busy practitioner finds necessary a deliberate individualization of each child, a projection into the future of the results of the child's current experience, and a use of time to learn what kind of illness the sick child has, what he needs, and how the family and physician can be helped to change or minimize any social circumstance that will impede complete recovery or aggravate trauma.

The Child as a Whole, or the Unitary Concept of Man—
The Psychosomatic Approach in Medicine

The concept of the "child as a whole" has gained ready acceptance. However, the phrase has come to connote the importance of emotional and social factors. During the first half of this century, gains in scientific medicine were so rapid that physicians tended to immerse themselves in objective and laboratory findings. Many of them fell into the error of thinking of sick persons as disease entities. Social workers, rejecting this practice, fell into a counterhabit of equating "wholeness" with another part, the emotions or the social circumstances.

Somehow, during the years of emphasizing the importance of the emotions, the obvious became overlooked. We have tended to ignore the reality of the biological basis of man's functioning. Possibly because the biological aspect of man leads toward the physical sciences, whereas the emotional is ramified by the social sciences, the biological aspects of man may seem more formidable than the emotional. We may have tended to avoid the difficult without realizing it. Understanding the biological base of human functioning creates a true appreciation of the intensity of psychological needs that grow out of biological helplessness or biological drives; in addition, it anchors us to reality, the framework for social services.

The unitary concept, that man does not and cannot function in separate pieces but as a total, dynamic, biopsychosocial entity, leads to consideration of the *psychosomatic* approach in medicine. The word combines *psyche* with *soma*, the Greek words for mind and body. Common parlance persists in using "psychosomatic" to invoke symptoms without organic cause, or a disease brought on by emotions. Even in medically sophisticated circles, certain disorders are characterized as "psychosomatic" if they have a heavy emotional component. For many years, however, those especially concerned with the field of psychosomatic medicine have made clear that they use the term to mean a comprehensive approach, not a category of diseases.[4]

Roy Grinker, an eminent neurologist, confirmed this in systems-analysis terms: " 'Psychosomatic' connotes more than a kind of illness; it is a comprehensive approach to the totality of an integrated process of transactions among many systems—somatic, psychic, social, and cultural."[5]

Pragmatists and mystics from earliest times accepted the unity of mind and body; lacking scientific medicine, they evidently relied for healing upon means they observed to be most efficacious. Witch doctors used incantations and rattles; the early Greeks used baths and fresh air. Mary Baker Eddy developed Christian Science healing. Two great physicians of the seventeenth century, Thomas Sydenham and William Harvey, observed that mental upset or excitement affected the circulation and acted upon viscera and heart. Since early in our own century, physiologists have experimented on countless animals to demonstrate the methods by which emotions affect the mind.

In the modern era no one questions the psychological component in certain diseases such as ulcers, rheumatoid arthritis, and hypertension. Equally accepted is the ill effect of worry or upset in precipitating flare-ups of preexisting disease, as in diabetes or thyroid conditions. Some persons believe that *all* accidents and diseases are caused by inner conflict. Whatever the range of acceptance, the psychic component in illness seems universally accepted.

Intellectual acceptance of theory must be based on an understanding of physiology, if it is to hold up under negative feelings. Otherwise it is easy to believe that clients deliberately or consciously become ill, or are in some fashion reprehensible because their emotions have caused the body functions to fail. Such an error results in the attitude that the client can be "healed" by words, whether by psychological interpretation or by confrontation.

The channels by which the emotions act upon the body are through the involuntary (not the voluntary) nervous system, which acts upon smooth muscle, the capillaries, and the glands. The hypothalamus, that part of the brain which mediates emotions, perceives a "danger" and readies the body in ancient, instinctive fashion for fight or flight, sending commands through the pituitary to the adrenal cortex, which in turn changes the chemical composition of body cells in accord with the physiologically perceived need. Prolonged stress thus creates exhaustion of the body's adaptive mechanisms. Tissue changes occur, causing inflammation and bleeding. Tension creates blood-vessel and muscle changes, clamping off normal activities and initiating others. Pain, vomiting, weakness, pallor, and so on, may result.

As indicated earlier, the most common obstacle in understanding the psychosomatic concept is a tendency to overlook the obvious, the contribution of organic or physical factors. Selye pointed out long ago that the physiological response to stress is identical whatever the nature of the stress. Hunger, cold, pain, shock, bleeding, exposure—any stress produces the same bodily reaction as emotional upset.[6] Anna Freud gently chided that most humane and intelligent group, the English pediatricians, for the same error that social workers sometimes fall into:[7]

> I always wonder why you are not equally interested in the other side of the picture, namely, what repercussions the truly organic disturbances which you treat have on the mind of the child. I often regret that pediatricians care more for the psychosomatic side and are less interested in the psychological after-effects of physical illness. There are questions such as the following: take for example a digestive disturbance in the first year of life, with a great deal of pain and discomfort, and which cuts out the pleasure in nourishment which belongs to that age. Will this have a lasting effect on the child's personality? There has been an overemphasis on the digestive tract; there have been times of revulsion against food or unsatisfied hunger. I think whenever you handle a physical disturbance of this kind, you should ask at the same time what it means in psychological terms. Whenever you interfere with the body of a child in some massive way, you should ask yourself—what will the child make of this?

Chapter 3 deals with the question Anna Freud raised, that of the effects of physical trauma on the emotional life of the child. The modern focus on reality gives equal weight to biological, emotional, and social factors in the child's functioning, and approaches the sick or handicapped child as a truly whole being.

Social Systems Theory—Its Implications for the Practitioner

While social workers and physicians, including psychiatrists, have been forging the psychosomatic or unitary approach to the individual, sociologists and social psychologists have forged a social systems or unitary approach to groups of individuals. Though the unitary approach to man has a biological base and the unifying approach to groups a sociological base, these corollary movements have much in common.

Social systems theory focuses on the dynamic, interreacting relationships of man with other men.[8] This is not new to social work, which has always concerned itself with the relationship of man to his human environment.

However, it has helped overcome the preoccupation with man's emotions that developed during the 1940's and 1950's. "Relationship" had taken on the connotation of the relationship between the individual and the counselor almost as if the two existed in a vacuum; relationships of the client with other significant persons were undervalued.

The swift changes of recent years have forced us to consider intervention with groups and whole societies. The population explosion and the proliferation of its attendant problems make extravagant a sole focus on the individual. Out of work with groups have come observations about relationships between peers and between the child and his family. A sharpened awareness of the interactions between individuals, or their "transactions," has turned us toward a stream of ideas from the sociologists and social psychologists that serve as correctives and enrichment to practice.

Social systems theory emphasizes that whether one considers only two persons (such as a sick child and his mother) or a large group or number of groups (such as the family, the hospital, the social agency, the school, the church, the ethnic group, etc.), the interactions between them mutually affect each individual and all who are involved. The relationships are circular, or mutual and interdependent. Not only is there a two-way street, but if any part is touched, the whole system is affected. For example, a baby's temperament, appearance, and behavior affect the mother's reaction to the baby, just as the mother's feelings about the baby affect her behavior and therefore the baby's personality.

One individual belongs to the many systems that impinge upon him and to which he contributes in some way. A sick child belongs to his family system, the ethnic system, the clinic or hospital system, his parents' church system, his father's employment system, etc. Someone remote can affect what goes on in the family, for one system affects another.

Though it should be obvious that we are all caught up in interacting networks of human events and relationships, we do not always remember the implications of this fact. We tend to forget that what affects the child affects the whole family, and that only as the family is changed can the child be changed, unless he is removed from them; a social worker, for example, may fail to interview a father because it is inconvenient for the worker to see him after he comes home from work. And we have been especially prone to forget that when a worker enters the picture, he or she becomes a part of the picture and changes the social system involved.

Without exploring the intricacies of social systems theory or venturing into its varied vocabularies, we can readily find useful two concepts that stem from social psychology's contribution to social systems theory. The first is the emphasis upon cognitive or rational aspects of behavior; the other is the importance of communication. Social systems theory calls attention to the importance—in the shaping of behavior—of cultural traditions, customs, social norms, beliefs, and learning. These ideas provide balance for the earlier emphasis in social work upon needs, feelings, attitudes, and emotions. They restore facts to their proper perspective.

Instead of assuming that individuals act in response to inner needs, some exponents of social systems assume that individuals act as they do entirely as a result of feedback from others and from their desire to achieve certain ends, such as approval or power. The emphasis is upon learned or patterned behavior resulting from social controls and the interplay of personalities within the group.* In fact, both concepts operate together.[9] Man acts in response to inner needs and also in concert with feedback and interaction with others.

The focus on interreaction that ensues leads to a focus on communication. Social systems theory describes communication as a "master process" whereby information is transmitted and received.[10] The person believes or "knows" what he has experienced to be true. What he has been "told" may be incorrect, not perhaps because something goes wrong with his perception, which is a very common reason for an incorrect belief, but because the communicator gives a partial or incorrect impression.

For example, an ill child hospitalized over a long period of time "knows" that a beloved physician no longer cares about him, because the physician no longer visits daily but passes the door with only a casual nod. The child is not told that the resident has changed services and therefore has transferred his clinical interest elsewhere. Free communication about the impending change in service and why the physician no longer visits would alleviate the child's loss of self-esteem as a result of "knowing" that he is no longer important to an esteemed person.

Today, nonverbal communication also receives more attention, since social psychologists have pointed out that "actions speak louder than words."[11] The tone of voice, posture, gestures, care taken in grooming or dress, and other aspects of behavior tell the person addressed more than what the other person says. Thus arises the confusion in the cosmetically handicapped child whose mother assures him she loves him but shows by body tension or coldness her own feelings of depression and disappointment in him.

The special sensitivity to what individuals communicate to others comes

* The outstanding exponent of patterned behavior is B. F. Skinner, who has revived and expanded the early twentieth-century theories of the Russian Pavlov and the Americans Watson and Thorndike. The conditioning of the dog to salivate at the sound of a tuning fork and the theory of behaviorism have been extended and expanded to embrace behavior modification of individuals. This is an important and widespread movement today. In addition, a bridge between psychiatry and social interactionism was built by Eric Berne in "transactional analysis." He put his ideas in popular form with the catch title "Games People Play," which so caught public interest that paperbacks appeared on drugstore racks and a song of that name was composed. An offshoot, "I'm OK, You're OK," has likewise placed elements of transactional analysis in the popular domain. As its author said, "The question has always been how to get Freud off the couch and to the masses."

from those who have studied the interaction of persons in groups, as in family therapy or group work. The sensitivity, however, carries over to human services workers in any form of practice, who become aware of what they "tell" clients with respect to keeping appointments, following through on promises, facial expression, tone of voice, and manner of dress. Those who work with children need to be especially aware of what they communicate in nonverbal ways. Working in behalf of chronically ill children requires constant communication with others in the helping professions. (This subject is treated in Chapter 4.)

The Determinants of Stress

A vast literature has accumulated about stress, much of it pertaining to research findings. Studies have been made of actual life situations, ranging from astronaut and submarine training to imprisonment, and of experimental situations, ranging from freezing and starving animals to shame interviews and observing the reactions of students waiting for examinations. Research has been physiological, psychological, and sociological. Out of the great mass of work done and interest in the subject have come cautions that many variables affect research results. The culture of the individual, his activity state, and the timing of the experiment are only a few of the multiple potentials for distorting results.

Definitions of stress vary, and, according to one source, "With the exception of extreme and sudden life-threatening situations, it is reasonable to say that no stimulus is a stressor to all individuals exposed to it."[12] However, despite the cautions about interpretation of studies and the difficulties of finding a definition that is more than a technical statement, such as "Stress occurs when an organism is forced into strenuous effort to maintain essential functions at a required level,"[13] some general ideas about stress have come from well-documented studies and/or seasoned observations. Certain well-supported hypotheses provide a starting point for consideration of the determinants and effects of stress.

The significance of these determinants is both physiological and psychological. As pointed out earlier, stress of any nature has the same physiological effect, and physiological reactions have their psychological correlates. Therefore broad general principles about the components of stress and its effects have practical application of special relevance in working with chronically ill children and their families.

Several themes have been identified regarding the determinants and effects of stress. These pertain to (*a*) the constructive nature of the right amount of stress, (*b*) the limit to which an organism can accommodate stress, and (*c*) the effects of other stresses upon the limit—duration of the stress and hope of release, and suddenness of the stress. These general themes may be amplified as follows.

Some stress is a good thing. A child develops, as does an adult, by opportunity to stretch his capacity to master challenge. For example, if a toddler falls down or an adult sees an automobile bearing down on him, a sophisticated neuroendocrine and neuromuscular chain of events occurs instantaneously. "Fight or flight" mechanisms of mind and body respond with an extra spurt of energy, and the extra energy enables the person to overcome the crisis. Having found that he could master the threat successfully, the child or adult is less afraid next time. He gains experience in how to walk, or drive on the freeway, as the case may be. Growth and adaptation have occurred.

Dr. Irene Josselyn has explained with special lucidity the importance of some stress in character development.[14] The handicapped child cannot develop mature behavior if he is deprived of the chance to meet challenges suitable for his age. An overanxious mother may prevent the child from taking necessary chances; normal siblings or peers may have defeated him so many times that he lacks the confidence to try something; weakness, crippling, or pain may have inhibited the physical effort necessary for growth experiences.

Everyone has a breaking point. War has provided grim laboratories for proof that even the strongest and best adjusted will collapse if stressed too much.[15] In short, any engine will stop if the hill is steep enough. (Thomas French, in describing the integrative capacity of the ego, uses an analogy of a picture thrown on a screen, in which the image—the stress—is larger than the screen—the ego.[16] There is not enough material to absorb the impact.) Looking first at the engine (and later at the steepness of the hill), we find the age of the person is of first importance. The nervous system of the infant is not complete at birth. During the first two years of life, fibers gradually develop a cover for the naked sheaths of nerves. During the preschool years, further refinement of nerve development takes place, until finally the child can throw a ball or perform a dance with fine coordination.

Incomplete physical development of the nervous system in infancy implies that the fibers cannot mediate as strong burdens of pain or stress as they can conduct later in life. Dr. Saul raises the question whether stressing an infant too severely in his vulnerable state will actually damage the vital nerve fiber.[17] This serious question raises doubts about the long-term effect of increasingly refined surgical capacity for protracted procedures on young children; whether the havoc to the nervous system of pain, fright, and maternal deprivation will need to be weighed against the technical capacity to ameliorate anomalies.[18]

The progressive experience of normal living results in correspondingly greater strength of the personality, and thus increases the individual's capacity to deal with stress. Negative or destructive life experiences, however, leave weak spots in personality development, or, if they occur early enough and are serious enough, they destroy "ego" capacity entirely.[19] The weak or vulnerable spot remains an Achilles heel for certain types of stress; the individual will collapse under a small amount of the stress to which he is vulnerable, whereas he may endure a large amount of other forms of stress.[20]

This concept of "emotional vulnerability" is well illustrated in a child who has undergone heart surgery at two years of age with good results, and then collapses emotionally at age five when a tonsillectomy is performed. The comalike reaction of this child to minor surgery is an illustration of the reactivation of old painful experience. Other weak spots are less obvious, but they remain like traps of quicksand in the personality and explain why seemingly strong persons of any age may react pathologically to a given type of experience.

The structure of the basic personality affects the way a person handles stress. Well-designed and careful research on college students has shown that persons with anxious temperaments who tend to blame themselves and to act in a "civilized" manner to unpleasant experiences suffer more adverse effect from stress than those who blame the other person and release their anger toward him.[21]

The number and severity of other stresses that a person is dealing with at the same time affect the amount of energy he has free to handle the new one. The multiple stresses of the very poor—the physical discomforts, poor nutrition, preoccupation with the next meal or next month's rent—diminish their capacity to rise to the needs of a deaf child or to projected heart surgery on the baby.[22] They raise the odds that the person will break under its impact—that is, that he will be apathetic, or ignore the problem, or meet it in a confused way—or that alcoholism or psychosis may demonstrate the collapse of his coping mechanisms.

Hope of freedom from pain or release from the threat affects ability to bear it. "It'll just last a minute," the classic reassurance when pain is administered, is soundly based, psychologically. Many studies, from those on the survival of Korean war prisoners to those of families of cancer patients, show that we can endure when we have hope of surcease; we go to pieces when we see no release. Hope increases human strength—or the size of the screen, in Dr. French's analogy—adding to the personality's usual capacity to cope with stress.[23]

The *suddenness* with which stress occurs, in addition to its nature, length, and severity, affects its impact. War studies of downed fliers showed that where the person has no warning, no way of mustering up defenses ahead of time, no physical and psychological adrenalin, his collapse is complete.[24] Warning gives time for the imagination to summon up ways of reaction, or psychological halfway houses before the catastrophe arrives.

Though the anxiety of waiting in suspense and the fear of future misfortune are regrettable, they cushion the blow.

The Concept of Crisis

Stress is distinguished from crisis, according to one of its earliest and outstanding exponents, Lydia Rapoport, as follows: "Stress generally is used to imply a negative or pathogenic state; it is considered to be some kind of a burden or load which presses down on the individual and creates a negative effect on his functioning. In contrast, the term 'crisis' refers to the state of the reacting individual. The state is one of upset."[25]

In a scholarly review of crisis theory that summarizes and interprets much of the earlier literature on the subject, Rosemary Lukton says, "Crisis theory rests on a series of assumptions that are in effect intended to explain, as well as to utilize preventively and therapeutically, some commonsense empirical observations. These observations concern the abrupt subjective as well as overt changes that occur in people at critical times during their lives."[26]

The traditional definition of a crisis is a stressful event in which the person's usual means of problem solving do not work. Among the characteristics of crises are that they are brief and self-limiting, lasting no longer than approximately six weeks, and that the person who is in a crisis is more emotionally accessible and open to help than at other times. It is also believed that a person who is helped with a crisis may carry over—to other problems—his strengthened capacity to solve the current problem.

Miss Lukton analyzes some of the contradictory and confusing ideas about crises that have appeared in the literature, and straightens out some of the tangles. She distinguishes between "normal" or developmental crises, which accompany changes in age or role, and "situational" crises, which occur as a result of some catastrophe such as illness. She says that some crises are dealt with by the person in a healthy way but that others, termed "active" crises for the sake of clarification, are those in which the person's coping mechanisms are insufficient.

Her thoroughgoing discussion reveals five points of special interest to those working with families of chronically ill children or with the children themselves: (1) that the amount of anxiety during a crisis is related to earlier similar experiences, which we recognize as Saul's concept of emotional vulnerability; (2) that there is nothing necessarily pathological about being overwhelmed and unable to cope; (3) that crisis can be an opportunity for growth; (4) that the worker must reach out actively and quickly and demonstrate practical help; and (5) finally, that instead of always thinking of crisis in terms of the interventive method, one may consider it a "task" crisis, which "refers to critical and demanding situations with which people must cope in order to achieve relative mastery of the tasks that these situations pose for them."[27]

It is the last, or "task crisis," that parents commonly refer to when they say life is one crisis after another during a child's chronic illness. However, the accumulation of stresses induced by repeated crises can indeed lead to situations of complete physical exhaustion and psychic depletion. Then the parent or child may be in an "active crisis," a situation beyond his own powers to cope with constructively. He is then subject to the characteristics traditionally ascribed to the need for crisis intervention. Rapoport defines the value of crisis intervention in these terms: "A little help, rationally directed and purposefully focused at a strategic time, is more effective than more extensive help given at a period of less emotional accessibility."[28]

Dependence and Independence

Man has two basic drives, described by various terms, but for practical purposes usefully characterized as dependence and independence. The presence of these conflicting instinctual needs determines the requirements for growth and development. They also reassure us about the reactions of clients, both parents and children. Saul says, "Growth, of course, is biologically predetermined and the organism has no alternative than to accept it as an unalterable fact and adjust itself to it."[29] This surge toward independence is a survival mechanism. As such, it constitutes powerful resistance against influences that might keep the person dependent.

The counterdrive for love and security is equally operative in a species that must have group cooperation for survival of the group. The need to be loved and cared for has its strongest biological rationale in infancy. Emotional security is necessary before the child can move appropriately into the next stage of development, for it is self-confidence that permits one to undertake a new venture. The needs for both dependence and independence are mutual and intertwined.

BASIC PREMISES IN CHILD DEVELOPMENT

The tenets of child development provide a baseline from which to consider the child's experience of illness or handicap. Out of the multitude of volumes and viewpoints about how children grow, the synthesis of a few basic concepts seems helpful in understanding the effects of disease or handicap. These concepts relate to the basic characteristics of child development: the importance of constitution, the inevitability of growth and change, the significance of change, the concept of ages and stages, emotional growth, fixation and regression, the development of the intellect, and the family as environment for child development. Factors affecting the human environment, such as socioeconomic status, ethnicity, and other aspects of culture, are omitted, since they are well known and because of the limitations of space.

The selected concepts attempt to set forth in plain language the key aspects of the so-called "epigenetic model," derived from biological observations about the sequential nature of maturation and the way in which environment affects development of innate potential.[30] The psychological application of biological principles has been set forth by experienced pediatricians, social workers, psychologists, and psychiatrists, including Gesell, Ribble, Erikson, Spock, the Bakwins, Goldfarb, Josselyn, Anna Freud, Fraiberg, Piaget, and Bloom.

Constitution as the Foundation for Growth and Development

Compromise has resolved the old quarrel about nature vs. nurture. Constitution has returned to a place of significance in the determination of personality. Genetic endowment is sometimes referred to as a "genotype," to signify that with certain exceptions hereditary potential is modified by environment. Two identical beans in different soils become large or small plants depending on soil and water. Nature may have endowed a child with the potential to become six feet four inches tall, but if his nutrition is poor he may become five feet two. Or he may have the gene potential to become a great musician, but with no opportunity to learn or hear music, he would perhaps do no more than whistle well. No man can exceed his hereditary potential; but neither does every man reach it.

A discussion of genetic transmission of hereditary defects will be found in Chapter 5, Prevention.

Body type, physical features, activity and vigor, bodily resilience, and sensitivity to both specific and general stimuli have been identified as genetic.[31] Intelligence is a notable characteristic in which the potential is genetic, although the degree of realization is determined by environment.[32] Whether the "nervous" baby, sensitive to all experiences, is the way he is because of genetic potential or intrauterine experience seems a matter of some controversy; certain researches have correlated long, thin, nervous babies with emotionally disturbed pregnancies.[33]

Thus the variants of physical constitution with which the child is born become the foundation on which personality is built. He is physically set to have an easy or difficult time. The placid baby may not notice at all what a sensitive baby will find upsetting. The experiences of early life and how the child incorporates them will further shape his career. The irritable baby makes the mother tense; her nervousness is further communicated to the child; he is unable to digest his food; his crying makes her more upset, etc. A child with a cleft palate or other physical deformity is also set for a stormy course. For example, not only is he deprived of the rewarding sensations of satisfactory feeding but regurgitation of milk through his nose will set up in the mother different responses than those brought forth by an attractive, satisfied infant.

This is not to imply that the child's constitution or physical characteristics determine his course. No matter how placid her infant's constitutional temperament, the mother will in the long run determine his future by her security, affection, and care. Her contribution or "input" is affected not only by the infant's nature and response but by her own emotional maturity, her experience during pregnancy and confinement, the feelings and actions of her husband and other children, and how the external world impinges upon her. She may be isolated and alienated, inexperienced and without relatives and friends who can guide and support her in meeting the child's needs. Or on the contrary, she may have strong family support that multiplies the nurturing available to the child and counteracts her deficiencies. Increasingly, fathers are providing direct nurturance and care. The parents, and to some extent the siblings, and, in some ethnic groups, the extended family determine the "soil for the bean."

The inevitability of growth and change. The child's growth is inevitable in all but the most severely damaged, for nature's lifesaving equipment "programs" the organism to become less helpless as quickly as possible. He will grab and put things in his mouth, crawl, walk, and run according to a sequential schedule for the human species. He will move through an equally inevitable sequence emotionally. Though modern authorities emphasize the flexible timing of the growth schedule, well-documented norms or averages exist.

The significance of change. Growth is change, not accretion. An adult is not a large child. This cliché of developmental theory warrants thought. Change takes place at an uneven pace, so that growth is a matter of peaks and plateaus. The periods of rapid change or "developmental crises" are uncomfortable for the child, because they are the times when previous personality is breaking down, new experiences are being incorporated, and new syntheses achieved. The child's discomfort creates annoying behavior. The parents face new problems to which their temperaments may or may not be adapted.

A biological base exists for the periods of psychological change. The baby is a satisfying, compliant being until he develops teeth; his ability to bite sets up a series of psychosocial changes and interactions. Later his neural and motor capacity to leave his mother on his own volition, to get into danger, to feel fright and insecurity and therefore the need to come running back sets up another series of circumstances. Repeated throughout maturation, critical episodes occur, periods of rapid change in which the child has new experience. These are not only difficult but vulnerable times, when either good or ill has special impact.

Vulnerability during times when old ways are disintegrating and new ways are being learned makes parental response to behavior especially significant. Accidents, illness or treatment that inflicts pain, and maternal deprivation are especially traumatic at these times. Elective procedures may best take place during periods of relative security, or developmental plateaus, and not during times of developmental crisis.

The "unitary" or epigenetic nature of growth refers to the psychological needs, and corollary demands upon and responses from the mother, which grow out of biological development and social circumstances. However, it does not mean that all aspects of physical, psychological, and social-system response keep in step. Circumstances or constitutional capacities will retard some physical and psychological factors and speed up others. A child may be ahead of the norm in motor skills and behind in communication for a period, then slow down in one area and catch up in others. A crippled child with inferior motor skills and inability to practice them might, for example, have superior social development because his mother has talked with him a great deal and because of superior mental endowment.

The Concept of Ages and Stages

Relative irreversibility is a further attribute of development that deserves special elaboration. The term grows out of the observation that the biological sequences of change create special needs, both physical and emotional, which must be provided for at the time they are needed. For example, milk is needed while the bones are being formed. Drinking a great deal of milk later will not cure bowed legs of rickets. The same thing largely holds true of psychological growth.[34] If needed resources are not provided, the growth thrust will take the child on past the stage to the next one, but with a weak spot in the fabric of personality. "Apparently there is a tide in the affairs of babies as well as men, which, taken at the flood, leads on . . ."[35]

Chapter 3 describes the stages in connection with their disruption by chronic illness. Only those specifics necessary for reference to the general concept are reviewed here. The idea is so central in child development and so complex, however, that both its foundations and its nature require some elaboration. Psychological development includes intellectual and emotional growth and change. Definite stages for each have been identified. They are inextricably intertwined, but pulling them apart for scrutiny makes possible a clearer picture of the combined thread.

Emotional growth. Thoughtful analysis of child development must lead to the idea that human life is much like that of the marsupials, in that the infant is not complete at birth but, like the joey in the mother kangaroo's pouch, is completely dependent upon a close relationship with the mother for many months before he becomes a separate and complete individual.

Measuring development from the time a child arrives in the outside world is artificial. Growth and development start at conception; birth, though it necessitates an instant, critical adjustment to the less protective environment, is actually only a stage in development. The great size of the human brain (in relation to that of other animals) requires nature to open the door to the outside world while birth passage is physically possible for the mother, but the lack of completion of the nervous system leaves the infant in a highly vulnerable state.

This vulnerability serves a purpose in ensuring a swift and determined start in the socialization process. Since life depends on the source of supply of food, warmth, and comfort, the baby attends the presence of the mother with literally life and death intensity. The same footsteps, the same smell and shape and softness, naturally associate themselves with a trustworthy source of gratification. When his eyes begin to focus and the blur becomes her face, and as she responds to his cries and efforts to communicate his needs, he watches and later grows to love her. Her love then becomes the central thing in his life, and fear of loss of this love becomes the source of greatest anxiety. Out of these early circumstances comes the potential for socialization.

An example of critical need during a stage of development, and of a task to be accomplished, is the critical need for security in mothering while the infant is so vulnerable to her love. If the mother is detached, ambivalent, preoccupied, or rejecting, or if the sounds and the sensations the child associates with food and comfort fail to arrive when he makes his needs known, or are always different, he cannot be sure; he is repeatedly anxious; he is often let down. He cannot achieve a sense of trustworthiness in the outside world or trust his perceptions of his own needs. Observations now are multitudinous enough to be sure that such babies become insecure grownups who can never really trust or love others.[36] The psychological resource for emotional growth was lacking at the time of critical need. Behaviors growing out of the needs may be subject to some modification through later positive experience. Periods of personality disintegration during situational or developmental crises offer opportunities for some new input. However, the basic weakness remains.

What hospitalization or institutional placement does to a young child will be discussed in greater detail at a later point; it is obvious that depriving the child of his mother during his earliest and most critical need of her is an adverse circumstance so serious in its later consequences that alternatives must be weighed very carefully.

The concept of ages and stages is related to the idea of surplus energy. Living things are endowed with energy, enough for life and for growth, with some left over for propagation of the race. The young organism utilizes surplus energy in pleasurable activities that lead to learning. The surplus of energy in combination with the myelination of nerve fibers during early life invests certain organs with a pleasurable sensation which ensures that the person will pay attention to them when their function is especially important. The mouth is invested with this surplus energy and heightened sensation during the first year of life. The mouth is in fact lined with fatty tissue and extra nerve endings during infancy so that the child will be impelled to seek to suck (which, among other things, prepares the throat muscles for chewing later on).

Infancy therefore has been called the "oral" stage. Because the gratification of oral pleasures is paramount during this period, current child-rearing methods welcome the use of the pacifier, encouraging the child to suck as much as he wants.[37]

Another concept closely related to that of psychological stages of development is that of fixations. *Fixation*, or the tendency to cling to one stage,[38] occurs when deprivation of gratification prevents the child from completing the stage and going on to the next, or when the next step seems dangerous—as when an excess of attention makes the stage so pleasurable that the child fears to yield it up. Thus the child with cleft palate could be fixated at the earliest or oral stage, when the mouth is important, if the defect were not repaired to the extent that he could suck satisfactorily, or if he were so painfully treated that he was traumatized at this stage. He might be fixated for lack of love and security, owing to his mother's reaction to his disfigurement. A child could also be fixated at the oral stage if he were denied an opportunity to grow by the mother's overprotective reactions.

Fixation is in contrast to *regression*, a falling back to an earlier stage when under stress. Typical examples of regression are seen in older children who start anew to suck their thumbs when worried or ill. Overeating may be another manifestation of regression under emotional stress. Regression always occurs during stress, and consequently always accompanies illness. It is a "normal" deviation, therefore, and concerns us only when it remains after the stress or the illness has disappeared.

The child who is not afraid to move into the next stage, and not prevented from doing what is biologically appropriate, will move ahead to the next step toward psychological independence. He never completely leaves behind the psychological characteristics of the previous stages but, unless he was severely "fixated," advances in his capacity for independence.

An outstanding exponent of the concept of stages of emotional growth, Erik Homburger Erikson, relates each stage to mastery of a task, which is necessary in achieving maturity. If the task is not mastered and a gain achieved, a defect occurs in personality development that is the opposite of the gain.[39] The tasks are increasingly complex as the child has wider social experience, and as his increasing physical maturity makes them possible.

The Development of the Intellect

The instinct of self-preservation propels the urge to learn. Powered by this great force, the intellect develops swiftly, 50 percent of it developing between conception and four years of age. By the age of eight, another 30 percent has developed, and the last 20 percent by the age of 17.[40]

Intelligence may be defined narrowly or broadly—narrowly as the comparative ability to answer test questions in relation to that of others of the same age, or broadly as the "degree of availability of one's experiences for the solution of immediate problems and the anticipation of future ones."[41] Though thinking and feeling affect each other, the intelligence is a separate constitutional capacity that has a large degree of independence from the instinctual drives.[42]

Piaget, a Swiss psychologist who is a recognized authority in the cognitive area of child development, defined six technical or three main stages by which intelligence matures. They begin with physical capacities, reflexes; then come imitation and play; and they progress to a systematic intelligence governed by awareness of relationships.[43] Essentially, in the preschool stage the child first makes the transition from sensory-motor to conceptual intelligence. In the lower grades the things he has learned become usable in terms of immediate, concrete reality. From the upper elementary grades through college, the child learns to operate on a hypothetical level, with gradual enrichment of the concepts of and capacity for abstraction.

Human services workers find intriguing, sobering, and of great practical importance the characteristics of the maturation of intelligence. Startling, perhaps, is the knowledge that little children cannot "think," as we customarily consider the word, however bright they are, until they are about seven or eight years old. That is to say, they are not capable of *conceptual thinking* until after they have accumulated multitudes of specific experiences from which to generalize.

For example, the child cannot understand "redness" as a concept, or "under" and "over," or "roundness," until he has seen, in the first instance, a red flower, a red hat, a red toy, and many other red things; or experienced, in the second instance, the spatial relationships of many things over and under; or felt, in the third instance, many round things.

"Percepts" are the building blocks of concepts. They are the stimuli of sensations we receive within the context of other experiences. They may be defined as what "we do mentally with what we receive."[44] First, the organic function of the brain itself is involved, and then the filter of emotions through which a sensory experience is conveyed to the brain. A brain-damaged child, for example, may actually perceive objects on a slant instead of on a level, and therefore writes words on the slant. More complex is the emotional filter through which stimuli pass that determines how they are "perceived" or recorded in the brain. A child whose earliest experiences with another person, the mother, demonstrated that others may or may not arrive when comfort is needed will "perceive" others as unreliable because the sensory image is received in context of prior emotional associations. He will also lack confidence in his ability to perceive correctly.

Intellectual growth, in other words, is *sequential and cumulative*, going through stages and depending on past experiences, just as physical and emotional growth are cumulative.

Moreover, we know that before the child can think conceptually, he first uses empiricism or "magic." Fraiberg describes the world of the two-year-old as "at times a spooky twilight world that is closer to the world of the dream than the world of reality."[45] All who are familiar with children know they associate what happens to them with good or bad behavior —it is as if they make it happen. Thus the pain of hospitalization is caused by having bad thoughts or having done a bad thing. Fraiberg tells of a bright two-and-a-half-year-old who had participated precociously in his parents' plans for a family trip to Europe, by plane, seeming to understand all that was said. Just before departure he began to cry, saying, "I can't go with you. I haven't learned to fly yet."[46] Little children have acute powers of observation but they cannot interpret what they observe because of lack of experience. The child who had not yet "learned to fly" could not conceptualize the necessary relationships between space, sizes, pictures, the airplanes he had seen, etc., and could think of flying empirically only by flapping his own arms. Reliance on a magical world in which only the empirical can be understood leads to many nightmares and misunderstandings.

Language is an important ingredient in the development of intelligence. Words serve as fixatives for mental images. They further make possible the understanding and incorporation of parental wisdom through parental commands. The ability to communicate and then to reinforce and extend understanding through reading gives enormous impetus to the capacity to learn.

Play is another important ingredient. From the reflexes, then, the pleasurable discharge of surplus energy through kicking, grabbing, and exploring, the child has experiences that lend an understanding of himself and his environment. The child imitates, and learns through imitation. He gradually gains ability to pretend that situations exist, at about age three, and both mentally and physically practices at mastering them in his play.

Out of intellectual growth comes *harnessing of the emotions*. Learning that things can exist, even though they cannot be seen, is a first source of reassurance, which comes at about six to nine months of age. If a mother exists, even though she is not in the room, anxiety is not so great. Later, when words arrive, language can be used to summon up mental images so that one is not so alone; words create an illusion of control. No longer is expression of frustration confined to kicking and screaming. One can channel anger into words and direct the emotion at a target, draining off some of the diffuse energy into the cognitive exercise involved. One can receive explanations that drain events of mystery or fear.

When *imagination* arrives, one can pretend invulnerability by being as big as the father or as fierce as a tiger. One can escape from the memory of hurt or the knowledge of helplessness into a soothing and pleasant world of fantasy, refurbishing inner resources to deal with the real world again. Playing helps build security and self-esteem by providing a degree of mastery over the frustrating and uncontrollable world.*

How sobering it is to realize the dependence of intellectual development upon the early social environment. Studies, including those of twins reared separately, show that "the effects of the environments, especially of extreme (abundant or deprived) environments, appear to be greatest in the early and more rapid periods of intelligence development," and that "a conservative estimate of the effect of extreme environments on intelligence is about 20 IQ points . . . the difference between life in an institution for the feebleminded or a productive life in society."[47]

The *environment* affects language, so essential to both intellectual and emotional maturity; it affects experiences out of which the "percepts" come that accumulate into concepts, problem solving and independent thinking, and motivations and expectations. The intellectual impoverishment of young children from culturally deprived homes who are neglected by preoccupied or working mothers and are lacking in opportunities for experience and play is directly attributable to the family's social circumstance.

The child who is physically deprived of full sensory-motor experience and stimuli from the environment creates additional concern. The blind, deaf, or paralyzed child needs substitute stimuli if he is not to be deprived of the perceptual accumulations on which conceptual richness and abstract thinking depend. Chains of ideas, further inquiry, and still further stimuli cannot begin unless someone is imaginative enough and cares enough to build in perceptual material especially during the time of most rapid

---

* The reader is referred to Erik Erikson's "Toys and Reasons" in *Childhood and Society*, and to Selma Fraiberg's *The Magic Years*, for both profound and entertaining illuminations of the significance of play in child development; and to Piaget on the subject for technical information (see notes 36, 42, and 43, pp. 501–2).

growth, that is, up to the age of eight. Through what filter of emotions will the deprived child's stimuli pass—that of frustration, hurt, and insecurity? Or can it be that of gratification?

Of special interest to adoption workers is the limited scope of intelligence tests of infants and young children. Tests can assess the general intellectual capacity of an infant as early as two months, and additional tests can determine the level he has attained at certain ages. However, these early tests are not always valid in predicting his future intelligence, since environmental and perceptual enrichment or impoverishment in early life affects the final breadth of his cognitive capacity. Not until he is about six can estimates be made of his true or lasting intelligence, and not until he is in the third grade can his school achievement be reliably estimated. When a child is struggling with the mastery of two languages, the problems of predicting achievement from early intelligence testing may be even more pronounced.[48]

The Family and the Transmission of Culture

The family, the small child's world, is a dynamic, ever-changing unit with a life cycle of its own. A young couple with young children grows older; different needs exist and there are different demands upon each member as the once helpless offspring prepare to leave the nest. Within the family system, relationships and interactions take on importance that transcends the individuals themselves. Today, in token of the unitary nature of the family, we refer to "sick families" rather than "sick individuals," or to families with varying degrees of strength.

The child learns from his family and ethnic group what society expects of him, how to pattern his drives, and what he can expect from the world. The family largely determines the materials for his percepts, and the emotional filters through which they pass. Margaret Mead narrated a film, "Four Families,"[49] which illustrates the way different cultures build into a child their expectations and transmit their ways of life by their different child-rearing practices. The American child is very early taught independence and initiative, in contrast with the preeminent value of obedience to family taught the Japanese child.[50] However, proliferating studies of the effect of social class on child-rearing practices show that in America the lowest socioeconomic class, tormented by financial insecurity and its multiple stresses, transmits a self-defeating way of life.

Kurt Lewin says, "culture is watertight," meaning that each piece is a bit of an interlocking whole that cannot be changed without changes in other parts. He describes the minutiae through which a culture is transmitted:[51]

in the way the mother treats a two- or three-year-old child, what the father talks about at the dinner table, how the worker talks to his foreman or the student to the professor, how the visitor behaves toward grown-ups and children, how the cookbooks are written, how opposing lawyers deal with each other after the court session, what type of photograph the candidate for political office uses for propaganda, and what religion means to a person in any denomination. A cultural change in regard to a specific item will have to be able to stand up against the weight of the thousand and one items of the rest of the culture which tend to turn the conduct back to its old pattern.

Fathers are assuming larger responsibilities in the home, and roles are less clear-cut than in earlier times. However, the mother remains the main source of nurture to the child. "The family" usually means the mother to the infant and toddler. In most families the father is primarily important as the key determinant in the mother's security. A secure wife is most likely to be a secure mother. When the child grows older, the father becomes directly important in providing a model for imitation and a demonstration of the masculine role, as well as someone whose love, and whose prohibitions, augment those of the mother. Siblings become important as models for behavior, as rivals for parental attention, and as givers of love or hate.

Complexity increases as the child matures and the life cycle of the family winds on. More relationships exist, quantitatively, more nuances sift through the perceptual screen as communication and abstractions can be understood, more opportunity exists for confusion in communication, and more opportunity arises for role changes and snags around which the currents flow. By the time of adolescence, the child's need to establish himself as a person separate from the family adds greatly to the potential for difficult interactions.

The Prevalence of Insecurity in Family Life

In the family, the infant finds or fails to find the security he needs for normal development. The family as an institution reflects the turbulent transition of the whole society. "There seems to be a general agreement that we live in a period of more critical transition, of revolution, and of more abrupt discontinuity in human and social affairs than ever before."[52] Profound changes are taking place in the structure and organization of family life, changes that inevitably create a shattering impact on child-rearing practices.

The number of married women who were living with their husbands and working rose from 24 percent in 1950 to 41.5 percent in 1972. An astonishing 60 percent of married women, with both preschool and school-age children and whose husbands were in the home, were working in 1972, according to U.S. Bureau of Labor statistics.[53]

Since the median earnings of both husband and wife were between $8500 and $9100 in 1972, the preponderance of families in which women worked were low-income families.[54] This correlates with statistics of the 1960's, which have been analyzed to show that the poorer the family, the greater the likelihood that the mothers will work, especially mothers of preschool children.[55] As might be expected, a larger percentage of non-White mothers worked than White, although in numbers they were less than a fourth of the total group. A number of professional women with preschool children were working outside the home to continue careers or fulfill personal needs or raise the family's standard of living, but the proportion in the total number of working mothers was small.[56]

The earlier figures had also been analyzed to show that by far the largest percentage, though by no means the largest number, of mothers who worked outside the home were those who had no husband—the divorced, separated, or widowed. Sixty-five percent of these mothers worked if their children had reached school age, over half with children aged three to five worked, and over a third with children under age three worked. Furthermore, most of these women worked full time, whereas only three-fourths of the women with husbands worked full time.[57]

Families of mothers without husbands are the poorest of all families. They form a third of the total group designated as "the poor."[58] With or without husbands, most women work for economic reasons,[59] although an increasing number are concerned with personal fulfillment, and an articulate group are resentful of their stereotyped women's roles as homemakers and mothers.

The sharp rise in the divorce rate in the United States reflects the unhappy, tension-filled world in which many young children live. One in every three marriages ended in divorce in 1972.[60] The divorce rate is substantially higher for those who marry young. (Current projections are that 25 percent of White and 46 percent of Black men under 22 and women under 20 will divorce at least once; that of those who marry under this age, close to a third of the Whites and half of the Blacks will divorce.)[61] Divorce rates decrease with length of marriage. The average duration of marriage is eight years, half of the divorces occurring within three to 15 years.[62]

Remarriage at a rising rate means that where there are two adults they increasingly include one stepparent. The latest figures available, those for 1971, show that 14 percent of all married women have been married twice or more, the percentage increasing with age.[63] In addition, many couples live together without marriage, so that the actual number of children who have stepparents cannot be known.

"One side effect of increasing divorce rates is that more and more children are growing up in fatherless homes."[64] In 1972, approximately 10 percent of all White children and 31 percent of all Black children lived with a mother only. There were six million one-parent families, most of them with a female head.[65] Despite these dismaying facts, or perhaps in recognition of their reality, the Children's Rights Statement proposed for the 1975 Delegate Assembly of the National Association of Social Workers included the right to "at least one parent... children are entitled to be raised by their biological parent(s)." The intent that children should have decent care and a stable, supportive relationship is well spelled out.[66] Nevertheless, the fact that social workers interested in children, and knowing from daily practice the impediments to child care that are built into one-parent families, should settle for a child's right to only one parent describes, as perhaps nothing else does, the dilemma of child rearing in today's world.

The information on how children are cared for while their mothers work is several years old, and there are no current nationwide data.[67] The child-care arrangements made by working mothers at the time of the last survey were not reassuring. About half of the children remained in their own homes, cared for by their father or other relatives, and another 15 percent were looked after in someone else's home. The statistics showed that 8 percent "look after themselves," including 1 percent of those under six years of age and 8 percent of those six to 11.[68] Only 2 percent were in day-care facilities. Less than $10 per week was paid in two-thirds of the cases where payment was made.[69]

The most obvious problem posed for the sick or handicapped child whose mother works is the adequacy of care provided. Does the caretaker provide the special diet, the supervised rest, the regular medication, see that the child puts on his sweater or rubbers before he goes out to play in cold weather, etc.? Does the caretaker have the creative capacity and motivation to devise means of stimulation and socialization for the child who is confined to bed or wheelchair? When the mother returns from office, factory, or service occupation, does she have the energy and patience to take care of his extra needs?

Equally important are the child's emotional needs. Since regression under stress of illness is inevitable, to whom does the chronically ill child turn for the mothering he needs? If he is handicapped, to whom does he turn when other children tease or ignore, or when frustration seems overpowering? If he is customarily well but becomes acutely ill, does his mother hastily arrange for someone else to take him to the doctor, transmitting her employer's annoyance that something is interfering with her work?

Many women remain in the home to care for their children if one is chronically ill. They cannot find adequate child care, and they are often too involved with medical care to be able to work outside the home. However, many mothers of chronically ill children do work. In these instances the helping person needs to know what happened that precipitated the mother's working. Was it the child's loss of his father, through desertion, divorce, or death? Was it economic privation? Did the mother find the child's condition too upsetting to tolerate? If the latter, does her employment outside the home transmit to the child a lack of acceptance and a perception that he is unwanted? Can she only be a mother at all if she has some escape? Does the child accept her working as token of the family's economic need? The interaction between the feelings of a working mother, caught between family and employment "system," and those of the child adds to the total strain, whatever the situation.

Those who specialize in marriage counseling have identified, among causes of troubled family relationships, the inability of the parents to change appropriately as the marriage matures.[70] For example, a husband and wife may get along happily while she can be his playmate, but when she becomes tied down and worn out with the care of children, he may be unable to mature enough to change his role, share part of her burden, and provide her with the emotional support she needs. He may be angry and jealous over losing his playmate, and she angry over his unwillingness to help her.

Pairing problems may also develop in a maturing family. For example, mother and son may develop a closeness that crowds out the father, or father and daughter become the pair against the mother. Children become confused if they see a child inappropriately receiving an excess of one parent's affection and the other parent jealous or retaliating, instead of the two parents acting together in discipline and affection. Later chapters will elaborate the pervasive and acute problems that chronic illness creates in intensifying the relationship between the sick child and his mother, crowding out the father and depriving the siblings of their share of maternal affection and attention.

The well-known *double bind* occurs when the parents say one thing but act another. The child is caught in the confusion. A family becomes entangled in insecurity and hostility because the members cannot be honest with each other. Frightened fantasies about what was really meant exceed the reality of the feeling or intended meaning of an action.

Scapegoating is another well-known attribute of unhealthy family relationships that deserves special note in work with handicapped children. All the festering unhappiness of some or all of the family members may be channeled toward one member. The equilibrium of the rest is maintained in this manner. For example, if a chronically ill child requires a great deal of energy and attention, the mother may feel that he is the reason she cannot give her husband the attention he needs, and that the husband's estrangement is therefore the fault of the child. The other children may concur as they feel the tensions and observe the interactions. They, too, may then resent the handicapped child, blaming him for the mother's preoccupation and perhaps the father's truculence or his absence from home. If the child has a cosmetic defect, it is the more natural that he should in truth become "the ugly duckling." The grandparents or aunts and uncles may reinforce this web of negative attitudes toward the child. The scapegoat need not be the handicapped child; any member around whom tensions swirl may be chosen.

Thus, in addition to the family problems created by lack of money and ill health, the family of a sick or handicapped child may be particularly prone to some of the unhealthy interactions that have been identified by marriage experts, because of the very way in which the incidence of some handicapping conditions occurs. These families have built-in vulnerabilities. A folk wisdom has developed among practitioners who work with the physically handicapped that marriages need to be unusually healthy to withstand the impact of a chronically ill or handicapped member; that a weak marriage does not hold up under the difficulties involved.

The Dilemma of Child Development in Today's Family

The unfinished organism that struggles down the birth canal into an environment with which he cannot cope alone requires for socialization—or, in other words, for development into a human being—security, love, protection, and opportunity for growth. If he is to progress normally through the sequences of development that have been programmed into him, he needs to incorporate into his personality layers of positive experience, which are the building blocks for his future contribution and well-being. The child is wholly narcissistic, needing everything, and giving in return only the love that rewards the very simple and the civilized. The child with a birth defect or illness of early onset needs even more and can provide even less in return.

Because emotional experiences are as self-perpetuating as genetic endowment, though taking a variety of forms, a growing number of children in our turbulent and increasingly impersonal society fail to find the family stability that their need for love and security requires. Nature has provided some insurance for maternal love, but the amount was evidently predicated on earlier societal forms. Fewer demands were made upon the capacity or emotional maturity of the mother, and she was enabled by the father to give nurturance to the children.

A sociologist has questioned whether in fact the present era has moved away from the child-centered society of the recent past:[71]

[There is] accumulating evidence that many American children are not being adequately cared for, but there are also indications of a general devaluation of children and child-rearing: ... [the] number of divorce cases in which neither parent wants custody of the children ... number of working women [testifying] they had left ill preschoolers unattended in locked apartments because they feared losing their jobs if they stayed home with them.... Even non-gainfully employed mothers may spend as little as 15 or 20 minutes a day in actual communication with their preschool children.... Many children have no other daily meaningful contact with adults.... Children not in school spend most of their time alone or with other children.... It seems fair to conclude that the status of children in our society is highly ambiguous.... There is less wanting of children.

The child takes his place in the family as only one unit of a dynamic group, the needs of all members requiring and receiving attention. In the group with whom most workers are concerned, the poor, the public welfare agency adds its demands to the system into which the baby comes. It attempts to buffer, but nevertheless reflects the taxpayers' demands that current economic self-sufficiency of the family take precedence over all else. In one-parent families, usually those headed by the mother, the implementation of this policy sacrifices the future capacity of the child to contribute his maximum to society.

Because human service workers develop the habit of seeing small children as important members of the families with whom they are working—the only members whose destinies they do, in fact, help to shape—they can speak for the child. They can work toward policies that sustain the family unit, enabling the family to give the child as much positive experience as possible. Where physical handicap adds its burden to child and parents, the need for prevention of unnecessary disability underlines the importance of effort in their behalf.

THE SIGNIFICANCE OF EXPERIENCE

The discussion of basic assumptions in the approach to sick or handicapped children is replete with references to the environment—social, emotional, and physical—or, in other words, to the child's experiences. Socialization is accomplished through experience. Principles regarding this aspect of life are not as comprehensive or well organized as we might wish, but by examining the many writings on crisis and stress, the particular kinds of experience, and the effect of environment on learning, we find a number of important generalizations.

Some of the principles have been referred to in previous pages, but they are summarized here because of the importance of the subject. Understanding the significance of a child's experience makes possible some prediction of his adult strengths and weaknesses. Prediction of the general effect of experience in turn makes possible selective planning of community effort, with greatest energy for development of programs that promise greatest gain and for combating circumstances that threaten serious hazard. Understanding the effect of experience also makes it possible for us to predict the probable effectiveness of differential treatment with given individuals and groups. We may estimate whether our work should have lasting results or provide only temporary relief.

Timing

Three closely related principles pertain to the time that experience occurs. Experience is most important that occurs early in life, that occurs during a time of rapid growth, or that occurs during a crisis or a change from one environment to another. A fourth principle relating to both timing and specificity is that experience is most significant at the time of a special need.

Substantiated beyond question is the fact that the earliest experiences are most important. The child grows most rapidly from conception to birth, and from birth to the age of four.[72] In addition to the factor of rapidity of growth, greater ease of learning exists when there is nothing to unlearn. Further, growth being cumulative, that which comes first shapes the rest. Modern psychological studies lead to this conclusion: "Less and less change is likely in a group or individual as the curve of development of a characteristic reaches a virtual plateau. We are somewhat pessimistic about the possibility for significant change in a characteristic once a plateau has been reached."[73] According to Publilius Syrus, "Each succeeding day is the scholar of that which went before it."[74]

Adolescence is the other time of rapid growth; this phase of life can also be considered a time of repeated crisis. The adolescent's vulnerability to good or ill is so well known that helping persons commonly say that one gets a "second chance during adolescence" to help a disturbed child. Deep concern over reinforcement of adverse preschool experiences during adolescence, as for example when a rejected child undergoes a later abandoning experience, is the negative side of the same coin.

The pregnant woman, mother of the children with whom we are concerned, or sometimes the female adolescent child of our concern, can be characterized as in a period of rapid growth, physiologically and emotionally, and also in a period that is a developmental crisis. The rapid maturation that takes place psychologically during pregnancy appears to be a corollary of the maturation accompanying rapid growth earlier in life. The special accessibility of the pregnant woman to help with emotional problems is expounded by Caplan, a psychiatrist well known for his interest in mothers and babies.[75] Conflicts regarding her sexuality and about the mothering she herself received are relived as she experiences the fruits of sexuality and prepares to become a mother. This special accessibility to help while half-buried problems are churned to the surface is characteristic of persons undergoing crisis.[76]

Another closely related principle relating to timing of experience is that the effects of a new environment are most meaningful during the initial period, or while the change is being effected.[77] This may explain in part the vulnerability during pregnancy, for the change creates a change in the way the woman is perceived by everyone, and thus in her personal environment. However, the principle is seen more clearly in the rapid orientation of a foreign child into a new group, or a new child in school. Every fiber is stretched to adapt, in order to find acceptance and security.[78] The intent listening and strained observation make it possible to pick up more quickly and receive greater imprint from experience than occurs later when one is less open to what is going on.

Specificity

A major point made by both skilled observers and research psychologists is that specific experiences affect specific characteristics. The anxiety roused by a threat that reactivates memory of an earlier painful experience has been discussed; the specific emotional vulnerability remains. Another aspect of specificity of experience is that of critical need during certain phases of development. The "phase-specific" need is part of the concept that environmental stimuli need to match physiological readiness if the child is to progress through sequential steps of growth.[79]

As mentioned earlier, the little baby needs to suck to develop muscles for chewing; he needs the chance to pull himself upright and room to crawl before he can walk. Similarly, there is an optimum time for learning words, which depends on hearing sounds and receiving encouragement and pleasure in the sounds he makes. In turn, learning words creates the ability to think about things. That the development of the intellect is dependent upon appropriate stimuli has come to be so generally recognized that programs such as Head Start receive massive federal funds and survive governmental economy moves.

Emotional growth is likewise dependent on appropriate response to age-specific, critical needs, as will be elaborated later, and deprivation or thwarting of these needs has been observed to create warping that is very hard to correct.

The studies of deprivation of a mother during her own infancy, in which absence of mothering was both early and prolonged, show that this experience affects specific characteristics. Speech is greatly retarded; consequently, the child is handicapped in the ability to think in abstractions and to form meaningful relationships with other persons.[80] One of the ironic tragedies of Nazi Germany was the experiment with "Hitler babies," where infants of the "best Aryan stock" were reared in scientific nurseries without indulgence or mothering, and grew to be severely retarded children.[81] The frustration that criminologists feel over the failure of everything tried thus far to significantly alter deviant patterns, the very limited successes in work with alcoholics and drug abusers, the long-accepted realization that sociopathy is relatively untreatable, all attest to the soundness of Josselyn's early dictum that "milk is a cure for rickets only when the bones are being formed."[82]

Intensity and Consistency

Bloom points out that the constancy and consistency of an environment affect its significance through the reinforcement and stabilization of the change that takes place.[83] It is the consistency of the experience that determines how powerful it is. Something that infiltrates every aspect of life, and from which there is no escape, has the greatest impact. "The effect of extreme environments is especially dramatic on young children, since they are unable to effect any escape."[84] A very young child who cannot even hide, run, reason, or protest, who cannot channel his misery into words or find relief through fantasy or play, is worse off than an older child; and an older child is more affected than an adult, whose accumulated inner resources can provide at least philosophical rationale if no other means of escape.

Intervention to prevent consistency in a child's feeling of abandonment by the parents while he is in the hospital is discussed in the voluminous literature on emotional aspects of hospitalization of children. Although not couched in the abstraction of consistency of experience, but rather as observations of behaviors, the works of pioneers such as René Spitz and Anna Freud urged parental visiting and relaxation of hospital visiting hours to avoid the anguish and despair that infants develop when they feel abandoned, as elucidated in Bowlby's well-known work.[85]

The consistency of experiences cannot be determined in most cases, for few exist in a vacuum, except in young children, where the simplicity of the organism makes either total gratification or total deprivation possible. The constant impingement of a network of forces, external and internal, that make life so individual and complex prevent any one force from being total in itself. A principle pertaining to experience is in fact that of its increasing complexity for the maturing organism. The older we get, the more experiences we have accumulated to influence the meaning of a current experience, the richer our concepts, and the broader and stronger our "ego span" (in the normal person). We perform more social roles, and we come in contact physically with more persons, ideas, and things. Consequently, a totally consistent experience, except for imprisonment or isolation in a nursing home, seems unlikely for an adult. We can, however, appreciate its possibility in an infant or in a child limited by sensory, motor, or mental incapacity, or in the gravely injured adult.

Reinforcement of experience is, unfortunately, easy to witness in a children's hospital ward. One may observe the child, bereft of his mother, spatially insecure through the unaccustomed height and lack of nestling covers in his hospital bed, approached by the white coats of frightening memory, and pinned down by strong arms while needles are placed in his body. His screams are to no avail while the intravenous is applied. It would appear that this experience of helplessness and rage under attack is, through a combination of reinforcement and the simplicity of the organism, total and consistent.

Preparation, Reaction, and Duration

The stress studies previously cited make plain that duration of stressful experience affects the individual's capacity to deal with it; American slang has incorporated the popular observation that prolonged stress always brings a breaking point—"he's had it!" One can observe painfully the breaking point approaching in a hospitalized child when the stress of maternal separation has been endured about as long as he can stand it; when the whimpering and tears show the demarcation point between despair and detachment, which Bowlby characterizes as the stage of grief in maternal deprivation.[86] Reinforcement of experience is but one part of the phenomenon. The capacity to withstand stress is the other. The infant's or child's immature personality may be crushed by a stressful experience that an older child or an adult could easily withstand.

Both stress and crisis observations show that the individual's behavior during the experience affects its significance in terms of enduring, lasting effect on the personality.[87] The person who channels his anxiety outside of himself, through actions, weeping, words, or anger and projection of blame, is less affected than the person who denies the experience or makes a show of rising above it. These observations come largely from the medical field, where social workers and physicians have worked with and recorded observations of persons confronted with bereavement, suicidal impulses, and anxiety over premature infants. In the same vein, adoption workers have learned that unwed mothers who give up their children are less disturbed later if they see the baby soon after its birth and go through the mental anguish of giving it up, rather than trying to pretend the baby never happened. Such terms as "worry work" and "grief work" have been used to describe the anticipatory preparation and conscious adaptation to loss which alleviates the adverse significance of painful experience upon later social functioning.

These theoretical concepts are of greatest practicality for persons concerned with sick and handicapped children, for they have positive as well as negative implications. They cue us in to services that will help modify the effect of adverse experience. That which seems most tactful or the easiest, that is, avoiding discussion of painful matters or helping the individual to "keep a stiff upper lip," is good manners but poor service to the individual faced with catastrophic experience, whether it be having a retarded child, losing a leg, facing a disruption of plans, or death itself. Helping the person talk it out helps avoid later serious effects. Helping the person take action to help himself is a related means of channeling off his anxiety and alleviating impact. The much criticized American funeral is an example of a positive means for discharge of anxiety in bereavement, through the countless details it requires the relative to perform and the opportunity it offers to express emotions.

We may also use our understanding of duration, with its component of reinforcement, as well as our understanding of consistency, in planning the length and variety of experiences the individual or group will have with the agency or counselor. Milieu therapy, so-called, with its consistency in a network of experiences, thus takes on a fresh rationale. The growing use of group members to help each other and the use of volunteers and paraprofessionals can be seen as important aspects of treatment or rehabilitation.

CHAPTER THREE

The Experience of Chronic Illness in Childhood

CHAPTER TWO attempted to establish a foundation for thinking of a chronically ill child as a child in a family. It set forth some general principles applicable to all human beings and all experience. This chapter will introduce the experience of long-term illness in childhood. Ensuing chapters will discuss specific psychosocial meanings occasioned by various medical problems; this one will attempt to isolate elements held in common from those that are unique. In effect it will present a synthesis of Chapters 6 through 18.

Child, family, and illness are intertwined in a dynamic, changing constellation. Attempts to separate the configurations cannot be entirely successful. They are artificial and often overlapping. For purposes of examining the meaning of illness, however, they will be divided as follows: effect of the character of the illness on family and child; effect of family structure, size, and relationships; effect of the child's age or stage of development; effect of the child's reactions to the stress of his illness; and the meaning of hospitalization, so frequent an occurrence during the course of chronic illness.

The purpose served by understanding what long-term childhood illness means to the child and his family is a finer perception of how to help. Lest the reader feel the presentation dwells too much on problems and ignores those strengths on which all help is built, the writer should comment on her awareness of the resilience of the human spirit, the astonishing strength children have, and how many times they come through difficult experiences scarred but nevertheless able to make a relatively satisfactory adjustment. However, in order to help, human services workers need to be sensitive to realities. No purpose is served by glossing over sadness and struggle.

The helping process depends on the agency's function, the practitioner's skill and philosophy, the availability of resources for relief of stress, other services the family and child receive, priorities, and other factors. Little is said here about the nature of helping, other than where it is generic and seems inseparable from consideration of the problem. Collaboration with other agencies and the resources that may be drawn upon to relieve family burdens are treated in a later section.

EFFECTS OF THE CHARACTER OF THE ILLNESS ON FAMILY AND CHILD

Among the similarities and differences of various diagnostic categories are the degree and manner of family burden; the distortion of family relationships, including the feelings of the siblings; the degree of financial burden; the need for housing adaptation; the pain component of the illness; the unpredictability of acute episodes with resultant disturbance in family life-style; the differences in school experiences; and the problems around dying and death in the illnesses that are fatal.

Degree and Manner of Family Burden

Asthma, arthritis, severe cardiac disease, sickle cell anemia, and muscular dystrophy often mean *sleep interruption* for the parents for long-continuing periods. Asthma attacks usually occur at night; the arthritic child is often awakened by pain and must be turned, soothed, or bathed; the child with severe heart disease may be sleepless and fretful and need to be held or propped up for easier breathing; the child with muscular dystrophy progresses to a stage where he cannot roll over and has to be turned.

Arthritis, cystic fibrosis, spina bifida, spinal cord injury, and muscular dystrophy usually create *physical burdens* such as lifting, diapering, dressing, feeding, giving physical therapy treatments, doing extra laundry, etc. If the child's upper extremities are involved, as in high spinal cord damage, muscular dystrophy, and some cases of arthritis, the child may not be able to wipe his nose or flick off a fly. The older child with muscular dystrophy who has become obese because of inactivity is particularly heavy to lift because he has no muscle tone and cannot help.

Asthma, diabetes, and advanced kidney disease require *complicated special diets*, which are time-consuming to prepare and call for thorough education in the principles of the diet and appropriate food preparation. Muscular dystrophy and spina bifida often require obesity diets that make the child feel deprived, depressed, and irritable. In order to eliminate conflict to the degree possible, the entire family should forgo fattening foods (unless contraindicated for health reasons), which adds to the burdens.

Asthma necessitates *extra housecleaning* on a continuing basis. Wet-mopping the floors and dusting are recommended daily, and cotton rugs, blankets, and curtains must be washed frequently.

Degree of Financial Burden

All chronic illness creates great financial burdens. Hemophilia imposes the most catastrophic, since the cost of blood plasma is staggering and often is not covered by insurance. Neither has it been covered by federal funds. Some federal coverage, however, is now available for help with the other financially catastrophic condition, kidney failure. Leukemia can be disastrous financially unless, as often happens, the child is a research subject and hospital and drug costs are reduced by research-project funds. Hospitalization is most apt to be covered in part by insurance, another alleviating factor. Head and spinal cord injuries are also very costly if the family is not covered by insurance, but since the injury often occurs in automobile accidents, liability insurance is a frequent resource. Spina bifida and arthritis require many periods of hospitalization, usually covered in large part by crippled children's services and insurance. Cystic fibrosis, muscular dystrophy, arthritis, spina bifida, and spinal cord injuries sometimes require extensive equipment. These cost less than hospitalization but are usually direct costs to the family. The Muscular Dystrophy Association is extraordinarily generous in alleviating the financial burdens of equipment for families of children with muscular dystrophy.

Need for Housing Adaptation

The crippling conditions that require wheelchairs, ramps, hospital beds, and lifts—spinal cord injuries, some head injuries, spina bifida, some cases of arthritis, hemophilia, sickle cell anemia, and muscular dystrophy—necessitate first-floor housing, sufficient storage for equipment, and hallways and doors wide enough for wheelchairs. Children with sickle cell anemia or arthritis need housing that is warm and has hot water and accessible bathtubs. Some children with asthma should not live in old houses with damp basements or in damp coastal areas where mold is prevalent in the woodwork.

Pain, Social Isolation, and Unpredictability of Crises

Physical pain is especially great in arthritis, sickle cell anemia, hemophilia, and advanced kidney disease, and in the treatment of leukemia and cardiac defects.

Continually isolated because of limitations in mobility are children with muscular dystrophy and spinal cord injury, and some with spina bifida. Those who may have few friends or be avoided because of stigmatizing characteristics are children with cystic fibrosis, spina bifida, spinal cord injury, and head injury. Fatigue often prevents social activities of children with kidney failure, cardiac disease, leukemia, and late-stage cystic fibrosis.

Children who have different dietary requirements, and for this reason cannot share fully in peer-group activities, are those with diabetes and asthma. Some with asthma may not be able to play outdoors at times, or visit friends who have pets. Children feel different and are sometimes regarded as inferior if they have, or are carriers of, hemophilia, sickle cell anemia, cystic fibrosis, or muscular dystrophy.

Children whose disease conditions subject them to unpredictable crises are those with hemophilia, asthma, and sickle cell anemia; they "live life with an if." Life is uncertain for children who are receiving dialysis or who have had a kidney transplant. All sick children with remitting disease such as leukemia, cystic fibrosis, or nephrosis may have unpredictable episodes because of exposures to infection that exacerbate their conditions, or for other reasons; and children with diabetes may at any time have insulin reactions or go into coma if their balance is disturbed.

Differences in School Experience

Children who most commonly attend schools or classes for the physically handicapped are the developmentally disabled, the head-injured, and those with limitations of physical mobility.

Among the major advantages of special schools or classes are the bus transportation, special attendents, physical arrangements, and high degree of individualization possible. Children with muscular dystrophy usually attend special schools even before they become confined to wheelchairs, because of the ease with which they fall down if brushed against or pushed. Not all children in wheelchairs but most children with muscular dystrophy, spina bifida, and spinal cord injuries attend special schools. Those with bladder and bowel incontinence find it easier to diaper themselves if they are among a group that does the same thing. Head-injured children also attend special schools if their learning disabilities are pronounced or their behavior too unstable to permit regular school attendance. Children with arthritis, hemophilia, and sickle cell anemia may attend special schools during flare-ups of joint damage in the lower extremities, and return to regular schools as the condition subsides.

Children with kidney failure receiving dialysis three times a week have serious school-attendance problems unless the treatment center is willing to adapt its schedule to permit them to receive dialysis in the afternoons and on Saturdays, so that they miss only two afternoons a week. Otherwise, they can attend school only two days a week, and consequently need to attend special schools or have home teachers.

Home teachers are needed by children with acute flare-ups of arthritis or nephrosis and in preterminal stages of leukemia and cystic fibrosis. Children with late-stage muscular dystrophy also require home teachers.

Factors Affecting the Manner of Death

A number of the disease groups described in this book have fatal terminations before adulthood in all but exceptional cases. Cystic fibrosis, muscular dystrophy, sickle cell anemia, and leukemia are fatal. Kidney failure is also, though life may be prolonged by means of dialysis and a successful kidney transplant. Heart defects cannot be categorized because of the wide range of severity of the different defects and their response to surgery. However, many babies and children die from heart disease. Many of the children with the myelomeningocele form of spina bifida also die. Death, then, is not an uncommon occurrence among children with the major chronic diseases of childhood.

The death of a child has many meanings in common with the deaths of other children. But the dying process is as individualized as any other experience in life. Many factors influence the experience for the child. How old is he—old enough to know what is happening to him? And if so, old enough to know that death is final, or young enough to have fantasies of fearful figures, or fear of going to sleep thinking he may not wake up?

Is his dying unexpected, or long anticipated and greatly feared? Is the death sudden or protracted? Is he at home or in the hospital? Has the great universal fear of abandonment, of dying alone, become a reality, or does someone he loves and trusts hold him or sit by his side? Does he expect an afterlife, and die thinking he goes to join his grandmother in heaven, or does he feel cheated that this is the end? Is he unconscious, is he drugged and half-awake, or is he fully alert when death comes? Does he die peacefully, with merely a cessation of breath, or does he die in violent pain, or vomiting, bleeding, or choking? Has his torment been so prolonged that he and his family come to welcome his death, or was life for him still sweet?

How will his parents remember the manner of his dying? Will they comfort themselves—"We did everything humanly possible" and "He had the very best doctors in this part of the country but they couldn't save him"—or will they go over and over in their minds their own or each other's acts of omission, and hate the hospital and the doctor for the impersonal, inhumane care the child received?

The constellation takes shape around several biological, social, and psychological factors. Chief among the biological factors affecting the dying process are the diagnosis, the child's age, and the physical treatment he receives.

Infection often brings relatively swift death to children with leukemia, muscular dystrophy, cystic fibrosis, sickle cell anemia, or kidney failure. Progressive weakness frequently precedes the terminal illness, and the infection constitutes merely the final event of the last day or two. Leukemia and cystic fibrosis are examples of two conditions in which death may be very different. In leukemia the child may die during a massive assault of poisonous chemicals, under investigation by a clinical research unit, and thereby die alert and in extreme misery. In cystic fibrosis he may die in a coma induced by administration of oxygen in response to his own failing supply. Although he knows what is going to happen, if he is old enough, his actual death usually occurs while he is "asleep." Some children with sickle cell anemia and some with heart disease die unexpectedly and swiftly in the midst of play or sleep; others with these conditions may die very frightening, painful, and protracted deaths. The child who dies now from heart disease often does so following surgery.

Children are described as having age-related feelings about dying. The youngest children are most filled with anxiety about separation from parents. The early-school-age child is horrified and fearful of death as a personified individual. Only the child of middle-school-age and older is capable of a realistic understanding of death.

Medical and surgical treatment has prolonged the life of many children who formerly would have died during early years. Many with spina bifida, cystic fibrosis, leukemia, heart defects, sickle cell anemia, hemophilia, kidney disease, and other threatening conditions now face death during adolescence instead of childhood. These children have invested more in life, and their families have invested more in them, than earlier. The children are intellectually more aware of the significance of their condition. They are almost pathologically sensitive to stimuli, and they are emotionally labile. Adolescence is a most unfortunate time to die.

There are some positive features. Adolescence is a time of high idealism and searching for meaning. Religious impulses are close, and many young people dedicate themselves to God or service to mankind in one form or another. An interesting facet is the manner in which their need for boundaries and anchorage leads many of this age-group to religions that emphasize discipline and certainty of belief. Some of these religious groups have comprehensive social organizations, a dedicated membership, and a strong paternal figure in the clergyman.

The clergy from such religious groups may be very helpful allies in creating support for the fatally ill adolescent. In addition to these groups are persons among the modern clergy who have loosened their ties to traditional theology and have substituted emulation of the life of Christ, using themselves in social service instead of traditional religious roles. These compassionate persons also constitute excellent potential resources for support to the adolescent facing death.

As will be elaborated in further chapters, especially those on leukemia and cystic fibrosis, an emphasis on communication with the dying person is gaining momentum. Experienced observers have pointed out that some children as young as four, and not infrequently by the age of seven, know they are going to die, but may maintain silence because of cues from their parents and others that the subject cannot be discussed. The wise and humane seem to agree that hope for cure should not be destroyed or imminence of death foretold, but that children should be permitted to ask questions about their outlook so their fears can be brought into the open and they can feel a sense of sharing instead of a hopeless nightmare of loneliness and lack of understanding. Drs. Solnit and Green have said that the child is really asking for reassurance that he will not be left alone or abandoned and that he will be taken care of and be all right.[1]

As in discussions of sex with young children, the adult should not introduce new material. If the child asks a direct question, "Am I going to die?," most experts seem to believe the answer should be truthful: that no cure is yet known for the disease in question, but the doctors are working on a cure and everything possible is being done to prolong the child's life. Turning the question around is a common interviewing technique: "What have you been told?" or "What do you think it will be like?"

The subject of how best to communicate with the child is so difficult that no one knows the answers, and there is some disagreement. One physician has said many practitioners feel that the child is attempting to manage his feelings, whatever ideas he has developed. "This is no time for deep psychiatric therapy, and if he is succeeding in abating his own tensions, let us assist him and not destroy whatever carapace [armor] is constructed as a defense against intolerable anxiety."[2]

In the increasing literature on the subject of dying, the feelings of the parents of a fatally ill child are commonly described as changing from initial shock, self-blame, and anger, to anxiety and an all-pervasive feeling of sorrow and mourning. Resignation or acceptance is sometimes achieved before the child's death occurs. The dangers of premature mourning, with a need for separation from and abandonment of the child, are described in the chapter on leukemia. This need to shield the self from unbearable pain by maintaining emotional distance may also be seen at the birth of a child with severe or multiple defects.

An awareness has emerged of the effect of a child's death on his siblings. Severe personality damage evidently is not infrequent. These children need a great deal more attention from helping persons, and more studies are needed in this area.

The literature also dwells on the emotional problems of the professional persons caring for the child. Death of a child is so genuinely terrible that everyone responds with great feeling. Managing one's own feelings is essential in order not to add unwittingly to the child's despair, abandonment, and/or horror. By no means can everyone manage his or her feelings about a child's death. The most common behavior of professionals, including physicians and social workers and some clergymen and nurses, is to postpone going to see the child, to neglect him, to make excuses to avoid him, or, in plain words, to abandon him at the time of his greatest need. No one wants to do this. Each person has to work out in advance how he will work around his own emotions. Audrey McCollum, who has amassed experience with deaths from cystic fibrosis, advises retaining a clear sense of purpose and of separate selfhood.[3] If it is necessary to find a substitute to perform the visiting and maintain the close relationships needed, the worker should be certain the substitute is indeed visiting the child frequently and meeting his needs.

EFFECTS OF THE FAMILY'S SIZE, STRUCTURE, AND RELATIONSHIPS

The effects of the child's illness on the family have been implied through the various ways it affects their lives as individuals, influences the family life-style, and affects relationships. These things reciprocally affect the ability of family members to nurture and care for the sick child. In addition, the size and structure of the family are among the factors that determine their capacity to meet his and each other's needs.

Family Size and Structure

The chronically ill child needs two parents. It takes two to cope when a child is sick at home over a long period of time. One needs to earn while the other stays home and takes care of the sick child; one may need to take time off from work and care for siblings while the other parent takes the sick child to the doctor or attends to the chores of living. Two may be needed to lift a child in a cast or to lift an older child who has become obese from inactivity. It often takes two to "spell each other" during long-drawn-out and physically wearing home care and treatment. When children are ill for weeks on end, needing to be turned or sat with, medicated, and comforted, exhaustion sets in if only one adult has the entire burden. And these things say nothing of the mutual support that parents need when fearful things are happening to a loved child, when worries mount, or when disaster strikes.

Because it takes two, certain elements become apparent. First is that the experience of the intact family differs dramatically from that of the precariously balanced partial family. The stage of the family life cycle has proved to play a large part in the greater stability of the family of school-age children. By the time one or several children are in school, most parents of chronically ill children have either separated or settled into a pattern of living together and caring for their children. Though gross distortion may have taken place and adverse patterns may exist in family relationships, there are still two adults and a home. The child has a buffering mechanism, an anchorage.

When there are two adults, a middle-class life-style is more apt to exist. Because two can earn, they are more apt to buy a house than move from apartment to apartment, and a certain stability develops as they live in a residential neighborhood and associate with similar families, and the children attend neighborhood school. Neighbors become allies; they can help with transportation to the hospital or doctor's office in an emergency or take care of the other children overnight. Some socialization pulls exist, to the PTA and to the church, and a circle of relative strength surrounds the family and thus the child. It will be recalled from Chapter 2 that the two adults in an increasing number of families include a stepparent, owing to the rising number of divorces and remarriages.

Second marriages introduce complicating elements into the family structure. The child may have three parents instead of two—one on the sidelines, blaming and competitive, or indifferent and resented as a noncontributor. The natural parent may be too fearful of losing the new partner to burden him or her with a full share of the load of caring for a sick child. Stepmothers have less investment in children not their own, and to this extent may be less prone to infantilize the sick child. They also tend to have conflicting feelings about the expense and inconveniences and hence about the child, and sometimes a feeling of "walking on eggs" with the child's father and with the paternal grandparents. Relationships become very complex, tenuous, and potentially destructive.

Young parents of preschool children also have special problems. The ill child will be one with either a congenital defect, such as spina bifida, or an illness of early onset, such as asthma, arthritis, sickle cell anemia, hemophilia, or heart disease, which creates special problems physiologically and psychologically. The parents' needs for good times and fulfillment are strong. They have not yet fully matured in either their marriage or parental relationships. With less job security, their financial status and general marriage balance are easily disrupted by an unexpected turn toward unhappiness and sacrifice. Often the mother has matured through the process of child bearing, and is more capable of sacrificing for a sick child. If life becomes too unpleasant and unrewarding for the husband, he may leave.

Other relationships exist in single-parent families or those in which there is a social-contract marriage. Drs. Podoll and Smith, of the University of Miami, who have recently summarized the literature on parent-child relationships in "partial families," point out that these children have greater problems with social adjustment, juvenile delinquency, sex-role identification, and—of special concern to those interested in the chronically ill child—problems of self-esteem. They also state that family disruption through divorce is more damaging to the children than that occurring from the death of one of the parents.[4]

Others who have remarked on this fact point out that "emotional divorce" may have occurred several years before the actual divorce. In the words of one youth, "It was no fun hearing them fight and wondering if you were going to land in an orphanage."

Not only do children suffer from what happened before the divorce, but the mother has a "diminished capacity for parenting," in the words of the leader of a group of single mothers, because of feelings of worthlessness, depression, and helplessness in controlling their own and their children's behavior. These women felt that their children were worried about their father's leaving and seemed to fear their mothers would leave also.[5]

The single parent cannot maintain independence and care for a chronically ill child at home unless child support is adequate and steady. The mother must either return to her family or lead the life of a welfare recipient. This adjustment may follow futile attempts at living with a friend or series of roommates while either or both of them work.

The single-parent family of lower class has been described as consisting of one or more women of child-bearing age, frequently related to each other. "Associated with this household type is a marriage pattern in which the woman has a succession of temporary partners during her procreative years."[6]

The woman's psychological dependency is heightened by the burden of caring for a sick child, and she longs for someone she can lean on who will help her. How frequently such mothers remarry is not known. A man may not wish to take legal responsibility for a burdensome child, and his relationship with the mother may be that of a nonlegal, temporary partner. Studies have begun of "divergent family forms," including social-contract marriages, multilateral marriages, and communal life-styles, but how the children will be affected is not yet known.[7]

If a single mother, divorced or not previously married, is living with a man to whom she is not married, the welfare department considers him a resource. A "man in the house" means that the mother may be in danger of prosecution for fraud, which adds greatly to the stresses she is under. Her desperation in trying to maintain the "love relationship," often in the futile hope that the man will marry and support her, creates tensions and disorganization, resulting in less free energy toward solution of problems and appropriate care of the sick child and other children. Serious counseling with her about potential resources in child care and relief of her burdens may lead to locating a relative who can help on an indefinite basis, especially if financial aid can be provided to the relative to attend to the child. It may lead to homemaker service by a mature person who can give the mother emotional support in addition to relief in managing her duties.

Foster day care for the ill child, or for other preschool children, may free the mother from some pressures. Practical help with transportation and clinic care by an aide or volunteer may offer additional partial relief from stress. However the problem is attacked, the mother's needs for long-term emotional support and partial relief from child-caring duties are vital elements in the plan.

The size of the family also influences its ability to mediate stress. An only child is indeed a lonely child when he is physically unable to reach out and maintain friends at school or in the neighborhood. Though sibling problems and resentments can be severe in families where a handicapped child is the mother's "special child," siblings bring in their friends and interests from the outside world. They require interplay and thereby force some socialization. They are natural outlets for emotion, as sources of affection or dislike. They are available for games or company, and, very important, they dilute parental concentration on the sick child. Observation repeatedly indicates greater normalcy of the sick child in families with other children.

Excessive size of family, however, usually means a physically exhausted mother, poverty, and inability to provide adequate care for the sick child. Exceptions are those families in which the oldest children are older teenagers or adults who provide help. The woman with many children who has produced a child with congenital defects may have an overwhelming love for the baby, and the child may be the pet of all.

Relationships Within the Family

Parental attitudes change over the course of time. When first confronted with a child's defective or life-threatening condition, the parents may be shocked, stunned, disbelieving. The early reaction is one of intense emotional turmoil. If they have taken an obviously ill child from doctor to doctor before a diagnosis is made, their first reaction may be one of anger at the medical profession, but if the diagnosis is entirely unsuspected, they first suffer from the universal reaction to catastrophe—guilt: "Why has this happened to us? What have I (or we) done to deserve this?" Then anger may begin to surface, as the hurt becomes unbearable and is displaced outward.[8] Rose Grobstein, Chief Pediatric Social Worker at the Stanford Medical Center, has pointed out that it is the social worker's responsibility to help families during this period of depression and anger, that although it becomes difficult when the parents lash out at everybody, it is nonetheless important to help them talk about the disease and to support them until they can face the future.

A concept that originated with a perceptive social worker, S. Olshansky, in regard to parents' feelings about retarded children, applies to attitudes that develop when a child has a severe physical handicap. He calls this "chronic sorrow," a feeling that is not acceptance and is not neurotic but natural, continuing, underlying grief.[9] Olshansky thinks release from chronic sorrow comes only when the child dies. One couple said that bursts of grief come unexpectedly when some small vent occurs—a child's question, or observing normal children at play—and sorrow gushes up. Then they return to matter-of-fact "acceptance."

Because life moves forward swiftly for the family, with repeated crises for the sick child and with new, important events for other members—pregnancies, job changes, accidents, promotions, school activities, housing changes—and because exhaustion sets in for the burdened mother and resentments and expenses and problems of interrelationships pile up, some families need repeated help throughout the lifetime of the child. Distortions—whether of the child's psyche or family relationships—often can be prevented or ameliorated if stresses are relieved through the use of resources and if the lives of all members of the family are considered.

A recurring distortion of relationships in families of chronically ill children seems to be the father's abdication of responsibility and increased absence from the home. Entwined in an abnormally close relationship are child and mother. The cause is in part induced by the mother's involvement in medical care while the father is working. She becomes an authority on what the doctor says and recommends, and the father is gradually left out. Also, the father needs his rest at night. By contrast, the mother's ability to nap when the child naps enables her more readily to get up at night; thus her nurturing function is heightened and the father's role minimized.

Several observers have also pointed out the disappointment that males often feel when boy children are physically weak. Fathers take pride in a little child's ability to throw a ball, and later to play baseball and football. Men who equate physical strength with virility, and virility with male worth, are especially prone to think of a weak son as a reflection on their own worth.

Class differences seem to exist. Males who take pride in mental capacity and place value on intellectual and artistic pursuits tend to be educated persons, and education is correlated (in general) with social class. The extent of distortion resulting from paternal abdication in spoiling the identity of the child and fostering too intense relationships between mother and son has led practitioners to emphasize the importance of intervention. Charles Hurt, who specializes in work with families with hemophilia, believes that distortion is not inevitable in middle-class families.[10] These fathers can usually take time off from work to participate in the child's medical supervision, and are articulate enough to profit from counseling.

However, the abdicating father and resentful mother are often found beneath the superficial garb of "normal," middle-class living. The harried expression, the weary, rigid, and tight nervous manner, often reveal something of the strain the mother is under in carrying the lion's share of the burden of the chronically ill child. The mother whose housekeeping standards are low, whose yard is neglected, and who has learned to greet continuing small household disasters without great distress, probably has made the best adjustment, except in the minority of cases where the father does share fully in the ever-present extra work and worries that the sick child creates.

The guilt of the mother in producing a defective child and the overprotection stemming from it are so often described as to create a stereotype. Self-blame does seem instinctive in Western culture as a reaction to any catastrophe—"What have I done to deserve this?" A vengeful God who sees every sin appears to have been incorporated in the personality of many persons. However, projection of guilt as anger—and felt as anger, not as self-blame—appears to be common. Many mothers blame the doctor who delivered the baby, or the spouse, or sometimes the child.

In all the genetically transmitted diseases, guilt in the parents is presumed, though by no means always evident on the surface. It is influenced by whether the transmission is sex-linked, as in hemophilia and Duchenne's muscular dystrophy, or recessive, as in sickle cell anemia and cystic fibrosis. The blaming or self-blaming attitudes of the parents also seem to depend on their prior knowledge of carrier status.

The tendency to medium or large families, when parents know they carry a genetically transmissible disease, is an enigma. No study is known of the motivation for repeated reproduction after carrier status is known. Religious reasons for failure to limit conception do not appear primary. In some instances, as in muscular dystrophy, the parents may not be aware of the full impact of the disease, because of its delayed crippling, until after several younger children have been born. This may be true also in cystic fibrosis if the first child is not seriously affected during early childhood. However, *the need to prove themselves normal* seems to be a strong motivating factor in some families. The shattering effect on self-esteem has been described,[11] and it seems probable that emotional havoc may play a large part in irrational decisions about further childbearing—whether to stop or to continue. Or, the desire to have at least one normal child may cause parents to minimize the meaning of known statistical chances. Only "one in four" chances of having a defective baby, as in marriages of two persons both of whom have defective recessive genes, may not sound ominous to a person driven by inner compulsion to prove his capability of producing sound offspring.

A two-way feeling toward the ill child seems almost universal. Most mothers love but also resent the child. The countless ways in which the sick child has inconvenienced, humiliated, burdened, frustrated, worried, and deprived her and the rest of the family cannot be overlooked. Overt rejection is not infrequent when the child has outward deformities from birth, as in spina bifida or other congenital malformations.

The relationships at special hazard in one-parent families have been the subject of a number of studies. Dr. Podoll has summarized research regarding the effect of the absence of a male model and the symbiosis of mother and child. Excessively dependent relationships between a child and parent, he states, result in retarded psychosocial development.[12] Persons working with adolescents with sickle cell anemia or cystic fibrosis have commented on the immaturity of a number of these young persons. These children are realistically dependent upon the ministrations of their parents, and are at double hazard of immaturity if reared by the mother alone.

The distortions generally found seem to have some specific applications. Though highly variable, they offer clues to problems created by various diagnoses. *Rejection* of the child with a cosmetic or outward defect at birth often occurs because of shock, grief, and feelings of loss (of an expected normal baby) and guilt. Though the parents may not discuss their feelings that the baby would be better dead, they may feel so, especially where the handicap is severe. This pattern is seen in spina bifida (myelomeningocele form).

In spina bifida and severe cardiac defects, the child's surgical treatment prior to release from the hospital means prolonged separation of mother and child. In premature infants this has been shown to impede development of normal mother-child interaction.[13] In any case where the child does not reward the parents with signs of gratification or response to care given, but instead cries and frets from pain, a barrier exists to the usual two-way flow of developing love.

Children with life-threatening illnesses manifested during infancy or early childhood arouse in parents extremes of concern, which may become mixed with resentment and sometimes an inability to provide appropriate discipline and guidance. This "vulnerable child syndrome" is frequent in cases of serious heart defects, kidney defects, asthma, sickle cell anemia, and hemophilia. It may occur in cystic fibrosis if the child is ill in infancy.

The *overprotective mother and abdicating father* are often seen in hemophilia and asthma. The *frequent absence of a male model* for the boy with hemophilia due to the abdicating father may also be found in other diseases of early onset, such as arthritis and asthma, which disturb early marriage relationships. The symbiotic or unhealthy *dependent relationship* between child and mother may be heightened in cystic fibrosis, because of the prolonged bodily contact in treatment, and in sickle cell anemia and asthma because of the child's physical dependence on the mother's help during attacks.

Maternal deprivation due to early, repeated hospitalization is most prevalent in severe cardiac defects, spina bifida, sickle cell anemia, nephrosis, and congenital kidney defects. *Lack of communication between parents* is characteristic when grief becomes intolerable, as in the early diagnostic and later terminal stages of leukemia, and has often been identified in asthma, when severe attacks in the young child threaten life or appear to.

Resentment, fear, and guilt among siblings have been identified in leukemia, asthma, diabetes, and hemophilia, and undoubtedly may exist in all other chronic illnesses of life-threatening nature or those of early onset in which the siblings are deprived of maternal affection and attention. Relationships among siblings are uniquely complex if the siblings are aware they are potential kidney donors.

The psychological effect upon siblings of the chronic illness of one child seems to depend on when, how long, and how much they are deprived of the things they want; the sick child's behavior and their retaliation with consequent guilt; and the strengths in the family, including parental attitudes toward them and the sick child. Some siblings develop a protective attitude toward the sick child, even when he is older than they. Deprivation of affection and attention from the parents, and deprivation of material wants because of the sick child's needs, create resentment that in some cases becomes very deep and destructive.

The ages of all the children are an issue, with respect particularly to whether the mother stays at the hospital with the sick child. If the sick child is of school age and can understand the mother's absence as only temporary, and a younger brother or sister is at a critical age in respect to maternal deprivation, it can be presumed the sibling needs her more than the sick child does, unless the latter is terminally ill. General policies that the mother should always be at home "because the other children need her," or vice versa, should be examined in terms of each child's special needs.

The general tendency of school-age and teenage siblings seems to be to go their own way and ignore the sick child, although there are obvious exceptions. The age differential affects their ability to do so with normalcy. Older siblings seem often to be protective of younger chronically ill children at school, and older girls may take on maternal roles.

The death of an ill child arouses fear in siblings who have the same disease. In cystic fibrosis, sickle cell anemia, and muscular dystrophy, two or more children in the same family may have the fatal condition. Often one child was very young when the other died, and he knows he had a brother who died but does not attach the death to his own condition. In other instances, notably in muscular dystrophy, the boys may be only a few years apart in age, and the younger can observe the older become gradually weaker and die, and knows he too has the same condition. In this disease, denial seems particularly prevalent, and a significant number are dulled by mental retardation. Lack of verbalization among the majority, or possibly lack of opportunity for communication, prevents us from knowing how much panic they feel. In sickle cell anemia, variations in the severity and manifestations of the disease allow more opportunity for realistic denial than in muscular dystrophy, where the same patterns exist.

Healthy children do not escape the fear of contamination by the disease that killed a brother or sister. Binger, who has made a study of siblings of children dying of leukemia, says, "We have noted their inner feelings of being responsible for the sibling's death, fears that they will be next, resentment that the parents spent so much time with the ill child, anger at the parents who 'allowed' the sibling to become ill, and preoccupation with inner fantasies around the death."[14] In Binger's study, children in more than half of the families showed later psychological difficulties after a sibling's death, even when they had earlier appeared well adjusted.

EFFECTS OF AGE AND DISRUPTION OF BASIC CHILDHOOD TASKS

What illness means to a child at the time it occurs, and the impression it leaves on his personality, are largely affected by his stage of development or, in other words, are age-related. Theories differ regarding the later significance of events of early life. A widely accepted formulation is that by Erik Erikson.[15] He has described the qualities man needs, and the stages during which their foundations are laid in the personality. He describes "tasks" to be achieved during each stage. Though he takes pains to point out that a task can be modified by later experience, his "eight stages of man" indicate a ladder of emotional growth that parallels the realities of physiological and social progression. Each stage serves as a building block for the next.

Serious disruption at any one stage averts normal progression and creates a distortion in the personality. We are concerned with the ways illness disrupts the "basic tasks" of childhood, and we shall use the Erikson formulation in the following discussion.

Basic trust, the first task, was described in Chapter 1, including ways it evolves from the infant's experience of consistent gratification of needs for comfort and nurturing. He learns to distinguish the outside world from himself, and to trust it through trusting that first object, his mother.

What of the child with a severe congenital heart defect or spina bifida who undergoes corrective surgical procedures during the first few months of life? If the child psychologists are correct, his mind has not formed; only the nerves at the top of the brain stem have sheathed themselves with myelin; he cannot distinguish whether the pain comes from outside or inside. He is completely vulnerable to the shock of pain and has no tools whatsoever to express distress except cries of rage. The surgery on newborns, the transfusions and innumerable punctures—do these things create such profound trauma to the incomplete nervous system that pseudo-retardation may occur? When the sick child receives, instead of one consistent set of touching, smells, heel clicks, and sounds associated with the pleasure of food and cleanliness, a myriad set from the ever-shifting teams of hospital nurses and aides, does he ever have the opportunity to incorporate basic trust in the outside world? Can he develop a sense of security if, at six months to a year, he begins to experience severe pain in his abdomen, feet, hands, from the vascular occlusion of sickle cell anemia?

The baby's mouth has special importance during the first year of life because it is the site of his main gratification, relief from hunger. Fortunately, few chronic illnesses affect the mouth in early life. However, inability to gratify hunger without distress, as in the allergic, colicky baby or the infant with a severe cardiac defect, or constant hunger, as in the baby with a voracious appetite due to cystic fibrosis, might be expected to have an effect on dependency, which is equated with satisfaction of oral needs during infancy.

Maternal deprivation through separation from the mother, for hospitalization or any other reason, is always a matter of concern and some controversy.[16] No one who has observed infants and small children in hospitals can doubt the classic formulation of mourning and despair the small child experiences when separated from his mother. Sula Wolff, in *Children under Stress*, says that between seven months and four years the emotional effects of separation and of the treatment of illness are at their maximum; that nothing has been devised to counteract the anxiety of these children. She advocates a parent's staying with the child, and refers to Anna Freud's formulation that "alone the child cannot master his anxieties. He may have fears of overwhelming attack and destruction because with his limited capacities he cannot understand what is going on. When his mother and father are present he leaves all this to them. He trusts them to put things right."[17]

Separation is only one form of maternal deprivation. Inconsistency is another. The mother conveys her ambivalence to this vulnerable organism if she holds her infant at arm's length, and tends him tensely, out of revulsion over his appearance, grief over her inability to bear a normal child, or fear that he will die. The infant's life depends on her mercies, and his psychic antennae are long. Therefore, preparation of the mother to receive her sick or defective child, and a great deal of emotional support while she is adjusting to his imperfection, are necessary and often hard to accomplish.

Beginning with the second year of life, the need for activity is as urgent as the need for loving gratification during the first year. When the child's growth impulses impel him to pull himself up in the crib, to crawl, walk, run, climb, and explore, disease may immobilize him; one wonders what happens as a result of immobilization for intravenous feedings, transfusions, casting, postsurgical treatment, or pain itself. Congenital defects that manifest themselves at birth or soon after, the respiratory diseases of infancy, and cardiac defects may create problems during the early part of the active period. The child with hemophilia, sickle cell anemia, nephrosis, juvenile arthritis, or leukemia may also suffer from activity limitation during the height of need for activity during the toddler period.

This is the time for development of *autonomy*, the beginning of self-confidence and the ability to stand on one's own feet. The child learns he can withhold or let go, since this is also the time of sphincter development. The child has a weapon for control, but he learns to relinquish it to gain love and praise, or by being shamed and whipped. How critical this weapon is in character development, and how hard-fought the battle, are revealed through many observations in later life.

Just as the mouth is most important in the first year, the bottom gradually becomes most important as developing sphincter control gives these nerves intensified feeling and the toilet-training struggle becomes the central issue between child and mother. Cystic fibrosis would seem to have serious impact on this stage of development. The frequent, foul, and bulky stools heighten the struggle, identify the baby with "stink" and "shame." The child with spina bifida who has no sphincter control has a different problem. Habit training involves longer periods of immobilization, more accidents, and uncertain success. Lack of sensation deprives the child of the weapon other children use.

The child's anxiety about separation from the mother is also thought to be at its height when the child is about two years old. The child who is running away, being very naughty, and exploring the world dares to do as he does because of his secure feeling that his mother will be there to run back to, to protect him against himself. A corollary is anxiety over absence of the mother at this stage of biopsychosocial development. Thesi Bergmann, an outstanding theoretician of child development, says the toddler has the "worst of two worlds" when he is separated from the mother by hospitalization.[18]

Initiative is the next stage of child development. The relative loneliness and social isolation of most chronically ill children and youth make initiative a vital determinant in both social and intellectual preparation for adult life. However, apathy, normlessness, and lack of motivation are terms frequently encountered in descriptions of obstacles to scholastic and vocational pursuits among handicapped adolescents and young adults.

The oedipal complex and its relationship to both initiative and its opposite, guilt, are abstruse. The very appellation of a Greek king's name to the complex reflects centuries-old knowledge of the child's competition with mother or father for the love of the opposite-sex parent. That this urge is strong in the four-to-six-year-old can be witnessed by any parent or careful observer. Erikson couples the childish drive for conquest with the earliest development of initiative, with exuberance and new thrust in mental and locomotor development.[19] Because children at this stage still think largely in magical ideas and fantasies, they easily develop guilt over "bad" thoughts. It is an easy step from guilt over such thoughts as "I hate you" to fear of punishment.

That illness punishes is unquestionably true. With some exceptions (muscular dystrophy, asymptomatic and unsuspected cardiac defects, kidney failure from glomerulonephritis, most spinal cord injuries, and diabetes), chronic illness in childhood tends to become established during or before the oedipal period. As surgical techniques have improved and diagnoses and follow-up utilize sophisticated, painful, intrusive procedures, "punishment" through medical care during this highly vulnerable stage of development becomes more frequent and intense. The fear of mutilation and the terrors of children are often not understood. Frequently the mother says, "He fought the doctors like a demon" or "You could hardly hold him down" during blood tests or biopsies. Apparently these children have had their fantasies confirmed by reality; that is, they felt guilt and feared punishment, and now it has arrived. Fixation at this level of development is a real possibility when this happens, with a resultant bent in the character toward guilt, fear, and hostility.

Some chronically ill children show a great deal of initiative during late childhood or adolescence and have few outward identity problems worse than those of the usual adolescent. No research is known that correlates onset and illness experience with later behavior. We can be guided only by what we know of child development in assuming that pain and "punishment" should be diminished as much as possible for the sake of the child's later capacity for initiative and establishment of a stable identity.

The task of the school-age child is the development of *industrious habits*; failure to master the task is said by Erikson to create a sense of inferiority. The schoolchild achieves his goal through satisfactory competition with peers and winning recognition for his successes. The chronically ill child particularly needs to develop industrious habits, since he will not be able to compete physically when he reaches adolescence and adulthood. And a seedbed for feelings of inferiority is especially unfortunate because the child's feelings of difference inevitably will be acute when he reaches adolescence.

Often children with a mild recurring illness or those who are small-sized from steroid medication or cardiac growth retardation pour all their energies into schoolwork and receive a great deal of recognition. Our concern is with the child whose leukemia, hemophilia, cystic fibrosis, sickle cell anemia, diabetes, muscular dystrophy, asthma, arthritis, spina bifida, head or cord injury, kidney failure, or other chronic conditions create major interference with his school career. He may miss school so often that he does not understand what the others are talking about, or for such a long period that he is below grade, or find himself isolated on the playground and without friends.

First grade, like junior high school, is a time of special insecurity, and a time when the foundation for all that follows scholastically is laid down. The child who gets behind then or whose socialization has been impeded learns to dislike school and starts to feel inferior. Onset prior to first grade, with interference to school entry and to satisfying peer relationships, happens most frequently in cystic fibrosis, sickle cell anemia, hemophilia, asthma, arthritis, spina bifida, leukemia, and head injury. Kidney failure, diabetes, and the immobilizing phase of muscular dystrophy usually do not appear until later in the school career.

The psychosocial problems of the chronically ill child peak at adolescence. The achievement of *identity* is the major task of this stage of development. Essential to the task is acceptance by one's peers, a definition of sexual identity as male or female, an occupational predilection or choice, and development of a value system through finding adults one can emulate. Inability to form a sense of identity or separate selfhood results in "role confusion," that is, bewilderment about what others expect and what one should expect of oneself.

Adolescence is the period when the self-image coalesces. If it incorporates hundreds of negative perceptions of self elicited by bodily limitations and negative reactions from others, the youth feels different, and inferior. Being different is the touchstone of identity problems in the chronically ill adolescent. This violation of the impelling urge to be like his peers is a torment with varying manifestations.

Early adolescence, or the period from approximately 12 to 14 years of age, is most difficult.[20] The onset of puberty coincides with entrance to junior high school. In contrast to a neighborhood school where the child knew the teachers and the rules, he now attends large classes where he is not known and where he must change classes, sometimes involving stairs or distance, in intervals too brief for comfort and in the midst of a jostling crowd. In contrast to a school that took for granted his appearance and limitations, now, during the height of his self-consciousness, he is subjected to stares.

Physical education classes frequently pose special problems. The youth may be ashamed to disrobe and shower in front of his classmates, particularly if he is sexually immature, wears an appliance, or has unsightly deformities. He may be required to sit on the sidelines while all the others participate in vigorous sports. The athletic coach, whom others can emulate and whose praise and encouragement provide an important constructive force, is not usually an available model to him.

Adolescence is not only a time when the accretions of childhood experience coalesce; it is a time of rapid growth. This means that it is a time of flux, when the personality is particularly open and vulnerable to experiences of every kind. The feedback from others has special significance. Stigmatizing characteristics, such as the irritating cough and foul flatulence of cystic fibrosis, the loss of hair from radiation for leukemia, the obesity and growth of facial hair from steroids for kidney disease, the smell of urine surrounding the incontinent youth with spina bifida, and the crippling of hemophilia or arthritis or muscular dystrophy—all these create the social situation of the stigmatized, described by Goffman:[21]

> The stigmatized individual tends to hold the same beliefs about identity as we do ... shame becomes a central possibility, arising from the individual's perception of one of his own attributes as being a defiling thing to possess.... [The physically normal person] feels on shaky ground ... showing familiar signs of discomfort and stickiness: guarded references, fixed stare elsewhere, artificial levity, compulsive loquaciousness, awkward solemnity.

The feedback the youth receives from others wounds his self-esteem. He longs for friends, to be like the others. His eagerness to be one of the group may desensitize him entirely to the burden that his physical dependency creates. In some instances his failure to make himself as acceptable as possible increases his social isolation.

Inability to attract the opposite sex is a part of the complex. The adolescent's obsession with his sexual attractiveness needs no elaboration. Sublimation of feelings of difference during school-age years, through successful competition in grades or hobbies, no longer forms a sufficient bulwark during adolescence. The bitterest cry of all is "Who would want to marry me?"

Those whose cosmetic defects are not severe, as is often the case in mild hemophilia or sickle cell anemia, and in diabetes and cardiac disease, not infrequently do attract someone from the opposite sex. They thereby overcome the worst of their conflict by what seems a successful resolution of their identity as man or woman. Although studies have shown their marriage rate to be lower than normal, a large percentage of some groups of handicapped adults do marry.[22] However, the severity of the handicap is an influential factor. In one study of the graduates of a special school for the physically handicapped, 36 percent of the women and 18 percent of the men were married.[23]

Inability to compete successfully with the parent of the same sex aggravates the problem of poor self-image of some chronically ill adolescents. Although adolescents traditionally seem to reject their parents, even to hate them, and look elsewhere for those heroes Erikson says they must search out and emulate, they in fact model after their own parents. The physically unattractive girl whose mother is pretty, well dressed, and petite is at greatest disadvantage. Reminders of her mother's sexual prowess are unbearable, if, like the girl with spina bifida, she may sit in a diaper leaking urine while her mother goes shopping and comes home with pretty dresses and cosmetics. The boy with hemophilia or severe kidney disease whose father takes his normal siblings fishing or backpacking but leaves him at home, or who ignores him while absorbed in watching the baseball games on TV, is in the same position. These children are defeated. They hate themselves and their bodies, and they project their hatred on their parents and the world around them.

Enforced dependence on the parents, primarily the mother, is a cause of heightened conflict in some chronically ill adolescents. During the psychological period when he should be liberating himself, the child with cystic fibrosis who needs to be "pounded," or clapped, in areas he cannot reach himself, the boy with hemophilia or sickle cell anemia who may be suddenly in acute pain and in urgent need of physical assistance, the young person who is gradually losing strength and knows he is going to die from leukemia or muscular dystrophy or kidney failure—in fact, all the physically ill in active phases of disease need the security of physical care that parents provide. Yet because of the psychological thrust toward independence, some are bitter. Others remain curiously immature and dependent, failing to grow up psychologically. In some instances the mother has encouraged immaturity, gaining perhaps unconscious satisfaction from keeping the child dependent, since she is denied the usual satisfaction of rearing a normal child.

Still another problem in establishing identity is that of those youths who have rapidly changing physical problems, as occur in hemophilia, sickle cell anemia, and asthma. The unpredictability and suddenness of bleeds in hemophilia and crises in sickle cell anemia mean that the child may be walking one day and in a wheelchair the next. He may go to school for the handicapped one semester and normal school the next. He does not know what to expect of himself—can he get his own drink of water or does he depend on his mother to bring it? Can he go to the basketball game or does he have to stay home and watch it on TV? The confusion is heightened by the feedback from his confused peers and parents. They do not know whether to regard him as adequate and competitive, as he is one day, or as dependent, as he may be the next.

A final problem that merits consideration is that of the chronically ill adolescent who has hitherto been well. He may be disabled suddenly by a long quiescent cardiac defect, unsuspected kidney disease, or a recurrence of apparently cured nephrosis, he may develop leukemia in adolescence, or incur a spinal cord or head injury during an accident. Nothing in his childhood prepared him for his new role. Depending upon the medical problem he develops and its duration and outlook, his expectations for liberation from parental dominance, for sexual conquests and career may suddenly disappear, or become objects of long, hard-fought battle. He is suddenly faced with a change in social role, body image, goals, and experience. He may be introduced to that greatest discontinuity of childhood, dying, an act undreamed of before old age.

These youths, like those suddenly blind, always suffer from depression. They have a loss to mourn, that of the old self, before they can accept their new self-image. The time for mourning cannot be foreshortened. (The topic of depression is taken up elsewhere.)

EFFECTS OF THE CHILD'S REACTION TO THE STRESS OF ILLNESS

The ways children react depend on what they are going through, their age level, and their previous experiences, or, in other words, by the degree of stress felt. Wide constitutional differences of temperament and intelligence also exist, as do other individual factors. Much depends on the degree to which the child is helped, or his trauma alleviated.

The Nature and Degree of Stress

It will be recalled from Chapter 2 that the degree of stress felt and the adaptive capacity determine the ability to cope. The several factors that generally determine degree of stress, such as its duration and suddenness, were described. In considering children, the developmental level is vital. An English psychiatrist has pointed out that the stage of development determines the stress the child feels. His social and emotional development determines what he experiences, and his intellectual development determines what he thinks about the experience.[24]

The degree of stress felt is also determined by earlier experiences. Saul's "Achilles heel" concept applies to infants and children as well as to adults. Reactivation of earlier painful experiences occurs when the child is threatened by a similar situation, which increases his anxiety and therefore adds to his pain. For example, the child who has been made insecure by previous separations from the mother, or by rejection, inconsistency, or painful treatment, enters a hospital with more fright and is more distressed by his current treatment.

Pain is a special source of stress in arthritis, hemophilia, sickle cell anemia, kidney disease, leukemia and its treatment, and cardiac surgery. Experienced nurses emphasize the need to reduce the amount of pain children must endure.[25] The adult can usually indicate that he has had as much pain as he can stand, but the acutely ill child who cannot speak for himself may undergo a crushing, intolerable burden of pain unless he is under the care of perceptive physicians and nurses who intervene with sedatives. Bergmann, the child analyst, says that, especially in early infancy, pain and discomfort "upset the delicate balance between pleasure and unpleasure which lies at the basis of mental development and determines the infant's positive or negative attitude toward life." She goes on to say that painful illnesses and painful medical procedures "are to be dreaded in the interest of mental development."[26] Anthony, an authority on disease and death in children, says, "Pain is the great problem for the sick child. The child in pain is a child maltreated, harried, punished, persecuted, threatened with annihilation."[27] (The effect of pain on little children is elaborated in the chapter on arthritis.)

Mattsson has reviewed some *other common stresses* specific to certain chronic disorders.[28] He points out the worries over coma or loss of consciousness and other fears and frustrations of the diabetic and epileptic; the fears of suffocation, drowning, and dying of the child with asthma or cystic fibrosis, and the embarrassment of the latter; the distress of children with bleeding disorders who fear they may bleed to death; the apprehension and depression that accompany a disorder of the heart; and the variety of fears of children on dialysis machines or those who receive transplanted kidneys:

The child with a serious, chronic disease has to cope with threats of exacerbations (flare-ups), lasting physical impairment, and at times a shortened life expectancy. Other common concerns of his and his family relate to mounting medical expenses and the interference of his illness with schooling, leisure activities, vocational training, job opportunities, and later adult roles.

Most significantly, this compassionate psychiatrist points out,[29]

The final outcome of the child's attempts at mastering the continuous stress associated with his disability *cannot be assessed until young adulthood*. Each progressive step in his emotional, intellectual, and social development changes the psychologic impact of the illness on his personality and on his family, and usually equips him with better means to cope. Changes in disease process and in family circumstances will also affect the adaptational process.

The Struggle to Cope

Mattsson emphasizes the positive. He points out that the child's increasing intellectual understanding, the progressively greater variety of ways he can express himself in language and activity, and his better judgment as he matures provide him with more assets with which to meet stress.

Social workers perhaps have a bias in the opposite direction, for they are geared to problems, and they hear and see the details of the strain that children and families endure. With gratitude and admiration for those who have surmounted severe long-term stress, the human services professions must direct most of their energy to helping children and their families

during struggles to overcome downward pulls, c[...]
crises.

Some signs of the struggle, with which the chi[ld needs] help, are denial, regression, depression, and one o[r more of] acting-out behavior. These, and observations o[f the] child, will be discussed.

Denial as a coping mechanism is described in d[etail.] It is a primitive psychological mechanism, used b[y all,] most useful in providing escape from intolerable [pain. It can] operate while a person is in the grip of great pa[in. It may re]minder of his disability, but it can spring forth q[uickly if it disap]pears. The daring, rebellious adolescent may be self-destructive by using denial of heart disease or diabetes and thus disregarding restrictions. Denial is often used by the fatally ill adolescent as a means of enduring what would otherwise be overwhelming depression. It is also used during the mourning period after loss of the old self, as in paraplegia or quadriplegia resulting from a spinal cord injury. During this period the person may nurse conviction of a miracle. He cannot be motivated to rehabilitation efforts that classify him as disabled, for he cannot endure the possibility that he will not someday be well. Escape can take many forms; if a person needs it, one should pause for very thoughtful evaluation of the purpose served before attempting to take it away.

Regression is inevitable when the organism is under emotional or physical stress. The child who runs crying to mother after falling down and the mother who "kisses away" the hurt are acting out the drama of an organism's return to an earlier way of securing comfort. The bed-wetting common after foster-home placement shows instinctive return to infantile behavior. The heightened dependency needs during pain or other forms of physical distress should be met. Just as the child whose finger has been kissed stops crying and runs back to play, the sick child who needs extra love and attention can relinquish his infantile behavior when he feels better.

The writer makes this point because of the sometimes mistaken application of behavior modification theory which fears that "rewards" will reinforce undesirable behavior. Counsel to ignore the child's cries of distress and instead to reward him when he smiles and is pleasant is inappropriate when a child is suffering. The dangers of prolonged infantilization are obvious and have been mentioned, for habits are easily formed and children will try to fill their psychological needs of unmet dependency in any way they can. However, it is deprivation of normal dependency needs that causes the problems. The inevitable growth urge that accompanies a young organism is so great that independence will carry him forward if he has not been overly spoiled or if he has not been traumatized. Sufficient trauma attends chronic illness that unnecessary deprivations should not be added.

The dangers of *infantilization* are most apparent in life-threatening or episodic illness of early onset, such as asthma, heart disease, hemophilia, sickle cell anemia, and nephrosis. The mother's memory of the attacks, her fright and fear of recurrence cause excessive solicitude. The interaction between child and mother between attacks, not her care during them, would seem to create the child's behavior. As indicated earlier, Green and Solnit coined a phrase, the "vulnerable child syndrome," to describe undesirable behavior stemming from a mother's solicitude after a child has had an illness from which he was expected to die—infantilization, bodily overconcern, difficulty in separating from the mother, and school underachievement.[30] Although probably most applicable to the child with a serious heart defect or severe asthma, the syndrome may apply to any child who has suffered a near-fatal episode in infancy or early childhood.

Prolonged infantilization often requires counseling for parents and/or child over a short or long period. Help to the mother in relinquishing the child is usually a key to helping the child. If the father has left, or is entirely inaccessible, substitute male models for boys such as Big Brothers may help. Physicians, nurses, and therapists are sometimes readily available as models if they are alerted to their importance in the child's psychological growth. The physical fitness programs for asthmatic children have enhanced self-confidence in some. Peer-group activities with adult leadership, such as the Boy Scouts, provide an opportunity for the child to feel some security and transfer some dependency to an adult outside the family while taking steps toward greater independence.

Helping persons who are accustomed to thinking in terms of psychological causation may need to remind themselves that withdrawal, depression, or severe acting-out may be the organism's normal response to severe assault from within.

The *withdrawn* child is often observed in hospitals or at home between intervals of hospitalization. His sad, quiet demeanor and lack of interest in his surroundings may trouble those who try to work with him unless they are aware that all his psychic energy is attending pain and exhaustion. He has nothing left over to invest in externals. The same phenomena are seen in adults after surgery. At first they are too exhausted to show interest in anything other than their own physical comfort. Later, they have energy for things outside themselves. The withdrawn child is often the subject of delighted response from parents and others after his pain and disability have receded: "He's a different child!"

Depression, like withdrawal, is a normal response to pain or immobility. Sadness is an expected reaction when one is in distress, unable to perform normal activities and dependent on or at the mercy of others. The chapter on arthritis elaborates this subject, as does the chapter on kidney disease.

Psychiatrists who have written about depression in childhood and adolescence point out that a critical element in depression is a feeling of hopelessness, belief that nothing can or will be done to rescue the person from the plight he is in. Episodic illness, such as nephrosis or recurrences of leukemia, can lead to hopelessness.

A certain amount of depression is normal for children in early adolescence, and a great deal more so for those who are suffering under threat of death or mourning the loss of an old self that will never exist again.

We are concerned when depression, in any of its guises, continues beyond the stage of active physical illness, pain, or the mourning period. Depression can be neurotic, and not "reactive" or normal to the situation, or it may be reactive to cosmetic disability and frustration of normal goals. As in any pathological mental state, careful diagnosis is essential. It is not easy to distinguish depression from retardation, or from the apathy that results from long-learned patience (as a child in a wheelchair learns to wait to be moved) and resignation. Whether depression is "reactive" or neurotic is also difficult to assess. As is frequent after spinal cord injury and among persons receiving dialysis, the worker may need to secure consultation or a referral to mental health experts.

Depression can be expressed in ways other than sadness: by restlessness, irritability, boredom, disorganization, acting out, and constant need for stimulation from loud music, alcohol, drugs, etc.[31]

Acting out among the chronically ill takes the form of reckless disregard of medical advice. Among diabetics, inoperable cardiacs, and youths with advanced kidney disease, hemophilia, or cystic fibrosis, occasional teenagers seem deliberately suicidal in flouting limitations. It is not always possible to ascertain whether they are testing how far they can go without incurring disaster—a "normal" adolescent tendency—or whether their anxiety is intolerable.

Acting out may also take the form of drug abuse. Use of narcotics for relief of pain creates a natural avenue to drug abuse in the painful diseases such as sickle cell anemia, hemophilia, and those cases of arthritis that continue into adolescence. More often, the use of marijuana or pills for highs begins in hospital wards, when the boredom and loneliness of evenings and weekends encourage one youth to share with or dare another and a group is formed around smoking or pill-taking sessions. Once the escape has been found, it is continued unless more constructive avenues are substituted.

Verbal abuse is another avenue open to the physically restricted child for the discharge of anger and expression of frustration. Sarcasm toward family members, peers, and nurses seems particularly used by intelligent, physically inactive girls. It is dangerous to the patient in destroying needed relationships, and to the siblings in creating a cycle of disharmony that adds to their guilt and resentment. This form of acting out warrants counseling and a sustained relationship quite as much as the others.

Treatment of Depression

The person who is depressed has no energy to use in devising constructive remedies for his condition, so that ideas have to come from the outside. The concept that depressed persons should be kept busy—do something, "get back to work"—is adhered to in some hospital wards where severe pain is characteristic, such as from treatment of leukemia or burns. Children are taken to schoolrooms and occupational therapy laboratories, or their work is brought to them, and they are expected to perform. Trying to concentrate on something other than their misery and on tasks expected of normal children may possibly reduce anxiety and thus pain.

A depressed child at home should be given something to do and have some kind of responsibility as long as possible. He needs the stimulation of changing scenes, whether going in the car on his mother's shopping trips or on other outings that can be arranged. He greatly needs games and fun, music, and pets, and to attend school or have a home teacher. The mother may be so busy and tired cooking, doing the laundry, caring for him physically, that a volunteer, neighbor, or relative may be needed to help keep the child as occupied as possible.

Treatment of reactive depression varies according to its cause. Teamwork with physician and nurse is necessary if causes are related to offensive smells, sounds, or sights. A common cause of depressed feelings in handicapped children and teenagers is inability to get around. It is normal for them to want to be on the go with their peers, but working out ways for them to get out of the house can be difficult. Partial solutions appropriate to some youth are membership in church groups, health agency clubs for handicapped, activities of special schools, and clubs around special interests such as photography or collecting. Some older teenagers find group activities and physical supports that enhance mobility in modified foster homes or boarding homes.

Chapters 9 and 17 elaborate the importance of keeping within the framework of reality imposed by the prognosis. Youths with fatal illnesses know their outlook. This does not mean they think about it constantly. They are involved in their own life situations, and the future may seem very far away. Activities that enrich, that offer pleasure and escape, that help the youth make some sense of his fate or arrive at a philosophy of acceptance or resignation, or enable him to make current contributions and secure a feeling of usefulness, are all appropriate. Vocational preparation is not. To the child or parent who says "What's the use of going to school? There's no future," the answer is that school is important because it provides avenues to self-enrichment and useful activity. It is a normal activity, and a major channel for socialization.

Some practical suggestions about ways to help youth cope with stress arose from observations of young adults under the stress of crippling from poliomyelitis at the Illinois Respiratory Center. Dr. Visotsky and associates there pointed out that patients who were visited frequently by warm friends or family were consistently best adjusted. "The presence of such people did much to prevent the patient from being overwhelmed in the acute phase."[32]

Community interest, as expressed in two-way radio participation in school, likewise helped them cope. These things tie in with the general principle that sharing a burden with someone who cares makes it lighter.

The poliomyelitis patients also demonstrated that the capacity to feel useful helped them. Their self-esteem rose when they knew they were important to someone. Staff reporting on helping burned children cope with stress pointed out that "someone must be on his side," and that this should be someone who can act as a friend, not someone involved in physical treatment.[33] This group commented on the importance of the mother's living in or staying with the child under five while he was in the hospital.

EFFECTS OF HOSPITALIZATION

Most hospital stays are short because of the high cost of care, the rapid effect of modern treatment, and increased knowledge of harm inherent in long institutionalization. Hospital care is used primarily for surgery and emergencies, and during acute severe disease or late terminal care. Some children with chronic illness may be admitted repeatedly during flare-ups. Those with arthritis or orthopedic complications, and children in late stages of kidney disease, cystic fibrosis, or leukemia may still require long periods in the hospital.

Shorter stays for most children help prevent the worst effects of maternal separation and family disorganization, and offer many benefits. However, the use of sophisticated technology and/or surgery guarantees painful and frightening experiences in the hospital. "The need for a specific diagnosis combined with technological advances and an increased knowledge of cellular chemistry have added test upon test... numerous machines, gadgets and instruments that have come to be considered essential," many of them developed during war and in space medicine.[34] The use of the tests and machinery means constantly recurring venipunctures, biopsies, casting, suctioning, catheterizations, surgery, forced coughing, anesthetics, many painful things. The intrusions, helplessness, fantasies, the crying or screams of other children, and the eerie equipment make hospital care especially traumatic for small children. Some children's hospitals have led the way to humane, psychologically protective care. The majority are dehumanized, where the child has no one person with whom to relate. The modern way involves teams of aides and maids, a multitude of technicians, and, in teaching hospitals, interns or residents and a score of white-coated specialists. Approximately 15 professionals, technicians, and aides exist in the hospital for every one physician.[35]

Fortunately, interest in the psychological components of care and in family-oriented medicine has seeped into most paramedical teaching and into an increasing number of medical schools. Some highly sophisticated, careful work is done in a few children's wards and hospitals to prepare children for surgery, encourage maternal support, and provide opportunity for children to play, draw, or talk out some of their anxieties.

Preparation of the child for his hospital experience is one of the measures that can reduce stress. Knowing something of what to expect ahead of time cushions the psychic shock (see Chapter 2, p. 19). Parents and helping persons should learn what if anything the hospital does to prepare the child for surgery. Some have brochures for parents, or comic-type books for children. Some conduct group tours regularly through the children's wards or for individual children a few days before admission, upon the physician's request. Others provide a highly individualized opportunity to learn what the child fears and knows and provide him with a reassuring preparatory experience.

A 1970 survey of 20 hospitals in the San Francisco Bay Area showed that eight made no provision for preparation, and that the other 12 ranged from one that offered weekly tours for all prospective child patients, encouraged questions and helped children to handle stethoscopes, etc., and then worked with each child individually on admission, to others that offered group tours for cardiac and tonsillectomy patients. Some tours were more frightening than reassuring.[36] If the worker learns that the hospital does nothing or very little and the child is to have surgery, she can be of some help to parent and child in regard to preparation by asking the hospital social worker (or liaison nurse, if there is no social worker) if a tour can be arranged for the child and his mother, with an explanation of what the surgery is to fix, where it is to be done, what the anesthetic will be like, and where and when his mother will be waiting for him after the operation. The amount and kind of detail will depend on his age.

Books for agency libraries that can be loaned to parents to read to their children at home, or that the worker can read with him, suggested at a San Francisco symposium on the effects of hospitalization, are Francine Chase, *A Visit to the Hospital* (New York: Grosset & Dunlap, 1958); Margaret Rey and H. A. Rey, *Curious George Goes to the Hospital* (Boston: Houghton Mifflin, 1966); and J. A. Sever, *Johnny Goes to the Hospital* (Boston: Houghton Mifflin, 1953).

Little children can be encouraged to play out their anxieties on their dolls. It is axiomatic that small children should take a favorite toy to the hospital with them, if the hospital permits, and that no child should be tricked into thinking that he is going elsewhere, or that his mother will be right back when she leaves. Often the worker can be of greatest help to the child by helping the mother articulate her own anxieties and to avoid feelings of panic, which would reinforce the child's sense that something dreadful is going to happen. She can help the mother bear hearing the child cry when she leaves after visiting him, and help her avoid the temptation to sneak out or to rationalize that he will be better off if she does not visit.

All literature pertaining to sick children emphasizes the importance to the young child of the mother's presence. *Despite the known need, many mothers in poor families do not stay* with their children after surgery or visit them frequently during hospitalization. This is in part due to lack of awareness in mothers and workers of the extreme distress small children experience during hospitalization.

The worker in the community should reinforce medical and paramedical staff in helping such mothers understand the importance of their being with the sick child and helping them make the necessary arrangements. The mother may not say so, but she may rarely leave her neighborhood and feel hesitant about exploring a new part of the city. A summary of findings regarding the life-styles of the poor says they are not only insecure and helpless but they "seldom participate in any activity that takes them out of the daily routine.... Socially, they seldom go beyond the borders of kinship and neighborhood groups."[37] The poor mother may feel inappropriately dressed and out of place in the big hospital, and have trouble finding her way around and be too insecure to approach the chatting, self-confident, or busy staff to ask directions. The worker may need to ask the hospital social worker, if there is one, or if not, the chaplain or nurse, whether a volunteer can meet the mother for the first time or two and help her find her way around.

Pictures, case vignettes, and descriptions that make the need for the mother's presence at the hospital come to life in a way textbooks often fail to do, and that may be profitably used for staff meetings of community agencies, are Emma M. Plank, *Working with Children in Hospitals* (Cleveland: Western Reserve University Press, 1962); John Robertson, *Hospitals and Children, A Parent's Eye View* (New York: International Universities Press, 1962); and *Red Is the Color of Hurting* (Washington, D.C.: Children's Bureau, U.S. Dept. HEW; Government Printing Office, 1967).

If a worker in the community is involved with the family, she can help bridge the gap and ease the trauma for young children entering the hospital without their mothers by preparing a summary for the hospital chart to help nurses, physicians, and hospital social workers to understand the child's home situation. The writers of a nursing textbook suggest including such family matters as ages and names of brothers and sisters; whether the parents live together, and if not whether one is deceased or, if separated or divorced, how recently; whether there were any recent important occurrences at home, such as the birth of a new sibling; what the child himself is called at home; what foods he likes and dislikes; whether he is trained for bowels and bladder, and what words he uses to make his needs known; whether he takes naps and how well he sleeps, and whether he says a prayer before he goes to sleep; what kind of play he likes, and whether he has a pet and what his favorite toys are; what he does when frightened or angry; and how much and what he has been told about coming to the hospital.[38] They also suggest that hospital ward staff should know what the child has been told about his parents' visiting, whether they will come to see the child and when, so that when he calls for them the members of the staff will know how to respond.

Children with chronic disease who have been in the hospital before may need psychological support when they know they will have to return. These children know how bad some of their experience is going to be, and may in addition have misunderstandings about why they are to go back. They may have guilty feelings that they have done something wrong and it is their fault that they are now to be punished. If the disease has a fatal termination, the child may be in a panic that this is the end. And just as "school phobias" are not phobias against school but resistance to leaving home for fear of what may happen when he is *not* home, he may have many reasons not to want to leave home at this time. If parents are fighting, or the mother has a boyfriend or a new baby, he may be worried about abandonment.

The adolescent who is returning to a long-term rehabilitation ward for treatment of a condition that began years before often has many positive feelings. He may know from experience that treatment will make him feel better, and be miserable enough to want professional help badly; he may have old friends among staff and patients whom he looks forward to seeing again; and if he is returning to a well-equipped, specialized hospital, he knows that electronic and motorized equipment and trained staff will greatly aid his mobility and thus his socialization opportunities. The hospital will be a place where he is among his own and safe from stares. He is not an ugly outsider there. For some, leaving the hospital may create greater conflict than admission, for life in a modern pediatric or adolescent wing often includes parties, school, games, and a group he belongs to. He may be going back to the loneliness of an ill-adapted home, apartment, or foster home where he has to sit alone because no one is available who can lift or push him around the community.

It is the disarray of feelings that needs to be talked out before hospitalization, with some sorting of the good and bad aspects of the experience and ways to make the best of the situation; most needed is an assurance of continuity of caring relationships while the youth is going through another critical and painful experience, with uncertainty about the future. Continuity of peer relationships, critically important to the adolescent, is jeopardized by a long hospital stay, especially in a hospital far from the home neighborhood. All possible effort should be made to encourage or arrange for visits from friends. An adult relative can sometimes bring a boy or girl from the neighborhood, or a schoolteacher can arrange for cards and visits throughout the hospital stay (not just the first week), or the worker can pick up a friend when she comes to see him.

Nights and weekends are particularly lonely times in hospitals. The therapists and technicians have gone home, the busy hospital activity, with constant interruptions through the day, has died down to emptiness, sounds of whimpering, boredom, and loneliness.

Social workers and other helping persons in the community want to go home, too, but if the most meaningful contact is to be maintained with a child in especially great need, after-five and Sunday afternoon visits are the most vital times to go (unless visits by others are ensured for those times). The writer has never forgotten a lesson from a seven-year-old facing an amputation in a hospital far from home. On a Sunday afternoon he was missing and was finally found crying, squeezed inside a dollhouse on a hospital porch.

CHAPTER FOUR

Community Resources

THE PRECEDING chapter discussed common psychosocial problems accompanying chronic illness in children. It is assumed that human care services, although varied according to agency function, follow an understanding of the problems, and that use of resources to relieve stress is a common practice. Accordingly, this chapter provides an overview of major public resources for relief of physical and economic stress; explores several pertinent services, including foster care and adoption for the chronically ill child; and describes strategies of collaboration. The last of these is central to effective service, for the child and his family require the help of a network of persons, not merely the help of a single individual.

Communities differ so widely throughout the nation that no two have identical resources. Furthermore, change is the order of the day. New services spring up, seemingly overnight, and others vanish. Purchase of services from a variety of private agencies; varying public resources and philosophies in different states and counties; shifting fads in counseling; diminution of old needs and the emergence of new ones as changes in demography and life-styles occur; the trend toward alternative services and peer-group organizations; and underlying all, the changing economic and political mood—all these make it impossible to encapsulate the resources for chronically ill children and their families.

Great expansion and proliferation of public programs for medical care, financial aid, and other social services took place during the 1960's. The services growing out of this forward surge are touched upon later. Their cost and complexities, and an abrupt change in political administration, reversed the direction and changed the provisions. Turmoil existed for several years, while trends crystallized and new legislation came into being. Major changes included a decrease in federal funding, separation of income maintenance from services, direct federal administration of income maintenance for all but the politically vulnerable group—families with children—and decentralization of services.

The changed approach to meeting human need had not fully formed when combined inflation and increased unemployment overwhelmed community agencies with applications for assistance. The added turmoil of overloaded agencies, staff shortages, and emergency measures obscures the shape of services to come. Thus the following descriptions in the sections on Medical Care provisions, Financial Aid, and Public Social Services must be read with these limitations in mind. The ensuing sections on Foster Care, Adoption, and Collaboration are less touched by the turmoil of the mid-1970's, though no human services will remain static in a period of such rapid change.

MEDICAL CARE

Two forms of medical care now exist, one sophisticated and personal for private patients, the other often hasty, discontinuous, and impersonal, for the poor. The main reasons that poor persons often receive inadequate care are maldistribution of physicians, fragmentation of programs, and the great size of public programs, which creates administrative difficulties.

Regarding maldistribution of physicians, Lesser says, "The increase in the numbers of low income families in the cities and the movement of the middle class to the suburbs have been accompanied by the departure of physicians in private practice to the suburbs.... The AMA News (March 16, 1970) reported that in 1945 the physician-patient ratio in cities was 1 : 450; in suburbs it was 1 : 2000. Now it is 1 : 2000 in the cities and 1 : 500 in the suburbs."[1]

The mass movement from rural areas to the cities has resulted in packing 70 percent of all Americans on 1 percent of our land, and most of the Black population lives, not in the rural south, but in cities.[2] As a result, in some inner-city areas, patients wait all day in county clinics, only to be turned away and told to return the next day, and we learn of women who choose midnight to take their children to the emergency room in order to secure medical care with the least wait.

These inequities and ironies have created deep concern over "health care delivery." The 1962, 1965, and 1967 Social Security amendments brought forth great nationwide programs for two groups, Medicare for the elderly and Medicaid for those receiving public assistance and for some other poor. Their very size created difficult administrative problems. In addition, many special health projects were created for families in target areas of greatest need.

Under their provisions maternity and infancy projects were located in cities and rural areas with highest infant mortality rates; children and youth projects came later, administered by teaching hospitals or local health departments, to provide comprehensive care for children in low-income areas. Neighborhood health centers, administered through the Office of Economic Opportunity (OEC), also provided direct service in target areas of ethnic poor.

Head Start health services, Health Services for Migrants, and Indian health service projects are among others that developed during the decade of the 1960's. Hospital and health department and privately sponsored family health care programs, family-centered pediatric clinics, multiservice projects for pregnant schoolgirls, and especially family planning clinics, burgeoned under vigorous federal leadership and the use of federal project money and Medicaid funds.

Greatly increased welfare caseloads, rapidly rising medical-care costs, and the many special projects increased the costs fivefold in two decades.[3] Alarmed, and aware that vast areas of need remained unmet, Congress and the National Administration concentrated on more economical and efficient health delivery systems.

A General Accounting Office study recommended prepaid group practice, expanded insurance coverage for out-of-hospital care, preventive measures, and, in general, moves to avoid the expense of hospital care.[4] Health Maintenance Organizations, or HMO's, on the principle of the Kaiser Permanente and Ross Loos plans in California and the Health Insurance Plan of Greater New York, which offer preventive and maintenance care in addition to curative medicine, were promoted by federal legislation and funding, and some believe they will be among the major health care vehicles of the future.

A more far-reaching move took shape. National health insurance gradually emerged as an answer to fundamental weaknesses in the system; Congress and the Administration have offered a number of proposals. At the liberal end of the spectrum is a comprehensive and wholly prepaid benefit system, financed and administered by the federal government with assurance of quality and cost control. At the opposite end is the Administration's proposal to rely on the private health industry to operate the program, build in heavy deductibles, and leave cost and quality control to the states. At the time of this writing, a national health insurance bill of some kind, though delayed, is on the horizon.[5]

Medicaid

The largest source of medical care for low-income families is Medicaid. It pays for much of the care they receive from hospitals, clinics, and private physicians.

Medicaid provisions vary among the states. Title XIX required that states that had provided medical care for the aged (most states) must also provide hospital, outpatient, physician's, and laboratory and X-ray services for other persons receiving assistance.[6] In addition, nonassistance recipients could qualify at the option of the states if the individuals were "linked by similarity of all eligibility requirements except financial provisions."

In fiscal 1972–73 Medicaid accounted for more than one-fourth of all public outlays for health services.[7] Rising costs have created growing resentment and congressional and administrative alarm. The attempts to change rules and tighten eligibility, though often creating waste, absurdity, and defeat of health measures, can be understood because of the vastness of the expenditures and rates of increase. The greatest increases have stemmed from rising hospital costs and physicians' charges.

No analysis has been found for Medicaid expenditures by age of recipient, but less than a nickel of every public dollar for personal health expenditures has been said to be spent on children.[8] Public funding accounted for only 30 percent of the spending for the younger groups and 64 percent for the aged. For persons under 19, 71 percent of the funds were from insurance or other private sources.[9]

A serious problem has been the unwillingness of physicians to treat individuals under Medicaid because of the inefficiency of the reimbursement system. The vastness of the program has necessitated computerized payment systems through third parties, which have been accompanied by frustrations and delays. Changes in eligibility requirements have compounded the administrative problems.

A disappointing review of the actual benefits of Medicaid to children in a New York community showed that, though the financial burden had been removed from the families, "little permanent change in amount or source of care had occurred after four years of the program. The program has reinforced the trend in our community toward two separate care systems, one of the private practitioner providing care for the well-to-do, and one of the health centers and public clinics providing care primarily for the poor."[10] Blame was placed on the apathy of poor families, and also on the refusal of private practitioners to care for their children.

Despite its limitations, Medicaid has enabled poor families in many communities to choose their own physicians and hospitals, has upgraded the care provided by local clinics, and, as experience accumulates, offers further potential to raise standards of care for children of the poor. Presumably Medicaid will continue to be the major financial resource for medical care of children receiving public assistance until national health insurance overhauls the system.

The early and periodic screening, diagnosis, and treatment program (EPSDT) of Medicaid. A Medicaid resource of potentially great benefit to children is the Medi-Screen or EPSDT program, through which children of AFDC families may receive medical and dental examinations and, if identified as in need of treatment, can be referred for care. The program has been beset by administrative problems, and the worker involved with a child who especially needs the examinations or treatment available may need to push to help him obtain its advantages. Though mandated by the 1967 amendments to the Social Security Act, the beginning program was not adopted in many states until 1972, and through December 1973 only 15 percent of eligible children had been screened.[11]

One negative and two important positive results have emerged from the Medi-Screen program. The negative has been voiced as follows: "HEW's performance is raising doubts on Capital Hill about the agency's ability to handle national health insurance and about the administration's insistence on a major role in health insurance for the states."[12] Since Medicaid is a state-administered program, and the states have varied widely in the degree to which they have committed themselves to make adequate medical care available to welfare recipients under its provisions, the fears of the states, their complaints and varying degrees of efficiency, raise serious question about what they would do with a still greater program, national health insurance.

However, another result is of great benefit. Statistics and information created in connection with the program are publicizing the health needs of poor children and forming the base for potentially great improvement in their care. In a three-year demonstration project in Portsmouth, Virginia, one group of children used as a control were examined and their families left to their own devices to find corrective treatment. The other group were given help by paraprofessional aides, transportation, health education, etc., in securing treatment. The latter spent a third fewer days in the hospital and made only half as many visits to doctors over the three-year period as those who were not helped, and the money spent under Medicaid for the latter was a third less than on the control group. This startling demonstration of the importance of accompanying medical examinations with help in following through on recommendations should have a far-ranging effect on the provisioning of auxiliary services.

Informational bulletins have been issued to medical and dental groups in an attempt to secure their cooperation. The involvement of official medical and dental organizations should in the long run help increase their interest in improved conditions for the children of the poor. A demonstration has occurred in California's Child Health and Disability Prevention program, officially adopted February 25, 1975.[13] This new law, a direct outgrowth of the Medi-Screen program, extends screening to all children before they enter the first grade. Although the provision does not offer treatment for the children found to have defects, it is a step in that direction, and meanwhile affords for the first time a means of learning how many children in the total population have physical defects, and where they are clustered.

Crippled Children's Services

The major continuing source of supplementary medical care for physically handicapped children, and in some states the major resource, has been a charter service of the original Social Security Act, the Crippled Children's Services. This agency, which was administered by the Children's Bureau, made a unique contribution by requiring a high quality of medical care through the use of certified specialists and approved hospitals. Each state has defined "crippling" in its own way; since the virtual end of poliomyelitis, state agencies have broadened definitions of medical eligibility to include cardiac problems and, increasingly, other chronic illnesses such as cystic fibrosis, sickle cell disease, and hemophilia.

In 1973, funding was reduced for maternal and child health, which includes Crippled Children's Services.[14] Because the costs of cardiac and orthopedic surgery are increasingly astronomical, and the Crippled Children's agencies often have run out of money before the end of the fiscal year, the future appears to hold increasingly tight financial eligibility and payback provisions until major changes in health care systems take place. Notable differences exist in the financial adequacy and the administration of state crippled children's programs.

Maternity and Infant Care Projects

Among the most objective achievements of the maternity and infant care projects have been dramatic reductions in the infant mortality rate and reductions in the number of hospital admissions of children cared for through the projects. Not so measurable but of great significance have been some demonstrations of unexpected enthusiasm for and cooperation in preventive health care among the poor.[15] Positive responses to highly personalized, dignified, and caring service, and ingenious methods of reaching out run counter to findings of the large-scale studies showing a general apathy among the poor toward preventive medical care.

Since state departments of health, not the federal government, will fund (through revenue-sharing monies) and supervise these projects in the future, agency staffs will need to join for community organization and decision making. Collaboration and increased communication should strengthen the bridges that are needed between health and community agencies.

Private Health Insurance

The blue-collar worker's family and the middle class usually have some form of health insurance so long as the breadwinner or winners are employed by organizations that offer group insurance plans. Extensive unemployment has undermined the extent of this safeguard against inability to receive medical care. Premiums for individual health insurance are too expensive for the poor and the unemployed. "A fifth of the population under age 65 has no financial shield against the hazards of illness. Still larger numbers have inadequate protection. Major deterrents are cost and non-accessibility of health care services."[16]

Until the unemployment of the mid-1970's, an increasing number of persons have had some insurance and, increasingly, a broader form. Seventy-two percent of the population had at least partial coverage of hospital costs and out-of-hospital X-ray and laboratory charges in 1972. Thus it can be seen that one of the first bulwarks against the cost of chronic illness in children is the father's insurance, and that motivation for the mother's employment often is to obtain or expand group insurance for her family.

Health Maintenance Organizations (HMO's)

Private insurance carriers, especially Blue Cross and Blue Shield, have been active in stimulating development and use of group-practice, health-maintenance organizations.[17] It is to be expected that Medicare and Medicaid beneficiaries will be encouraged to secure care through health maintenance plans and that private insurance companies will continue to encourage their use. The record of prototype HMO's, such as the Health Insurance Plan of Greater New York and the Kaiser Permanente plan, in reducing hospitalization days will make preventive care attractive to government and insurance companies alike.*

FINANCIAL AID

Confusion over the term "social welfare" has harmed provisions for public aid and services. The federal government lumps housing, health, social insurance, education, veterans' benefits and hospitals, and such other programs as vocational rehabilitation and child nutrition, together under the term "social welfare." However, "welfare" means public assistance to the common man, and possibly even to government officials. Total social welfare expenditures have increased greatly, until they now *account for 55 percent of all government expenditures* ($300 billion in 1973, about one-fourth of the GNP).[18] On a television newscast, the United States Secretary of the Treasury responded to questions from newsmen about spending for the war in Southeast Asia. He responded, "Defense spending hasn't risen; welfare takes fifty-five cents of every dollar. Cut welfare."

"Cut welfare" has been a general response meaning "Get the chiselers off relief" and give less money to the poor. The general public does not relate welfare expenditures to increases in educational benefits for Vietnam veterans, increases in Social Security and unemployment compensation, and the billion-dollar increase in medical care. The federal administration's budget proposal for fiscal year 1975 has asked that 45 percent of the total

* See note at end of chapter, p. 118.

budget reductions advocated be made in HEW programs, a very threatening proposal for low-income families.[19]

However, the actual increase in public financial aid has been very large in recent years. "Welfare," or public aid, consumed 3.5 percent of social welfare funds in 1965 and 6.7 percent in 1973. The percentage of income maintenance, or cash benefits through Old-Age and Survivors and Disability Insurance (OASDI), unemployment insurance, etc., decreased by 3 percent. It would seem that as Social Security and other cash benefits fail to keep pace with the cost of living, the number of welfare recipients rises. One important factor that cannot be overlooked is that the percentage of total funds available for all social welfare purposes from private sources is shrinking, and that which must be borne from taxes is increasing.[20]

Supplemental Security Income for Chronically Ill Children

Social Security amendments that permit severely disabled children to qualify for Supplemental Security Income are of special interest to those working with a chronically ill child and his family. The child's income benefit greatly exceeds the amount he would be allowed under Aid to Families with Dependent Children, and does not count in determining the family's eligibility for AFDC (though it reduces the AFDC grant by subtracting him from its computation).[21] Therefore, for low-income families, including those receiving public assistance, this measure merits close scrutiny and careful work to make certain the child's case is presented in such a way that he qualifies for the program if he is indeed eligible.

Public Law 92603, as signed in October 1972 and amended later, provided federal funds in monthly amounts of $146 to a single person or $219 for a couple, effective January 1974.[22] Most large states supplement these amounts. The law made Medicaid mandatory for recipients of SSI benefits, so that some medical care is guaranteed in addition to income.

The law removes the aged, blind, and disabled from public assistance and places them under the administrative aegis of the Social Security Administration. This great forward step for the groups covered unfortunately leaves vulnerable the unpopular category, that of aid to dependent children.

Age limits were removed for Aid to the Disabled, so that disabled children of any age now qualify for benefits without regard to the wage earner's social security insurance status.

Requirements for qualification are both financial and medical, and are determined in two separate steps. The means test is applied first, by the local Social Security office. If the child qualifies financially, his record is submitted to a regional disability determination office for decision regarding the severity of his disability. The methods are similar to those that have been used to determine eligibility for Aid to the Disabled (ATD), and identical with those used to determine medical eligibility for disability benefits under Social Security.

The provision is new at this writing, and the panels that adjudicate severity of disability have had no experience in evaluating child disability. The level of severity of impairment necessary to qualify has been determined on the basis of inability to work. Substantial experience will be amassed by the various state regional teams before the federal office arrives at satisfactory guidelines for the teams in determining child disability.

Meanwhile, the Social Security office has issued to the teams general guidelines pointing out that a child's normal task is *maturation*, in contrast with the adult's usual task of employment. Maturation is described as consisting of growth, learning, mastering basic skills, and emotional and social development. School attendance is not considered a satisfactory guide regarding the severity of an impairment.[23]

Social workers and other helping persons who are concerned with assisting a child to qualify for SSI income (and its Medicaid accompaniment) should emphasize the importance of full medical reports that contain objective evidence (laboratory and X-ray and physical findings) of the degree to which the illness has progressed. In addition, they need to provide full social reports to the Social Security office for the regional disability panel, describing the ways in which the child's maturation has been or is affected. Severity is not determined by eventual outcome in death but by what the illness is doing or has done to the child's growth, learning, skill mastery, and emotional and social development. These facts will enable the teams to visualize the extent of the disability and may swing the balance in their decisions.

If the regional panel disqualifies a child medically, when the worker knows that he is severely ill with a long-term illness or badly affected functionally, the family should be helped to appeal. The regional offices will vary a great deal, especially in the first few years, in their determination, and the appeal process probably will be necessary in many cases while they are arriving at sound guidelines. The greatest difficulty probably will be encountered in securing benefits for children with remitting disease, who may seem completely well between severe episodes, as in the case of cystic fibrosis, sickle cell anemia, leukemia, hemophilia, and juvenile arthritis. Health problems in which seasonal variations occur, as in asthma triggered by pollens, will also constitute adjudication difficulty.

Food Stamps

The food stamp program[24] was authorized in 1964, and amplified by the 1971 amendments. It is administered by the United States Department of Agriculture. Counties have varied widely in their use of this resource. Modification of the program is the subject of debate in Congress and the Administration at this writing.

Many low-income families other than those receiving public assistance may secure food stamps. The maximum income to qualify is set by the USDA. A few deductibles are allowed in computing the "adjusted maximum" monthly income to qualify. Of special interest to families with sick children is the deductible for medical costs, unfortunately "exclusive of special diets." Another deductible is payment for child care when such care is necessary to permit the mother to go to work. The maximum income to qualify goes up twice a year to permit some adjustment for inflation. An example of a current maximum was $475 net income for a family of four (after deductibles).

An offshoot of the food stamp program is called WIC (women, infants, and children). This program, for mothers with children four years of age and under, is intended to reduce malnutrition, one of the risk factors in pregnancy and child development, by providing high-protein supplements to the diets of those eligible. The USDA traditionally is more attuned to the interests of agribusiness than to the needs of the poor, and has been slow in implementing this program.

PUBLIC SOCIAL SERVICES

The shape of publicly funded social services to come can be projected sketchily from the present base, the provisions of the 1975 amendment to the Social Security Act, Title XX, and some attributes of General Revenue Sharing. The major portion of this section describes the services of greatest relevance to sick or disabled children as they are constituted at the time of this writing. They should be viewed with the revised legislative and funding provisions in mind.

The provisions of Title XX, which enables provision of the social services, were hammered out over a period of several years by representatives of the federal administration, Congress, and major social welfare organizations. The last welded themselves into a Social Services Coalition to protect the restrictive proposals of the federal administration and inject more effective and humane provisions; their participation is an example of the means by which helping persons at state and local levels may collaborate and work to secure funding for human care services under General Revenue Sharing provisions.

As described by the National Association of Social Workers *NASW News* in February 1975, Title XX grants "state governors broad discretionary powers and responsibility for public planning and public reporting of social service programs." Major changes will affect "eligibility, services planning, and accountability, but will not appreciably change Federal funding." The social services goals specified are "self-support, self-sufficiency, protection for children and adults unable to protect themselves; deinstitutionalization when appropriate; and institutional placement and services within some institutions when necessary."[25] The only mandated service for AFDC families is family planning. At least three services selected by the state must be provided for recipients of SSI. Thus a broader program of services may be possible for chronically ill children who qualify under the SSI disability provisions. Optional services include among others *child care services, protective services, homemaker services, health support services*, and "*appropriate combination* of services designed to meet the special needs of children, the aged, mentally retarded, emotionally disturbed, *physically handicapped*, alcoholics and drug addicts."

In addition to these and other provisions, the Amendment specifies that the 1968 Federal Day Care Requirements will remain in effect at least until 1977 "with certain modifications."[26]

The law also contains some undesirable features relating to a "parent locator" service that give HEW the right to use Internal Revenue Service records and that will force mothers to comply with district attorneys in finding absent fathers.

The coexistent potential for opportunity and danger inherent in Title XX is apparent. Competing lobbies for funds available at the discretionary power of the state governor will include those that are well organized and long-standing. Groups and individuals interested in "health support services" and "appropriate combinations of services designed to meet the special needs of children" and programs for the physically handicapped have an opportunity to build needed resources, but they will need to frame effective coalitions to compete successfully.

Two matters pertaining to revenue sharing are worthy of note. One is that services other than social welfare are included in the Revenue Sharing Act of 1972. These include public transportation, health, recreation, social services, financial administration, and libraries. Localities may spend federally allocated funds to states and localities for operating or maintenance costs for any activity on which they spend their own money. "A survey on the use of receipts for the first two entitlement periods indicated plans for spending relatively less for social welfare and more in other permitted areas."[27] Thus it is apparent that the areas of competition are not only within the field of social services but in the broad field of human services, and that, thus far, social services in general have not fared as well as such public concerns as transportation, recreation, administration, etc. Another basic aspect of revenue sharing is that the funds allocated do not equal those lost to the communities by the elimination of categorical assistance grants. Revenue-sharing publicity has emphasized the decentralization of benefits but not the cut in funding. Therefore effective competition is even more necessary and success even more difficult.

A county that organized to make sure that social welfare received its full share of revenue-sharing funds, San Diego, California, has recorded its experience.[28] Dr. Jack Stumpf, professor of social work at the San Diego State University, and some students estimated the total loss of funds and made their findings known. The official agencies, ethnic organizations, and alternative service agencies publicized the need for revenue-sharing funds to help compensate for the losses. Sufficient publicity and pressures were brought to bear so that an allocation board was formed of representatives from the city, county, and United Way. This board received project applications, formulated criteria, trained raters, and granted the funds accordingly. As a result of intensive and continuous efforts and the pooling of staff, expertise, and community pressures, the county has allocated a much higher proportion of General Revenue Sharing funds for human care services than the national average.[29]

The Existing Base of Child Welfare Services

The Child Welfare League of America issued a statement in 1971 pertaining to goals and needs for child welfare services: "The basic needs of millions of children are unmet; these children lack in their families and communities the essentials for maturation and fulfillment of their potentialities. Thousands of other children could benefit by the kind of assistance that many parents today need and want. Child welfare services are inadequate, fragmented, poorly financed, and in many communities, nonexistent."[30]

The League defined a comprehensive system of child welfare services as including (a) services to support and reinforce parental care, (b) services to supplement parental care or compensate for its inadequacies, (c) services to substitute in part or in whole for parental care, (d) preventive services, (e) regulation of agencies and licenses, and (f) community planning of services for children and parents.[31]

The first three categories are in daily demand by persons attempting to help chronically ill children and their families, and their underdevelopment creates need for concurrent ingenuity and community organization.

Services that supplement parental care, such as day care and homemaker service, and that substitute for parental care, including foster care and adoption, have received more recognition than other basic services to strengthen family life. The latter have received official lip service in legislation providing for financial support and services to dependent children but have suffered from lack of sufficient financing to a level of decency and professional staffing for the counseling needed.

In the study of protective services for neglected children, "which have been identified as our most important child welfare problems," Bernice Boehm pointed out the high proportion of reported cases from one-parent, public assistance, low-level education, minority-group, large-sized families. She said the "stress is almost overwhelming. However, little attention has been given to the alleviation of stress in such families, even though their prevalence in neglect caseloads marks them as a group of high vulnerability."[32] This and other studies of protective services have shown that children whose problems were physical or medical showed higher success rates than other groups, probably because of the specificity and visibility of the problem and the relatively greater ease with which physical problems can be ameliorated.

The 1967 Social Security Amendments eliminated Child Welfare Services as a separate title and transferred them to Title IV-B. New federal regulations implementing Title XX have not been issued at the time of this writing. The federal regulations for child welfare services have stated, "Child welfare services will not be limited to AFDC cases. Child welfare services will be available on the basis of need for services and shall not be denied on the basis of financial need, legal residence, social status or religion."[33] However, fiscal and administrative regulations, which provided federal financial incentives if child welfare services went to AFDC recipients, and which placed child welfare and AFDC in the same state agency, brought about a decline in child welfare expenditures other than those to AFDC recipients, and seemed to result in a division of labor within public assistance agencies in which child welfare workers focus on children in need of placement and on protective services.[34] Service to children in their own homes tends to be confined to that which can be provided by the AFDC "service workers" to recipients and potential recipients.

Separation of eligibility from service in public welfare further diminished the provision of services to children in their own homes. Whereas workers formerly were required to make quarterly visits to maintain financial supervision, they now go to the client's home only if an eligibility worker or other person refers the case and the client wishes service. When they went to homes, they saw the conditions and could observe the children. Now that this entrée to service no longer exists, new means are needed to identify children who need the services of the AFDC service worker. Eligibility workers are too overwhelmed with processing grants to observe behavior and write out referral forms, and are thus poor vehicles for service requests. Clients most in need of help may not recognize their need, or may fear the children will be taken away if a worker discovers the true circumstances. Workers in other agencies will need to take more initiative in calling to the service worker's attention the situation in which help should be offered.

Federal funding of social work scholarships during the 1960's and the reduced number of social work jobs have upgraded the quality of staff and greatly strengthened the public agency's ability to provide competent social services. Staff of other agencies involved with families receiving public assistance or SSI do well to push past the barriers and secure the help of the service worker. The public agency worker has great advantage in tapping financial, medical, homemaker, and day care resources of the agency, which, combined with counseling, provide excellent opportunity to alleviate stress.

There is great variation in the availability of public children's services to nonassistance families. Greatly to be regretted is the practice of providing child welfare services on the basis of income level or assistance status, unless the children are in need of protection. "Protection," however, is a word that can be stretched to cover more than abuse or overt neglect. Needed services for chronically ill children can sometimes be included.

The protective services worker will not give unwanted service, which weakens as well as strengthens her approach, in that at times service must be demonstrated before a family knows whether it is what they want. However, the worker does make home visits, and therefore is accessible to families who cannot or will not go to a mental health clinic. Child care and transportation arrangements, fatigue, and inconsistent patterns constitute problems that sometimes prevent effective use of mental health services by poor families. A substitute becomes available to them to the extent that service workers in public welfare agencies have the necessary skills.

HOMEMAKER SERVICES

The mother of two children with cystic fibrosis lay down on the floor in a sleeping bag and zipped herself in. When she refused to get up, emergency homemaker service was provided and the mother was taken to a hospital for rest. In another instance, a homemaker took charge and cared for the siblings while the mother stayed at the hospital with a dying child. By contrast, in a family where the children were left alone while the mother spent most of six months with a child who died, one girl said when grown, "I was ten years old at the time. We children felt so alone. Although we got by, somehow the family just didn't seem to get back together. We were never the same after that." Homemaker/home health aide service has great potential in alleviating trauma and stress in the families of chronically ill children.

Homemaker services are part of the array of in-home services that, by definition, can be brought into the home, "singly or in combination ... [for use] therapeutically, or to prevent or arrest disability, to supplement limited function and to protect and support those whose capacities for optimum development, function and participation in family and community life are threatened.... They are described as key services in preventing family disintegration in periods of family crisis, where the physical and psychological health of children is threatened," among other uses.[35] Homemaker services are often combined with those of a home health aide, under supervision of a social worker or nurse.

Over the years, homemaker services have been developed in an uneven and meager fashion by a variety of health and welfare agencies. Some have been designed to serve only the clientele of the agency and others to serve the entire community. Although the main thrust in recent years has been in the development of services for the aged, some public welfare agencies maintain homemaker services for children or contract for them, primarily to care for children when mothers are psychotic, on drugs, or in the hospital. Other agencies, such as the Visiting Nurse Association, and some hospitals that have home care programs also provide homemaker services for families with children, as do a growing number of nonprofit and profit-making private organizations.

Ten times as many homemaker and home health aides as now exist are said to be needed—300,000 instead of 30,000.[36] The scarcity of the service is a serious obstacle, and, compounding the problem, homemaker service is very costly. Though private homemaker agencies are willing to provide care for nonassistance families, the hourly charge is so great that the average family cannot afford it, except on a limited basis. Even when a sliding scale is available, few families can be accommodated at the lower end of the scale because of limitations in agency funds.

In acknowledgment and defense of the cost, the National Council for Homemaker Health Aide Service, Inc. has explored the relationship to the cost of foster home care. The salient fact of their report should be underscored: "The decision to place a child in a foster home because the alternative of a 24-hour homemaker home health aide service is more costly than a day of foster care is poor economy if, as frequently happens, the 'day' of foster care extends to a childhood of days in foster care which could have been avoided by the use of a few days, weeks or months of homemaker home health aide intervention to hold the family together."[37]

The mother of a chronically ill child should not have to zip herself into a sleeping bag before some human services worker becomes aware of her exhaustion, or to get to the point where she refuses to take the child home from a hospital and forces foster care. The helping professions should exert greater effort in tapping the potential of this valuable service.

DAY CARE

Day care as a resource to relieve stress in families of chronically ill children is feasible in only a small proportion of cases. Nevertheless, it should be considered in the repertoire because respite from care of preschool siblings and, in some cases, supervised care and socialization of the affected child may hold the family together during a critical period.

Day care usually denotes supervised all-day care of children between the ages of three and six whose mothers are working. It differs from nursery school care, which is usually provided for only a short period each day and is focused on education and socialization. Day care may be commercial or administered by a public or private social agency, and may be in foster homes in accordance with the licensing laws of the state, or may be in small nurseries. Some agency day-care programs have been provided for children whose mothers are not working outside the home but who are under tension, ill, or overburdened, and who are unable to provide adequate mothering.

In a historical review of day care provided under public auspices, Mary Lewis has pointed out that the original goal was to "provide adequately for the care and protection of children whose parents are, for part of the day, working or seeking work or otherwise absent from the home or unable for other reasons to provide parental supervision."[38]

Since the law placed child welfare services in the same agency with AFDC, and since Congress and the Administration focused on trying to get mothers off welfare and make them work, funds for day care were channelled through public assistance. Miss Lewis says, "the entire program became virtually embedded in public assistance."[39]

The single greatest obstacle to effective use of day care is the high cost. The fees charged are too high for the majority of persons who have extra expense for the care of a chronically ill child. In September 1974, the Quaker legislative organization in California reported, "in 1974, about twenty years after child care in California took its first big steps forward, child care programs are floundering. There are not enough funds. The rosy promise of the late 1960's has faded."[40] Whether local initiative of child advocate groups will be effective in securing revenue-sharing funds to assist day care programs is unknown. The implementation of Title XX, as it affects day care, is also a question for the future.

Supervision of day care centers is another problem that has been met in only partial fashion. In the county of the author's residence, a private contract agency is employed to provide technical consultation to the group care centers, approximately 50 of which are public and another 450 private, profit or nonprofit organizations.[41] The publicly subsidized centers must meet certain standards and utilize technical consultation, but the private nursery schools, ordinarily run by individuals without training, "do not wish to be bothered." Their licensing standards are minimal; they have no supervision; yet they provide custodial care for the majority of children whose mothers work.

In a study of "Unsupervised Family Day Care in New York City" the mothers preferred group to foster family care "because it is reliable."[42] However, the foster family homes visited (which the research staff thought were probably better than the average) ranked high in the characteristic thought to be the most significant index of the quality of a day care program, namely the quality of adult-child relationships.[43]

Head Start is spearheading a significant move in expanding the benefits of day care to handicapped children. Probably stimulated by the energetic lobbying of parents of the mentally retarded and other developmentally disabled, the 1974 Amendments to the Economic Opportunity Act call for at least 10 percent of the nationwide enrollment in Head Start to consist of children who are handicapped and require special services.[44] The handicapped are defined as "mentally retarded, hard of hearing, deaf, speech impaired, visually handicapped, seriously emotionally disturbed, *crippled, or other health impaired* children who by reason thereof require special education and related services." In its second annual report to Congress, the Head Start administration described its achievements in modifying physical facilities, purchasing special equipment, and securing diagnoses of handicapped conditions (through a cooperative arrangement begun with Medicaid staffs), as well as its "widespread efforts to develop skills of Head Start personnel in working with handicapped children."[45]

FOSTER HOME CARE

Foster care has come under increasing attack. Designed to provide temporary care for children until they can return to their own homes or be adopted, foster placement has proved a limbo for many. The services that their families needed in order to improve their capacity for child rearing have not been funded or emphasized. In many instances, the parents have no capacity for parenting or desire to care for the child. But their parental rights have not been terminated, and the child is not available for adoption.

Realistically, foster care has proved a vital service for thousands of children, and will continue to provide their only avenue for life other than institutional care. However, greater emphasis should be given to services to children in their own homes, so that families may remain intact.

Physically handicapped children may need foster care from birth. Children with massive birth defects may be rejected by their families, who refuse to take them home from the hospital. An unwed mother may decide on relinquishment before she knows the child will be defective, but ambivalence about keeping the child may be tipped toward relinquishment by the presence of the child's defect. Children who are separated from their mothers for prolonged hospital treatment may not seem to belong to the family—the maternal "instinct" has been impaired by physical separation.

Frequently, older children with physical problems need foster care. Family disruption may occur owing to the desertion, illness, or death of the father or mother; severe problems with alcoholism, drug addiction, or psychosis may develop in one or both parents. The mother may not be able to cope with a child who needs a great deal of physical care.

A family decision not to take the child home from the hospital may come at any time in a long career of repeated hospital admissions. The decision may not be that of the family but of the medical and nursing staff, who cannot in conscience return a child to a home that has proved physically harmful or repeatedly unable to cope with the child's medical care needs. In such instances, the families may resist the suggestion of foster placement. Although they may feel incompetent or unwilling to care for the child themselves, they think or rationalize that he continues to need the specialized services of a hospital. They are threatened by the suggestion that some other family could take care of him. Instead of overriding this feeling, greater effort should be made in some instances to understand the root of the family's insecurity or inability, and to provide resources that will make it possible for the child to go home, even though the plan may represent a compromise. Foster home care does weaken family ties and the children who have been separated often never go back to their families.

Finding and funding foster care for the chronically ill child. If foster care is essential, an attempt should be made to adhere to the Child Welfare League's basic standard that "A foster home should be selected for a particular child on the basis of the suitability of the family and child for each other."[46] The goal is not met in many instances. The child is hard to place, and an extensive recruiting campaign is usually essential to find any relatively acceptable foster home for him. "It is surprising how many people have a hang-up against physically handicapped persons," according to Mary James, supervisor of a special unit for foster care of physically handicapped children in the Los Angeles Bureau of Public Assistance.[47]

The "hang-ups" Mrs. James referred to extend not only to potential foster parents but to some child placement workers. Some show special interest in handicapped children. These workers appear to be outnumbered by those who are lukewarm, silent, or openly negative about their feelings of revulsion toward physical abnormality. One worker was honest and said frankly that he always feels a tension when he is with a handicapped person. He feels that handicapped children should not be allowed to live. Although such an extreme view is not usual, workers may feel so overwhelmed by the child's needs and the difficulty of caring for him that they may project their attitudes on the prospective foster family and thus interfere with their ability to find a suitable home.

That great difficulty exists in finding suitable homes for the severely handicapped is unquestionable. However, as in all instances, the child and his needs must be individualized. The amount of extra physical care needed may be minimal or not seem overwhelming to an experienced parent. A child suffering from fatigue and waiting for heart surgery is, for example, very different, and needs a different type of foster family, than an incontinent child with spina bifida or spinal cord injury who walks with braces and crutches.

The characteristics in foster parents that have been suggested as helpful are experience in parenting, a general feeling of security about taking care of children, and the ability to see each child as a child, not a handicap. One placement worker with special interest in physically handicapped children said the best foster mothers in her experience had been those who like to have children dependent on them, and who need the child's affection and feedback that they are good mothers, but who are still able to let the child grow.

Foster parents are sometimes young idealistic persons who have decided not to add to the population growth and are looking for ways to be creative and giving. Often those who are willing to consider a child with a handicap have had some experience with illness, either in the family or professionally. A couple who have had personal experience with one condition such as asthma may consider an asthmatic child, for they feel they know from experience how to cope with the attacks. It has been suggested that foster parents can "work up" to more difficult problems as they master a few crises.

Foster parents who have been located by one agency to care for severely handicapped children are said to be aggressive women unafraid of crises, medical personnel, special school staffs, or caseworkers. They may have been practical nurses or in some instances registered nurses.[48] Some women have disabled husbands at home; the higher board rate represents for the husband an amount above his pension, and he is available to help the foster mother with lifting, chores, and round-the-clock supervision of children and paid attendants.

Foster parents often have children of their own. When they are near the age of the physically handicapped foster child, frictions are frequent. The foster child cannot but perceive the difference in warmth the foster mother feels for her own, and thus his longing for his own mother and his feelings of loneliness and rejection mount. These feelings can be expressed in a variety of self-defeating ways—attention-getting mechanisms that bring on punishment and overt rejection. If the foster child has been made dependent by hospital staff, the task of the foster mother is even greater in helping him become independent.

The foster parents' own children express resentment over the ramp that may have been put at their front door or other signs that advertise to the neighborhood that the family is taking in a boarding child, and they get less attention from their parents than they did before. The neighbor children may say "Your baby sister's got no hands," or they may be teased at school. Thus, though mature, experienced foster parents are desirable, and applications come from couples who, being tied down with their own children, want to take in foster children as a way to make money, foster parents with young children of their own bring risks.[49] Foster parents whose children are grown, by and large, would appear to be more suitable.

Just as group homes have proved more satisfactory than foster family homes for many physically normal adolescents, they would appear to have merit for the severely handicapped. Group homes in which teenagers can participate in management, decisions, and rules help build judgment and independence. They do not, as do foster homes, set up situations where handicapped youths are placed in child-parent relationships that torment them with reminders of their own parents' seeming lack of devotion, and jealousy of the secure relationship between the foster parents and their own children.

The group nurseries for "atypical infants" and for normal infants seem a regressive step. Despite the many difficulties, foster family care seems important to the young, handicapped child who cannot receive warmth and security in his own home.

Extra funding is essential for foster care of children with severe physical problems, because attendants are necessary to help with the extra laundry, lifting, feeding, and other physical care, and to relieve the foster mother at night or when she goes shopping.

The limitations created by need to secure extra funding are illustrated by the practice of one large agency. Although it maintains generally high standards, it places physically handicapped children in nurseries for the retarded. This unfortunate practice takes place because foster mothers who qualify to take crib cases can receive a negotiated rate of pay. Though the agency is aware that a child who is normal mentally must live with a group of severely retarded siblings, no administrative provision has been made for his care elsewhere.

Two funding sources available are those for children with neurological disabilities such as spina bifida who qualify under Developmental Disabilities programs, and those for children who qualify under the Supplemental Security Insurance provisions. The latter source is restricted by the provision that a child in his own home shares the income of his parents. Therefore he must be already placed or still in a hospital in order to qualify unless the parents' income is very limited. As elsewhere indicated, this new program is still in the process of creating appropriate regulations.

A maneuver sometimes resorted to in order to obtain extra funds for foster care of children with special needs is encouraging removal from parental custody by the courts in order to secure the higher board rate the court system can pay. This strategy, which takes advantage of federal funding for children removed by the court, runs contrary to the interest of the child by weakening the family ties.

Because higher board rates can be paid by county agencies if the administration authorizes them, determined staff workers can prevail on the agency—and sometimes do. Foster parent associations have been organized

Preplacement and placement problems. As much attention as possible should be paid to the placement process and to features that will prevent unnecessary replacements. The chronically ill child is especially vulnerable to the terrors of separation and placement so aptly described by John Bowlby, Therese Benedek, Ner Littner, and others, by virtue of his separation experiences for hospitalization and the trauma he has undergone.[50] The tendency of the small child to think of another separation as punishment for being bad was illustrated by a seven-year-old boy who called urgently for the worker, ran and threw his arms around her leg, and said desperately, "I've been a good boy, I've been a good boy," when he knew that replacement in another foster home was under consideration.

In that case, the foster mother had been unwilling to hold a place vacant for the child during the time he was rehospitalized. This not unusual problem creates a feeling in the child that the foster family does not care about him; it is perceived as another rejection.

In the Los Angeles special project, careful preplacement work is done to prepare both foster mother and child. All equipment instruction is performed and household modifications made (such as ramps installed) prior to placement, so that the foster family will not feel insecure about this part of caring for the child. The child's preplacement visits to the foster home culminate in a weekend visit to the foster home if possible.

Once the placement is made, the foster mother is often confronted with behavior that frequent and long-time hospitalization and family rejection have created. The child may not have learned normal family give-and-take but have been waited upon by hospital staff who were paid to pick up his toys if he dropped them. Those who were there while he was acutely ill saw his fright, knew of his pain and loneliness, and tried to compensate. More than one foster mother who spoke at a Child Welfare League meeting on foster care of physically handicapped children mentioned their embarrassment over the neighbors' reactions to hearing the child scream while being disciplined.[51] They indicated long, painful sessions in teaching the dependent, long-hospitalized child to function as independently as possible in a family setting. It is believed that foster mothers may need more and repeated interpretation and support in regard to the degree of stress the child has had. The tendency to regard dependent behavior as "spoiling" is natural; extraordinary patience is required to live with an infantilized older child, especially one not your own.

The greatest area of overt difficulty discussed by foster parents and by adolescents who had been in foster care pertained to recreation. The foster parents told of the physical difficulties of transporting children in wheelchairs or on gurneys to amusement centers or even to the grocery store. The adolescents described the dullness of staying at home and of feeling left behind when physically normal children went with the foster family on errands or outings they could not go on. Since they were accustomed to the constant activity in the hospital and the many recreational events arranged for them, normal family routine seemed dull at best. Most important, severe mobility problems stand out in their full panoply of psychosocial meanings in a home environment, whereas they are muted in an institution geared to minimize them.

The school bus and the opportunity to be with other children most of the day five days a week provide a channel for the socialization so desperately needed by handicapped children. Thus school placement as soon as possible after foster home placement alleviates the conflicts and unhappiness created by mobility problems.

A perceptive and severely handicapped young adult who had been in several foster homes said that unhappiness over inability to go home is projected on the foster home relationships. Awareness of rejection by parents, or, at best, failure to understand why the mother cannot provide needed care, comes to the fore through comparison of other children in a foster home neighborhood. A recurring complaint of hospitalized children is the feeling that persons paid to take care of them lack real feeling for them. They hunger to be cared about.

Relationship of foster parents, workers, and natural parents. Three potential areas of hazard need special attention in the relationship that exists between foster mothers, caseworkers, and natural parents. Natural mothers of normal children in foster placement are easily crowded out of their children's lives. Medical problems add a source of tension to the inherently tenuous relationships. The natural mother may feel overawed and resentful of the woman who seems so able to do what she cannot do in caring for her child; her guilt is magnified. The foster parent who takes the child to the doctor hears what he says and becomes an authority on what is wrong and what to do about it. The location of the foster home may be so far from the natural mother's work and environment that it is difficult for her to get there. If the foster parent feels angry or contemptuous of the seemingly neglectful, ignorant, irresponsible parent, her attitude shows. The mother visits less and less often, and when she does come, she may be loaded with expensive "foolish" toys or come with a new boyfriend. If she takes the child home for a weekend, the foster mother may feel he has been badly neglected when he returns.

The foster parent potentially can teach the mother and strengthen her capacity to care for the child. She can make it plain that she is only taking care of the child temporarily until his condition improves or the mother's situation improves. She can emphasize the improvement he is making, the simplicity of his care, if this is the case. What is unfortunately often a destructive force can be reversed. However, this requires a good deal of reinforcement and participation by the caseworker, because the foster mother sees the child's disappointment if his mother does not visit as promised. Identifying with him, she finds it very hard not to blame the mother and shows it.

The relationship between the foster mother and the caseworker in regard to physician contacts should be made clear in the beginning, and the record should make the relationship evident, so that change of workers does not invalidate a good beginning plan. Because a foster mother's role is that of substitute parent, and parents take children to doctors or clinics, the foster mother becomes the repository of the medical recommendations unless the worker has been careful to avoid this unsatisfactory situation. The pressures of practice make it easy for the worker to ease herself out of time-consuming clinic visits and conferences with the physician and let the foster mother do it all. When this happens, the worker gradually loses track of the child's medical needs, and all she knows of his progress is what the foster mother says: "Johnny is doing all right," or "His medicine has been changed," or "His brace has to be fixed."

Particularly because long foster care placements are usual and the medical picture changes over time, the agency, not a series of foster mothers, must retain responsibility for the child's medical care. "The agency should assume and retain responsibility for the child's welfare," the Child Welfare League Standards point out.[52] The physician, as well as the foster mother, should know what the worker's responsibility is and how she plans to keep in touch with him. Depending on what is feasible, the worker may meet the foster mother and child at the clinic for the examination, and go in with them to hear what the physician says, or she may arrange for periodic conferences with him. If the agency has a pediatrician, the worker may keep in touch with the medical recommendations and progress through him.

If roles have not been clarified and the worker virtually abandons medical responsibility to the foster mother who is caring for the child, two serious results occur. First, the agency has no medical record, and a dichotomy exists in the running record between what is happening to the child socially and what may be going on medically. The worker thus cannot know what is realistic from an emotional standpoint, what is practical in relation to school, whether the foster care is indeed adequate for the child's needs, and how soon the child may conceivably go back to his own parents. She must be able to correlate medical information from a primary source with the other facts forming the constellation.

The second problem is the confusion in role between foster mother and placement worker, both in the mind of the foster mother and in that of the doctor. The latter gains the impression that he has done his part in imparting information to the foster mother, and he thinks of the worker as an interloper in the relationship built up between himself and the foster mother. The foster mother may enjoy having access to the medical information, with consequent feelings of importance, so she too may come to feel the worker is an interloper.

An aggressive foster mother who is able to deal with crises, ignore stares when, for example, she wheels a child on a gurney through the state fairgrounds, can intimidate a young worker, or a worker who is unsure of her function. She can easily crowd out the worker as well as the natural mother. If this happens, the worker is in an untenable position when the child's medical problem changes, or when the foster family situation changes and the child must be replaced.

The current trend to consider adoption for any child whose natural parents do not remain actively involved with him, and to consider any child adoptable no matter how handicapped he is, underscores the need for the foster care worker to remain fully cognizant of the child's total situation.[53] The agency needs direct access to medical information from a physician. The damage of role confusion between worker and foster mother can be avoided if the worker takes it into account in the beginning.

ADOPTION

"Unwed Mom Selected as Miss World," the newspaper reports, and the title winner declares, "I'm proud of my baby. I'm not married, but I'm not ashamed."[54] Her selection, even more than her attitude, explains part of the reason one agency, the largest private adoption agency in California, placed only 449 children in 1973, in contrast with 1,900 in 1968.[55] The shortage of white infants pushes adoption agencies into finding homes for the "hard to place," including physically handicapped children who would have been deemed unadoptable a few years ago.[56] "Adoption should not be ruled out for severely handicapped children," wrote a Missouri child welfare supervisor 13 years ago.[57] Today, adoption agencies are saying "No child is unadoptable." A long step forward has been taken in recent years. The Child Welfare League of America issued a news release in 1969: "Today, agencies plan adoption for children who would have been unplaceable three or four years ago. Adoptive families are being sought for the thousands of children who are older, handicapped, or nonwhite."[58]

Sober reflection makes clear that a great deal of difference exists between "Adoption should not be ruled out" and "No child is unadoptable." What chronically ill or handicapped children are suitable candidates for adoption, if relinquished by their parents, and under what circumstances should adoptive placements be made? Available follow-up studies throw little light on the situation, since, as one of the major recent studies on adoption outcome has pointed out, handicapped children usually were not placed in adoption at the time children were placed who are now the subjects of follow-up studies.[59] Fortunately, at least one major study in depth is available, and some experience has been gained that provides insight into the areas that warrant exploration.

The criteria against which successful outcome of adoption can be measured should be held in mind while considering the suitability of a child for adoption. What are we seeking in adoption? A home, for every child who needs one, that offers him a reasonable opportunity for healthy development, and parenting satisfaction for the persons who adopt him.

Kadushin, one of the authorities in the field, uses parent satisfaction in lieu of child adjustment as the criterion against which success of adoption can be measured, on the basis that if the parents obtain satisfaction from the child, his behavior must be such as to indicate that he is getting along relatively well. Parent satisfaction is easier to study than child adjustment, in light of the temporary stresses children undergo that make adjustment an unstable characteristic for purposes of measurement. The four major studies on adoption outcome of the last decade, however, look at the child's adjustment.* From about one-half to two-thirds of the children are adjudged to have made fairly good, good, or superior adjustments.[60]

It would appear, therefore, that one way of looking at the relative success of the adoption of physically handicapped children would be to use the newer model of parental satisfaction as a criterion, and to assume that if one-half to two-thirds of the children make a satisfying adjustment, their adoption is as successful as that of physically normal children.

An in-depth study in California of the outcome of adoption of children with medical problems satisfies this measurement.[61] Three out of four families who were willing to take part in the study and who had adopted children with a "moderate or severe handicap had attained a sound, resilient, fulfilling family life, as evidenced from comments the parents made about the child's development and achievement, his way of coping with unusual difficulties, their own satisfactions with and love for the child."[62]

The investigators' conclusions that agencies can place "children with medical conditions of all degrees of severity" with confidence deserve a closer look. Statistics are poor comfort for those on the wrong side of the mean. Studies in the social sciences are valuable primarily in illuminating areas for further concentration, and this one is no exception. The child welfare worker involved with one chronically ill child whose family can never be expected to care for him is concerned not with statistics but with whether this child is adoptable. One cannot lump "medical conditions"

---

* The four studies are by Witmer in 1963, Lawder in 1966, McWhinnie in 1967, and Ripple in 1968, described in Alfred Kadushin, *Child Welfare Services* (New York: Macmillan, 1970).

into one entity. Parental burdens and ability to attain satisfactions are not measured alone by "severity" of the handicap. A blind child has a severe handicap indeed, as does a child with congenital absence of one or more limbs, but these are static conditions. They create sorrow, but not constant crises; skill and wisdom, but not getting up at night for weeks on end or periods of anxiety over the child's life. In other words, *"handicap" must be distinguished from "illness" in considering a child's adoptability,* and consideration given to each condition's unique meaning.

In Kadushin's study of the adoption of older, physically normal children, factors negatively related to outcome were the age of the child at placement (the younger, the better), the number of placements prior to adoption (the fewer separation experiences the better), and the child's capacity to develop interpersonal relationships.[63] Outcome was positively related to

parents' acceptance of the child, in their perception of him as a member of the family, and negatively related to self-consciousness by parents regarding adoptive status. . . . Parents derived satisfaction from many areas: the child himself—his personality, temperament, mannerisms, and disposition; his achievements—artistic, athletic, social, educational—at school, in the community, with his peers, and in the home; the parent-child relationship, companionship from the child, affectional responses from him, his obedience to, respect for, and sympathetic understanding of the parent, as well as the child's pride in them, identification with and sharing of confidences. In addition, there was the occupation of parenthood itself as a lifelong interest, in the pleasure it affords, in helping a child grow and develop, in successfully handling the problems of child rearing.

The study of adoption of children with medical problems showed that the investigators considered the study biased in favor of positive adjustment by the refusal of 38 couples to participate, some for frank reasons of problems within the family, including divorces in three cases, and persistent refusal by 19 of the 38 to even give the reason for refusal. Of those who did participate, the study showed that the adoptive parents were older, less well educated, and in a lower socioeconomic class, as a group, than those who received physically normal children. The interviews showed that some of these parents were well aware that they had to take a handicapped baby or none at all, and one woman described how she "just sat down and cried" when the caseworker telephoned and told her that the baby available was blind. However, instances were cited in which severe handicaps (deafness and cerebral palsy) revealed themselves for the first time some months after placement, and these families wanted to keep the child.

A very wide range of handicapped children were placed for adoption, many with correctable defects and the majority with static conditions such as deformity of a finger or wry neck, but the children included a few with very severe conditions including complete deafness, amyotonia congenita, severe heart defects including tetralogy of Fallot, and even spina bifida of the myelomeningocele type. Unfortunately, the body of the study does not reveal what kinds of conditions the children had whose adoptive parents refused to participate or were divorced and those where an unsatisfactory adjustment had been made. However, a conclusion of the study was that the severity of the defect was the most important variable.

The parents did not seem as concerned about the medical problem, however, as the behavior problems, which were found more often among the children who were severely handicapped. The adoptive parents' lack of comprehension of the relationship of the medical problems and treatment experiences to the behavior problems was poignantly illustrated by some of the case examples. The investigators commented on the need of some of the families for service after adoption. However, they evidently did not connect the emotional problems of the child with his physical handicap or treatment, for it was stated, "The study parents who continued to struggle with some difficulty reported that their problems were infrequently related to the medical conditions. Parents were more apt to consider serious behavior problems the chief area of difficulty."

The most startling find of the study was that only a few couples remembered anything more than mild concern, if any, when told the child had a medical problem and were given the diagnosis. In one instance where a baby girl had a serious heart defect, the father did not want to adopt the child when told of her condition, but upon seeing her, he was so captivated he said, "We're taking that cutie home." Obviously he had so little comprehension of what lay ahead that seeing an attractive baby girl led him to decide an issue of great magnitude on impulse.

Since the study reports a practice of many years ago, when placement of physically handicapped children was just beginning, some parents were given the diagnosis merely by telephone and told to think it over and let the agency know if they wanted the child. The investigators' recommendations include greater attention to the interpretation of the medical problem. The contrast between these parents' reaction to first knowledge of serious medical problems and that of natural parents is so great that one can only conclude that a number did not understand what they were hearing and had little inkling of the implications.

What should be discussed with the prospective parents? First, *what should the worker and her supervisor learn about the medical problem* from the pediatrician and other sources? In light of the goal to be achieved by adoption, parenting satisfactions, and the insights into the attributes that provide these, one can list some of the things to be gone into thoroughly. The answers will affect decisions whether the child is indeed a suitable candidate for adoption, and if so by the family under consideration or another family; or whether subsidized foster care and/or guardianship should be considered as a long-term plan. If a family is not affluent but otherwise eligible, the issue of a subsidized adoption may also need to be weighed before the prospective adoptive parents are drawn into any discussion. The following conditions need exploration:

1. In what ways will the condition limit the child's physical functioning (mobility, sight, hearing, coordination)? Does the family have any special negative sensitivity to this limitation, for example, an athletic father who would want a son to do well in sports; or, on the contrary, are they perhaps especially equipped to relate to this limitation?

2. In what ways will the condition affect the child's appearance? His growth? Is this a family in which outward manifestation of difference would be particularly important, or not?

3. What kind of home care does this condition require? Will the parents need to perform exercises that are physically strenuous or that are painful for the child, or give injections? Will frequent transportation to a therapist be a major factor in treatment? If so, does the prospective father participate in household and parenting responsibilities, and if not, is the mother strong physically and emotionally?

4. Does the medical problem characteristically create social isolation because of the treatment demands or the differences it creates, and if so, is the prospective family one that has a strong kinship network or church network that would offset tendencies to isolation?

5. Is the condition correctable? Do children frequently outgrow this condition? Can helping the child through the medical and related psychosocial problems offer opportunity to the prospective parents for needed fulfillment and self-actualization?

6. Is the condition one that will require many hospitalizations? If so, is a subsidized adoption possible or needed? Is the condition one in which expenses usually are covered by insurance, or, as in hemophilia, does insurance usually exclude an important needed ingredient, blood?

7. Is the condition progressive—does it get worse, and if so do the downhill stages occur at predictable ages?

8. Will the child have multiple handicaps? If so, as in myelomeningocele, do these handicaps include lack of bladder and bowel control? Is there a significant possibility that the combination of handicaps will include mental retardation? If the child will need a great deal of medical supervision and care at home, does the family have the resources necessary?

9. Is the condition likely to be fatal, and if so, at what age do most children die from it? If, as in a severe heart defect, the condition is grave but not necessarily fatal, and the outlook depends in great part on whether the child can be helped to survive until he is large enough for surgery (perhaps at the age of two years), does the family have relatives, finances, physical stamina, etc., to provide the necessary care? Or should the child be cared for by a specially equipped foster mother until the most serious risk is over?

Examination of these questions leads to the obvious conclusion that such statements as "No child is unadoptable" or "Agencies can feel comfortable placing any physically handicapped child for adoption" are oversimplifications. Each child's condition merits thorough consideration. Agency pediatricians are not able to predict the future in many cases, or to answer all the questions that need to be explored before a child is considered adoptable, or considered for a specific couple. Some infants will have to remain in foster care for a period of observation before valid conclusions can be drawn.

Prolonged observation is sometimes necessary because of the difficulty of arriving at a diagnosis. A child may fail to thrive, but the exact nature of the reason remains unknown. Fortunately, most adoption agencies have the resources to permit study of the child by experts. Nevertheless, a year or two may elapse before final decisions can be made.

Greater attention to relinquishment offers one potential for eliminating some of the difficulty. Pressure for relinquishment at birth creates problems. Natural mothers often say they know little of the father's background. However, in some cases the mother may be able to learn from him something of his family's medical history if she is told this is important. Among Blacks, the high incidence of the sickle cell gene creates the possibility that the recessive gene in the mother will be matched by the father, and the child may have sickle cell disease. If the history the mother gives includes deaths of siblings at an early age or undiagnosed illness among siblings, special effort and attention should be made to learn about the father's medical history. In reading one case record, it was found that a mother relinquished her infant reluctantly, and only because she was convinced that he would have the advantages of a good adoptive home. The child soon revealed medical problems of such severity that the agency justifiably considered him unadoptable.

A fortunate coincidence exists if the California study of the outcome of adoptions of children with medical problems can be extrapolated to the practice of other agencies.[64] This study, it will be recalled, showed that placement workers tended to place babies with special medical needs in homes of less desirable adoptive parent applicants—among them, older couples. Experience with natural parents of physically handicapped children indicates that an intact family which has been together for a number of years weathers the stress of caring for a chronically ill child better than a young couple in the early stage of the family life cycle, when social activities and physical satisfactions are more important than later. It may well be that older adoptive-parent applicants are especially well suited to parenting a child with medical problems if their age means they have been married longer, and providing they understand what they are doing and have had a chance to think through all the implications.

Experience with children has been shown to be important in satisfactory foster care of the chronically ill or severely handicapped child. In Kadushin's study of the outcome of adoption of older children, a third of the adoptive parents had other children and almost all had experience as parent surrogates.[65] Although the presence of other children in the home can be a complication, it would appear to be a favorable factor in attenuating anxiety over health crises that are common to all children.

Also in the California study, a second fortunate coincidence occurred. The physically normal babies went to couples with no children or only one child, but over half of the children with medical problems went to applicants with one or more children, 20 percent of the severely affected going to couples with two or more children. The workers thought of these applicants as less desirable, in that agency policy usually prevented placement of children for adoption in families with two or more children, but by accident they utilized a positive feature.

Experience in adoption agency practice shows that adoptive parents are indeed resilient, able to undergo great stress in order to secure the satisfaction of being like other families and having the enrichment of children in their lives. The agencies themselves are among the best in the social work field, ordinarily well endowed financially, well staffed professionally, and highly motivated. Yet they have concentrated primarily on placing children, with only a minimum of follow-up even during the year that ordinarily follows placement prior to completion of legal adoption.[66] Some feeling has existed that families have not wanted any continuing supervision, and the fewer follow-up visits the better.

As with other social agency staff, absence of information or inner revulsion about physical abnormality has created a tendency to shift full responsibility for understanding the meaning of a medical problem to pediatricians and nurses. A good look at the adoptive placement of children with medical problems makes clear that both the preplacement and postplacement processes require careful, highly individualized social services. The psychosocial problems created by chronic illness in children are compounded by the problems of separations, discipline, feelings about adoption status, etc., that are inherent in adoption and correlate with the child's adjustment.[67] The many happy experiences that adoptive parents have with chronically ill children can be increased if preventive work is done.

COLLABORATION WITH MEMBERS OF THE HEALTH TEAM

"We fractionalize families to death with our helping practices." The White House Conference on Children in 1970, where this statement was made, set forth the principle that all children have the right to high-quality health services that are "family-centered, coordinated, comprehensive, continuous, compassionate, personalized and accessible." Yet the report characterized preventive health services as "grossly underdeveloped, poorly organized, and fragmented."[68] Remedial services, too, are "fragmented, inaccessible, impersonal, full of discontinuities."[69] Fragmentation is inevitable, for it is the corollary of specialization, and specialization is a necessity of expertise.

Social services are among the fragments that must be welded into this "family-centered, coordinated . . . service." The practical problems created by fragmentation of social services

are especially detrimental in the care of a chronically ill child. . . . Responsibility for a child's long-term care rests not with him but with his parents, who are often burdened with the care of other children; . . . the impact of long-term illness in the family often exacerbates many existing psychosocial problems that in turn interfere with the ability of parents to care adequately for their chronically ill child.[70]

The authors of this statement, who set up a family pediatric clinic in Baltimore, said further:[71]

Families with a chronically ill child often appeal to various community agencies for help with their complex social problems. In many communities, services are compartmentalized and, therefore, do not deal with the total family as an integrated unit. Since each agency sees only its part of the family problem and since communication between agencies is often inadequate, a family not infrequently receives conflicting, and at times diametrically opposite, advice from different sources. As a consequence, the parents of chronically ill children often become suspicious or completely alienated toward all health and welfare agencies.

A teacher, talking to a group of social workers, said, "You are part of the front line in the nation's war against ill health and the dependency related to, and deriving from, ill health. In this role, the demands made upon you for new knowledge and skill are considerable, and in many instances, your education has not prepared you for this role."[72] Some of the skills she referred to had been spelled out in a report on helping the handicapped by the Council on Social Work Education. They include "a capacity to coordinate social work concerns and operations with those of colleagues in other disciplines who provide services to the same clients, skills in the analysis of the nature of the setting and the impact upon professional practice, skills in understanding the concerns, procedures, and operational status of colleagues in various professions (including social work), and skills in assessing the dynamic characteristic of teams and in evolving viable team working relationships."[73]

Practical Considerations in Collaboration

Social workers, like physicians, tend to work alone or only in their agency milieu. Therefore, the individual must be conscious of process. And the team play necessary, if total attention to the patient's and family's needs is to be achieved and sustained, and if the natural tendency to fragmentation is to be circumvented, means that someone—usually the social worker

—must monitor the overall process. The skills referred to in "evolving viable team working relationships" are both the high-level planning and coordination of health and welfare systems and the day-to-day operations in working effectively with persons in other agencies. Often the day-to-day relationships are thwarted by bureaucratic rigidities that can be modified only by high-level intervention. Usually the modifications come about because workers at the operating level have been frustrated in trying to help clients take advantage of resources theoretically available within another system. Workers who have accumulated case material for ammunition, and who are able to communicate effectively with supervisors in their own agency as well as with relevant outside groups, can achieve these high-level policy changes in agency relationships. However, this means much patience, strategy, and stamina.

Some Common Obstacles

Human services workers find nothing so difficult as working with colleagues in other agencies. A student, reporting back on her summer work experience, said, "It was wonderful, marvelous, all except working with people in other agencies—they're terrible!" Not infrequently, one hears physicians or clergymen say, "I'm a social work hater." Still more frequently, attitudes of contempt and anger permeate social-agency conversations about physicians and hospital staffs.

Anger arises from frustration and hardens into stereotyping. Frustration comes, in part, because each tries to "use community resources" instead of to collaborate with others. Treated as objects to be used rather than as clusters of persons to be understood, the staffs of other agencies react as one would expect. The telephone is a malevolent tool of stereotyping. Too busy to set up a conference, where personal contact would permit liking and understanding to develop, the worker hears a voice over the telephone suggest that she call back later, or that the agency cannot supply the service requested. Stereotypes develop that others are "impossible to work with"; distrust and expectation of defeat then become self-fulfilling prophecies.

Some serious problems do exist. The fragmentation necessary to permit specialization in large hospitals and welfare departments creates bureaucracies of complicated structure. Workers must learn so many rules and jurisdictions and accommodate themselves to such rapid changes that psychic mechanisms come into play to protect them from collapse. Some of these mechanisms are destructive, and may be transmitted—especially by telephone—as indifference.

The public welfare department is especially vulnerable. Werner Boehm has pointed out the relationships between societal values and the social work profession. Social work (in public agencies) is exposed to public scrutiny; it has a lower level of professional education than some (for example, medical or legal); it has lower socioeconomic status and, in public welfare departments, suffers from a higher degree of bureaucratization.[74] In respect to societal values, a former U.S. Under Secretary of State, George C. McGhee, has written, "To most Americans, *welfare* is a dirty word. It connotes wangling and weaseling for public dollars. It has been made to seem that our welfare system is somehow at odds with the national character.... We tend to take a stereotyped view of welfare as a system in which lazy loafers who refuse to work are supported by those who do." (He later remarks in the same article that 73 percent of persons receiving assistance are the aged, the infirm, or dependent children.[75]

The public welfare worker is tarred with the brush of welfare, in the view of her social-work colleagues as well as the general public. Like physicians and nurses who have learned to carry on objectively and compassionately in a leukemia or burn ward despite the harrowing environment, many unusually able social workers in the welfare-department structure carry on amid the limitations they cannot change. Yet they may be looked down upon by hospital and private agency workers of less emotional maturity because of the telephone manner of some eligibility clerks, and the maze of contradictory regulations within which they work.

The hospital social worker is subject to a different but similar set of negative forces. Where others in the setting have concrete, understandable functions to perform, she talks and listens. The business of the institution is to admit critically ill cases or clinical material helpful in research or teaching, whereas the hospital worker is trained to see the patient as a person and to make others aware of him as an individual, often prolonging his stay until he has a place to go or until relatives are found who can take care of him. The business office may demand payment of old bills before provision is made for further care, even taking liens on property and sending reminders to the bedside concerning bills of catastrophic proportions, whereas the social worker pleads the person's inability to work and the effect of worry on his health.

Social workers, inside and outside of hospitals, unknowingly commit gaucheries or mistakes that irritate others and serve to remind them of their outside status. One hospital social worker who had been a registered nurse said that the most valuable aspect of her nursing background was that it had socialized her into the institution. She meant she had learned the hierarchical rules, how to get along with doctors, nurses, and sick persons, and behaviors and terms appropriate and inappropriate in a medical setting. Social workers who enter hospital social-service departments with no prior experience in a medical institution need to become aware of the subtleties of professional interaction and the etiquette of the hospital society. As with anyone in a new setting, the worker needs to learn when to be forthright and when to avoid confrontation, when to stand for a principle and when to compromise.

To the physician, whose interest is in treating the patient, social information relevant to the patient's utilization of medical care is welcome, but other social data may seem only gossip. The worker may use medical terms inappropriately or ask questions at inconvenient times. The worker may fail to perceive herself as she appears to the sick person, family, or physician, and may offend both patient and staff by dress or behavior not expected in a medical setting.

Thus the hospital social worker, like the worker in the welfare department, is functioning within a setting that demands all her psychic energies. In order to learn the complex world, and to accustom herself to the physical and emotional pain of the patients, she too may develop mechanisms that are destructive to collaborative relationships. Insecurity may be masked by identification with the authority of the physician or the prestige of the institution.

Despite the obstacles, effective collaboration does take place between staffs of health and welfare agencies. Those who have described projects that in effect bridged the two systems for the sake of help to a specific group talk about means to improve (1) communication, (2) knowledge of the services and limitations of others, and (3) clarity of roles.

Communication

"Where usual or special barriers to communication exist, it is the social worker's responsibility to know his own communication ways and his own communication biases if he is to understand and successfully work with communication problems in others," writes Frances Feldman in discussing communicating with families.[76] The popular sensitivity and encounter sessions have helped many persons understand better the way they seem to other persons. The nonverbal ways of communicating, the middle-class biases, the differences in cultural background have become well known through the angry writings and speeches of representatives of ethnic groups.

Yet in the sensitive area of building bridges between professional groups who have stereotyped each other as hostile, "We communicate what we are. We communicate attitudes and feelings as well as ideas."[77] Especially on the telephone, which is used so much in interagency communication, these things come across through tone of voice, noncommittal attitudes, or silence. Remarks meant in jest, or culturally loaded words, may be misunderstood. The context of what is said affects the message given. Beyond her own intent in communicating a message, the worker must maintain an awareness of the other's perception of her attitudes.

Knowledge of Others' Services and Limitations

The hospital worker in a specialty service, with patients from a wide geographical area, cannot know all the social agencies, or all their functions and restrictions; the community is too vast and varied. She may have worked closely with a child and his family over several years, when he is hospitalized or attends clinic, but have no knowledge of local agencies that could be of help. The family may, in fact, be known to one or more local agencies, in connection with that child or other children or family problems, but if the mother does not mention the fact, the hospital worker may continue in ignorance of the potential services the agency offers.

The local worker in a public welfare department, family counseling or probation office, health department, or school may be in a similar situation. If she has never visited the medical center, and has not had occasion to inquire about the social service department there, she too may be working without knowledge of potential help from hospital social service staff.

The social worker or other helping person should take the responsibility of determining whether the medical center has a social work staff and, if so, whether any worker is assigned to the specialty service providing care to the child. Because the parent or child may not know that the person who takes an interest and talks with him is a social worker, an inquiry to the family is a preliminary step, but the answer may be inconclusive. The local Crippled Children's Services office should know, however, if the medical center has social workers, and if the workers perform only eligibility functions or services.

Letters of inquiry that open the way to telephone contacts and to conferences as soon as possible provide a way of learning what the hospital social worker's duties are and how best to begin a continuing working relationship. Letters addressed to the center asking for "diagnosis and prognosis" about a given child are usually directed to the record room and are eventually answered by an intern; they must be directed to the social service department. The letter should explain why the agency is interested, and ask specific questions related to the agency's interest.

The public welfare worker may not receive an initially cordial response from the hospital worker. She may not trust the worker to treat information confidentially if she has had negative experiences with workers from other welfare departments. Unless a conference has been scheduled at a time she is least prone to be called away, an urgent matter may preoccupy her.

An invitation to the hospital worker to visit the county area, to see its resources and environment, and to pay a joint visit to the family may be well received. If a hospital-based worker becomes acquainted with the local agency staff and learns of the services the agencies provide, along with all the potential resources here, she may come to understand both the services and the limitations of the community.

Large urban areas pose some of the same problems as distant smaller communities. With freeways bypassing residential areas, the hospital worker may never have seen many of the neighborhoods in her own city. Agency workers may know the medical center's location but may never have visited it because of time, traffic, and parking problems. Attendance at pediatric grand rounds and less formal staff discussions are often open to outsiders with special interest in a given patient or subject. The rounds, which are sit-down conferences, offer the agency worker an opportunity to observe the relationships and hear the discussion of hospital, professional, and technical staff.

Committee work is another channel frequently used to permit knowledge of other agencies' functions. Official agency representation on case committees may be confined to top-level staff and their comments restricted by set agency policy. However, in San Mateo County, California, for example, working-level practitioners often participate in committees and the interaction has been largely effective.[78] NASW, Community Council, and other social service, social action, or private health agency committees, in which the worker is functioning as an individual, permit a refreshing exchange of ideas about agencies and acquaintances with staff. Staff-meeting program committees may welcome suggestions for speakers from hospital social service departments.

In describing the knowledge needed about other agencies and methods of obtaining it, Fern Jaffee, of the Health Insurance Plan of Greater New York, described the collaborative work done in connection with the Upper Manhattan Maternity Project. She said that (a) it is important to know the "life-style pattern" of other agencies ("With some agencies I always write a letter to request a conference, knowing that staff members require clearance from top administrative personnel; with other agencies, I make an informal telephone call, knowing this is the accepted precedure"), and (b) one must know who the key people are, since the top administrative personnel may not be as helpful as someone in the agency who is particularly interested in your program and who knows how to gain his agency's collaboration.[79]

Learning whether an agency can expand its services to assume new responsibilities obviously requires participation of top-level staff of both or all the agencies involved. Of the many special collaborative projects, some that have been described include those for the unwed pregnant schoolgirl, comprehensive health care for preschool children, rehabilitation projects for the disabled, and a major project in Los Angeles that created foster home care for disabled children without homes to go to at time of discharge.

In the latter project, staff workers of the hospital social service department accumulated data regarding the harm done and expense caused by lack of home care resources for rejected handicapped children; through supervisory staff the directors of hospital and public welfare department met and involved county commissioners, and then the appropriate intermediate-level department heads worked out the details of the program.[80] The new program required the public welfare department to provide additional funding for foster home payments, extra staff, training for the staff, prolonged recruitment of foster home applicants, office space, travel and clerical expenses.

Yet it was accomplished through demonstration of its fiscal soundness to the Board of Supervisors and its humanitarian value. Cox and James, who have described the project, like Mrs. Jaffee in New York, have brought out the *commitment* that is essential in developing collaborative progress. Collaboration requires energy, creativity, flexibility, and willingness to do a little extra.

Clarity of Roles

As more social content has been introduced into the education of paramedical personnel, a blurring of roles has occurred in many settings. A general tendency exists to determine primary relationships with child and/or family not according to the traditional role of the profession but according to the opportunity for counseling and related services, and according to the rapport that may have sprung up between the therapist and the child or family. This tendency to utilize natural or spontaneous liking and trust has also arisen in determining the extent of responsibility of paraprofessional workers.

The loosening of rigidities is welcome, and common sense dictates the direction. Warmth and good listening, the elements of emotional support, are not the sole property of social workers. Nevertheless, the pitfalls are evident: there is an invitation to casualness, to allowing decisions about responsibility to fall upon such extraneous factors as skin color or the worker's emphasis on counseling in contrast to less interesting duties. It is easier to sit and talk than to perform exercises, give baths, iron clothes, or trudge up and down looking for housing. It is easy to confuse talking and interviewing.

The most serious problems arise from the patient's or family's confusion concerning whom to talk to about what, the unwarranted invasion of privacy by persons not trained to perceive or deal with roused anxiety or hostility, and the waste of a crisis opportunity by someone who does not know how to exploit its advantage.

The tendency does, however, serve to underscore the need for action inherent in these situations, for careful assessment of the needs of the family and/or child, and for determining who has the best equipment to meet them. A conference between the workers or therapists involved should be held, with decisions reached about who will do what, and for how long, until reevaluation. With help or consultation from the social worker, the therapists or homemakers going into the home during a given period may be able to accomplish much of what the social worker would do in observing relationships and reinforcing certain behaviors, or lending support to a mother under stress.

Three areas are subject to special hazard. The first is in relation to an indigenous aide who, because of language facility or color and subculture, is expected to carry the main thrust of counseling. The paraprofessional may be related to the family, or may be among their widened circle through church or other connections, and be caught up in conflict between agency identification and personal identification. Subprofessional staff members may feel conflict about their limitations and feel the need to refer to professional staff when the situation becomes complex. Busy workers who have learned how helpful an aide can be may thrust more upon her than is fair, or grow careless about the need for alertness to tension or conflicts in a given case situation. Special problems also exist between some hospital staff and workers from outside agencies. The hospital staff worker, who regularly sees the medical staff on rounds and in conferences, who is accepted as part of the institutional team, and who is aware of the daily situations on wards or in clinics, usually is in the best position to secure medical advice and to interpret medical need to outside agencies. However, if the child has been in the hospital so briefly that the hospital social worker has had no opportunity to become acquainted with him and his family, the worker may prefer to arrange a conference directly between the agency worker and the most appropriate physician. Since hospitals vary widely in staffing patterns and relationships, the most effective or preferred mode of intra-hospital communication should be agreed upon by the supervisors of the hospital and by the community social service departments.

Another area commonly requiring clarity of roles is that of the relative responsibilities of the public health nurse and the social worker or workers. A potential for overlapping and even competition has grown up because social workers in family and public welfare agencies have tended to avoid the needs of the ill; because hospital social workers have saved themselves time by asking a public health nurse to evaluate the home and provide them with information; and because the training of the public health nurse has emphasized the need for understanding the social and psychological components of patients' problems. Public health nurses have tended to step into the vacuum created by the absence of social work services in the families of the ill.

A nursing background equips the nurse to give nursing service; the public health nurse has the added responsibility of training the family in health care. In a model developed by the staff of the California State Health Department, the function of the nurse was defined as identifying physical and emotional needs of patient and family *that require nursing intervention.* Further, the statement continued: "The nurse provides direct nursing care; helps the patient cope with illness or maintains health by giving support, health teaching, supervision, and coordination of health care services. She sustains the patient during times of stress." The model described the social worker as assisting the patient and his family in "maintaining psychological and social stability in the face of illness and treatment. In relieving psychological and social stresses that affect treatment, the social worker utilizes knowledge of the psychosocial implications of the illness; [she] utilizes insights into feelings, motivations, adaptive capacity, family relationships, role, and socioeconomic and cultural influences of the patient's usual environment."[81]

In many communities, public health nursing and the visiting nurse service of the private agency have been combined, or they distinguish their services by geographical area. Traditionally, the visiting nurse service has offered bedside nursing service, in contrast to the health education emphasis of the public health nurse. A study conducted by the Visiting Nurse Service of New York in 1967 stated, "Typical nursing care offered by the field staff nurses included giving an injection to a diabetic woman, exercising the muscles of a man who had had a stroke, teaching an expectant mother how to care for herself and her baby, helping an orthopedically handicapped youngster to become more independent, and helping the psychiatric patient and his family to adjust to his illness. In other words, almost every kind of patient has been seen by the visiting nurse."[82]

Of special significance in this report were statements that "emotional support was the preferred nursing function . . . least preferred was community referrals," and that "patients, though satisfied with the care they received, wished nurses had more time to perform direct nursing care."[83] The average hospital patient also would probably prefer that the nurse give him more nursing care. Two insights into potential problems emerge from this statement. The preference for "emotional support" that some but not all nurses feel can lead to confusion with the social work function if there is a social worker on the case.

The second problem, the dislike for "community referrals," points up the common experience of persons attempting to secure help from a worker in a public welfare department. Telephone service is frequently so inadequate that many attempts are necessary before getting a call through; and the fragmentation is so great that several persons are talked with before the right worker is located. No wonder, then, that students said, "Workers from other agencies are awful." Or that a nurse wrote many years ago, "Teamwork comes to fruition only when individuals who are themselves reasonably emotionally mature have sound professional knowledge and recognize the necessity of working with others toward a common goal. It involves mutual respect for the contribution of each member of the team, and the acceptance of responsibility for one's full share—and more—of the load. We cannot demand respect or force cooperation; this is reciprocal behavior and we will receive both as we prove ourselves worthy."[84]

Working with Physicians

Communicating with physicians involves the same elements as collaborating with hospital social work staff, therapists, or public health nurses. Some further considerations deserve note, however, including those previously described that affect the hospital social worker's relationships with medical staff.

Effective work with physicians on behalf of the client requires of the social worker that she become sensitive to the impression she is making—again because we "communicate what we are... our attitudes and feelings." Anger and fear are probably the greatest obstacles to effective working relationships, with a lack of knowledge adding its own problems. Anger toward the medical profession in general rarely carries over to one's own physician, nor is it prevalent in adoption agencies that work with selected pediatricians. Its source in public welfare agencies lies in the unfortunate circumstance in some communities of physicians refusing to accept patients receiving assistance because of the paperwork and the delayed payments inherent in third-party intermediary pay arrangements. Specialists who schedule one or two hours for first examination lose valuable time and money if the patient misses an appointment without notice, which is not infrequent among AFDC families. Too often the result is that less qualified and less scrupulous physicians provide medical care for most of the agency's clientele; and justifiable anger arises in the agency over what the agency staff observes happening. Anger over one episode or one physician's practice can infect the attitude toward the entire medical profession.

Less worthy feelings of anger may exist among some social workers. Particularly among workers who work best alone and resist any authoritarian, supervisorial, or even mutual sharing of responsibility, feelings of competition color their attitudes. They feel defensive about the higher social status of the physician, and are intolerant of his authoritarian ways.

Defensiveness is closely related to fear. Fear of the physician's contempt or discourtesy, or of his prestige and knowledge in an area where she feels ignorant, may so immobilize a worker that she cannot explain her interest in the client sufficiently or ask intelligent questions. As the late Charlotte Towle expounded, "Knowledge changes feelings." Getting acquainted with a few good physicians can counteract the tendency to paint them all with one brush.

A serious shortage of physicians exists, especially among general practitioners, and the cost of medical education is very high. Though much of the cost is subsidized, the still-high cost to the student, the heavy scholastic demands and stiff competition, and the traditions of the profession yield an individual prone to certain characteristics. He (or she) is frequently from a well-to-do family; because his studies exacted his total energies, he may have learned little else; he is above average in intelligence; he has worked under intense pressure for a prolonged period; he has been socialized into an aristocratic group; he has high standards of exactitude, proficiency, and efficiency for himself and others.

He often works very long hours and is conscious that others do not; and he often practices on a high plane of intensity occasioned by the life-and-death nature of his treatment and decisions. Although the increased trend toward group practice shelters him from some of the loneliness of decision and around-the-clock demands, the physician is essentially a "loner." No one tells him what to do; not only must he make up his mind swiftly, knowing his mistakes may cost the patient life or limb, but he must simulate matter-of-factness and calm, or dissimulate optimism and good cheer. He sees the most base, and the most noble, among both his patients and his colleagues. He also puts up with boring chronic complainers, and, if he is a pediatrician, with boring, repetitious dietary instructions and immunizations. Like others, the physician is influenced by feedback from others, and from their expectations. Current attitudes toward doctors reflect the distrust of authority that has come from the extensive corruption in modern life, but the usual patient still vests his physician with godlike attributes. His associates, neighbors, and tradesmen treat him as someone rich, powerful, and authoritative.

The physician, then, is not bred for team play. But if the compassion that led him into the practice of medicine remains, he is grateful for all that helps his patients and helps him help his patients. He becomes a richly rewarding person with whom to work if the social worker will help him overcome his stereotype of her as either a snoopy, hardboiled individual or a vague, fuzzy-minded do-gooder who is wasting his time. The parent and the worker have a right to know what the child's condition is and what to do to prevent unnecessary disability. The physician will respect this right if relationships have been established and communication is adequate.

In a conference of cardiac-center social workers, a pediatric cardiologist known for effective cooperation made suggestions about attributes that promote effective relationships with physicians. He emphasized relevance of social data and succinct reporting. These require selectivity and restraint; the most interesting aspects of the case may not be pertinent to the medical objective, which is helping the child and family utilize medical care or adjust to limitations. Selectivity and relevance have been emphasized elsewhere as important to team relationships. Among other benefits, these attributes promote confidentiality, help narrow the focus, and save the time of the group.

In working with private physicians, a brief letter, asking for a conference at his convenience, stating why the agency needs medical information and suggestions, and enclosing a release of confidentiality signed by the client, helps to further relevance and brevity. It also gives the physician an opportunity to review the patient's record, refresh his memory, and anticipate the worker's telephone call for an appointment. Flexibility in hours is necessary in holding conferences and making or receiving telephone calls from a physician. Often the doctor makes his telephone calls after office hours, and also schedules conferences after the last patient of the day has been seen. If the worker has left word with the physician's secretary asking him to call back, the worker should be prepared to remain at her desk until well after five o'clock. By asking the secretary when the doctor usually makes his telephone calls, the worker can anticipate the probable time.

A suggestion made by Dr. Leonard Linde is that the worker use appropriate language.[85] This means avoiding social-work lingo, as well as medical terms (which one may mispronounce or use inappropriately). Since the physician often uses terms the worker does not understand, a preconference review, sometimes with the help of the office medical textbook or consultation with an agency medical consultant—if one is available—can facilitate understanding and cut down the many interruptions otherwise necessary for clarification of the physician's meaning.

One or more well-prepared, focused conferences with the same physician about different clients may make it possible to maintain further relationships with him by telephone. The guardian of his telephone calls and his time, the office receptionist or nurse, is an important person to get to know. She may want to know what the call is about, and may prefer to ask him the questions and relate his reply to the worker. When a direct question needing a brief answer is involved, such third-party involvement may be satisfactory. If, however, the worker needs to relay information about the family's circumstances that affect the child's care and to secure a thoughtful discussion, direct communication with the physician may be necessary. In seeking it out the worker will want to avoid offending a receptionist or nurse who is trying to be helpful or who is closely identified with the busy physician.

Before the worker calls the physician, she should determine whether the agency has failed to pay him for care for which it is obligated, or whether the clients have been carelessly missing appointments without notification. If medical payments are badly delayed, she should express her concern but state her lack of jurisdiction, pointing out to the physician that the worker in a large agency has no control over financial procedures.

The Clergyman as Member of the Health Team

The clergy is an appropriate and needed segment of the health team but one insufficiently utilized. Clergymen take the initiative in visiting active members of their churches or parishes if someone informs them of family illness, but otherwise they must depend on requests from the family or member of the helping group involved.

Clergymen vary widely in their ability to be helpful to a child or family during serious or terminal illness. Individual differences in personality and approach, in theology, and in experience with illness should be taken into account. Some pastors are very busy because of lack of adequate assistance within the church and their various community involvements; some see their duties as extending only to members of their own parishes; others, no matter how busy, always have time to meet need, and keep to no boundaries.

Some of the younger clergy have received seminary training in pastoral counseling and working with the sick and dying. Others have never attended a seminary and may even have received no formal training toward ordination. Because no licensing or uniform standards exist for clergymen, some unfortunate deviations have occasioned unjust criticism of the entire group.

Because of the relatively small number of chronically ill children in the population and the relatively large number of church members beyond the child-rearing age, the number of seriously ill children or youth any one clergyman has seen is small. Unless he has worked as a hospital chaplain, he will be inexperienced in attending on the illness and death of children, though he will usually have had considerable experience in counseling troubled families and helping older persons when death is near. Clergymen may not be able to relate comfortably to the child at the time of death though they may be able to sustain the family and indirectly the child. The modern trend among Protestant clergy is away from direct spiritual guidance and toward general emotional support. This can be superficial, or it may demonstrate that someone does care and is available, a true source of support.

Members of the congregation known to the clergy may help the family by attending a child at the hospital, and some may be cheerful, adaptable, steady persons. Others may cover their own distress by stilted or inappropriate comments. Church members can be thought of, by and large, as a substitute "extended family" and a valuable source of support for lonely, exhausted parents.

The way the family and the child perceive their own clergyman, or if they have none, the clergy in general, will affect his ability to relate to them and to know how best to help.

In situations where the family has no pastor but where they indicate a struggle over the meaning of catastrophe, or philosophical and religious questions, the worker can ask if they would like to talk with a member of the clergy. If the answer is not in the negative, the worker should try to find someone who matches the family in religious background (Catholic, fundamentalist Protestant, modern Protestant, Jewish, agnostic); the hospital and campus chaplains, the Council of Churches, the Archdiocese, and some agency directors and supervisors are possible sources of information. The worker should then arrange to talk with him about the family.

The worker can learn from his attitude whether he would be comfortable counseling with the family, and also whether it might be helpful for him to get acquainted with the child. In an interview, the worker will gain some impression of whether the clergyman seems to be a flexible, supportive, and relaxed person who would have enough time to sit and listen to a distressed mother or child, and the sensitivity to relate to their needs. If he shows reluctance or discomfort, he can be asked if there are other clergymen he knows or members of his congregation he can suggest. If he does visit the family and/or the child at the worker's instigation, an early follow-up with the family will reveal whether the worker should encourage further contacts.

Many hospitals have chaplains. They vary in their work and relationships. An experienced chaplain who is active on the wards may be of great help to parents and child while the child is hospitalized, and may be able to suggest a clergyman who can visit in the home if this seems indicated.

As technical advances occur in saving life or prolonging existence, more dilemmas arise of a bioethical nature. The chaplain tends to be part of the group called in to help make decisions, or to help the family bear to make a decision that life should not be prolonged. When the worker is involved with a family undergoing an agonizing ordeal of this nature, she should attempt to learn if the hospital has a chaplain or the family has a minister on whom they can call, and should help to promote participation of such a person, unless it is definitely known the family would not want this kind of help. Usually, life and death do call forth religious impulses.

The worker needs to safeguard the client from her own religious biases, including a view that religion is meaningless or is a form of escape. The client may share this view, but well may not when he is faced with intolerable grief or anxiety. Among workers who are themselves religious, a temptation exists to offer their own philosophy. This can be unfortunate if the family has a childhood religious background that is theologically different from the worker's.

NOTE: Since this chapter was written, Congress passed over the President's veto (July 26, 1975) a Special Health Revenue Sharing Act of 1975 that authorizes, but does not appropriate, two billion dollars for continuance and expansion of some existing programs, changes in other programs, and provision of some new services that will affect families and children. The extent and nature of its funding and implementation will determine its impact. A new feature included is provision for beginning aid to families with hemophilia (see note to Chapter 11, p. 319). The special federal funding for persons receiving dialysis and kidney transplantation and for persons with hemophilia points in the direction of federal aid for persons with catastrophic illness. (From Bills and Resolutions S66, A18 and A19, and House Bills HR 2925, 4114, and 4115, pp. F438, E437–500 *passim*, Democratic Study Group Report for the week of July 28, 1975.)

CHAPTER FIVE

The Unborn Child and the Mother

THE CHINESE determine age by counting the child one year old when he is born. His first "Chinese year," the time he is in utero, is his most important. This is the time that determines his constitution, the soil in which all life experiences will be planted—the time that the very characteristics and circumstances of the mother are molding the kind of person he will become more profoundly than the mother as a person will ever do again. And no outsider, however beneficent or skillful, will influence his life to the extent his parents do. This, then, is the time for helping persons to exert their greatest effort, by providing the mother and father with the services they need.

The remainder of this book is about services to minimize disability, enrich life, and delay death, those services that public health personnel call "secondary" and "tertiary" prevention. This chapter is about primary prevention, or "prepathogenesis," the prevention of illness or handicap. Chronic illness in childhood unfortunately is not entirely preventable. The present stage of medical knowledge does not permit prevention of juvenile arthritis, leukemia, or many other conditions. But there are disabling conditions that need not occur. These include some of the birth defects, including those that may not be apparent at birth but show up later, such as cystic fibrosis or sickle cell anemia. The National Foundation estimates that 6 percent, or one in 16 children, are born with a significant birth defect.[1]

Tools are at hand for primary prevention, some of them of very recent origin. Obstetricians, pediatricians, and public health personnel have identified the "mother at risk," and a parallel group, "infants at risk." The majority of defective children come from a small group of mothers, said to be about 20 percent of the total.[2] All pregnant women have special needs; more will be said about this and about the social obligations to them.

However, *all pregnancies are not equal.* Helping persons who must give priority to certain clients because of the size of their loads, or who need to identify categories of clients to refer for special social services, must know how to define the high-risk mother. Services can then be provided according to the needs of the mother, the function of the agency, and the skill of the workers.

In addition to the tool of identifying mothers at risk are scientific advances in genetics—chromosomal analyses and enzyme assays that have begun to permit identification of carriers and fetal cellular characteristics. Great social advances have occurred, including public acceptance and support of family planning services, and continuing refinement of contraceptive techniques. There is wider acceptance of male sterilization and, the most dramatic social change of all, the legalization of abortion. Mothers who are known to be at risk can now prevent or terminate pregnancies if they wish.

However, mothers at risk have formidable problems, social and emotional. Despite the startling advances, many of the mundane but critical preventive problems require long-sustained, patient, often ingenious effort. Some problems are insoluble. In no field does the recent emphasis on "advocacy services" find greater need for expression. This chapter will describe high-risk mothers, preventive tools, prevention of genetic disease, and the social needs of all pregnant women. The goal of all reproduction, healthy children, and the right of all children, good health at birth, can be more nearly secured if social measures implement the knowledge of prevention that now exists.

HIGH-RISK MOTHERS: DEMOGRAPHY AND DEFINITION

"When we speak of mothers at risk, we are thinking most of all about the relationship of the course of the pregnancy to the outcome; or in other words, the risk to the infant."[3] A high-risk baby has been defined as "one that stands a greater than average risk of developing neonatal, life-threatening disease or sequellae due usually to maternal disease or complications at birth. These high-risk babies have 'high-risk' mothers, for it is the maternal condition that usually determines the outcome of the pregnancy."[4]

The decline in the birthrate is a positive influence on the number of infants at risk of chronic illness and disability. The fertility rate has steadily dropped to below 2.1 per family, as has the actual number of births, in spite of the increased number of women of childbearing age.[5] The U.S. birthrate was 23.7 per thousand in 1960 but only 14.8 in the 12 months ending May 1974.[6] A June 1974 newspaper item quoted pollster Gallup as finding that the percentage of Americans who favor large families is the lowest since he began polling 38 years ago.[7] Only 19 percent said that four or more children were ideal; the most popular number now is two children.

The large number of women of childbearing age could cause the decline to be reversed. However, the increase in the number of women working, the older age of marriage and childbearing, the increased efficiency of contraceptives, and the availability of legal abortion, combined with the expressed desire of women for small families, are encouraging for a continued low birthrate.

The greatest cause for optimism is the decline in births among poor families. In the late 1960's the birthrate in families with less than $5,000 annual income declined so sharply that the group produced one million fewer children than if the rate of the early 1960's had continued.[8] The decline in birthrate was more pronounced for the poor, 21 percent in contrast to 18 percent for the more affluent, and, in absolute numbers, fell about twice as far in poor families as it did in more well-to-do families. Births to poor women fell by 32 per 1,000, compared with 17 per 1,000 among the others. For poor Black women, the fall was even greater; they produced 49 fewer babies per 1,000. The availability of government-sponsored birth control clinics is credited with this decline. In one New Orleans hospital, a study showed that of 30,000 women who came for birth control advice, 75 percent had not been using any contraception or had been using inefficient methods. They were offered birth control pills or the intrauterine device (IUD), and 85 percent said they would use them.[9]

Although the decline in the birthrate among the Black poor is a cause for hope that proportionately more children will be wanted and provided with a better chance for a good start in life, it should be noted that continued growth of the non-White population is projected, from 12.8 percent of the population in 1965 to 14.6 percent in 1975–80, and to 20.5 percent in the year 2000.[10] It is from the Black poor that the largest proportion of physically disadvantaged babies comes. However, the rapid upward mobility of the Black population lends hope that the proportion of disadvantaged children will continue to decline.

Another demographic cause for optimism is the recent decline in fertility among older married women (over 35), if the California experience is typical. The greatest decline in legitimate live births between 1969 and 1972 occurred in this group: since they used legal abortion least of any age-group, it is to be assumed they have benefited from the general availability of effective contraceptives in limiting the size of their families.[11] Among Black women, the dramatic drop in fertility also occurs in the third- and higher-order births, both legitimate and illegitimate.[12] Thus, as becomes clear from the ensuing discussion, we can expect a much better record in regard to infants at risk. The major problem area will be discussed in detail later, namely, the rise in fertility rates among teenagers. This is indeed an alarming phenomenon, creating health and social hazards for both mothers and babies.

Obstetricians designate high-risk categories in terms of age (excessive youth [under 16] or obstetric old age [over 35 years]); parity, or number of children in excess of five or six, as well as frequency of pregnancies; socioeconomic and psychological conditions, including poverty, excessive fatigue, illegitimate or unwanted pregnancies; medical problems, including exposure to rubella, syphilis, Rh incompatibility, heart disease, diabetes, chronic kidney disease, thyroid trouble, and a condition most prevalent in poor mothers, toxemia (preeclampsia); and prior history of premature delivery, stillbirths, or obstetric problems. Smoking, malnutrition, drug usage, twinning, attempted abortion, and radiation are other adverse factors linked to prematurity and/or impairment in the child.[13]

PSYCHOSOCIAL RISK FACTORS

Examination of risk factors reveals quickly that many of them are social. Excessive youth or age and large number of pregnancies, excessive fatigue, and illegitimacy, malnutrition, smoking, the use of drugs, and especially poverty are described as adverse many times in the literature of maternal and child health. Typical is a statement of Arthur Lesser, former chief of the now diminished Children's Bureau, who said, "In the administration of the maternity and infant care program we are responding to the fact that serious differences exist in the amount and quality of care received by poor expectant mothers and their infants, as compared with middle class children, *resulting in an excess of preventable deaths, illness and handicapping conditions among the poor.*"[14]

Poverty

Dr. Lesser further states, "Poverty reflects many unfavorable associations with childbirth which affect infant survival. Women living in poverty become pregnant earlier in life, are pregnant more frequently and at shorter intervals, and continue childbearing until later in life than do middle class women. They also have more complications of pregnancy and have a poorer reproductive history. All of these are associated with a less favorable pregnancy outcome, especially as represented by premature birth."[15]

The size of the problem of poverty declined during the 1960's and early 1970's; the unstable economy and inflation of the mid-1970's threaten the gains, but how seriously is unknown. In 1969, Goldstein placed approximately 10 percent of all families in the United States below the poverty line, with more than twice the proportion of the nation's Black families (about 12 percent of the population) below the poverty line in all sections of the country. Poverty is distributed unevenly in different parts of the country, the most prevalent being among both Whites and Blacks in the Southern states, and, as is well known, poverty tends also to cluster in inner cities.[16] Most unfortunately, the poverty rate is higher among families with children—14 percent of all families, and 40 percent of all

Black families with children.[17] Intertwined with the problem of poverty is that of family size. "The larger the family, the greater the risk of poverty, the less likelihood of escape; a third of all 5-child families are poor."[18]

Social services directed toward poverty as a risk factor in pregnancy must have more specific targets than the global concept of poverty. Poverty is not a matter of income alone, but a multifaceted state. Though searching questions have been raised about the validity of a "culture of poverty," those familiar with it are well aware that poverty has many common aspects. Therefore, we need to know *why* poverty causes prematurity and preventable deaths and handicaps. The answers are not yet definitive; some disagreement exists, and various aspects are examined in detail throughout this chapter. A brief statement is nevertheless pertinent here.

Dr. Frederick North categorizes the reasons as three: (a) hazards to the fetus physiologically that stem from nutritional deficits, lack of medical care to the mother, ill effects upon her of crowded living quarters, etc.; (b) indirect influences springing from the kind, or lack, of health care of mother and newborn; and (c) influences on the child's later development.[19] In considering the physiological effects, he refers to the short stature of women deprived of adequate nutrients in their own childhood, and the well-known association of the mother's stature to childbearing capacity, as well as the problematical matter of direct nutritional effect on the fetus of inadequate maternal diet.

Delay or absence of prenatal care among the poor has been associated with poor outcome of pregnancy, but the reasons why poor mothers do not avail themselves of resources is in some dispute. Is it ignorance or lack of motivation, or is it difficulty in making arrangements, and impersonal, inadequate health care? Dr. North argues for the latter: "The experience of many anti-poverty programs indicates that when the realistic barriers are removed, utilization by poverty groups approaches or exceeds that of the more affluent population."[20] Social workers may find this simplistic; a later discussion deals with the complex factors hindering utilization of prenatal care.

Prematurity

Prematurity, officially designated as *low birth weight,* is the most common risk factor, and one in which medical or social reasons may constitute the major cause. The newer term is intended to clarify reference to an objective measure—weight—in contrast to gestation, which depends on the mother's memory regarding the time of conception and is therefore statistically unreliable. Low birth weight is defined as 2,500 grams or under, or, in other words, a birth weight of five and a half pounds or less. Weight is customarily lower in certain groups of infants, particularly those of non-

White mothers; consequently, these babies are not "prematures" in the gestational sense. However, they do belong in the category of babies at risk because small babies are especially frail. The blood vessels in the head, small and fragile in any newborn, are even more so in the tiny baby, and thus more easily ruptured (creating brain damage). The respiratory system may be less ready to cope with the hazards of life outside the womb. The premature baby's temperature control system may be even more unstable than a normal infant's, and the baby is susceptible to feeding difficulties and infections.[21]

Dr. Lesser comments on prematurity and low income as follows: "These mothers [in low-income groups] give birth prematurely to an alarming extent, low birth weight being commonly 15–20 percent, or 2 to 2.5 times the expected rate. *This is the principal group of so-called high-risk infants.*"[22]

The premature infant not only is subject to greater risk of illness and major permanent crippling, but is more apt to die.[23] Prematurity is by far the leading cause of death among infants under one year, and in the first month of life the death rate is 20 times that among infants of normal weight. The smaller the baby, the more subject he is to illness and death; however, non-White babies and girl babies (often classified as "prematures" because of their weight) are less subject to hazard than are White boys, for actual length of gestation is also important to survival.[24]

Nutrition

Of the several factors associated with poverty and known to lead to low birth weight, one needing serious attention is nutrition. Precise effects of poor nutrition in the mother of the human infant have not been established, although conclusive animal studies have been performed for many years. Controlled studies on humans are difficult to perform. Enough is known, however, about the relationship between poor prenatal diet and incidence of underweight and frail infants to render the subject not a dull academic matter but one basic to the behavior of the pregnant woman and the future of the child.[25] As such, it deserves a hard, new look.

Pregnant women need about 200 extra calories a day, extra protein, extra calcium, more vitamins A, B, and C, and extra iron.[26] New tissue and nerves come from protein synthesis—the fetus requires protein to grow into a normal child. Meat provides the best source, offering not only protein but some essential minerals and vitamins. Prenatal iron deficiency, from lack of meat and other iron-rich foods, has serious consequences for the baby as well as the mother. Milk, which is the infant's major food, does not contain iron. Nature's growth plan expects the baby to arrive in the world with several months' iron supply in his liver to last until he can begin building up his own iron stores.[27]

Without iron, both mother and baby develop iron-deficiency anemia. Anemia in the mother causes fatigue and apathy. The anemic baby gets off to a poor start, is subject to diseases, and may become acutely ill. Low hemoglobin in pregnant women was found, in an extensive English survey, to be related to increasing age, parity, low socioeconomic class, and small stature. It was "associated with a stillbirth and neonatal mortality rate which was nearly twice the average."[28]

Low-protein, high-carbohydrate diets are associated with greater risk of toxemia. Both overweight and underweight, if excessive, are associated with this hazard.[29] Whereas overweight traditionally has been regarded as the common prenatal nutritional problem, underweight recently has been found to contribute to prematurity or low birth weight.

One obstetrician writes that the premature rate is three times higher in clinic than in private patients.[30]

Even when we could account for a number of the prematures associated with severe toxemia, abruptio placentae, multiple pregnancies, etc., we were still left with quite a large number of premature deliveries with no recognizable causes. It is among these women that I suspect that malnutrition is playing a fundamental role in causing premature labor and delivery. The premature rate of less than 2% among my clinic patients at Richmond shows what good prenatal nutrition can do even in the present state of our ignorance of the exact mechanisms. Good prenatal nutrition thus can play a role in the prevention of many of the common permanent complications of the premature infant including cerebral palsy.

"The Policy Statement on Nutrition & Pregnancy" of the American College of Obstetricians and Gynecologists, issued on December 1, 1972, said that weight gain should not be "restricted unduly nor should weight reduction normally be attempted." Dietary supplements including iron and vitamins were recommended.

Overweight from the use of carbohydrates to relieve hunger, with lack of good protein sources due to lack of money, is often encountered among the poor, and notably among Mexican and Black women. The beans and tortillas of the former and the high-fat, high-carbohydrate diets of the poor Black do not provide the iron and vitamins needed. Culturally acceptable diets based on ethnic food patterns can, however, be made nutritionally sound with the advice of nutritionists who know the elements in the various ethnic diets and how to improve them.

Concern about hunger in the United States has produced many studies documenting the financial inability of low-income groups to purchase nutrients essential in a pregnancy diet. In September 1969 the Sacramento, California, County Department of Public Welfare presented findings of a survey of their AFDC clients.[31] Though their sample consisted of a group in which 60 percent had White Caucasians as heads of household and 70 percent had at least a tenth-grade education, 44 percent, or nearly half of the total, had been without food or money at least once during the previous year. One-fourth of the group had been without food or money up to five times during the year. When they ran out of food, they had to borrow from friends or relatives, most of whom could be assumed to be in the same socioeconomic class.

This preinflation study pointed out that though there had been a 25 percent increase in the cost of living in the previous ten years, the AFDC grant from the state had not changed. The chronic inadequacy of the AFDC family diet even at that time was revealed by the study in several ways, including figures showing that two-thirds of the group were spending less than three-fourths of the United States Department of Agriculture low-cost food plan, and 10 to 20 percent, less than one-half the cost. Of special note for those concerned with toxemia and anemia was the finding regarding which food the families stop buying first: 67 percent responded that they first stopped buying meat. In response to questions regarding the food they would buy if they had more money, 80 percent said meat.

In actual dollars, 75 percent of the group spent between $15 and $29 per month per person on food. The California Public Assistance grant, one of the highest in the nation, allowed at the time 22 cents per meal per person in an AFDC family. When a number of social workers' families lived on this amount for a week in December 1969 to find out for themselves what it would buy, they discovered that by careful budgeting they could live on peanut butter sandwiches for lunch, oatmeal for breakfast, and spaghetti with meat sauce for dinner with a small apple or small orange for vitamins. Bread became the mainstay. In 1972, one study showed that the average payment in all but four states was below the poverty level of $331 per month for a family of four, and that the typical payment for the total expenses of each child was $35.

Public assistance budgets traditionally have included a small extra food allowance during pregnancy. In California, recent AFDC budgeting practice effected by court action permits a small additional amount of money for the baby's nutrition as soon as the mother brings medical verification of pregnancy. This now means an extra sum of approximately $20 per month, depending on the number of children in the family. The total budget is so low in comparison with the current cost of living that the additional allowance sinks into a great hole of debt and unmet need. Furthermore, medical verification of pregnancy often occurs so late that the mother has not had the intended advantage during the critical early months of gestation.

Teenagers and food faddists are known to have outstanding nutrition problems. Women who live on "Zen macrobiotic" diets, high in rice and sunflower seeds, may develop serious deficiencies affecting the whole course of pregnancy and delivery, and hence problems for their infants. Mixtures of plant proteins that contain the enzymes necessary to trigger and supplement other enzymes have become fashionable substitutes for meat since inflation, and dwindling food supplies have encouraged creation of other complete proteins. However, the cost of the ingredients, the complexities of most of the enzyme-adequate recipes, and the time required in their preparation make them impractical for most poor mothers. The use of Zen diets for infants, using "Kokoh" or other health foods, has caused serious malnutrition in some babies and is a cause of concern where communal living or other alternative life-styles promulgate ideologically based but often nutritionally inadequate diets.

Smoking and Drugs

Excessive smoking has been proved to be associated with low birth weight.[32] "There exists a proven tendency for smaller infants to be born of cigarette-smoking mothers; indeed this tendency can be related to the number of cigarettes smoked, to a two–three times higher prematurity (by weight) rate, and to a statistical difference in term–birth weight. The smallest infants are born to mothers smoking twenty or more cigarettes per day in the antepartum period."[33]

Drug addiction also is associated with low birth weight and, in addition, creates a high mortality risk to the infants owing to fetal addiction and withdrawal symptoms after birth.[34] In the author's county of residence (near San Francisco, the city with the highest rate of overdose deaths), three babies were admitted to the county hospital on one weekend in May 1974 because of withdrawal symptoms, which are very painful as well as life-threatening. One authority says that habitual use of LSD, heroin, or other narcotics may cause congenital malformations or a withdrawal syndrome.[35]

Drugs taken by the pregnant woman that may threaten a baby's well-being include those taken for medical purposes, as in the well-known thalidomide tragedy, with its many gross birth deformities. All drugs and vitamins can be harmful during pregnancy, even aspirin, constituting one reason why good family-life education in schools and the earliest possible medical supervision during pregnancy should be promoted.

The extent to which teenagers contribute to the drug abuse problem during pregnancy is not known. In California, one of the most severely affected states, drug arrests of adolescents under 18 years of age increased over 2,000 percent during the decade of the 1960's.[36]

The Teen Years as a Risk Factor

Teenagers, with their snacking and irregular eating habits, constitute another important group of pregnant mothers with special nutritional problems. Diet as a risk factor in teenage pregnancy can best be understood against some background of other risks facing the pregnant teenager. However, confusion results from lumping all teenagers together, and from combining teenage pregnancy and illegitimate pregnancy. These subjects overlap but are not synonymous. Though statistical groupings blur the issues, they are treated separately here to the extent possible.

Pregnant teenagers received a great deal of attention throughout the 1960's, when the Children's Bureau promoted comprehensive service projects for them, combining educational, health, and social services, and sponsored many meetings for the sharing of information among professionals. Concern rose from the mounting problems. Despite the steady decline in the birthrate as a whole for the past 15 or more years, "studies indicate that young unmarried women are not only beginning sexual intercourse earlier but are also engaging in it with more partners than before—hence women in the young childbearing ages today are probably more exposed to the risk of pregnancy than before."[37] In addition, the actual number of girls entering and swelling the reproductive age is greatly increased because of the effect of the "baby boom" after World War II. Among illegitimate births between 1969 and 1972 in California, the largest number have been to girls 15 through 19, and the rate of decline in births has been less than that among older married women. Among reported illegitimate births in California, there has been a "startling rise among White teenagers," a rise of 3 percent between 1971 and 1972. The rate is four times as high among Blacks.[38]

Unfortunately, these figures do not help us understand as much as we would wish in regard to the magnitude of the risk to mothers and infants. The juvenile mother, 15 or under, is obstetrically and psychologically different from the girl 18 or 19 years of age, and her home circumstances tend to be different. A professor of obstetrics, quoted at the National Conference on Parenthood in Adolescence, said that a girl reaches biological maturity five years after beginning menstruation.[39] Biological maturity would usually be reached at about age 18. Therefore, the statistical grouping lumps the juvenile, at very high risk medically, with the girl who is entering the optimum age of childbearing.

The very young girl is still growing, so that her own body is utilizing food that would later go to the development of her unborn child. Her pelvis has not reached its maximum size. In commenting at the conference, one professor is quoted: "A child of eleven simply does not have the pelvic capacity to pull through the situation."[40] The juvenile mother is more prone to premature delivery and prolonged and difficult labor, and also to toxemia.[41]

Consideration of toxemia, mentioned earlier as a particular risk to low-income mothers, leads back to diet. This serious medical condition, discussed in detail later (see pp. 136–37) is related to poor nutrition.[42] However, its special prevalence in young mothers leads some researchers to believe that youth itself causes toxemia in pregnancy.[43]

Control of toxemia requires avoidance of salt, which waterlogs the tissues. This means elimination of frankfurters and potato chips and various TV snacks and drive-in foods high in preservatives and sodium, customary teenage foods. Weight control also requires avoidance of pastries, milk shakes, and other similar teenage comfort items. Young teenage pregnant girls of low-income families who are anxious to conceal their pregnancies, and therefore go without prenatal care and education, subject themselves to the risks of toxemia by following these diet patterns. Osofsky and Renga, after reviewing many studies, say, "In sum, most authors have found significant increases in the incidence of excessive weight gain, toxemia, fetal-pelvic disproportion, prolonged labor, prematurity, perinatal loss, and of ominous portent, have reported increases in maternal loss in very young mothers."[44]

The older married White teenager who receives good medical care, prenatal education, and good low-cost food (as in the case of wives of service personnel who shop at the post exchange) is potentially as capable of delivering a healthy baby as the older woman, or more so, according to a Navy obstetrician and researcher, but he says that, like all teenagers they require intelligent obstetric management because of a greater tendency to prolonged labor, with the risk of death or damage to the infant as well as trauma to the girl.[45] He states also that precipitate labor and prematurity are additional hazards to the infant more commonly found in even this favored group of teenagers, especially with their second or later pregnancies. Other physicians have reported that the outcome for the infants of mothers under 20 is clouded by higher death rates, as well as prematurity and neurological and other handicapping conditions.[46]

The health and well-being of the pregnant teenager, whether married or unmarried, cannot help being influenced by the psychological immaturity of the mother, who has not yet completed the "tasks" of adolescence. The separation from parents, the finding of identity as a person and a woman, the completion of education and preparation for career, the need to work through personal dependency needs before readiness to meet dependency needs of others—all these are interrupted. The girl who has a baby thinking "I will have somebody to love *me*" is indeed ill-equipped to care for a child whose life and health depend on her ability to love him.

Marriage, which an earlier generation saw as a solution to teenage pregnancy, has proved an illusory one. "Young parents are more likely than others to have low educational and occupational advantages and skills, with occupational choices and income expectations restricted accordingly; to come from low rather than middle or high income families, to live with in-laws, possibly in cramped quarters, possibly with attendant frictions, but in any case, not on their own."[47] One out of two teenage marriages ends in divorce.[48]

Because the mother will frequently become the wage earner, her education assumes special importance. A number of experimental or demonstration projects have been set up in different parts of the country, some connected with school systems and others with health agencies. One goal has been to continue the girl's schooling, if she has been excluded from regular classes, so that she may keep up with her grade after the baby is born. Some persons with experience in these special projects believe that it is better to keep the girl in her regular classes, with the hope that more lasting success may be achieved.

Whether the teenage girl is married or unmarried, she is at great risk of repeated pregnancies and school dropout. All authorities seem to agree that repeated, closely spaced pregnancies place the girl at very high risk of having damaged or high-risk babies. The spacing of pregnancies at short intervals is thought to increase the danger of low birth weight and other complications for both mother and baby. Whether the follow-up reports come from educational or medical sources, they indicate that even the best comprehensive services, given for a relatively few weeks or months, do not interrupt long-term negative influences, which result in the girl's continued sexual activity and childbearing. This finding is in keeping with Bloom's reports on experience (see p. 40) and has major implications for the kind of social services that are provided.

Illegitimacy as a Risk Factor

Illegitimacy as a term receives disparagement, both because of its association with stigma and because current life-styles affect the validity of statistics on illegitimate births. The word is clearly understood, however, and is therefore useful, and the state of illegitimacy remains a legal, health, and social hazard to the child.

Illegitimacy spans the entire age-group of childbearing girls and women, many of whom have entirely different problems than the pregnant teenager. Until recently, out-of-wedlock births occurred more often among older girls and women, with the peak rate among women in their twenties. Four-fifths of the reported illegitimate births in 1960 were to women 18 years of age and older.[49] The particularly large increases in illegitimate births between 1940 and 1960 occurred in women over 20.[50] The upsurge of illegitimate births at teen ages gradually changed the picture during the 1960's, and by 1968, as the *Statistical Abstract of the United States* shows, the number of illegitimate births was greater in the age-group 15–19 than in the group 20–29.[51] "The proportion of out of wedlock births among 15 to 19 year olds rose from 15 percent in 1960 to 27 percent in 1968."[52] However, in California, the rate of illegitimate births in the early 1970's remained higher in women in their twenties,[53] although it declined in older groups, thus narrowing the gap.

The extent of the problem of illegitimacy is unknown, but according to Goldstein, about one-third of all first births are conceived outside of marriage, and in 1968, one in ten of all births was out of wedlock (5 percent of the White and 31 percent of the non-White).[54] Income statistics on the "lately wed" show the highest rate in the lowest-income group. Despite the high proportion of illegitimate births occurring in the optimal child-bearing age-group, the Children's Bureau quoted a maternal death rate four times as high for unmarried as married mothers, twice the rate of premature deliveries, and twice the infant mortality rate.[55]

The reasons for such high risks are influenced by the age and racial composition of the group of mothers and, until very recently, by the hazards of illegal abortion. California statistics show that illegitimate births are more frequent in the young, Black, and poor.[56] Furthermore, many are not first births but as high as fifth or higher. All of these attributes are risk factors in themselves. In addition, delay in securing prenatal care, or not securing it at all, has been implicated.

The New York City Department of Health stimulated a study by the Community Council of Greater New York and the State Department of Public Welfare which explored the hypothesis that delay in seeking prenatal care might be a causative factor in the high mortality rates of illegitimate infants and unmarried mothers, and that it might point to special needs.[57] The researchers concluded that

> the women see no need to get care earlier or at all (20%), that they try to conceal their pregnancy as long as possible (18%), that they find it inconvenient either because they are caring for children at home or for other reasons (16%), that they are reluctant to give up or take time off from their jobs (12%), that they do not know they are pregnant (9%), that they cannot pay the costs of care by a private physician (7%), or finally, that clinic intake requirements at the clinic where service is requested make them ineligible (6%).

The authors of the report commented that the reasons differed among groups—the young girls were more apt to wish to conceal their pregnancy or were unable to face it, and the Black and Puerto Rican women were most apt to see no need for care and to be caring for children at home. Of special cause for dismay, this study showed that unwed mothers receiving public assistance had the poorest record of prenatal care in comparison with the rest of the group. "Though the social investigators may see these women several times during the pregnancy, they are generally not informed of the pregnancy until late in the second or until the third trimester."[58]

In his account of the very poor social situations of pregnant teenagers, Osofsky quotes a study "which indicated that the typical girl who became pregnant out of wedlock in her teens and required welfare assistance might be expected to deliver nine out of wedlock pregnancies during her reproductive years and that the cost to the social welfare department over the course of the girl's lifetime would average $100,000."[59] He quotes a New Haven study to the effect that girls pregnant under 15 who were followed five years had an average of three and a half pregnancies, almost all out of wedlock, and only 5 percent did not become pregnant again.[60] The New York City study attempted to learn why the girls so seldom used social services (only 19 percent used specialized services); the interviewers concluded that most girls knew of agencies but that the major deterrent to use was seeing no need for service.[61]

Because of the diversity of the group, its lack of homogeneity, there is no single approach to the services needed. Some generalizations do arise from the negative aspects of the studies and demonstration projects, and from the experiences of those who have involved themselves with various segments of the unmarried mother population. Those helping persons who work in agencies that have peripheral contact with unwed mothers, such as Social Security and public assistance offices, schools, and hospitals, are in key positions to reach out to them. The illegitimately pregnant girl or woman has been bombarded by society with the concept that sex is splendid and fashionable, but when her body swells, she may well hit a wall of puritanism; contempt in the eyes of an eligibility worker who thinks immediately of "man in the house" and a referral to the district attorney; exposure and red tape when she tries to get Social Security benefits for her unborn; smirks or at times callousness at the hospital from staff with the attitude "Let her suffer, that will teach her a lesson." If she is a school girl, she often is excluded from class, and if not, she is exposed to the comments of her peers that she has been dumb to get caught. Most wounding, her mother may be enraged, scathing, or jealous, and her father, if she has one, caught in a violent emotional tangle about her sexuality.

Replacing agency attitudes of indifference or contempt, if they exist, with desire to help obviously is required, as is taking time to establish a relationship of warmth and concern. Those responsible for staffing policies may need to be made aware of the needed time, and the preventive pay-off, of reaching-out services. Specialized agency personnel have pointed out that unwed mothers often are greatly in need of housing, jobs, money, and social opportunities. The barriers to early prenatal care may be manifold, yet it too is a vital need. The barriers to medical care may require negotiation of financial eligibility requirements, or location of prenatal facilities closer at hand, or provision through a specialized agency. The problem may be a requirement for parental consent for medical care, and the girl's inability to face her family.

Urban communities, where most of the population reside, have a host of specialized agencies. The helping person in a peripheral agency often needs to build a bridge to the specialized agency or agencies, and to make certain that some coordination exists between the several that may eventually be necessary in providing adequate services to the girl or woman and her infant. A referral is not enough, for unfortunately many agencies unwittingly think inwardly of their own functions before the needs of an applicant who may not fit into their requirements.

Those girls who come to attention early in pregnancy now have the option of continuing or terminating their pregnancy. Many wish to have and keep their babies, and this appears to be more often true of the immature, emotionally disturbed girl than the more sophisticated. They deserve the opportunity for counseling, to learn from an experienced and, hopefully, warm and concerned expert of the options. The referring agency worker or teacher may have learned what to expect in regard to the objectivity of different agency personnel. Ideally, all specialized agencies, whether adoption, maternity home, family planning clinics, or abortion clinics, have staffs capable of objectively helping the girl to decide what option she wishes. In reality, most will be identified with the function of their agency, and therefore the referring person needs to sound out the services of the agencies she uses as well as to try to learn what appear to be the inclinations of the girl or woman, before taking her to the agency for counseling.

Over and over again, warnings have been sounded in regard to the risk of repeated pregnancies of the unwed mother. It would be naïve to expect that any helping person is going to change a girl's sexual behavior pattern in light of the societal emphasis on gratification of sexual needs. However, the only barriers to prevention of pregnancy are psychological. In communities where family planning clinics are not publicly funded or readily available, private clinics exist or a private physician's aid can be enlisted. Parental consent may still be necessary for birth control services for minors in many states, a condition that increases the problems of psychological interrelationships. If the psychological barrier is in the helping person's mind, not the client's, a transfer of the case is indicated; if the conflict is in the client's mind, the worker needs to intervene actively in seeking the best possible counseling and advice for the client. There is no place for passivity or neutrality in preventing the births of children who are at high risk and are soon unwanted.

The Older Mother

The older woman may not have a large family, but she often is the mother of several children. She does not receive the attention given to the teenager, though her pregnancy too is at high risk for several reasons. Having a number of children usually places her in the lower-income group; she is more apt to have had obstetrical and personal health problems, including hemorrhoids, varicose veins, high blood pressure, kidney or heart disease, and possibly a history of delivering prematurely or having a still-born child. Yet she is the mother least likely to seek out prenatal care because she thinks she knows the answers, having amassed such substantial experience, and she is most likely to face difficulties in getting to a clinic or physician's office because she is needed at home. She may be from a minority group with religious proscription against the most efficient birth control methods, but she may be rejecting her pregnancy.

If she receives public assistance, the chances are four out of five that she does not want more children, according to a study reported by Podell in 1968.[62] However, the Rainwater study of contraceptive and sexual behavior of the working classes brought out that, though they were as a whole interested in family planning, many tended to be sporadic, inconsistent, and ineffectual in regard to contraception, largely because the father did not wish to wear a condom and the mother disliked the messiness and handling of genitals necessary in using a diaphragm and jelly.[63] Dr. Rainwater concluded then (in 1960) that the contraceptive pill would not be widely accepted, primarily because of the inability of many to follow a consistent routine. Fortunately his predictions have not been borne out.

In California in 1971–72, the total of illegitimate births among women over 25 declined much more sharply than among those under 25, and even more sharply among older married women. It will be recalled that birth rates among the oldest married women evidenced the greatest relative decline;[64] also that they utilized abortion services less, and thus must have used effective contraceptives more. The *Family Planning Digest* reported that in New York City the average mother receiving public assistance has three children, and that the birthrate is declining.[65]

Multiple Psychosocial Risk Factors

The foregoing discussion of biopsychosocial risk factors makes clear that they do not exist singly. The mother at high risk for one reason is prone to risk for others. Michael Harrington pointed out a marked correlation between mental health and multiple stress factors, citing a Cornell study showing that "the sheer number of stress factors was more important than the quality of stresses."[66] Lack of proper food, lack of prenatal care, and lack of emotional security (which may be translated physiologically into lack of rest) constitute a triad that follows lack of money.

Graduate social work students at San Diego State College explored the social situations of 25 mothers receiving public assistance.* They found that some mothers did not appear at great risk despite their low socioeconomic status—those in the optimum childbearing years, having a first or second child, resourceful personally, and receiving help from their middle-class families. But a number of other mothers suffered from a variety of concurrent risks—poor housing, illness, use of drugs, apathy, too

---

* Mrs. Marlo Caruso, Mrs. Sue Mogle, Mrs. Joyce Lam, Mrs. Hazel Brown, "Master's Essay, 1970."

many preschool children. More significantly, these mothers existed at a point on a long continuum of adversity. There were women who came from broken homes or poverty, had incurred damage to their capacity for meaningful relationships, had attended school irregularly, had had brushes with the law, became pregnant early in life, and had had a series of pregnancies. They were currently in poor health, had a record of one or more abnormal pregnancies, and *despite their need for medication and its availability, paid little attention to the doctor's recommendations.*

One could speculate that their *negative attitudes toward authority and slowness to trust* were as important as the apathy of ill health in preventing them from utilizing available medical care. It should be pointed out that these mothers had access to private medical care through California's Medicaid provisions, so that one cannot blame crowded, uncomfortable clinics for their disinterest. Although there were more Black and more unwed mothers in this group, neither education, ethnicity, nor lack of resources distinguished them from the other mothers. Their backgrounds and history of early multiple pregnancies did.

Helping persons can recognize such women as in need of a great deal of reaching out. They are identified by the larger number of children or pregnancies beginning in adolescence, and by their records of deprivation and behavioral problems. These are the women who do not have sufficient inner resources and who need a supply from outside to help compensate for their lacks. They need long-continued, multifaceted help, not crisis service or aid during pregnancy only.

Basic services are needed by the socially high-risk mother: homemaker service that lifts burdens and educates in child care and home management, child day care that continues the educational process and provides respite and opportunities to get out of the house, contraceptives that will lengthen the interval between pregnancies and give her a chance to recover physically and perhaps to enjoy the children she has, and housing that is located close enough to public transportation to make possible the use of public facilities for medical care and recreation. These provide the framework around which long-term emotional support is given. The importance of such support cannot be overemphasized, for many of these women are depressed, feel worthless, and greatly need evidence that somone cares and is willing to help. Granted, the service needed is costly and it will not remake the mother's personality. But preventing the births of high-risk or disabled children requires that we at least try; if we do not, "prevention" remains a pretty word.

MEDICAL RISK FACTORS

Medical risk factors include those that seem to be entirely physiological and others that are influenced by the social circumstances of the mother. The latter include toxemia, diabetes, and heart disease.

Toxemia

Toxemia of pregnancy is of special concern to social work because it is a major cause of maternal death and is particularly associated with deprivation. Prematurity, stillbirth, and neonatal death are excessive in mothers with toxemia, so that the hazard of this poverty-related disease extends to the infant as well. "Pre-eclampsia [a term synonymous with toxemia] and its severity are factors of considerable importance in determining the fate of the fetus," according to British authorities, who cited a death rate for babies of severely eclamptic mothers of over twice the overall rate and a rate of nearly twice for babies of mothers who were moderately eclamptic.[67]

The medical literature defines toxemia as a composite group of diseases occurring during pregnancy that cause swelling (*edema*), high blood pressure, albumin in the urine, and, if not brought under control, convulsions, coma, and death. When the disease begins early in pregnancy, it is said to be a complicating factor of an already existing tendency to high blood pressure or kidney disease. These cases are differentiated from the classical "metabolic toxemia of late pregnancy," in which symptoms do not develop until the latter half of pregnancy and subside within a few days after termination of pregnancy.[68] It is in this latter kind of toxemia that the causative factors are linked to poor nutrition and social circumstances.

Statistics show that the high rates are in non-White mothers. Although there has been a dramatic decrease in maternal deaths from all causes including toxemia, and in both non-Whites and Whites, the condition still is associated with race and diet.[69] One authority, Dr. Thomas Brewer, who feels very strongly about the association between lack of good diet and the human waste caused by toxemia, quotes from an earlier work by another author: "The disease prevails among the underprivileged and is seldom seen among well-fed and well-cared-for patients."[70]

For many years the cause of toxemia was a medical mystery. Widespread studies and analysis gave conflicting clues regarding the importance of diet. Some early studies showed low figures where the diet was low in protein; on the other hand, strong evidence associated lack of protein and vitamins and high rates of toxemia. Dr. Brewer says, "Popular theories of the pathogenesis of this disease . . . have totally ignored its obvious relationship to poverty, malnutrition, ignorance and socio-economic deprivation." He emphasizes "the simple direct relationship between poor nutrition in pregnancy and the development of toxemia in late pregnancy," and defines the cause as "fundamental disturbances in metabolism, primarily in the metabolism of hepatic (liver) cells, brought on by malnutrition."[71]

Those especially concerned with pregnant girls and unwed mothers must be particularly alert to toxemia. Although the authorities differ on whether teenage is in itself a cause of toxemia, there seems to be agreement that young girls do have an excessive rate of toxemia, and also that more women develop toxemia in their first pregnancy than later.[72]

Symptoms that indicate a special and urgent need for medical supervision include swelling of the ankles or lower legs after bed rest, headaches, disturbances of vision, nausea and vomiting, and reports of high blood pressure. Swelling of the face and/or hands is also considered abnormal.[73]

Women who have toxemia in mild form may develop a severe case in a short period of time. Evidently excellent results can be obtained by good prenatal supervision and adequate diet, with hospitalization if necessary. However, if severe toxemia (eclampsia) develops, the mother is at great risk and requires highly skilled obstetric care. Pregnancy is terminated as quickly as feasible.

Classical medical treatment has been to restrict sodium. Medical ideas differ in respect to the place of salt in the diet. Dr. Brewer feels that an unpalatable, low-salt diet inhibits good nutrition.[74] His great emphasis is on the need for plenty of lean meat, eggs, and milk. He is critical of sodium restriction that extends to avoidance of milk.

Another discrepancy that may be confusing to those working with pregnant women is the changing medical position in regard to obesity in toxemia. The classical approach has been that obesity must be avoided at all costs; some physicians have placed such great emphasis on holding weight down that some mothers tend to starve themselves or are placed on near-starvation diets in an attempt to bring down excessive weight. Dr. Brewer believes that "it is much more important for the obese woman to eat a good adequate diet than it is for her to lose weight during pregnancy." He distinguishes between obesity from overeating nutritious food and the harmful obesity that arises from lack of protein and excessive carbohydrates to stifle hunger.[75] The National Research Council's Committee on Maternal Nutrition "found no evidence that excessive weight gain ... causes toxemia or that caloric restriction had any influence on toxemia."[76]

High blood pressure and kidney disease, which cause the same symptoms as classical toxemia or "metabolic toxemia of late pregnancy," have different consequences. Clients with certain kidney conditions not only are at risk during pregnancy but develop more severe high blood pressure as they age and undergo additional pregnancies. Chronic kidney conditions such as glomerulonephritis are thought to be contraindications to pregnancy—"The patient with chronic glomerulonephritis as a rule cannot go through pregnancy without serious danger to life and has very little chance of obtaining a living baby."[77] These chronic conditions should be distinguished from acute kidney problems such as pyelitis, which do respond successfully to drugs and are not incurable, although a small percent of women who have acute kidney infections can be seriously ill.[78]

Diabetes

Diabetes, though not common, is one of the greatest hazards to mother and baby. The social worker should learn whether the mother has had long-standing diabetes from childhood or has acquired it recently as an adult, since the implications are much more serious for the former.[79] All diabetic mothers need meticulous care throughout pregnancy. Their insulin requirements become unpredictable, and common problems such as morning sickness throw off their regimens.[80] The diabetic mother, especially the long-time diabetic, is prone to toxemia as well as to diabetic acidosis.[81] Physicians therefore frequently order sodium (salt) restriction, which adds practical complexity and emotional deprivation to the diabetic diet.

The last three months of pregnancy afford a critical period when the baby may die if the mother's diabetic condition goes out of control. Hospitalization must be immediately available, especially if symptoms such as nausea indicate that the mother's insulin needs and supplies are out of balance.[82] Physicians often recommend cesarean section or induced labor a few weeks before term in order to reduce the hazards of death to the baby in the uterus.[83]

Popular literature reassures the lay public that the diabetic mother now has an excellent chance of safe delivery of a normal baby under modern medical conditions, but the medical experts agree that the "fetal waste" from miscarriage, fetal death, stillbirth, and infant death is very high (about 40 percent).[84] Congenital anomalies were found in 9 percent of the infants in a sample from a large Boston clinic.[85] However, it is only recently that enough diabetic mothers to provide material for studies have been able to deliver live babies, so that the extent and nature of the risks to the children are not agreed upon. A review of the literature gives the impression that major differences occur according to the length of time the mother has had diabetes, whether her body has incurred degenerative complications as a result, and possibly according to the resources for good medical management during pregnancy.

The child is said to inherit diabetes on a Mendelian recessive basis. Dr. Priscilla White, an American specialist, reported in the early part of the 1960's a study showing that of 82 children born after the mother had diabetes, five developed manifest diabetes and the tests on six more showed latent diabetes; in her total study of 102 children ages one to 20, 9 percent of the children had either latent or overt diabetes and 14 percent were borderline.[86] This contrasts with a 20-year study in Copenhagen showing that of 91 children who survived the neonatal period, 83 developed normally and only one living child had diabetes.[87]

Dr. White added a grim footnote to the kind of hazard maternal diabetes poses for the child. She wrote, "Maternal parental morbidity represents a problem. Late maternal mortality is 10 percent. There is no evidence of resentment on the part of the children but they have questioned the relationship of their own birth to their mother's shortened life span."[88] She is referring to the adverse effect of pregnancy upon the life span of the mother. However, the Danish specialist quoted insists that diabetes has not been shown to shorten the life of the mother in Denmark.[89] The difference in American and Scandinavian resources for medical care come to mind, adding to the urgency of social measures to ensure that pregnant women have medical advice available.

Heart Disease

Heart disease is one of the major causes of maternal death, though not ranking as high as toxemia, hemorrhage, or illegal abortion.[90] Dr. Curtis Mendelson, specialist at a New York hospital, states that most of the pathology is from rheumatic heart disease and most of the deaths from acute heart failure.[91] The danger is to the women who have substantial heart damage, described clinically as class III or class IV heart disease. Deaths occur primarily after the fifth month and after delivery. The statistical incidence is low, but because social factors bear a direct relationship to prevention of catastrophe, social workers should attempt to understand the problem and give priority service to these mothers at risk.

Prevention of pregnancy (through choice of a reliable means) and therapeutic abortion in case pregnancy occurs and is detected in time are described as part of medical management of the woman with severe heart trouble. In instances in which the social worker's religion prevents her from helping the client in the wholehearted, active fashion that may well be necessary, the worker should refer the client to a social worker of another religion. Dr. Mendelson states that sterilization is unnecessary now that open-heart surgery is available, if the woman does become pregnant. However, the clients of social agencies may be better candidates for successful sterilization than for heart surgery, especially if the choice rests between a simple vasectomy for the husband and a life-threatening, highly complex, and expensive operation for the wife.

In case of accidental pregnancy too late to terminate, or pregnancy in a woman whose religion prevents contraception and therapeutic abortion, social work efforts will be guided by the aim of medical management, namely, reducing contributory burdens upon the heart. Mendelson states that "the major cause of maternal death is due to the burden of pregnancy" and "the outcome depends on preventing heart failure."[92]

The heart pumps more blood during pregnancy because an increase in circulation and more oxygen are needed for the growing baby. Thus the mother's heart is taxed for the greater circulatory demands. In addition, the baby tends to retain more fluid and sodium.[93]

Obvious ways to help relieve the burden on the heart include avoiding heavy housework, stair climbing, lifting, and exposure. Particular care is necessary to avoid the strain on the heart imposed by upper respiratory infections. Hospitalization is advised if a high-risk cardiac mother does contact a cold or the flu. "Respiratory infection is the most important contributory cause of severe heart failure."[94] If the mother is obese, she is advised to reduce. She is also placed on a sodium-restricted diet to reduce water retention.

These prosaic, commonplace, and deceptively simple-sounding recommendations may have much greater social complexity than more dramatic measures, as is apparent to anyone who has tried to help rehouse large families on welfare budgets from upper-story apartments to first-floor housing; or who have searched for housekeeping relief for mothers who were lifting heavy babies; or who themselves have undergone the depressing burden of dieting in the absence of money to buy lean meat and salads. Among the most difficult, from a practical standpoint, may be prevention of colds, especially if the house is drafty and the family does not have sufficient bedding and warm clothing in winter. The cardiac mother's need for rest and other precautionary measures remains for several weeks after the baby is born; thus the housekeeping aids and extra budgetary items must continue.

The management of the cardiac mother is complicated if she is an unwed teenage girl. Since a significant number of girls attending the adolescent rheumatic fever clinic at Johns Hopkins Hospital became pregnant, a researcher there conducted a study. Almost 20 percent of the girls became pregnant over a two-year period: 12 percent of the White and 22 percent of the non-White female patients. The only variable the researcher found that distinguished the pregnant from the nonpregnant was heart damage (not all children with rheumatic fever sustain heart damage). The study showed that while only 10 percent of the noncardiac patients became pregnant, one-third of the total with heart disease did become pregnant. The researchers speculated that "Such pregnancies may represent the rebellion of adolescents who because of their heart disease have been restricted on physical activity over a period of years.... The data do indicate that at least so far as the patients we have studied are concerned, the presence of a physical handicap is associated with significantly higher risk of one major sociomedical problem, adolescent pregnancy."[95]

The number of girls who might be expected to have heart disease of life-threatening proportions is doubtless small. For these, a joint conference of the professionals involved would seem indicated, regarding advisability of and facilities for abortion and sterilization if the pregnancy is discovered in time. If the girl is unwilling to terminate pregnancy or if it is too late, institutional care in a maternity home or hospital would appear to be needed to ensure the diet and supervision necessary.

If a mother goes into severe heart failure, immediate hospitalization is imperative. Warning signs, symptoms of impending severe failure, are paroxysms of shortness of breath and coughing up of blood. Social workers should help cardiac mothers to see their doctors quickly if they have problems with vomiting, nausea, coughing, shortness of breath, or coughing up blood.[96] If the mother recovers, hospitalization for the remainder of the pregnancy is advised, despite the difficulties of this expensive, inconvenient care for someone who looks and may feel well. However, the danger that she will go into another episode that she will not survive is so great that the patient and her family should be helped to accept its necessity.[97] The degree of social work involvement necessary to create such a plan under the circumstances in which most families find themselves is immediately apparent.

Dr. Mendelson states that women with mitral valve disease from rheumatic fever may be able to undergo heart surgery as a means of surviving pregnancy. If the mother has access to an experienced cardiac team that is able to evaluate her as a surgical risk, and to a hospital that provides the highly specialized services necessary, she may have a *mitral commissurotomy* with minimal risk of death. However, social agency clients may not secure the skilled evaluative procedures and surgical care without assistance in locating a suitable medical resource and financing the care. Fortunately the mother will probably be "a good teaching case" and therefore her admission to a university hospital may be expedited by the intern and resident on the service, or the private physician may refer her to a teaching hospital or to a heart center. In regard to the risk of death, "the importance of case selection cannot be overemphasized ... complete diagnostic facilities are prerequisite,"[98] which underlines the importance of helping the client get expert medical service if she is to have heart surgery during pregnancy.

Dr. Mendelson advises that heart disease in the mother does not create defects in the infant, except as a woman with congenital heart disease runs a higher risk of having a child with a congenital deformity, and as lack of oxygen in the mother's bloodstream from heart dysfunction is a potential cause of anomalies or fetal death. He states that loss of the infant occurs more often as the result of some other condition such as toxemia or an obsteric complication.[99]

Rubella and Rh Incompatibility

Two additional medical risks a baby incurs during intrauterine life are those from maternal infection, such as German measles (*rubella*), and from Rh incompatibility. Both are minimized by early qualitative prenatal care and medical supervision of the mother. Those who work with pregnant girls and women can help prevent serious damage to infants by helping them get to a doctor or clinic early in pregnancy, ascertaining whether the mother knows if tests have been performed, encouraging her to ask about results and to follow any medical recommendations made.

Among the special risks of poor women are contraction of infection due to overcrowding. No one is exempt from virus diseases, but persons in continued close contact with others, especially schoolchildren, are at greater risk of having influenza and such childhood diseases as measles and chickenpox. Many maternal viral infections including influenza have been proved dangerous to the fetus, capable of creating stillbirths, prematurity, mental retardation, seizures, blindness, and various other physical defects.[100] Of particular hazard is *rubella*, a mild disease in the mother but potentially lethal to the child. "The specific teratogenic [fetus-crippling] effects depend on the gestational age at time of infection; in general the earlier the infection the more numerous and severe are the defects."[101]

The first three months of pregnancy are the most dangerous period, particularly the first two. The estimated percentage of children who will have congenital rubella or the "rubella syndrome" has been reported from a high of 80 percent to a low of 10 to 20 percent, depending on the type of research performed, its location, and degree of understanding of the disease.[102] One study in the Baltimore-Washington area showed that 50 percent of the women with rubella in the first three months of pregnancy miscarried, or gave birth to dead or handicapped babies.[103]

Many babies die soon after birth. Others may have only one handicap such as cataracts, deafness, or heart defects, whereas many are multihandicapped; they have severe mental retardation, are growth-retarded, have various abnormalities of bones and organs, in addition to cataracts, congenital heart disease, or deafness.[104] Of special note is the continued infectiousness of some of these children after birth. As a result, their own conditions may worsen and cataracts develop, and the babies may expose others to rubella. The "virus shedders," as these infants are called, may remain infectious for over a year.[105]

Lesser says that more than 20,000 babies were born with defects after the 1963–64 epidemic.[106] Since another epidemic was predicted for the early 1970's, great effort was made to perfect a vaccine. One was developed, but it was a live-virus vaccine, which could infect the fetus if a woman vaccinated happened to be pregnant or become pregnant shortly thereafter. A great deal of discussion resulted in a decision by the United States Public Health Service to inoculate, not the group at risk—girls and women who might become pregnant—but schoolchildren. The rationale was to wipe out the source slowly—rubella among schoolchildren who might infect their mothers or older pregnant girls.

According to Lesser, only four out of every ten children between one year of age and puberty have been vaccinated. The vaccination problems have varied in different communities, in part because controversy still exists about the target population. Some have raised questions about the wisdom of vaccinating schoolchildren as evidence has accumulated that vaccinated children can shed the virus without showing symptoms of rubella, thus becoming even more hazardous as carriers. More work is needed on the vaccine.[107]

Fortunately, women who had rubella as children are protected against contracting it later. *A serum antibody test has been devised* that can be made from the same blood drawn for the test for syphilis at time of first prenatal examination. Its use is routine in good obstetric practice. The percentage of women known to be susceptible has varied from 30 percent in California to only 5 percent in one county in Maryland.[108] If a susceptible woman is later exposed to rubella during early pregnancy and a test shows she has contracted it, she can consider an abortion. If the test is negative, the mother can be immunized immediately after the birth of the child, before the possibility of another pregnancy occurs. California law now makes testing for rubella susceptibility part of the required premarital examination. "Such certificate shall also state whether the female applicant shows evidence of immunological response to rubella (German measles)."[109]

"Social-contract marriages" or "shacking up," some of the communal life-styles, and the frequent delay in marriage until after pregnancy often defeat the benign features of the law in protecting the child. Where social practitioners have contact with pregnant women following alternative lifestyles, rubella susceptibility testing should be arranged if at all possible to persuade the couple or head of the commune to provide the coming child with this maternal protection.

A mother can be "allergic" to her baby in utero if she is Rh-negative and the child's father is Rh-positive.[110] Most persons do have the Rh factor in their blood and are therefore "positive." Women can have their blood tested before they marry, to see if they are among the small group of "negative" persons. If they have not been tested, good prenatal supervision will ensure that the mother's blood is tested at the time of her first prenatal visit.[111] If the fetus has inherited the Rh factor from the father and is therefore Rh-positive, the woman's blood will develop antibodies against Rh-positive blood, or she becomes "sensitized." The condition is irreversible. She may have become sensitized through a blood transfusion of Rh-positive blood or during an abortion.

First babies are rarely affected. In succeeding pregnancies, however, the baby will usually develop *hemolytic disease of the newborn*, formerly called *erythroblastosis*. This condition, manifested by jaundice and increasing symptoms of the disease, creates mental retardation, cerebral palsy, deafness, and other severe defects.[112] An exchange transfusion, a drastic measure referring to total exchange of blood, can be used to save the baby.[113]

A human blood product has been developed, an anti-Rh immune globulin under the commercial name of Rho-Gam. Rho-Gam is given to Rh-negative mothers within 72 hours after delivery of each child, or after she has an abortion, to prevent the "allergic" reaction or formation of antibodies against the next Rh-positive fetus. Good maternity hospital practice has incorporated this feature.[114]

The National Foundation has expressed concern that the use of the serum has been impeded by its high cost and apparent lack of knowledge of its importance and availability. States may use federal maternal and child health funds to purchase and administer it in health department clinics or make it available to physicians.[115] In a national conference in 1969 on infant mortality, one obstetrician participant said that infant mortality from hemolytic disease has dropped sharply since 1965, and commented that excellent care that takes into account the many influences on maternal environment (intrauterine) and heredity can do much to assure a favorable outcome.[116] This condition has continued to drop.[117]

A negative influence of unknown proportion is the growth of alternative life-styles that may include no prenatal care and home delivery. When children are not born in hospitals and mothers are not attended by obstetricians, the recent progress in testing for Rh incompatibility and administration of Rho-Gam is not available. Social workers and other practitioners who are involved at least peripherally with pregnant girls who are planning home deliveries and ignoring prenatal supervision should attempt to make sure that the girl has at least one thorough prenatal examination with laboratory work. Follow-through with the girl and her physician or clinic on the possibility of Rh incompatibility is important.

PREVENTION OR TERMINATION OF PREGNANCY

High-risk mothers, and others, now have tools available for the spacing of pregnancies, for absolute prevention, or for termination of an unwanted pregnancy. These methods, or tools, include contraception, sterilization, abortion, and amniocentesis, to be discussed later in a special section on prevention of genetic disease.

Social workers and other helping persons should be clear about their own responsibility when counseling with parents at risk who are weighing choices about reproduction. The worker needs a clear knowledge of the facts, not in order to dispense them, but to understand the issues.

The first issue the parents face is whether they wish to conceive a child in the light of the particular risks they face. The issue is not a clear-cut matter of the individuals' constitutional rights to pursue "life, liberty, and happiness" in their own ways, but constitutes a conflict between their own rights and emotional needs versus the well-being of their unborn child. Three persons, not two, are involved, but one of them cannot act in his own behalf.

In the author's experience, parents of genetically defective children may conceive again several times, as if to reassure themselves and prove to the world that they can create a normal child. However, a study in the early 1960's reported to the contrary, that families and their extended families ceased having children when a genetically defective child was born.[118] Sylvia Schild, a social worker who has counseled with parents of children with phenylketonuria and is familiar with the reactions of parents to diagnoses accompanying mental retardation, emphasizes the emotional havoc that occurs when a genetic defect is diagnosed.[119] She states that parents suffer from a "shattered self-adequacy syndrome," and that "the knowledge that one possesses a defective gene causes a momentous insult to the ego structure of the affected individual."[120]

Because parents are in such turmoil, and because the decision they make about bearing more children has such far-reaching results for themselves, their other children, and the unborn child, the situation is one of unusual complexity and skilled help is of the utmost importance.

The social worker's responsibility in regard to their childbearing is to help the parents arrive at a rational decision, on the basis of facts, not blurred by emotion or lack of information. This means the worker should be as free of personal bias as possible, or ask for a transfer of the case. She will need to help the parents air their feelings and, after this, to sort out the issues. Parents frequently will need the advice of one or more experts who can provide the best possible forecast of medical or genetic risks, once their feelings have been dissipated and conflicts resolved. The worker should also learn the medical facts from the professional source, not from a parent, who may not have heard all the facts, or may have misunderstood or so sifted them through an emotional screen that they were not accurately perceived. A common misunderstanding pertains to statistical chances; the parent may believe that "one in four," for example, means that one in four children in his family will be affected by a genetic defect, not understanding that statistics apply to each *pregnancy*, rather than to each *family*.

Genetic counselors and/or other physicians vary in the kind and amount of information they give. Some provide medical and statistical information only, and at times in highly technical fashion, whereas others discuss the kind of burden a handicapped child will impose, and extend the conference into an individualized counseling session. If, after the initial conference with a knowledgeable person, further medical or technical information is needed, a conference with a pediatrician may be advisable. If parents want to weigh the various factors—contraceptive methods, possibility of sterilization, or pregnancy with amniocentesis and abortion if indicated—a conference with a gynecologist is needed. In no case should the worker either (a) provide birth control information or (b) thrust her views on the parents. The worker may, however, discuss the need for birth control information. She will probably help to find the best possible sources and be a supportive link in the use of experts in the field and a sounding board for parents who need to sort out facts and feelings. In work with juveniles, active intervention is often needed to help unwed, sexually active teenagers secure reliable contraceptives.

Contraceptives

Contraception is no longer controversial in the United States. Referred to as "family planning," it has been endorsed by the executive branch of the federal government and funded by the legislature in behalf of persons unable to afford birth control services.[121] The Catholic Church does not object to family planning, but endorses only abstinence and use of the rhythm method. The U.S. Department of Health, Education, and Welfare has issued a publication, DHEW Publ. no. HSM 73-16002, that describes current methods according to reliability, problems, side effects, advantages, and whether a prescription is needed. Planned Parenthood associations in every community supplement this bulletin with many pamphlets.

"The pill," or the oral contraceptive, is "highly effective" if consistently used. It cannot be used by all women, and requires a medical examination before prescription in order to determine if conditions exist that would make it unsafe. The pill is not used for women who have or have had epilepsy, migraine, mental depression, heart or kidney disease, asthma, high blood pressure, and diabetes.[122] The American Medical Association says, "There are some women, in addition to those with tendencies toward blood clotting disorders, who should not use oral contraceptives. These include women who have cancer of the breast or womb, serious liver conditions, or undiagnosed vaginal bleeding when cancer has not been ruled out."[123] Side effects can include spotty darkening of the skin, weight gain, clotting, or internal bleeding.[124]

The pill may be medically acceptable but not feasible psychologically. Recent packaging improvements have overcome the problem of the need to count, to ensure three weeks on and one week off, as most schedules require. Packages are available that include placebos or "sugar pills" for the days contraceptives are not to be taken, so that the person who is mentally or emotionally incapable of counting can still use this method.

For persons whose life-styles are incompatible with consistent use of the pill, or who are entirely incompetent, the IUD, or intrauterine device, is often tried. This very effective method cannot be used by approximately 10 percent of women who attempt it.[125] It may cause cramps or bleeding, and be so uncomfortable that women who have used it do not wish to use it again. It is, however, of such significance as a contraceptive method that refinements are constantly under way. A new device is the CU7, in which a copper wire is wrapped around an IUD; another is the Progesterone T, a plastic device with progesterone, which is slowly infused into the uterus instead of into the whole system (as happens when the pill is used). The CU7 has been found satisfactory for women who have not had children, and thus represents a great advance.[126] Some IUD's need to be replaced by a physician once every year or two.[127]

Other methods include diaphragm with jelly or cream, condoms, condoms and foam, and the rhythm method. The last, which incurs no religious objection, is also least effective, because of difficulty in determining safe time if the menstrual cycle is irregular.[128]

A long-acting progesterone administered by injection every three months has been developed called "Depo Provera," which can be used for women unable to utilize other methods. The drawback is that it may interfere with the ability to become pregnant at a later date; given that possibility, sterilization may be preferred, since it is a one-time-only procedure.[129]

Unwanted Pregnancy

The widespread availability and use of effective contraceptives would seem to eliminate unwanted pregnancy. However, unwanted pregnancies or ambivalent feelings toward becoming pregnant have by no means disappeared, as is evidenced by the large number of abortions, the number of parents who continue to produce genetically defective children even after experiencing the suffering and burdens the disease creates, the number of mothers who batter or seriously neglect their children, and the failure of the illegitimacy rate to decline in keeping with the total live birthrate.

A member of the Psychiatry Department at Stanford University School of Medicine, Dr. Warren Miller, has described various stages when women are psychologically vulnerable to unwanted pregnancies.[130] Early and mid-adolescence, when girls are first becoming fertile and first learning to take responsibility for themselves, a time of transition and of anxiety about sexual activity, is one such stage. Another is the end of the reproductive cycle, when, again, the ability to have children is in transition, and conflict creates inefficient use of contraceptives. Most significant, it would seem, are crises in relationships with the sexual partner, times of quarreling and making up, or of separation and brief reunion, or of fear of loss of the partner. In addition, Dr. Miller outlines psychological vulnerability at times a girl first leaves home, moving into an apartment or living with other girls, or moving into a social setting with different standards and pressures.

Loss of a child is another time when precipitate action may result either in ill-advised and regretted pregnancy or in sterilization.[131] The Stanford pediatrics staff have reported their observations of pregnancies occurring when a leukemic child is dying or has died, and other social workers have commented in a similar vein. Experience has shown that many women having abortions had suffered personal losses, either because of death or incurable disease in the family, or through termination of a long romantic relationship.[132]

Abortion

Dr. Alan Guttmacher wrote in a popular magazine article:[133]

Abortion should never be used casually, or as a substitute for mass contraception. ... I decry the necessity for so large a number of abortions, for each abortion bespeaks medical or social failure. If every act of intercourse in which pregnancy is not the desired result were protected by effective contraception, few abortions would be performed. The first line of defense against unwanted conception must be contraception, which is both medically safer and socially preferable. Legal abortion can only be justified as the second line.

Abortion is a controversial issue: the opponents advocating the right of every fetus to life; the proponents that legal abortion is preferable to the unquestionably horrible and dangerous procedures women secure or perform on themselves if trapped into unwanted pregnancy with no access to legal abortion. The Supreme Court declared in January 1973 that state statutes limiting abortion are unconstitutional on the ground of interference with the right of privacy guaranteed by the Constitution. In addition, the Court ruled that it was illegal for a state to place any restrictions on abortion except that it be performed by a licensed doctor during the first three months of pregnancy, and after that only such regulations as were necessary to protect the woman. In the article quoted, Guttmacher states that legalization has "corrected the mix," racially, of legal abortions in New York City. The ratio of White to non-White had been more than 5 to 1, and of White to Puerto Rican 26 to 1. After two years of the liberalized law in New York State, 47 percent of abortions were performed on Blacks, 42 percent on Whites, and 11 percent on Puerto Ricans.

The reasons women seek abortion may be categorized as medical, psychiatric, or socioeconomic. *Therapeutic,* or medically indicated, reasons for abortion are cancer of the cervix, severe heart disease, severe high blood pressure, nephritis or severe kidney disease, or breast cancer. Before abortion became legal for all women in this country through the Supreme Court decision in January 1973, abortions for women with these medical problems were generally permitted on the basis of the pregnancy's threat to the mother's life.[134]

A second group of women with medical reasons for termination of pregnancy are those at risk of having deformed, mentally defective, or physically ill children. These are mothers who have genetic or multifactorial constitutional defects (see the following section on prevention of genetic disease), or mothers who have been exposed to infection such as rubella, irradiation, or *teratogenic* (fetus-crippling) drugs.

However, the majority of abortions are sought for psychiatric or social reasons. Sloane describes therapeutic abortions as needed for psychiatric reasons when there is "danger of, or exacerbation of, an existing psychosis, or the precipitation of one, including a post-partum psychosis; suicidal risk due to the exacerbation or precipitation of depression; potential exacerbation or precipitation of serious neurosis or emotional instability; mental retardation in the mother; the threat of fetal abnormality; and exposure to rape or incest."[135] After a discussion of these conditions, and a review of the literature pertaining to incidence of psychiatric problems and to the effect of abortion on emotional instability, Sloane states: "The risk of exacerbation or precipitation of a psychosis is small and unpredictable, and suicide rare. On the other hand, emotional instability is alleviated (for a time) by interruption of the pregnancy." He further states that psychologic ill effects of abortion because of mental retardation in the mother, or exposure to rubella or rape, are negligible and that "termination seems beneficial."

In a large California county that provides access to a high quality of medical and social service, and in which legal access to abortion is not impeded by administration attitudes, 28 percent of the abortions in the county hospital in 1971 were performed on *married women*.[136] In the absence of statistical data regarding reasons for abortion among married women in the United States, a reported Swedish experience may hold true in this country, that the "strength of women with large families is often already tried almost to breaking point"; furthermore, that whether married or unmarried, conflict between the parents is often present.[137] The number of women having abortions for medical reasons doubtless is very small in relation to social reasons, although in the country mentioned amniocentesis is performed on every pregnant woman over 35 (because of the danger of Downs syndrome in older mothers) and it is known that some older mothers seek abortion after amniocentesis and genetic counseling.

In a newspaper article about husbands accompanying women to abortion clinics, the feature writer commented that the men seemed anxious about whether their wives would withstand the procedure satisfactorily but showed no remorse about the abortion, which seemed to have been agreed upon because the couple had enough children or because of a health or financial problem. The article further said that women often came without their husbands, either because the men were at home babysitting or because the wife did not want her husband to know she was having an abortion.[138]

The chief counselor in the large clinic mentioned reported that the abortion rate coincides with the illegitimacy rate in respect to age. There the latest statistics show the largest age-group delivering illegitimate babies is 20–24, which is the peak age for abortions.[139] Statewide statistics confirm the county experience, that the highest rate of abortions takes place in women of ages 20–24, and also that unmarried women utilize abortion much more than married women. In 1971–72, four times as many unwed women had abortions as married women in California, according to official statistics, and two-thirds of the *recorded* pregnancies of unwed women were terminated by abortion in that year.[140] It is of note, however, that the same statistical report comments on the "startling rise of illegitimacy among white teenagers despite the availability of legal abortion" and that the statistical phenomena suggest that "despite the availability of legal abortion many women are choosing unwed motherhood."

Because the subject of abortion is almost bitterly controversial, its psychological effects are variously reported, depending on the source. This author has concluded from studies seen that definitive information is hard to find, but that most reasonable is the conclusion that prior psychological stability determines the reaction; that obvious, severe, immediate disturbance is infrequent.

Abortion procedures vary with the length of the pregnancy. Until 12 weeks of gestation, the fetus is removed by vacuum aspiration, which can be performed in a clinic or office. The amount of pain depends on the skill of the medical staff and the tension of the woman; in the county clinic mentioned, all girls under 17 are given an anesthetic, though the procedure is described as relatively painless in the majority of instances. After 12 weeks of gestation, abortion is performed by saline injection, which induces labor, similar to that in childbirth, usually within 24 hours. This method, which is very painful, is also less safe, being "only twice as safe as having a baby, not 10 times as safe, as in the case of vacuum aspiration."[141] In the small percentage of persons who have complications, they may be very severe, so that saline abortion is a hospital procedure and may mean several days in the hospital.

This aspect of abortion has special relevance to mothers who abort after amniocentesis and genetic counseling regarding risk of having a defective child. Culture of the amniotic fluid requires two weeks, but the fluid is not diagnostic until 14 weeks. The timing of the parents' emotions about abortion, their social circumstances, and the circumstances of the medical procedures ideally should be close. However, women who abort to avoid having a genetically defective child cannot take advantage of the safer, less painful procedure of vacuum aspiration. Especially in the instance of sex-linked defects, where the decision to abort is based on determining the sex of the child, the final decision may need more time than medically desirable after the results of the amniocentesis are known, unless the decision has been crystallized firmly at some earlier time.

Sterilization

Sterilization of either of the parents may be performed if they know definitely they want no more children, or are certain they wish to avoid pregnancies. This most certain contraceptive measure usually bears the hazards of irreversibility, and in some instances emotional repercussions. However, it may also bring great peace of mind and promote greater marital satisfaction. No legal barriers exist to voluntary sterilization except in Connecticut and Utah, where it is limited to reasons of "medical necessity."[142]

A class action suit resulting from abuse by physicians in a Southern county of welfare recipients' civil rights to voluntary sterilization, concurrently with sterilization nearby of two mentally retarded girls, resulted in highly restrictive HEW regulations against use of federal funds for sterilization of mentally incompetent persons. The obstacles were made so great (see *Federal Register*, vol. 39, no. 26, February 6, 1974) that they virtually prohibit sterilization. A federal judge later permanently enjoined the HEW from providing federal funds for sterilization of minors and mentally incompetent adults.[143] Because the current situation discriminates against the right of parents to protect mentally incompetent children of childbearing age against unwanted pregnancy, further legal action may occur. Meanwhile, physicians may be afraid to perform sterilization procedures on severely retarded girls or women even when no federal funds are involved.

According to the Association for Voluntary Sterilization, sterilization should be considered when "there is the probability of transmission of an hereditary defect," when pregnancy may endanger the well-being of the mother, or parents cannot fulfill the responsibilities of parenthood, or choose to limit the number of children they have. The organization points out that sterilization is not indicated when there are temporary financial difficulties, physical or emotional problems that may respond to treatment, or a couple merely wishes to delay parenthood rather than terminate its possibility permanently.[144]

Male sterilization, performed by *vasectomy*, or the closing of the sperm tube called the *vas deferens*, is a minor operation usually performed in the doctor's office under local anesthesia, and creates no physical aftereffects. It is not castrating and does not affect sexual potency. The American Medical Association said in 1968 that it is "safe, quick, effective, and legal."[145] Some recent studies have suggested that males have developed antibodies to their sperm following vasectomy. The significance of this is not clear at the present time.¹⁴⁶ Increasingly popular among the educated middle class, vasectomy is still resisted by many men because of misunderstandings and fear of anything even vaguely threatening masculinity. Many articles in the literature point to its beneficial results.¹⁴⁷ In the few instances reported of adverse effects on sexual potency or psychological stability, the consensus has been that the men had prior problems of potency or serious pathology.

Female sterilization, created by *hysterectomy*, is a major operation. It requires several days in the hospital and a substantial convalescence. Depending on the extent of the operation—that is, whether the ovaries are removed—and the personality of the woman, glandular changes may occur that result in depression unless medication is prescribed to lessen physiological upset. Sterilization may also be performed by *tubal ligation*, which is frequently performed a day after childbirth. A new technique permits this operation to be performed as an outpatient procedure, sometimes without anesthetic. An instrument called a *laparoscope* is inserted through the umbilicus, and forceps inserted or cautery performed through the laparoscope, which is then manipulated to permanently scar the tubes.¹⁴⁸ This new method requires that the physician have skill, judgment, and special training. Furthermore, the instrument is expensive. Accordingly, laparoscopy is not simple, but where available it offers a great advantage over hysterectomy.

PREVENTION OF GENETIC DISEASE

(This section, pp. 152–57, is by Doris Harvey, with consultation from Howard M. Cann, M.D., Associate Professor of Pediatrics, Stanford University School of Medicine.)

As infectious diseases become more preventable and responsive to treatment, genetically determined diseases account for an increasing proportion of illness and death in children. About a third of all pediatric patients admitted to Montreal Children's Hospital during the year ending July 1970 had diseases of genetic or combined genetic and environmental origin.¹⁴⁹ A comparison of causes of death at a London hospital for 1914 and 1954 showed that deaths from genetic disease rose from 16 percent to over 33 percent.¹⁵⁰ More recently, a compilation of causes of hospital deaths in Newcastle from 1960 to 1966 showed 10 percent due to chromosomal or single gene defects and an additional 31 percent to probable but complex genetic etiology. Only 41 percent could be counted as definitely nongenetic.¹⁵¹ With regard to the economic impact of genetically determined disease, the Montreal Children's Hospital study found 32.4 percent of total hospital days used by patients whose disease was wholly or partially genetic.¹⁵²

The suffering caused by genetic disease is impossible to measure. Perhaps it is sufficient to point out that, of the diseases discussed in this book, four (cystic fibrosis, hemophilia, Duchenne's muscular dystrophy, and sickle cell anemia) are wholly genetic. Diabetes mellitus and spina bifida are partially genetic and so also may be arthritis and asthma. Some kidney disease—although a small proportion of the total—is wholly hereditary. Some congenital heart disease may be genetic. It is not known whether there is any inherited component in leukemia.[153]

A Review of Rudimentary Genetics

The many Nobel Prizes for chemistry and medicine and physiology awarded since 1940 for work related to *biochemical* or *molecular genetics* illustrate the recent explosion of knowledge in this area. George and Muriel Beadle point out in their book *The Language of Life* that genetics was not a subject heading in the 1910–11 *Encyclopaedia Britannica*, but by 1965 15 pages were devoted to it. Another excellent book on genetics for nonscientists and beginning students is Isaac Asimov's *The Genetic Code*.[154]

While the current revolutionary change in basic knowledge of genetics is in biochemical genetics, a minimal understanding of *classical* or *transmission genetics* is essential for one who is working with families and children with genetic disease. In the late nineteenth century, a biologist named Walther Flemming noticed that a cell contains material that is readily stained by a red aniline dye. During cell division, this material, *chromatin*, collects into pairs of threadlike bodies called *chromosomes*. Before the actual division of a cell, each chromosome forms a replica of itself and the pairs of chromosomes pull apart. Each new cell has an equal full set of chromosomes, now known to be 46 in man. The only exception is in the formation of egg and sperm cells. These cells contain half-sets of chromosomes, so a fertilized ovum contains 23 pairs of chromosomes (one of each pair from each parent) just as do other human cells. A chromosome is thought to be made up of a string of *genes*, each of which determines a different characteristic. Genetic material is passed on with remarkable accuracy and precision. Very rarely, an error occurs in the self-copying process and a new transmissible characteristic arises (*mutation*). There is usually no observable change in chromosomes to account for this, but sometimes, because of incorporation of both members of a pair of chromosomes during egg or sperm formation, there is a resultant imbalance in all the cells of the newly conceived fetus. An example of this is the 47 chromosomes per cell in *Down's syndrome* or *mongolism*.[155]

Mendel, the Austrian monk who discovered the first laws of heredity, called traits *dominant* or *recessive*. In dominance, a single gene is sufficient to determine a characteristic. This usually means the characteristic will be seen in more than a single generation in any one family. Once an individual carries the gene and therefore has the characteristic, he or she can pass the gene on to the offspring. This gives rise to a characteristic family pattern, generation after generation. Since, like the chromosomes, the genes occur in pairs, a parent who carries an abnormal gene (herein used to mean a gene with the potential for producing disease or defect) has a 50 percent chance of passing that gene along to an offspring and a 50 percent chance of passing along the normal partner gene. Therefore, not all offspring of an affected parent need be affected.

In recessive inheritance, an affected individual must have two of the same genes for the particular characteristic. Since he receives one from one parent and one from the other, this is inheritance from both parents. The parents each carry only one abnormal gene and will not be affected. Such a couple will be at risk for conceiving affected children and the risk is 25 percent *at each pregnancy*. In the relatively rare instances where one parent is affected with a recessive disease and the other is an unaffected carrier, the risk is doubled. A person who carries two identical genes dealing with the same characteristic, be they normal or abnormal, is called a *homozygote*. A person who carries two different genes for the same characteristic is called a *heterozygote*.

Diseases such as hemophilia and Duchenne's muscular dystrophy, which are almost always transmitted from mother to sons, are labeled *sex-linked* or *X-linked*. The two sex chromosomes of the human female are designated X and the genes for these diseases are passed on in the X chromosome from mother to children of both sexes. These diseases occur only in the sons because the male has only one X chromosome. The other sex chromosome in males is designated Y, and it is slightly different and smaller. Half the spermatozoa transmit the Y and half the X chromosome. The genes in the Y pass from male to male only. Genes in the X chromosome for which no equivalent alternatives exist in the Y chromosome exhibit full effects in sons.[156]

Multifactorial or *polygenic* inheritance is involved in about half the major malformations found in newborn infants, including cardiac anomalies, cleft palate, pyloric stenosis, congenital dislocation of the hip, and certain major neurological maldevelopments (*neural tube defects*). A number of genes may contribute to the defect. Environmental factors play an important role, determining the threshold at which malformations occur in genetically predisposed individuals. Defects may occur before pregnancy is recognized, so sexually active women of childbearing age should avoid unnecessary drugs and other environmental influences suspected of being harmful.[157]

In the case of two of the neural tube defects, *spina bifida* and *anencephaly*, Naggan and MacMahon have shown that marked differences in prevalence between ethnic groups probably stem from environmental rather than genetic factors. Regardless of ethnic group, they found decreased socioeconomic status to be associated with increased prevalence.[158]

Methods of Prevention

Prevention of genetic disease has been an objective of genetic counseling from the time when it was possible only to inform a family of a bare risk figure to its present sophisticated state. Genetic counseling today involves confirming or proving the diagnosis of the disease in the family, analyzing the pattern of occurrence in the family, testing certain family members for the carrier state, and applying genetic principles to the determination of recurrence risk for the couple or family member being counseled. Information about the disease and recurrence risks must be presented to the couple in terms that are meaningful to them so they can make intelligent decisions about conceiving offspring.[159] They should be encouraged to discuss with the counselor what they know and feel about the disease involved, what religious pressures they are likely to experience, how much they want a child, and how they would feel about interrupting a pregnancy to avoid having an affected child.[160] There is almost always need for follow-up and reinforcement. Some families need extensive counseling and social service assistance.[161]

Counseling is done by personal physicians, some subspecialists, and medical geneticists. Recently, persons in a number of professions related to medicine (social work, public health nursing, and psychology) have become involved in genetic counseling and, in a few institutions, special training has been offered to nonmedical genetic counselors. The previously mentioned study at Montreal Children's Hospital suggested an apparent gap between the available resources in medical genetics and the demand for them.[162]

Many couples, particularly those at high risk for conceiving children with a disease where the burden is great, choose to avoid having further children. They achieve disease prevention through what Kaback has called "enlightened fear and restricted rights."[163] This choice may become easier as parenthood becomes less the expected norm, but these families will still deserve counseling about all alternatives to reproduction such as adoption and artificial insemination and all methods of preventing conception.

Appropriate Mating

Techniques that limit freedom of mate selection on the basis of the "quality of one's genes" are not usually an accepted form of prevention. Objections can even be raised to *compulsory* methods that restrict carriers of the same deleterious gene from marrying. Legal statutes prohibiting cousin marriages, accepted for many years in a number of states, exemplify the attempt to prevent genetic disease through limiting selection of a mate.

Prenatal Genetic Diagnosis and Selective Abortion

It is possible to diagnose some genetic conditions in the unborn fetus. This gives the parents the option of terminating the pregnancy (selective abortion) provided the diagnosis is available early enough in pregnancy. *Amniocentesis* is a widely used technique that can be done early enough to be useful in decision making. A small amount of fluid is withdrawn from the amniotic sac by puncture through the abdomen. The procedure is carried out at about the fourteenth to sixteenth week of pregnancy on an outpatient basis under local anesthesia and aseptic conditions. Physicians attempt to minimize pain but there may be some discomfort as the needle enters the uterus. A feeling of pressure and cramping may be present. Most patients accept a second tap when it is necessary, but there is an occasional refusal on the basis of discomfort. Major complications of the procedure to mother and fetus probably do not exceed 1 percent. Some of them are maternal bleeding, infection of the amniotic cavity, induction of labor with inadvertent abortion, puncture of the fetus, and puncture of the placenta with resultant fetal bleeding.

Amniotic fluid contains cells of the fetus which can be stimulated to grow in tissue culture, i.e. outside the body. The cultured cells are used for chromosome examination and certain diagnostic biochemical tests. Growing cells for chromosomal analysis takes about two to three weeks. It takes four to six weeks for growth of enough cells to make enzyme assays.[164] These time factors are important because the whole process of prenatal diagnosis—the preliminary counseling, the decision for or against amniocentesis, the procedure, the wait for analysis, the decision based upon it—must all be fitted carefully into the time schedule of pregnancy. The procedure must be done late enough to obtain amniotic fluid safely but not so late that selective abortion cannot be performed. Even these relatively long times for analysis are minimal, and technical problems in laboratories may necessitate second taps or otherwise make the time element more crucial.[165] In California, the law states that abortion cannot be performed after the twentieth week of gestation. In a recent (1973) Supreme Court decision, it is the twenty-sixth week.

Amniocentesis is most frequently used in women at risk for having children with Down's syndrome because of advanced maternal age or occurrence of the syndrome in a previous child. Diagnosis is by chromosome examination. A second use of the procedure is in families at risk for inherited metabolic disease. Diagnosis is based on enzyme assay, and it is now possible to detect an affected child in a growing list of metabolic diseases. Unfortunately, this is not yet possible in cystic fibrosis[166] or in sickle cell anemia.[167] Most sex-linked diseases cannot be diagnosed prenatally, but determination of sex and selective abortion of males can be used to assure an unaffected child. In one sex-linked disease, classic hemophilia or Hemophilia A, it is now possible in a limited number of cases to distinguish between affected and unaffected male fetuses because of the closeness of the genetic locus for Hemophilia A to that of another inherited X-linked condition that is recognizable in cultured amniotic fluid cells under suitable conditions.[168]

Prenatal genetic diagnosis by amniocentesis is not a routine matter undertaken anywhere. Because experience is important to the successful accomplishment of all the procedures involved, only certain centers with well-equipped facilities offer this service. The number of centers has increased recently, from 121 worldwide in 1971 to 251 in 1973.[169]

Carrier Detection plus Prenatal Diagnosis and Selective Abortion

When a reliable, inexpensive method of carrier detection for a recessive disease is available and, for the same disease, early prenatal diagnosis is possible, couples at risk for that disease are in a relatively advantageous position. If they wish, carriers can avoid marriage to other carriers. If two carriers do wish to marry, they need not forfeit their right to reproduce, since each pregnancy can be monitored to be sure the child is not affected with the disease determined by the genes carried by the parents. In this way, prenatal diagnosis and selective abortion can be employed without waiting for a first tragically affected child to identify the risk of the parents.

The only disease now qualifying for a practical program of this type is Tay-Sachs disease, a relatively rare disorder involving cerebral degeneration and death before age four. Tay-Sachs screening programs take advantage of the fact that this disorder occurs with relative frequency in a small, well-defined population group, Jews from Eastern Europe.[170]

It is unfortunate that there are so few genetic diseases for which both carrier detection and prenatal diagnosis are possible at this time. For the pregnant woman, the preventive method of choice, limited as it is, remains prenatal diagnosis and selective abortion. Society must concern itself with the ethical questions involved and remain flexible, because we can expect continuing advances in carrier detection, prenatal diagnosis, and treatment of affected children. At any given moment, the current status of each of these factors for the disease in question must weigh heavily in decision making.

NORMAL NEEDS DURING PREGNANCY

When Mrs. Doe or Susan Jones announces her pregnancy to the worker at the welfare department (social security office, juvenile court, family counseling agency, adoption agency, church, school), she does not present herself as a young primipara or grandmultipara at high risk, or even as the normal prospective mother of someone with a 70-year life span. She appears to the worker behind the desk as a juvenile delinquent, "acting out sexually," or as a tired, shapeless woman unable to care for the brood she has already, or perhaps just as another woman whose husband has left her (is in jail, is unable to work, etc.).

A stretch of the imagination is necessary to visualize the medical, social, and psychological needs that pregnancy has placed upon this client. The worker's professional commitment requires her to make this stretch and, further, to consider the action her agency can take to improve its services to her. The worker has to rise above a human reaction, "Oh, not again!" and above her own mound of paperwork, if the child in Mrs. Doe is to have a fair start in life.

The welfare department will authorize MediCal funds, in California, for a verification of pregnancy before providing Mrs. Doe with an allowance for the unborn child. The worker cannot tell the doctor to order laboratory tests for rubella susceptibility, syphilis, and Rh status, and to take a chest X ray. But it seems possible that a welfare department could give the client a slip for the doctor authorizing him to order these tests and providing him with the address of the agency person to whom to report his findings. It is believed that, if workers used their knowledge of agency resources and concerned themselves with the special needs of pregnant women, they could in some instances stimulate their agencies to policies necessary to implement needed services. Decisions about counseling and the time to provide it, training of staff, for whom and by whom, are among other administrative policy decisions that social agencies must take if pregnant women are to receive special consideration in behalf of the coming child.

The high-risk mother has been described in previous sections. The needs of all pregnant women are reviewed briefly here, as the last aspect of prevention of "infants at risk." Needs to be described are those for prenatal care, education, nutrition, and psychological and material support.

All pregnant women improve their opportunity for normal delivery and a healthy infant if a physician has recorded their pelvic measurements, ordered tests for rubella susceptibility, Rh status, syphilis, and tuberculosis, and has noted problems of blood pressure, kidney function, or other abnormalities, and instituted remedial measures well before the expected confinement. Ideally, prenatal care should begin as soon as the mother suspects she is pregnant.

The first examination should include a thorough physical examination and beginning instruction of the mother.[171] Possible danger signals the woman should know (and the helping person also) are shortness of breath, headaches, persistent nausea and vomiting, pain in the stomach or lower abdomen, swelling of ankles or hands, puffy eyes, bleeding, and cessation of fetal movements after they have once begun.[172] A telephone call to the physician or public health nurse is necessary. Depending on the advice given, the mother may need to be examined by the physician at once.

Traditionally, the follow-up examinations have been scheduled once a month during the first six months of pregnancy, every two weeks during the seventh and eighth months, and weekly during the ninth. Special attention is given to weight, blood pressure, urinalysis, and listening to the fetal heart beat, in addition to any special problems of the mother.[173] Recently some doctors have questioned the desirability of routine scheduling of examinations and have suggested individualizing the frequency of follow-up according to the health and other needs of the mother.

Prenatal care varies greatly in quality, ranging from excellent medical treatment, supportive discussion of the patient's concerns, and measures for alleviation of both major and minor harassing physical discomforts, to impersonal service hastily provided after the mother has endured a long, uncomfortable wait.

Long waits in bleak surroundings still serve as deterrents to prenatal care for the largest group at greatest risk, the poor. Private physicians' refusal to treat Medicaid patients because of delay in receiving payments from the intermediary insurance companies, unrealistic requirements for partial payments for care, large bills, and credit office harassment regarding unpaid bills for previous confinements make technically available public facilities actually unavailable in many instances. Helping persons should seek to negotiate unrealistic bills and support the patient in determining to get prenatal supervision. Otherwise the chasm between concerns of the professional staffs and those of the business office defeats many community attempts to provide care to the underprivileged. The special maternity and infant care projects begun in 1964 and jeopardized ten years later, described earlier, rose from concern over the polarization of prenatal care available to the two segments of society, the medically independent and the medically indigent.

One of the great advantages of good, comprehensive prenatal care is education of the prospective mother in care for herself and her coming baby. The education women want is from individual conferences with their physician and reading materials.[174] Obstetricians who provide qualitative service do take time to discuss each woman's concerns and provide her with advice. However, a substantial part of the instruction generally received is in groups led by nurses and dieticians. Usual education includes information on bodily changes during pregnancy, the growth of the fetus, and details of labor and delivery, as well as many aspects of infant care, including feeding and bathing.[175] Frequently, clinics provide individualized instruction from dieticians and follow-up by public health nurses. Some of this intended help is meaningless if communication is impeded by a mutual lack of understanding of the other's perception, as when a dietician talks about ounces and grams of protein, and recommends menu plans that have no relevance to the economic and cultural circumstances of the client. However, a great deal of potential emotional support comes from paramedical services that constitute an important part of prenatal care, and although some of what is relayed is not received, some is by most mothers.

Various studies of the very poor have shown that exposure to education, even that on subway cards, and particularly that in magazines and from the radio and television, has an impact on the person's capacity for positive action. Women who at an earlier period in history would have learned folk wisdom may be devoid of information in an urban, impersonal society. This need can be met by small group meetings of pregnant women. Effort may be necessary to inform women about resources and to help them secure transportation and child care.

Nutrition was discussed in the previous section regarding the high-risk mother, so that its importance and the problems it creates need not be repeated, except for emphasis on the changed philosophy regarding weight gain. No longer is overweight almost an obsession among obstetricians, and strict dieting a constant cross of the woman hungry because she is "eating for two." Rather, underweight is of greatest concern, because of the studies showing a relationship between an underweight mother and a small baby.[176] Iron supplements are available in pill form, and are almost universally needed.[177] If welfare department formularies do not permit them, the worker who is concerned with a poor mother should explore other resources. This small, tangible item is of great importance, and fortunately lends itself well to an appeal to club groups that want charitable projects.

PSYCHOLOGICAL NEEDS, OR THE FOUNDATION FOR MATERNAL CARE

Literature describing the emotional aspects of pregnancy generally agrees that pregnant women tend to be introverted, passive, dependent, childish, concerned with themselves and their fantasies, and even apathetic about the external environment.[178] Helene Deutsch, whose classical work *The Psychology of Women* was written 30 years ago, considers this changed psychological state to be triggered by the physiological changes, and to constitute a bridge to motherliness. There is speculation that the increased need to give after the child comes requires a period of self-reinforcement.

Pregnancy is also described as a time when the woman's feelings about her own mother come to the fore, as she begins to think of herself as a mother, and that as a consequence of these feelings she retreats into her own childhood.[179]

Among the fantasies are those of inadequacy, and fears of inability to have a baby and of death; unreasonable fears are so common as to be "normal." During the last part of pregnancy the fears turn toward inability to stand the pain of labor, and of having a defective child. Dr. Caplan, a psychiatrist whose insights have also created a major contribution to this field, describes pregnancy as a time of crisis and growth, when the turmoil of feelings brings to the surface otherwise buried conflicts (see p. 37).[180]

That pregnancy is a crisis period has major significance for those attempting to be of help to the mother and her family. Crisis is well known as a time when a little weight tips the balance in either direction; and as brought out in Chapter 2, experience of any kind is most influential during a period of growth and disequilibrium. The pregnant woman is likely to be more open to help during this period than earlier or later.

And conversely, because a woman's dependency needs are so great during pregnancy, marital disharmony is especially disruptive. She may well find her husband unable to gratify her needs to cling if any of several common phenomena exist. He may be immature and not ready to be a leaning post; he may feel crowded out of her affections and resentful of her absorption in herself and later in the baby; neither the woman nor her husband may be prepared for the various changes, physiological and psychological, that can take place in her, ranging from irritability to crying spells, unusual food interests, and changed sexual behavior. She may seek out a dependent relationship with her mother, and in-law friction may develop.

In attempts to prevent common problems of the past, modern maternity care seeks to involve the father in prenatal classes and, increasingly, in the delivery of the child. The trend toward blurring of male and female roles, women's liberation, interest in the natural, etc., that exists among elitists and in the counterculture can be expected to seep into working-class mores. Involvement of the father and education in the gestation and birth of his child may possibly reduce the number of desertions during pregnancy or soon after childbirth.

However, when disharmony or desertion occurs, some helping person needs to be available to the mother for the emotional support she requires. If the worker is too busy to give this support, she should find someone else to do it. The reason for meeting the woman's needs is not simply a matter of kindness but of helping her to be a good mother when the child arrives. If her own "cup is not filled," it cannot overflow. Psychological preparation for the baby and the foundation for maternal care begin during pregnancy.

Dr. Caplan has pointed out that the mother's attitude toward her pregnancy changes over time—that, commonly, women do not want the pregnancy at first. Many practical reasons exist why the newcomer will inconvenience or seriously disturb the family situation. Since many women work, they think of lost workdays and income, missed installment payments, and material losses; housing plans need to be changed to allow for more room; the parents do not want to be tied down. Some of the clients often known by social workers may have even more serious reason for dismay, including harassment by the district attorney's office, multiple trips to welfare offices and clinics to arrange for maternity care of a perhaps uncertain quality, and, above all, how to support a baby or another child. The unwed mother has even more conflict to face.

Rejection of the pregnancy is not the same as rejection of the child. The initial reaction changes, and even under the most adverse circumstances, most mothers of first babies want their babies by the end of the pregnancy, Dr. Caplan says.[181] Attitudes toward later children are not known. In the author's personal experience in hospital and public health service, initial reactions to physically normal babies are generally warm and loving while the mother is in the hospital being taken care of, but when she gets home, much depends on how burdened she is and whether she has enough diapers, a washing machine, etc., and how soon she gets pregnant again. If she is in physical and mental misery, the constant demands of an infant can curdle maternal love.

Thus, the mother's state of mind is determined by reality when the child arrives. During the woman's pregnancy, helping persons should concern themselves with the facilities the mother will have to care for the baby. The number of diapers is highly significant: constant washing, wet diapers hanging near the stove or radiator, a smelly, crying baby who cannot be changed—all these get in the way of love. Babies that must be cribbed in grocery boxes or dresser drawers may soon be crying with earache and stuffy noses.

Welfare department budgets technically may include amounts for baby clothes prior to the child's delivery, but the total AFDC budget is so low that the mother often uses the money for rent or food. Furthermore, the time lapse is substantial between the request for funds, their authorization, and receipt of the check. The latter part of pregnancy, not the arrival of the baby, signals the need for sound advance planning. It has been pointed out that the normal mother begins to prepare for her infant after the quickening, for it is then that the fetus seems like a real baby to her; and it is a bad sign if the mother fails to prepare. However, in countless instances, it is learned in public hospital maternity wards that the new baby has not so much as a dozen diapers or a blanket in which to leave the hospital. These children are not all rejected; they are merely the infants of apathetic mothers who had little psychological support and no funds for baby clothes.

Whether rejection of the pregnancy can affect the baby physically, or the course of the pregnancy and delivery, was carefully investigated in a Swedish study of the pregnancies of women who had applied for and been denied a legal abortion.[182] There were no significant differences between the study group and the control group; however, there was a small but surprising increase in the rate of children with malformations in the unwanted group. Authors of the study speculated that the state of stress and attempts to induce illegal abortions and drugs might be responsible.[183] Several authors who have written about the effect on the child of emotional disturbance in the mother during pregnancy have concluded that the infants are likely to be thinner and more irritable, to cry more, and to have feeding and sleeping difficulties.[184]

CHAPTER SIX

Asthma

ASTHMA IS the most common chronic disease of childhood. The National Health Survey showed that 26 per thousand, or more than 1,500,000 children in the United States, suffer from the disease. It accounts for approximately one-fourth of the days lost from school because of chronic illness.[1] The size of the problem alone merits serious attention by those concerned with human services.

The significant role played by psychosocial factors in this complex and often disabling condition commands even greater need for consideration. "In no disease does the parent so often undergo the fear his child is dying," one specialist has observed, and perhaps in none is the child more frequently subjected to a gravely frightening experience. In addition to the undesirable psychological effect of the symptoms, the triggering mechanism for the attacks is in many instances related to disturbed emotional states. Because of the importance of this characteristic, a special section on severe, emotionally triggered asthma has been contributed by Miriam Pachacki, A.C.S.W., whose private practice specializes in work with families of children with this condition, and who at one time worked extensively with parents and children with intractable asthma hospitalized at the Children's Hospital at Stanford.

Asthma is predominantly a disease of early and middle childhood, its severity often tapering off at adolescence; for a few, however, the disease is lifelong. It is most frequent among Caucasians and twice or half again as common in boys as girls.[2] The predisposition to asthma is inherited. Just what the disease is, or how to define it other than in terms of its symptoms, is not yet entirely understood, according to the specialists. Most children with asthma, however, are generally agreed to have an allergy, or state of hypersensitivity to one or more substances in the environment. An understanding of the disease therefore proceeds from an acquaintance with its allergic base.

THE MEDICAL REALITIES

What Is an Allergy?

Allergies are found in all social groups and in a variety of manifestations, and so commonly that, according to studies reported, from 10 to 24 percent of the population have serious allergic diseases and 20 to 50 percent have minor or evanescent allergic conditions. Children are particularly affected, because most of the allergic conditions begin before the fourteenth year of life.[3]

Medical sources describe allergy as a hypersensitive tissue reaction to factors in the environment that for reasons not completely understood create special stress for that individual.[4] Hypersensitivity is another way of saying that the body's normal barrier to invasion by an allergen has been lowered. The lowering of the barrier may be caused by constitutional changes, illness, trauma, age, or emotional disturbances.

The hypersensitive person remains "atopic," or abnormally sensitive to the environment over a continuous period; his particular manifestation is only a symptom, and both cause and symptom not infrequently shift—thus allergy has to be thought of as a continuous and shifting process. The specific antigen or substance to which the person is overreactive usually seems to depend on what he may have been heavily exposed to over a long period or to whatever substances are especially prevalent in the environment at the time. Some persons are allergic to only one or two substances and others to a myriad; some become immune to substances that have been noxious and other hypersensitivities develop.

The part or parts of the body that react to the allergen are also specific but subject to change over a period of time—e.g. the skin as in eczema or hives (urticaria), the bronchi as in asthma, etc. Why one organ is affected rather than another is not understood. Heredity is thought to play a part, affected by the anatomical geography. The response consists of a neuroglandular, neuromuscular, and neurovascular reaction that creates spasm, inflammation, and swelling; in organs affected by mucous glands, there is an increase in secretions.

The allergens, or substances in the environment to which people may become allergic, include almost everything. They are classified as (a) ingestants, such as foods, toothpaste, and lipsticks; (b) inhalants, such as pollens, dusts, molds, animal danders, and chemicals; (c) injectables, or medications, and the poisons of insects; and (d) infections, although the exact mechanism of infections in producing asthma seems to be subject to disagreement.[5] Young children are most susceptible to food, house dust, and molds, in contrast to pollens, because of their circumscribed environment. The infant's diet exposes him to very large amounts of a few foods proportionate to his weight, such as milk, eggs, grains, legumes, citrus fruits, beef, and pork. In addition, some lesser used foods are highly allergenic—shellfish, chocolate, nuts, and cinnamon.[6]

Inhalants most commonly affecting little children are house dust, molds that live in damp and old houses, feathers, animal danders, tobacco smoke, and household supplies such as ammonia, pesticides, and varnish. Most allergic persons are said to be sensitive to house dust; this is different from outdoor dust, being composed of a variety of substances including minute particles of deteriorating cotton from furniture, upholstery, and clothing.[7] Pollens may be responsible for seasonal asthmatic attacks or for additives to the allergenic pool. Of greatest significance are the wind-borne pollens that occur in great frequency or concentration in a given locality. Ragweed is notorious (east of the Rockies), with a dozen members of the large family of grasses also providing difficulty for some persons.[8] The weather may be a factor, with chilling or heat or humidity triggering an otherwise dormant difficulty; and emotional difficulties are frequently implicated as complicating factors.[9] Some psychiatrically oriented persons believe that emotional problems or disorders are contributing and perpetuating in some patients.

Diseases commonly believed to be allergic are asthma, hay fever, rhinitis, eczema, hives, migraine, and gastrointestinal allergic reactions. Eczema is often a forerunner of asthma.[10]

Allergy is generally conceded to be genetic, a hereditary tendency that coexists with exposure to allergens.[11] The heavier the inheritance, the earlier the child will show signs of becoming allergic. A child who develops eczema and/or asthma in infancy or early childhood has a more serious disease because the input of constitutional factors is greater in relation to length of exposure. Small children are in greater hazard from the disease, as will be discussed later.

Nature and Symptoms of Asthma

"Bronchial asthma is a common capricious disorder of respiration affecting persons of all ages with repeated attacks of difficulty in breathing; this may develop into continuous respiratory embarrassment. Its characteristic features are wheezing, labored breathing, an irritative tight cough and tenacious sputum."[12]

Asthma is not a single disease, some authorities believe, but a variety of diseases; Dr. Minoru Yamate, Consultant in Allergy at the Stanford Department of Pediatrics, calls it a "response," often to lung infections, that continues by reflex action. Many children respond to allergens outside themselves. A few are thought by some physicians to be reacting primarily to emotional tensions. Those who are reacting primarily to internal causes are said to have "intrinsic" as contrasted with "extrinsic" asthma.[13] "They all wind up looking like the same thing but the range of precipitating causes is very, very wide, so that the program good for one child is not good for another."[14]

Many children manifest their allergies early in life: they have eczema as infants; rhinitis, which seems to be colds; and sneezing and wheezing in response to a great variety of irritants. They are said to be severely affected and difficult to treat. Another group does not develop asthma until they are older and are allergic largely to pollens and other inhalants; these children, who have specific sensitivities, are easier to treat.[15] A summary of recent studies of age of onset shows that "well over half" develop asthma before age five, placing them in the first, or early and difficult, group.[16]

The difficulty in breathing that asthma creates is caused by edema or swelling in the bronchial tubes, with increased secretions of mucus and spasm of the tubes, which interfere with the passage of air and exchange of gases in the lungs. As the child gasps and labors, he takes in air; but owing to the swelling and secretions, not all the air can be expelled. The trapped air further prevents the intake of fresh air; and as the oxygen–carbon dioxide balance is thrown off, the child develops a systemic or generalized illness.

Asthma usually starts with sporadic, mild episodes of wheezing, the child being entirely well between times.[17] In the early stages the episode may end abruptly. Later the attacks increase in frequency and severity. As the disease progresses, they can become continuous. Although attacks can occur at any hour of the day, Blanc, a physician who is himself asthmatic, says acute attacks usually occur in the early hours of the morning, beginning with a sense of impending suffocation, a short irritating cough, itching, chilling, a runny nose that is an allergic manifestation, and what he calls "profuse diuresis," which in children often means bed-wetting:[18]

> Sooner or later, the stage is reached where the patient has to sit up in bed, elbows on knees, and gasp for breath. The noise of his wheezing can now be heard some distance away.... Asthmatics adopt many different attitudes in order to get a little relief. The commonest one is to plant the elbows on the knees. Others kneel beside the bed with the elbows fixed on the bedside and the head supported by the hands. In this uncomfortable position they doze and fall, regain their position, only to doze and fall again. This miserable sequence lasts the whole night through.

It should be noted that by no means are all attacks as long as those described by Blanc; some are relieved quickly by medications. However, they frequently last several hours, and stretch into a long, tapering period in which both child and parent are worn out. If the attack is not relieved by medication, and continues for more than 24 hours, the child is said to be in *status asthmaticus,* commonly referred to as "status." This condition varies in severity but is always hazardous, and requires continuous supervision and a physician's care. *A child in "status" should be regarded as an emergency.* In an acute attack the child's breathing is so badly impaired that his heart pounds, he turns blue, and he coughs in a desperate attempt to bring up mucus. He may become unconscious, and even suffer heart stoppage or "cardiac arrest." However, the danger is less from death during an attack than from permanent damage to the lungs, although death is possible, especially in young children.[19]

A pre-attack period is described by physicians who see many asthmatic children. Harvey lists physical as well as emotional symptoms that can warn of attack in different children, headaches, gastrointestinal symptoms including abdominal pain, constipation or diarrhea; Blanc and Harvey each describe mood changes, with depression, restlessness, and whining among them.[20] Often families can recognize the imminence of an attack by the child's behavior.

Cause of Attacks

Among asthma's frightening and frustrating features, discouraging to parents and physicians alike, is the elusive nature of the triggering mechanism. Treatment can be symptomatic only, and often ineffectually so, until the cause is found; the cause is often so difficult to determine that a baffled young physician has called it "witchcraft." Some children have direct reactions to known allergens; let a dog walk through the room and the child begins to wheeze. But far more patients seem to maintain a balance between resistance and a mass or accumulation of allergens or stressors; the scales tip and cause an attack when one more stress is added to the number the body has been able to cope with. One experienced social worker describes the situation as being like a "pool" of allergens; when one additional factor is added, displacement occurs and the pool overflows. A detective quality to diagnosis and treatment is required in unearthing the nature of the pool and of the additive triggering or final stressor. Because immunities develop to old allergens and new sensitivities arise, the detective work needs to be very shrewd indeed.[21]

Caplin, who like Blanc is an asthmatic physician specializing in treating persons with asthma, says that many substances trigger attacks but are not substances to which the person is truly allergic. He cites the irritation with which normal persons' mucous membranes react to paint, smoke, hairsprays, insect sprays, and even powders and perfumes. "How much more must they bother the person in whom there are sensitive membranes which are easily provoked to swell and pour out fluids?"[22] Cold wind, exertion, changes in barometric pressure, and strong emotions are other nonallergic "triggering" mechanisms.

Psychological Origins

From earliest times, emotional components in the pool have been recognized. The classical authority on allergy, Vaughan, states, "It is generally agreed that emotional reactions do influence vascular reactions which are basically involved in allergic reactions. The difference in opinion comes in the questions whether frustration, anxiety, feelings of insecurity, rejection . . . can cause asthma."[23]

The exact role of emotions has fascinated the psychiatrically oriented and baffled many parents and clinicians. Harvey, like Caplin, includes it as a triggering mechanism:[24] "Once asthma has been established, acute attacks may be triggered by emotions. There is a physiologic basis for some emotionally precipitated attacks, particularly when the emotional upset is accompanied by shouting, crying and rapid breathing . . . it becomes impossible after a time to separate problems which are precipitating asthmatic attacks from those that are secondary to the asthma. The secondary gain can become a significant problem." Some persons have pursued emotion as a primary cause at great length.

Exponents of emotional causation seem to fall into three groups, the psychoanalysts, the behaviorists, and the stress theorists. The latter, like the analysts, link psychology and physiology in a biological unitary manner, but emphasize the physiological mechanisms by which psychosomatic manifestations occur. The analytic group considers the cause unconscious, with symptoms representing attempts at resolution of conflicts. Desires that are not completely repressed or sublimated find expression physiologically. A great many analytically oriented studies have been made, with general agreement that in the case of asthma a disturbance exists in the mother-child relationship. The child is insecure because of the mother's overprotection, rejection, or inability to be consistently giving for a variety of reasons.[25]

Some studies give weight to narcissism in the mother, with her conscious or unconscious feelings that the child is a burden; some point to outright rejection by the mother, who has rigidly high standards and who nags and punishes the child for lapses in behavior; others emphasize overprotection, with development in the child of dependent fearful traits. The asthmatic attack is seen as a repressed cry upon threats of or actual separation from the mother. Threats include birth of another sibling and any form of rivalry for the mother's affection.

The behaviorists cite research of the Russians and research with guinea pigs. The widespread resurgence of interest in behaviorist theory in recent years has amplified the notion that protective reactions of an organism can be aroused by a conditioned reflex. The overanxious mother who "rewards" her frightened child during an asthma attack by solicitous behavior "conditions" the child to have more attacks to gain her solicitude.[26]

The stress theorists point out that the hypothalamus, upon receiving stimuli, mediates the emotions physiologically via the adrenocortical route; or that biological energy travels via the autonomic nervous system to the organ systems involved and creates the abnormal neurovascular, neuromuscular, and neuroglandular reactions.

These various psychological approaches are not as far apart as they seem at first glance; certainly they complement each other and at least build the foundation for an understandable way in which the emotions do channel themselves into the allergenic pool. The behaviorists merely amplify and focus on two elements compatible with analytic theory, the pain-pleasure principle and the principle of inertia. Saul, an analyst who traditionally avoids esoteric overtones and keeps his ideas rooted in the unitary concept of man, says, "The child's longing for the parents and its anxiety when left alone are deeply biological. They are concerned with the individual's very existence and when such deep seated emotions are aroused they produce far reaching biological change. It may be that the allergic response is part of the organism's equipment to adapt itself to survival in its environment... may well be a response conditioned to certain emotional aspects of that environment as well as or in addition to certain physical and chemical changes."[27]

In recent years, the Children's Asthma Research Institute and Hospital in Denver, an institution that works on the assumption that severe, intractable asthma stems from the family environment, and thereby removes the child completely from his parents for one or two years, has released some interesting studies. These pertain to two subgroups of children in the institution, those whose asthma improves rapidly after removal from home, and those who continue to have severe disease. Purcell, the chief investigator, repudiates earlier, widespread assumptions that all asthmatic children are neurotic or are from unhealthy family environments, but he does point to evidence that at one end of a bell curve is a group of asthmatic children from specific kinds of family constellations, on which he is working.[28] Both his studies and one by Dubo et al., at the University of Michigan, show no statistical difference in severity of personality disturbance or personality profiles according to severity of asthma.[29] The latter did find a significant difference between the degree of family disturbance and the child's emotional disturbance (which serves to validate their methods).

In keeping with the Denver findings about subgroups, a study by an Oakland psychologist who used psychological tests on a group of 62 asthmatic children found a number of differences, not in severity of disease, but in parental attitudes and children's perceptions. The children of one group were more pessimistic and angry, felt less able to rely on their parents for support, and were more preoccupied with oral needs and aggression; and the parents had more friction, with the wife being domineering and perceiving her husband as irresponsible.[30]

The largest study, from Johns Hopkins, raises some questions from a research viewpoint, but its size makes its findings especially interesting in light of other works on subgroups.³¹ Almost 4,000 mothers of wheezing children were interviewed; Blacks were dropped (evidently because of difficulty of finding the mothers at home during the interviewers' hours). The findings showed that boys from small, Protestant, middle-class families had higher rates of asthma except in those families where the father plays a major role in support of the child. The investigators' discussion of their findings and assumptions include the hypothesis that boys, as contrasted with girls, are forced to renounce their initial dependence on the mother and identify with the father; that conflicting expectations about independence arise in the process of socialization; that asthma is related to the intensity of these dependency conflicts. Another finding of interest was that there are significant sex differences in favor of boys in small, lower-class families, described as those where the mother gives major emotional support.

Experienced social workers and clinicians repeatedly observe the presence of anxiety and tension in asthmatic children. Their comments include generalizations about the prevalence of disturbed families and children when this disease occurs. However, no personality profiles or specific emotional syndromes have been validated by studies, and clinical experience testifies to a great variety of family constellations.

An obvious complication in understanding causative psychological factors is the inevitable presence of secondary psychological reactions. Kaufman states that asthmatic children with food allergies are guilty when they eat forbidden foods, fear punishment when they do so, develop patterns of anger, fear, anxiety, and depression. He describes the children as irritable and prone to regressive behavior such as thumbsucking, or conflicted behavior such as tics and stammering.³²

Treatment

Treatment of asthma frequently baffles and frustrates because finding the cause is so difficult. An intelligent mother's close and continued observation, after she is instructed what to watch for, is the basis on which the physician begins his determination. He may request that she keep a notebook with careful charting of foods the child eats, his activities, behavior, the wind, the weather, etc. The mother alone may be able to report the usual precipitants of an attack. However, because the pool may "run over" as a consequence of one of a number of precipitants, she may be discouraged about identification of any one cause. Some authorities believe that certain allergens will react only in the presence of one another; some believe that a child will only react if he is emotionally upset at the time he is exposed. Weather has an effect on a number of children. At this stage of knowledge, diagnosis and treatment of each child remains a highly skilled, frequently tedious, and even mystifying task. No two asthmatics are alike.

The goals of treatment are said to be relief of distress, avoidance of further complications, and development of immunity to allergens.[33] The general procedure consists of medication and sometimes oxygen and intravenous fluids or other lifesaving measures during and after acute attacks, identification and elimination of inhalant and food causes, and hyposensitization therapy.[34] The emergency may be taken care of in an emergency room or may require hospitalization. However, the long process of avoiding further emergencies and helping the child avoid crippling lung complications rests primarily on the care the child receives at home and in the physician's office. One physician categorizes treatment in two parts—what you can do for yourself and what the physician can do for you. The first part includes *avoidance* of allergens to which the child is known to be hypersensitive and of those irritants that generally excite a bronchial reaction.[35]

Hyposensitization therapy, or injection of extract designed to decrease the bodily reaction to the offending antigen—part of what the doctor can do for you—is a long-standing and widespread method of treatment. The treatment is of temporary value, giving relief during the season of maximum exposure and for a few months afterward. In other words, it does not confer an immunity as vaccination does. Injections are employed for allergic responses only to inhalants, not to food, and these are of course limited to substances that are not poison, as would be the case with chemical sprays or pesticides. The customary hyposensitization series of injections are for seasonal, co-seasonal, or perennial pollens. These series frequently take from four to five months to complete and consist of weekly injections.[36]

Controversy over the value of hyposensitization therapy exists owing to the many instances in which it does not seem to help, and owing to its probable abuse by less than conscientious physicians who exploit prolonged treatment by injection for profit. In addition, studies by reputable investigators have arrived at different conclusions. One study published in the *Journal of the American Medical Association* in 1966 declared, "No justification was found for promising any greater benefit to children treated with allergens than they would obtain from placebo injections."[37]

Despite the impediments to assessment, immunologists and pediatricians point to successful employment of hyposensitization therapy and proof of its value through studies by reputable investigators, when the dosage is correct, the antigens employed are the right ones, and the timing is related to the period recommended. The effectiveness of the treatment should not be taken for granted, however, and whether the child improves should be explored. Adverse reactions are not rare; competent medical care is of utmost importance.

When asthma is very severe, the steroid drugs, such as ACTH, cortisone, and prednisone may be used. These drugs are different from others in that their action is not specific to the attacking agent of a disease but, rather, increases the body's resistance to the attack. How they accomplish their "wonder drug" effect is not entirely known, except that they catalyze the adrenal cortex secretions. Their prolonged use has been found to create serious irreversible damage to vital body structures. Intractable asthma may be treated with steroids for lifesaving reasons. If the treatment continues, the symptoms return in greater severity when attempts at discontinuance are made; this is a serious dilemma, and the process of weaning away from steroid drugs is itself a major medical goal. Hospitalization is usually necessary, in order that skilled observation and immediate care can be provided.

Infection is said to be a frequent precipitant of asthma, especially in infants and young children. Therefore antibiotics may also be used as specific drugs against the agents of infection.[38]

Drugs given to bring children out of an acute asthmatic attack are *bronchodilators* named epinephrine and aminophylline, or their derivatives. Both are dangerous drugs and should be given by a physician or under his supervision. Both are also literally lifesaving and without substitute for relief of a severe attack. No delay for any reason should be permitted in getting a child to the doctor for an injection when he is having an attack that has not responded to home treatment. Home treatment includes oral or nebulizer preparations of epinephrine, various expectorants, steam or moist air, and in some instances oxygen. A relatively new drug, Aarane or Intal, has achieved some remarkable results when used several times daily as a preventive procedure. Tranquilizers may be used to avoid or reduce the vicious circle of fright and spasm.[39]

When a food allergen has been identified, it must be eliminated completely from the diet. Because of the probability that the child will be allergic to the most common foods, considerable ingenuity may be necessary to avoid all products that incorporate them while still providing adequate nutrition.[40] The mother needs a chart that describes the "food families" as a supplement to careful instruction by a dietician or nurse. (Although some physicians are competent in providing nutritional and dietary details, many are not.)

Artificial substitutes for milk have been developed for babies' formulas, but the creation of satisfactory foods that completely eliminate milk, eggs, or particularly wheat are extremely difficult to prepare. Because a child will remain chronically ill if he continually eats a food to which he is known to be allergic, the provision of a suitable diet is as important as medication or equipment or provision of medical care.

Avoidance of allergens includes environmental control of inhalants. Children with asthma should sleep in a dust-proofed bedroom. Sleep occupies such a large proportion of the hours spent in one place that the avoidance of common allergens during this period takes on major importance. A dust-proofed room is one in which carpets and drapes have been removed, mattresses and pillows have been covered with plastic covers, and cotton or wool spreads and blankets have been replaced with those made from synthetics. The room is then kept clean by daily mopping. Needless to say, cigarette smoke and other pollutants should not be introduced; air conditioning should be installed where practicable and where outside air pollution is a hazard. Like the special diet, these requirements are obviously difficult, especially for families of limited financial, physical, or emotional resources.

Another frequent problem is allergy to mold. Like house dust, the spores of this allergen are widespread, especially in old houses, for the type of mold in question, "Monilia," inhabits damp basements, old underflooring, moldy wallpaper, etc. Since dampness and age are the two facilitators of mold, children of assistance families are particularly subject to this allergen. Hyposensitization therapy can be attempted.

Outlook

In many instances, the asthmatic child "outgrows" the disease even when it appears that irreversible lung damage has occurred.[41] Reasons include a literal outgrowing, or growth in size of the bronchial passageways, with relative increase in size of the passageway in relation to the size of the swollen tissue. Larger airways permit more room for swelling and mucus while still permitting air to get through. In addition, the child who is allergic to foods learns what he cannot eat and usually cooperates in avoiding it. Since he can be reasoned with and becomes capable of conceptualization, he is more capable of mastery. The emotional balance between mother and child is changed as the child goes to school and peer relationships take on more importance in the total scheme. Boys, who it will be recalled are more prone to asthma, are also more prone to outgrow it.

Dees warns, however, that outgrowing asthma is less common than the public has been led to believe; that despite a positive outlook for the majority, asthma is a terrifying, long-term condition with constant threat of death or invalidism. The death rate from asthma is statistically small in children in the United States (about 0.3 per 100,000), but for individuals the danger always exists.[42] Children with asthma need the best medical care available.

PSYCHOSOCIAL IMPLICATIONS

The psychosocial impact of asthma is highly variable. "Life is a battle," in the words of one mother, but elements of the battle differ and the war may be contained or extensive. In the families of asthmatic children one sees in living form the medical dictum that asthma is not a single disease

ASTHMA

entity but a "syndrome" or "response": a group of symptoms arising from various causes. The child with mild asthma has a different life than one who has severe disease. Asthma in the preschool child means something different than asthma in the school child, and asthma due to allergies to common foods creates different problems than asthma due to inhalants. Certainly the child whose asthma has a strong emotional component presents different problems to himself and others than one whose precipitants are primarily physical.

Family Adjustment

Constant fear besets the parents of a child who has had one bad attack, especially if the child has been in "status" or near death until he receives emergency medical care. Many families have said that the worst time is when the child is small. The infant or toddler cannot understand or cooperate; his breathing is most severely affected and he is in fact in greatest danger because of the small size of his bronchial tubes; the parents are least experienced and most prone to panic; the precipitants have not been identified or the case has not been fully diagnosed; and perhaps the family has not yet found a helpful physician.

Asthma's unfortunate predilection for nighttime attacks has rippling effects. The mother usually gets up when she hears the child coughing or wheezing, and often the father sleeps on, or "plays possum," as one father said. Notable among the nine intact families I interviewed in connection with manuscript preparation, three fathers brought out their inability to bear listening to the child suffer. In two cases, the father had a relationship of unusual intensity with the child, and in the third, he identified the child's suffering with that of his own father, who died in an asthmatic attack. This father said that he sometimes has to go out to the garage when the child's attack begins so he will not hear her gasp.

The frequently heard phrase of the mother, "I felt so alone," is easy to understand as one visualizes her sitting up while the rest of the world sleeps, succumbing to feelings of helplessness and panic if the wheezing child fails to respond to medication but progresses to terrified gasping. One mother said, "Pretty soon you become so identified with the child it is as if you have no self of your own." "It has always been just Jimmy and me" sets the stage for some of the common strains on the father-mother-child relationships.

One or two weeks' nightly sleep interruption is enough to create fatigue and irritability. How great, then, the fatigue, and how constant the irritability, when lack of sleep continues over a period of months. In some cases the father takes turns with the mother, giving the child his medication, putting on the vaporizer, giving the child a drink of warm water or weak tea and comforting him. In the majority of cases, however, it appears that the father is fully roused only when he must rush the child to the emergency room for an injection, or if the mother becomes beside herself with worry. Thus the irritability of the mother finds her husband the natural target: "He is so immature," or "He's irresponsible," or more frequently, "He's too selfish."

The stage of the family life cycle creates an interlocking aspect of parental relationships. In most cases of preschool children, the marriage is young and its balance therefore precarious, and relationships are based less on mutual parenting than on opportunities for shared recreation and physical satisfactions. Other young children, pregnancies, inexperience, and financial struggles add to the picture. What percentage of marriages break under the strain is not known, but many do. "We each built up a wall, against each other and the rest of the world," one couple said in telling of the storm they had weathered with the aid of counseling. This word picture of a "wall," like the word "alone," recurs in discussions with parents of asthmatic children.

Frank resentment against the child may also grow out of the sleeplessness, fatigue, and frustration. One mother said of her husband, "He acted as if Bobbie's attacks were a personal vendetta against him." Not only may the father's deprivation of normal family life turn into resentment toward the child, but the mother also may resent the creature who refuses to yield to ministrations and creates such havoc in family life. The resentment may be overt, and lead to angry shouting at the child who is wheezing and gasping. Probably in more instances, resentment is buried. This can lead to distorted perceptions of the kind of care the child should have. Mothers may permit the child to expose himself repeatedly to known precipitants of asthmatic attacks, or they may persuade themselves that the child has attacks deliberately, to get attention.

Quality of Medical Care

Because the mother often does feel so alone, she particularly needs an understanding pediatrician or pediatric allergist. She needs someone who will listen to her frustrations and who can help her keep some perspective. A physician who is interested in "the whole child" and is sophisticated in family relationships is a bulwark against preventable family damage, especially if he utilizes counseling for families who need more than he can supply. The physician needs to be a person who has treated enough children with asthma, and kept up sufficiently with modern drugs, that he has the capacity to treat the child medically with skill. If he places the child on steroids unnecessarily, or keeps him on these dangerous though life-saving medications too long, he can create greater physical damage to the child than the asthma originally caused. The asthmatic child can die from inadequate care. Management of asthma is frustrating in the extreme to professional and parent alike. Moreover, the physician must be that rare person who can be called in the night and on weekends. He has to be willing to pull on his clothes at two in the morning, over and over again, and go to the hospital to give the child emergency care.

Finding this paragon is very difficult. Many families do not have such a physician. Some have a pediatrician who meets part of their needs, and an allergist who acts as consultant to the pediatrician and whose office administers skin tests and hyposensitization treatments. Other families attend clinics, where an intern on duty at night can administer injections, but they see different doctors at times of clinic visits, or they may see physicians who are impersonal and disinterested in the individual family.

Consequently, the helping person—social worker or other practitioner—should be alert first to the parents' account of the medical care they receive. If they are satisfied, or if they find in their physician an unusual source of help, the first requirement has been met, and the worker can lend his energies to other aspects of their problems. But if their account of medical care is one of frustration, the worker is in the delicate position of helping to guide the parents toward better medical care. In urban areas, pediatric allergists exist who meet the unusual requirements necessary. The agency medical consultant, the crippled children's division, or the local tuberculosis or respiratory disease association knows the specialists and can often make helpful suggestions. The worker may be able to steer the parents toward securing consultation from a skilled and caring physician. If the consultation begins a relationship that the parent wishes to continue, the worker should help the family to do so. Bearing in mind that a marked difference exists in the way two persons relate to each other, the worker should not be surprised if one family enthusiastically responds to a physician and other families do not.

Dietary and Housekeeping Problems

As stated earlier, little children suffer primarily from food allergens and from house dust. Dietary allergies may express themselves in eczema, colds, runny noses, and abdominal pain and diarrhea prior to the development of asthma or, in other words, in an unattractive, itching, crying, fretful baby or whining toddler who requires a great deal of attention. The eczema may be so severe that the child's eyes swell shut; his scratching and the restraints necessary cause additional problems.

Caplin states that with children under one year of age, asthma is due usually to infection or foods or both; that it is simple to manipulate the infant's diet; and that the child's symptoms often disappear quickly when the child is taken off cow's milk, eggs, orange juice, or wheat.[43] Middle-class families with access to adequate medical care should have no substantial problems with substitutions. However, misunderstandings, lack of specificity by the physician, in-law interference, baby-sitter carelessness, or maternal lack of respect for authority (the physician) can occur in any household, especially if the mother is a teenager, unwed, or a poor mother with many children, deprivations, and distractions.

Food allergies of children who are over a year old, when additional allergens become apparent and more complex foods become usual, often pose serious difficulty. Diagnosing which food causes the attack may take a long time, much experimentation, and shrewd observation. According to Caplin, 12 foods cause over 90 percent of the problems—milk, wheat, eggs, chocolate including cola drinks, peanuts and legumes, cinnamon, citrus fruits (mainly oranges), tomatoes, corn, berries, fish and shellfish, and food colors.[44]

The shifting nature of allergens frustrates the family, especially if the child ceases suddenly to be allergic to one food item and develops an allergy to another. The conscientious mother may blame herself, or wonder how her child secured a forbidden food, until an unmistakable episode demonstrates that something hitherto harmless has become an offending substance. Understanding the food families requires special instruction. Who of us would know that a peanut is not a nut but a legume? Or that frankfurters and lunch meat contain corn syrup? Only a tiny amount of the allergic substance produces the explosive tissue reaction that causes symptoms. This may be difficult for the mother to understand, or for her to convey to indulgent grandparents, neighbors, immature baby-sitters, or even to the child's father. Well-meaning caretakers may have no idea that something in the juice or cookie may cause the child's eyes to swell shut or cause him to choke in the night.

Mothers who work, or who have many children, and are unable to devote all their time to supervision of one child meet defeat in keeping the allergic child from even those foods she herself knows will cause him to have an attack. When the child reaches the climbing stage, his agility in reaching sweets containing food coloring or flavored with peanut butter may seem unbelievable.

Corn derivatives are among the most ubiquitous products in the so-called convenience or prepared foods that modern housewives buy. Corn syrup or corn meal appears in such surprising foods that very detailed food lists are necessary for mothers of children allergic to this member of the grain family. One mother told of seven years of miserable existence, with a scratching, wheezing child, countless hours in doctors' offices or driving to them, months of sleepless nights, and feelings of guilt induced by allergists who made her feel she was not observing their instructions, until a dietician gave her a food list that detailed all brands of foods containing corn derivatives and those that did not. "It was like a magic wand—as if someone waved magic over us!" she said. Other mothers have told of the hours they spend reading labels, and of their frustration because labels do not include all ingredients.

As in kidney failure and diabetic diets, much depends on the mother's aptitude and time taken to prepare foods from the beginning, without recourse to the canned soups, mixes, helpers, tinned stews, and frozen dinners that make up much of the modern diet. The mother who lacks sufficient intelligence, energy, or motivation to adapt her cooking to the child's needs requires a great deal of supportive instruction. A homemaker may be able to teach and help her; a patient public health nurse may be a resource, or the clinic dietician if she has been drawn into the helping process, or a grandmother, or aide. Among the most difficult to help are those with cultural and language barriers—where foods customary in the diet have not been analyzed by the clinic dietician and where the father may be the master of the household and ignorant of and impatient with minutiae of diet. Other families in need of long-term assistance are those in which no regular mealtimes exist and children help themselves to any food they can find when they feel hungry. The obstacle of a mother's need to work to support the family can usually, though not always, be overcome. If a parent is alcoholic and the child is untended for hours, an outside source of supervision is essential.

The most conscientious and knowledgeable homemaker may fail with an allergy diet if the child has become allergic to household dust in addition to the offending foods. Neither the mother nor the physician can determine what is causing the child's attacks. Therefore, the "dust-free environment" is recommended. The child should sleep in a separate room and not be allowed to crawl in bed with the parents. Keeping the child's bedroom dust-free is more practical than trying to keep the entire house free from dust, and in addition it protects the child for at least half the time.

In addition, the sick child's night attacks are less disturbing to other family members. Also, the vulnerable asthmatic child is less prone to catch infections from others if he has his own room. Great variation exists in the degree to which families are able to maintain a separate room; sometimes the child may have a crib in the parents' bedroom. In such cases every effort should be made to help the family find housing or modify conditions to create a room for the asthmatic child.

A dust-free room is a barren environment. The preschool child is less affected by the cell-like atmosphere of his room than an older child, and is more apt to be satisfied to play there than the older child. Feelings of banishment, lack of stimulation, and loneliness can occur if the mother overdoes the protection of the room and keeps the child there. However, if he has his own television, and a plastic-covered "bean-bag" chair, and toys enough to keep him occupied, the main problems may narrow down to those encountered at night. He may want to sleep with his parents, and cry when he cannot, thus disturbing their sleep, or the mother may accustom herself to wakeful listening. She may be uneasy about closing the bedroom door for fear of not hearing him start to cough and wheeze.

One mother commented that maintaining a dust-free room "is a drag" and her feelings and burdens are important. This mother referred not only to the daily or twice-weekly wet-mopping and frequent washing of the woodwork but to preventing an accumulation of possessions in the child's room. She said that if the child could have two rooms, one for his possessions that mount up into dust catchers, and one to sleep and play in, it would be much simpler.

The extent to which mothers maintain the recommended dust-free environment depends on their housing potentials, how worried they are about the child's illness, how driven they are to try everything, and also how tired they are and how hopeful that something they do will help. The mother who is completely frustrated because nothing seems to prevent her child's attacks may give up. Additional factors seem to be the extent to which the family understands the recommendations, and whether they have the money or are willing to spend it to replace all dust-producing equipment and purchase substitutes. Father and mother may disagree about where the money should go, when there is not enough to buy many things they need. In cases of real poverty or limitations of public-assistance income, private agencies such as the Respiratory Disease Association may be willing to finance plastic covers, an electric blanket, a plastic-covered chair, and in some instances locate a secondhand television set for the room. Creative mothers with income and energy can make a dust-free room relatively attractive, with bright-colored vinyl, washable synthetic-fiber throw rugs, plastic valances, etc.

When a social worker in the community is involved in helping a family achieve a recommended dust-free environment, she needs specific guidance from the child's physician or clinic. Detailed knowledge of housing requirements is vital if money and time are to be used economically.

Moving

Moving to a different town or area in an effort to avoid noxious inhalants is controversial. Some physicians do not recommend it, on the basis that after a period of time the child will develop sensitivities to substances in the new environment. However, when a child is allergic to molds, and the family lives in a coastal area where these are unavoidable, serious consideration should be given to moving. If he is not subject to molds but is to pollens, the coast may be preferable. If a child is subject to allergy from pyrethrums (insect spray) and the family lives in a truck farm area, moving the family or the child away seems indicated. In many cases, a high dry area does relieve the symptoms of severe allergies including asthma; at times, moving to a different part of the city makes a difference because of the pollens. In a small child, a year or two of relief from asthma may be a vital factor in the physical and mental health of child and family.

Pets

Pets create common sources of difficulty for the child allergic to inhalants. Allergists disagree about appropriate disposition of the family cat or dog. Some will tolerate no fur-bearing animals in the household of a child they are treating. Others suggest trying to keep the pet outdoors as much as possible, and always out of the child's room—keeping the pet but not replacing it when it dies. Pediatricians who are aware of the sorrow the loss of the pet may bring to the asthmatic child and his siblings try to balance emotional and physical factors. Dr. Yamate believes the child's happiness and harmonious family relationships are transcendent goals. "If I could be sure the pet was causing the asthmatic attack, I would say remove it, but if one is not sure what is causing the attack, perhaps it should stay."[45]

Siblings are especially prone to resentment if their pet is destroyed, or if they are deprived of a pet. One mother of a quarreling household told of a family conference she called in desperation, hoping differences could be negotiated. Instead, a sibling said, "Can't we get rid of Jimmy instead of Pal? I like Pal lots better." In households I have visited, pets are common, and in one instance each of six children had his own cat or dog. Some children are only mildly allergic to dander, and some are said to be allergic to one dog but not to another. Caplin, who represents the restrictive view, states that although an allergic individual may not be allergic to animal dander when tested, being atopic, he may develop it later if heavily exposed. By and large, all asthmatic children are thought to be better off if the family keeps no furry pets, because the fewer irritating particles breathed the better.

In a few instances, children are so highly allergic to animal dander that they cannot visit the home of a relative, a neighbor, or family friend because of the animals. One mother blamed this situation for social isolation: "We have no friends." Another described the heartbreak of grandparents who, though they boarded their dog when the family visited, found the child still so allergic to dander in the furniture that he could no longer visit them. It seems possible that the mother's fear of what may happen during the visit may reinforce the negative influences and trigger the attack, or the child may be highly suggestible as well as allergic.

Financial Problems

The two-parent family with good health insurance and at least one automobile in running order, does not find asthma an overwhelming financial burden, in comparison with other major chronic illnesses. Particularly if the father's group insurance has a major medical feature that includes cost of drugs, the costs to the family are limited to those for drugs not covered by insurance, and for replacement of blankets and rugs, plastic covers for the child's mattress, and gradual replacement through the house of overstuffed furniture and rugs made from wool with those made from synthetics. However, if a move is necessary, or if air conditioning or radiant heating is installed, great expense is encountered.

In these intact, middle-class families, cost problems are those of inability to keep up with friends or neighbors who have the material benefits of two incomes, where the wives work, and cost problems due to the siphoning off of extra funds that would go to luxuries or a higher standard of living. How these problems affect feelings toward the child was indicated by one mother who had disclaimed any sibling or family difficulties, but who said bitterly, "One week of every four of my husband's work goes to support Jimmy's asthma." Resentment becomes more serious when insufficient funds exist to meet all real needs. One mother spoke openly of an older sibling's resentment of the asthmatic child. "It isn't that she thinks I'm lying when I tell her there isn't money for a new dress. She sees the figures there in black and white. But when I have to stop at the drugstore and pay $40 for his medication, there just isn't that money left for the things she wants."

The one-parent family, or the large family on an inadequate income, or the family whose insurance has run out finds asthma a serious financial burden. A severely affected child may be hospitalized from a half-dozen to two dozen times, especially during the early stages of asthma. A car in running order must be available at all times to take the child to the hospital emergency room or the doctor's office twice a week for injections. Transportation thus becomes a major financial problem. A family receiving public aid on a flat grant requires outside assistance for gasoline and upkeep of an automobile, unless some unusually reliable relative is always available, night and day, to take the child to the doctor for emergency care. Equipment necessary to create a dust-free bedroom can cost $150 and more, if all bedding must be replaced and the mattresses and springs covered with heavy plastic.

The parent with insurance that does not cover drugs is in trouble if the child does not respond to usual medication and is placed on new and/or expensive drugs. A relatively new medication found highly valuable for severe cases, Intal, currently may cost $30 a month. Children on such drugs are the children who need frequent, regular trips to the doctor's office, so that their families have high transportation costs. Food costs may be higher than normal, especially if the child is allergic to foods commonly used by low-income families and busy mothers—frankfurters, bologna, beans, TV dinners, hamburger supplements, etc.

Thus, cost is by no means negligible. The problem is relative to the resources available and the margin above necessities. It spills over into feelings about the asthmatic child.

Foster Care

Respite may be needed by the most conscientious family—six weeks of relief may save a marriage. In an earlier era, convalescent homes for severely affected children were used for a child's care away from home over extended periods. Such institutions have dwindled and are near extinction owing to the high costs of medical care. Protective services for children should be expanded to include foster home care for seriously ill children who do not need hospitalization but whose well-being requires close supervision and extra care.

In social situations that do not prove amenable to change, as in those where parents are alcoholic, irresponsible, or retarded, or the family is so large and the income so small as to frustrate any major, prolonged housing and dietary modifications, foster care may need to be considered while the child is small. Removal of custody and court action, initiated by physicians or other concerned persons if children are frequently hospitalized as emergencies due to lack of home care, can be avoided if the community provides remedial preventive resources.

School-Age Problems

By the time the child reaches school age, the child and his family usually know what foods to avoid and have adapted to substitutions. Most of the continuing incapacitating asthma is due to exertion, cold, wind, inhalants (grass and weed pollens, etc.), and nervous tension.

Exertion, cold, wind, and play in grassy places as precipitants of attacks create the dilemma of maternal protection, with dangers of infantilization, versus vesting a child with responsibility for his own actions. Competition with peers is the dominant thrust of this stage of development, and in the excitement of competition he forgets his restrictions. However, by the age of 11 or 12, he should be responsible for determining his own activity, according to Dr. Yamate, whose goal is to make the child "a participant, not a spectator in his own care."[46]

This general guide obviously is subject to modification according to the intelligence and stability of the child. In practice the mother's feelings also influence the degree of responsibility she relinquishes to the child, as does the general discipline exercised in the family. Children who must come in the house by a certain time to avoid the evening chill, who are permitted no boisterous play, and who carry notes to the teacher asking that they remain inside during recess run the risk of greatly limited socialization with their peers. If, however, they are not restricted and have repeated attacks in the night that cause them to miss school frequently for two or three days at a time, exhausting the parents and disturbing relationships with siblings, not only are they centers of tension in the family but their school-peer relationships are disturbed also.

The child's ability to play at other children's homes, and to participate in such activities as slumber parties, seems an important part of normal peer relationships in the middle class. Most families currently have dogs and/or cats. If a child begins to sneeze and wheeze when he comes in contact with animal dander, he cannot visit his friends. A child who is subject to night attacks cannot stay away from home overnight unless the friend's mother is unusually attuned to his needs and the friend lives near enough that the parents, after telephoning the child's parents, will bring him home. These limitations are of variable importance, of greater significance to the only child or the shy child who has begun to feel left out and different or very dependent on his mother.

The extent to which the child should be given responsibility for his own activity and medication can only be determined by other impinging factors. The severity of the disease is a primary influence. If the child is "steroid-dependent," or, in other words, if his life is in balance, every precaution seems valid despite the danger to the child's social adjustment. This also applies if he is exhausting himself in play, ignoring his wheezing as long as he can and then using an aerosol spray as often as he wishes in order to keep up with his peers. Again, his life is in danger.

The underlying attitude of the mother is another determinant. Instances are seen where excessive permissiveness appears to be occasioned by rejection, not by rational decisions in behalf of the child's wholesome development. When a mother allows a child allergic to animal dander to sleep with a dog on the bed, the possibility of rejection warrants exploration. Defeat is another attitude that can lead to excessive permissiveness. The mother who is completely frustrated by inability to determine causes of attacks, and who has struggled unsuccessfully with a variety of inconveniences, from elimination diets to wet-mopping every day, may have decided to let the child do what he wants to do, come what may.

The intelligence and temperament of the child are of great importance in determining a sensible course for the school-age child with asthma. The normally intelligent, stable child does not want the distress of an attack, or to miss school and play, and if he receives intensive medical care he soon learns a great deal about allergies and about how far he can go without bringing on an attack in the night. Children learn from experience when to stop, or when to come in the house, except for times when peer competition or unusual excitement spurs them too far, or unless a neurotic element exists.

Intelligence affects school performance to an unusual degree in the asthmatic. Like the hemophiliac, the asthmatic child often misses school for two or three days, too short a period to have a home teacher. If he is a bright child, whom the teacher likes and approves, and if he has siblings or neighbor children who can bring home his assignments, he can make up the work he has missed. He therefore is spared the bewilderment of ignorance regarding class discussion when he returns, with consequent feelings of shame and disapproval of peers and teacher. If, however, he failed to learn to read in the first grade, either because of dullness or hospitalization or repeated absences, he may appear stupid, dislike school, not try, and earn the teacher's disapprobation. Such a child, who does not make up the assignments he misses during frequent absences, gets farther behind each year. If he has native intelligence, he will still earn a low score on the IQ tests that test learning content. When "tracks" or divisions in classes occur, he will be placed with the slow learners. "Ma, they always put me with the dumb kids."

The importance of school as a socializing influence in the child's life is second only to that of the home; and in asthma, because of the frequent absences, intelligence sets off a chain of circumstances that not only affects the child's ability to manage his own activities but plays a major role in personality development. During school age, the child needs badly to succeed, to win recognition from peers and teachers by getting at least average grades and excelling in something. If he is intelligent enough to "win" in spite of school absences, he can overcome, at least in part, the handicap of the illness.

The teacher's attitude is often the crux of an asthmatic child's school adjustment. Parents frequently complain that teachers seem to have no understanding of asthma, despite its prevalence. Some teachers panic, and are unnecessarily protective. However, in junior high school the most frequent complaint is that the teachers hardly know the children, that they are not even aware that a child has special needs. One mother who served as a teacher's aide said that prior to this experience she blamed the teachers, but after seeing how difficult it is for them to cope with large classes, she understands why they resent anything that adds one more responsibility or burden. She had found that notes sent to school were disregarded; now she understands why.

Teachers in elementary schools in stable residential areas usually seem to be understanding and helpful if the child is normally intelligent and the family shows an interest in school. Some mothers go to see the teacher before school begins to explain that Jimmy has asthma, tell the teacher that he knows what to do if he has an attack, and to assure her that the mother will always come if called. They thereafter usually find teachers very cooperative. Schools that have school nurses are most fortunate, in that the teacher has the reassurance of help from a specialist if she needs it. Some principals take major responsibility for children with special needs. The child who is permitted to use aerosol sprays may leave his nebulizer in the principal's office, if there is no nursing office, and go there to use it.

Physical education classes can pose problems, for sustained or competitive activity is frequently prohibited. Physicians may not appreciate the difference between the desirable mild physical activity that keeps the child's muscles in tone and the competition and overexertion sometimes required in physical education. If physical education class is recommended and the child has attacks because of overexertion, the school may put him in a substitute class where he does nothing. Most children with asthma seem to particularly enjoy and be able to cope with baseball and swimming, short-spurt action activities. The American Academy of Pediatrics has recommended that asthmatic children should not be unduly protected and that individualized plans be worked out by physician, parent, child, and school.[47]

One study of the school achievement of severe cases of hospitalized asthmatic adults, most of whom were in the 17–21 age bracket, showed that only 14 of 68 had completed high school, and that their school careers had been characterized by irregular attendance.[48] The modal grade of completion was the 10th. This study is obviously skewed in the direction of persons who would have had most reason to miss school because of severe illness, and though the record is below the average for all persons in the United States (about three-fourths finish high school), it seems surprisingly good in light of the skewed sample.

No solid findings in regard to school achievement are available. Modern educators seem to pass children to the next grade despite poor achievement, to avoid stigmatizing the child. In the asthmatic, school levels may be much the same as those of well children. Whether social-class factors tend to provide cultural and therefore educational advantage to asthmatics is in question. The popular notion that asthma is more prevalent in the upper classes is not borne out by accumulated studies, which are contradictory. One study of Denver children showed more upper-class mothers responding that their children had allergic histories. A study in Aberdeen, Scotland, showed more mild asthma in upper classes and more severe cases in the lower (which could reflect the results of treatment or lack of it).[49]

The Child's Personality

Despite the long, intensive effort to prove that asthma is caused by emotional problems, no solid evidence exists. Gordis summarizes the studies as follows:[50]

> In summary, the psychiatric studies indicate that there is a higher frequency of emotional disorders in asthmatics than in the normal population, but that this frequency may not be higher than in other groups with chronic disabling conditions. The observations thus suggest that the emotional disturbances may be the result rather than the cause of the asthma; the dyspnea experienced periodically or frequently by the asthmatic may be a particularly important determinant of emotional disorders in such patients since the breathlessness reminds them of their life threatening disease.

Asthma's effect on the child's personality affords a classic example of how one facet of life interplays with others. No two children are alike. The relevancy of the disease is determined by the way other factors relate to it. The four variables that seem most important are the severity of the asthma and the substances to which the child is allergic; the child's native intelligence and degree of sensitivity; the father-mother-child relationship; and the quality of medical care. Many other factors count also, but the interactions of these four with each other recur as seeming determinants in the child's personal development.

The severity of the disease determines how the child feels physically. If the child is taking medication that gives him a stomachache, or if he is losing sleep and also taking medication that makes him drowsy, he is prone to be abnormally quiet and/or moody. One mother described her boy as "spooky quiet" when he feels bad. Asthmatic children who have had many fear-producing experiences including trauma during hospitalization may be withdrawn and sensitive. It is not uncommon to find shyness and fear of strangers in little children who have asthma. Boys whose growth has been retarded by steroid drugs have self-esteem problems as they approach puberty and become adolescent.

The precipitants of the attacks have some bearing on personality, depending upon the way the parents manage the child. Children whose asthma seems particularly related to infections, and who must avoid being around other children with colds, stay indoors during inclement weather, miss school frequently during "flu" season, and develop solitary interests with concomitant loss of opportunity to develop social ease. Wind, barometric change, and exertion, as precipitants, similarly limit the child's opportunity for normal play activities and thus his chance for recognition, success, and happiness. However, a few asthmatic children who are allergic to these same precipitants are resourceful, outgoing children and even leaders among their playmates. They have attributes that outweigh their disability. Good intelligence, drive, imagination, and talents can bring the successes they need and place them in front. One example is a high achiever with excessive drive, whose class project was called "WHEEZE," and who created intriguing quiz games to go with it.

In contrasting such a child with children at the opposite end of the range of personality, who become upset if they fail to make a basket in basketball or have to stand in front of the class to present a "Show and Tell," it is obvious that two factors outside the child have direct bearing. One factor is a permissive pediatrician, who is willing to come out at night if the child does get into serious trouble by overdoing, and who believes the child's happiness comes first. Such a physician guides the parents into a relatively relaxed attitude toward the child's activities, while educating the child to find a reasonable line between overdoing and invalidism. Such a course places greater responsibility on the parents and the child than a strict medical attitude, and it can create problems for parents who think concretely and lack flexibility. It also creates problems for children who are in conflict over parental authority and can play the doctor against the parent. Perhaps most difficult is the dilemma when the child abuses the freedom and responsibility placed upon him, and lives by constant recourse to medication. A child who can take a Tedral tablet whenever he feels the need, or has an aerosol spray at school that he can use at will, may keep himself just under the edge of acute episodes, stretching his physical limits to suit his recreational activities, and incur permanently damaged lungs.

The other element that affects the child's personality is the parental attitude, described in detail on p. 191. Dr. Rhyne says, "Atopic children view their physical disability very much as their parents do."[51] A perplexing observation I have made may be explained by a study reported in connection with the large Baltimore study referred to earlier.[52] In several instances I observed that children of overtly or covertly rejecting parents seemed emotionally "stronger" children than those of mothers who evinced greater sensitivity, compassion, and love. A study by Bronfenbrenner attributes negative effects to what he calls "love-oriented techniques."[53] He says that they undermine capacities for independence and achievement, particularly in boys. By "love-oriented techniques" he means the use of reasoning, appeals to guilt, and withdrawal of love to bring about the desired results in the child. "Power-assertive techniques," by contrast, rely on physical punishment.

Although one may expect that children who have been rejected, especially during asthmatic attacks when physical incapacity and fright require an extra amount of emotional support, will be maladjusted and probably become hostile persons, it was notable in several instances that they seemed more self-reliant than children who were treated lovingly. Dependence and fear of being away from the mother seem relatively common in asthmatic children; in two instances the mothers described first onset of asthma when the child was separated from the mother because of the mother's hospitalization or illness in other members of the family, and ensuing attacks at times of separation. In a third case, a child relinquished by the mother as an infant had his first attack at time of first foster home placement, and when he was placed in a second foster home, he had another asthmatic attack.

Severe, Emotionally Triggered Asthma

(The next four sections, pp. 189–94, are contributed by Miriam Pachacki, A.C.S.W.)

Identification of wheezing triggered by emotional factors is difficult to differentiate from wheezing triggered by exposure to allergenic substances. In my work with asthmatic children I have learned to look for certain clues that indicate the existence of emotionally triggered asthmatic attacks. The first is year-round, constant wheezing, although testing has demonstrated that the child is allergic to substances that are seasonal. The second is patterns in wheezing not related to exposure to allergens, wheezing that consistently occurs around certain stressful holidays or events such as Christmas, birthdays, or periods of family stress. Stress is not always negative. The joyous anticipation of a birthday party can be as stressful to a child as worried anticipation that mother will be angry when she discovers her best lamp has been broken.

Wheezing triggered by emotional stress is just as dangerous as wheezing caused by an allergenic substance and requires the same appropriate medical attention. One of the risks in demonstrating to parents that their child's wheezing is emotionally triggered is that the parents will become angry and assume that the child is wheezing deliberately. Psychotherapy or casework intervention does not cure asthma. It helps the child and his family to identify the stress that triggers wheezing much as skin testing helps to identify the substances to which the child is physically allergic. I consider asthma or wheezing both a physical disease and a form of behavior.

Psychodynamics

As a behavior, wheezing and/or asthmatic attacks can be used in the service of one's emotional or psychological needs both consciously and unconsciously, just as symptoms of other chronic diseases can be so used. Children in therapy have revealed many uses for their asthma: simple avoidance of school on a day when a test is scheduled; believing they are holding their parents together by nearly dying (parents can't desert dying children); resolving their own conflicts by withdrawing into illness; punishing hated or resented parents by keeping them awake at night; preventing arguments between parents by forcing them to focus on the child's wheezing; etc. There are as many uses for wheezing as there are children with asthma and situations in which they find themselves. One may ask, do all children or people wheeze for emotional reasons? In my opinion, they probably all do occasionally. Many adults who had mild or relatively mild asthma as children will recall instances when they wheezed or even brought on an attack of wheezing deliberately, in order to avoid some unpleasant event or to make their parents feel guilty for having punished or deprived them.

Why would a child use a dangerous illness as a coping mechanism? If we knew the answer to that question, the process of treatment could be altered. What we do know is that human behavior is not always rational. We tend to use what is available to us to influence our environment or to solve our problems. Children with asthma have asthma available to them. Wheezing is a behavior that elicits certain responses from the environment. One must recall that behavior, not verbalization, is the language of childhood. Words are gradually substituted for behavioral language as one matures, but even adults use behavior to communicate. Many adults don't say, "I feel grumpy and irritable today," but instead act grumpy and snap at everyone. Wheezing can be used in the same way as any other behavior: to express feelings, to avoid and solve (or cope with) problems.

When a person has only a single important means of expressing himself, he is in trouble. The emotionally healthy person needs an extensive repertoire of ways to communicate, to express, and to cope. The child with severe intractable asthma always, or almost always, uses wheezing to express, to communicate, and to cope. This child has discovered that wheezing is his most effective way to deal with the environment. He never develops a healthy repertoire. The use of wheezing as a mechanism operates at different levels of consciousness. Children vary in the degree to which they consciously use wheezing. Some are aware of what is happening but are not in control of what they are doing. Surprisingly, the risk, the actual threat to life is secondary, and at times not important. This suggests that one of the mechanisms operating in severe, emotionally triggered asthma is the need to have impact on the environment at any cost.

Rarely is the child so self-destructive that his wheezing is suicidal, although frequently it is a symptom of depression. Children substitute wheezing for appropriate behavior because parents cannot for various reasons tolerate the appropriate behavior. For example, an asthmatic child may have learned to wheeze as a substitute for crying when he perceived that crying distressed his parents or earned disapproval from them.

Substitute mechanisms in an emotionally disturbed or emotionally deprived child are not unusual, but the asthmatic child has available the dangerous weapon of wheezing, which he can use in a maladaptive manner. Another child might have resorted to bed-wetting, stealing, or lying.

The Parent-Child Relationship

It is extremely important for parents, if the family is intact, to develop at least a reasonably satisfactory marital relationship. The reasons for this will be discussed later. The family as a whole needs to keep the asthmatic condition in perspective, neither ignoring nor underestimating its seriousness, but at the same time not allowing it to dominate. There are families where literally nothing is ever planned or even considered as a family activity because "Johnny might wheeze and then we couldn't do it anyway." The child who is allowed to create this kind of situation comes to be regarded as a kind of family affliction, a second-rate citizen who reflects on the adequacy of the parents and interferes with the reasonable satisfaction of the social and emotional needs of his siblings.

I have observed certain repeated patterns in the families of severely asthmatic children. When these families have been referred for therapy or counseling at early stages, it has become possible to identify the symptoms that could contribute eventually to the severity of the disease. Every severely asthmatic child I have known has been in some way undesired or undesirable, although not necessarily totally rejected. Sometimes he was born too soon after a previous sibling. Sometimes the sex was wrong. Sometimes the child was born at a time of family crisis, economic or emotional. Or he looked like a hated relative. "He looks just like his father," a divorced mother may say. Or "She reminds me so much of my sister and I couldn't stand her." That there would be marital problems either caused by or resulting from chronic illness in a family is a common and probably valid presumption. The remarkable thing in the families of severely asthmatic children is that the problems seem to be quite specific. In many families the mother has been either physically or emotionally abandoned by the father. The syndrome of the absent father (divorced, deserting, child born out of wedlock, etc.) is self-evident. The physically present but emotionally abandoning father is more difficult to recognize, since some of these men are hard-working (married to their jobs), involved or even overinvolved with their children, and at least on the surface responsible family men. Some husbands who are alcoholics, sexually inadequate, or abusive fit the usual descriptions of emotionally abandoning husbands and fathers.

There was one interesting exception to this picture in an intact family with children. The father was very much involved and concerned. The mother's previous husband and baby had died. In the mother's fantasy life, her asthmatic child was the child she had lost. She eventually realized that instead of accepting her present husband's love and devotion, she was holding him off, particularly in relation to the asthmatic child. She was unconsciously following the pattern of "abandoned" mothers who lean heavily on their asthmatic children for emotional satisfaction. This leaning can vary from requiring rather simple social attention to lover-like relationships in which mother and child frequently sleep together. The sex of the child seems to make little difference in this pattern. The fathers in these families tend to be rigid and passively controlling men, frequently with histories of extreme dependency on their own mothers.

Most severely asthmatic children live in constant fear of being abandoned, partly because of their helplessness and dependence during an attack and partly because of the unconsciously communicated fear and resentment of the mother toward her own abandonment. In some instances, the retreat into illness, especially *status asthmaticus*, seems to be an unconscious effort to regress into nothingness (or death, which *status* simulates) in an effort to "begin again."

It is startling to me to learn that even very young children know what is happening in their families and to themselves, in other words, why they are wheezing. This awareness, if not conscious, is very close to consciousness. The children often confuse sickness with punishment or "badness" (not just in asthma) and confuse parental fear and concern with parental anger and disapproval. A climate of trust and acceptance is needed to permit children to reveal that they know why they are wheezing and that they might even have started wheezing deliberately.

The Treatment Approach

The medical component of severe asthma in the child requires the highest degree of cooperation between the child, the family, the doctor, and the social worker or therapist. The wheezing behavior can sometimes be controlled by medication, but as a method of expression, communication, or coping, it must be replaced with behavior that accomplishes similar results more safely, realistically, and appropriately.

The treatment approach that has been most effective in my experience is basically simple, but not easy to accomplish. First of all, it is necessary to help both the child and the parents to identify a specific instance when wheezing has occurred without the presence of allergens, infections, or whatever physical substance is known to trigger wheezing in the child. Both child and parent then begin learning how to discover when and how the child uses wheezing to communicate and to cope. The goal is to substitute appropriate behavior and/or verbalization depending upon the age of the child.

A crucial period in treatment occurs when the child is ready to give up wheezing in favor of less dangerous and more appropriate ways of coping and reacting. He can do this only insofar as his parents will permit. This can be difficult for even the most cooperative and concerned parents, who need to tolerate periods of undesirable behavior in the child. The therapist also provides constant reality-oriented feedback to the child about what he is doing and why.

One common pitfall is parents' and doctors' pride in a child who is a model patient, never fusses no matter what the doctor does. It should be recognized that this child feels just as strongly as the child who is openly negative about his medical treatment. Sometimes the child who doesn't let you know how he feels is in more trouble than the one who does. A child's reaction to medical treatment depends a great deal upon his age. A very small child perceives it as punishment simply because it hurts. The older child is intellectually capable of recognizing that medical treatment is intended to help him, but he nevertheless perceives it as an assault or aggression on his person. This is further complicated if in the child's fantasy life he has perceived his asthma as a kind of monstrous being (a common fantasy in asthma) that inhabits his body and sometimes takes possession of it.

Parents and physicians feed into this fantasy unwittingly by talking about asthma as if it were a separate entity that must be gotten rid of. The child knows that in the process of getting rid of the "monster" he himself could be endangered ("gotten rid of"). If the fantasy of the monster is incorporated into the self-image of the child as he grows older, he begins to see himself as different from other children, a kind of hard-breathing monster whom others are afraid of. In reality children are often fearful of the child who wheezes and they tend to stay away from playing with him.

Medical treatment is also related to control, to the child's need to control what enters and leaves his body, which is seriously interfered with in the allergic child who is placed on diet restrictions and medications and is bombarded periodically with shots, intravenous injections, etc. There is a great deal of concern expressed over the problem of overprotection of the asthmatic child. I am inclined to be concerned less with overprotection than with overcontrol. Parents are, and should be, protectors. Children require protection. However, the degree of protection should vary with the child's stage of growth and development. One protects a child from being injured by a car by controlling his behavior in relation to the street. When the child is able to internalize the control and keep himself from running into the street, it is important and healthy to relinquish the control to him. This relinquishment of control to the child when he is ready to take over is very apt not to happen when a child has a chronic illness. There are enormous ramifications to this problem, and it is an important area when one is working with the emotional component of asthma.

I wish to stress that I have been discussing the severely asthmatic child and his family, in which the emotional component is very marked. Where does mild, medically controllable asthma end, and severe, emotionally triggered asthma begin? At present it seems almost impossible to determine. By studying the families of children with severe, emotionally triggered asthma, I believe we can identify certain symptoms, patterns, and dynamics that exist in special identifiable syndromes. Because certain clues are recognizable, a psychological assessment is warranted early in the history of the asthmatic child; the potentially pathological family pattern can then be interrupted and the use of asthma as a coping mechanism can be avoided or prevented. In families where these patterns do not exist and where there is little or no potential for them to develop, the allergic child will prosper under programs of increasingly effective medical management, including social adjustment. It is the predictability of the difference between the two that is vital and that deserves further study. No amount or quality of medical care is sufficient to compensate for the emotional components of asthma, just as no amount of psychotherapy will compensate for inadequate medical care.

● ● ●

Mrs. Pachacki's comment regarding the difficulty of determining where medically controllable asthma ends and severe, emotionally triggered asthma begins is typical of all aspects of this disease. The Purcell research team's conclusion that there are two groups of asthmatic children seems to be substantiated, but in a practical sense the finding may be only academic: the medical and emotional problems of the two groups are not mutually exclusive. The relative influence of psyche and soma varies among individuals, and a comprehensive approach is essential in every case.

The social focus may be upon concrete problems such as diet, housing, or a parent's need for respite, or on complex family relationships. Withholding judgment, careful assessment, and a shift of emphasis when indicated are basic to the helping process. A sustained supportive relationship, where possible, permits significant nuances to unfold while helping the mother feel less alone. The physician plays an unusually important role in the treatment of asthma, for a comprehensive approach to the disease involves him in all aspects of family life. The presence of his influence extends the usual triad of father-mother-child to a father-mother-child-physician group with whom the worker must relate.

Help to young parents with a small child is particularly important. The preschool child by and large is the most ill, his parents the most upset and worried, and intervention at this early stage probably has greatest significance to the marriage and the child.

CHAPTER SEVEN

Chronic Kidney Diseases

KIDNEY (*renal*) disease is not a single entity; many kinds exist and their import varies widely. The kidneys are vital parts of several intricate mechanisms that sustain life. Because of their relation to the heart and circulation of the blood, they are part of the *cardiovascular-renal* system; and because of their excretory function and anatomical relationships, they are part of the *genitourinary* system. Kidneys affect, and are affected by, the condition of other organs.

The National Kidney Foundation estimates that kidney disease is the fourth leading health problem in the nation today. Urinary tract infections are a common cause of children's admissions to hospitals and next in frequency to upper respiratory infections.[1] Four thousand children between the ages of one and six are stricken with childhood nephrosis annually, according to the Foundation, which has also identified kidney disease as the top cause of work loss among women and the second cause of absenteeism among men under 25. Over eight million Americans are said to suffer from kidney-related diseases; about 58,000 die each year from terminal kidney disease.[2]

Good care is necessary during acute kidney disease to save life. The family's ability to obtain adequate medical care, and to adhere to the doctor's instructions during the follow-up period, influences the development of chronic kidney impairment. As the latter creates great misery and may terminate life, the social components create important differences in outlook for the individual.

Serious kidney disease or abnormality affects the personality of the child and the life of the family. The many ways the influences develop become clear as one begins to understand the diseases or conditions and their treatment. Frightening and very painful bodily changes occur in some, such as gross swelling and bloody urine. Hospitalization may be required, sometimes repeatedly. Diagnostic and treatment procedures often involve the external genitalia. They require numerous intrusive procedures, with needle insertions and sometimes catheters, the latter particularly in girls. Medical treatment may bring its own serious hazards, including severe retardation of growth. Finally, if uremia, or the end stage of kidney disease, occurs, that most fateful of all questions arises—whether to permit a child to die, or whether he should enter the long, painful course of life on dialysis, with the hope of an eventually successful kidney transplant and a period of useful life. Those who work with the family and the child cannot divorce their work from these implications.

THE MEDICAL REALITIES

Children's kidney problems include *infections* of the urinary tract, *kidney inflammation* following streptococcal infection, *congenital anomalies* in the structure of the kidney or urinary tract, *tumors, stones,* and *obstructions*. To be discussed here are urinary tract infections, including *pyelonephritis*; *congenital anomalies*; *glomerulonephritis*, which in its chronic proliferative form is most apt to lead to *uremia*, or *renal failure*; *nephrosis* (sometimes called *nephrotic syndrome*), which occurs either as a stage of chronic nephritis or as a separate condition; and renal failure, this at some length, for though it is rare, the psychosocial implications are massive.

The Kidneys and Their Function

A pamphlet prepared by the National Kidney Foundation, "Your Kidneys," describes the two bean-shaped, fist-sized organs that lie below the back of the rib cage, and consist of two outer layers, an inner sac or pouch, and a drainage tube.[3] The outer layers, *cortex* and *medulla*, are made up of perhaps a million tiny identical units, called *nephrons*, that drain into the *pouch* or *kidney pelvis*. The large tube from the pouch, the *ureter*, in turn drains into the bladder.

The kidneys are part of the *cardiovascular-renal* system, receiving blood from the heart through a branch of the aorta. Their functions include maintenance of chemical balance in the body. In complex ways not fully understood, "the kidneys regulate the internal environment within narrow limits through varying the volume and concentration of the urine produced. They also remove metabolic wastes and various substances ingested, such as medications and poisons. The kidneys also have an important role to play in the regulation of blood pressure and the production of red blood cells."[4]

Blood is filtered through the nephrons, water and wastes removed, and much of the water returned purified to the blood. The amount needed of body chemicals such as salt, sugar, nitrogen, potassium, and some proteins also passes back into the bloodstream via the membranous walls of the nephrons. The excess water and wastes are drained out of the nephrons to collect in the pouch, or pelvis, and then pass out through the ureters into the bladder for storage and emptying.[5]

The *glomerulus* (the term derives from Greek) is the functioning—in contrast to storage—part of the kidney. In conjunction with *nephron* (Greek for kidney), it produces the disease term *glomerulonephritis*, a variety of nephritis characterized by inflammation of the capillary loops in the glomeruli. The prefix *pyelo-* refers to the pouch or collecting sac, the kidney pelvis, and *pyelonephritis* is thus an inflammation of the sac. Problems can come from two directions, either from the bloodstream, in a process that scars the nephrons so that their filtering function cannot take place, or up from below into the kidney pelvis. Typical of the latter are infections, often from feces via the rectum or introduced by a catheter. Tortuous scarring of the ureters occurs from repeated infection, so that drainage is impaired. If this happens and infected urine backs up into the sac and the nephrons, destruction of kidney function results.[6] Because there are so many nephrons, thousands of them can be destroyed and the kidneys still function without giving any warning sign of trouble. Then, when all but a relatively few are gone, the kidneys fail. *Uremia* occurs, or waste products back up into the bloodstream, which is fatal unless the artificial kidney machine is used and/or a kidney transplant is provided.

Tests of Kidney Function

Various tests have been devised to determine kidney function; these are often seen on medical reports or are referred to by physicians or medically sophisticated parents. The well-known urinalysis shows whether there is blood (*hematuria*) or pus (*pyuria*) or albumin (*proteinuria*) or sugar in the urine, and also provides a measure of *specific gravity*, which indicates how dilute or concentrated the urine is. Another test, involving injection of dye and measurement of excretion rate, is the PSP test, the initials referring to the dye used (phenolsulfonphthalein, or phenol red).

Blood tests are also used to indicate the kidneys' efficiency in clearing wastes. One of the most common is referred to as the BUN, or blood-urea-nitrogen test. A more sensitive test often used as a definite indicator of approaching failure, or uremia, is the *creatinine* test.[7]

Collection of clean urine in an infant or small child, especially a girl, is not easy, sometimes involving immobilization and often in girls the use of catheters. Like needling, these intrusive procedures are resented or create terror in the child, especially one in conflict during establishment of toilet training or in the age of fantasies of guilt and punishment.

Cystoscopy, a notably painful procedure designed to illuminate the internal structure of the ureters and bladder by introduction of a lighted tube, is usually performed under anesthetic on a child.[8] X rays include an *IV (intravenous) pyelogram*, in which dye is injected into the bloodstream as in a blood test; and a highly uncomfortable procedure called a *retrograde pyleogram*, involving a combination of cystoscopy and X rays.

Recurrent Urinary Tract Infections

Urinary tract infections, as indicated previously, are common in children. Unfortunately, they often recur. One study showed an average of 11 episodes per affected child.[9] The incidence is four or five times higher in girls than boys, and most often begins in infants or preschool children. The disease is very hazardous in newborns and frequently results in death, especially in boys.

A bacillus transmitted from feces is responsible for most of these infections. Because a girl's urethra, or tube from the bladder to the outside, is shorter and more easily accessible to process of infection, much less concern is felt when a girl has an infection than a boy. Some malformation of the tract is often the cause of repeated infections in a boy. If the infection is confined to the bladder, as happens in many instances especially in girls, it is termed *cystitis*, and is readily treatable with sulfa drugs.[10] "Although acute infections within the urinary tract may be confined to the bladder, the majority involve the ureter and kidney as well."[11]

According to Rubin, "The seriousness of urinary tract infections in children is best appreciated when its long-term effects are known. For over a quarter of a century investigators have emphasized the recurrent nature of the disease and its tendency to become chronic, distorting the anatomy and function of the kidney and leading to renal failure and its complications." He supports his statement with studies showing significant percentages of children who later died or had persistent infections or obstructive problems or severe renal damage.[12] Stealth of the disease and complacency of parents and some physicians or inadequate follow-up evidently account for the serious effects over the long term. Just enough treatment to relieve the child's discomfort and clear up the pus in the urine during each flare-up may leave the bacilli at work unnoticed in the urinary system, until serious damage has been done.[13] *Pyelonephritis,* or infection of the kidneys by microorganisms from below as described, or from the bloodstream, is very uncomfortable during the acute flare-ups. The child has chills and fever and frequent and painful urination, and usually has other signs of a general infection such as nausea and vomiting, weakness, and headache.[14] Well-known drugs such as *Gantrisin* clear up the immediate problem. Hospitalization for several days is often necessary during the acute stage, and continuation of the drugs at home for a brief period.

The conscientious follow-up urgently advocated to prevent later disability consists of prolonged rather than brief drug treatment,[15] and meticulous, repeated examination of the urine to determine whether bacteria remain and what kinds of bacteria are present.[16] The physician must know whether the same bacteria are causing relapses when additional flare-ups occur, or whether some new strain is creating a separate recurrent problem. Relapse, or discovery of the same persistent bacteria, indicates that the infection has not been eradicated by previous treatment and may continue to destroy kidney function.[17]

The literature indicates that prolonged, silent infectious kidney disease is hard to study and that much is yet to be learned.[18] One authority states that progressive pyelonephritis is very rare, and believes that urinary infections alone, without complicating factors, do not lead to renal failure.[19] "Host" factors are implicated as well as bacterial; that is, there may be autoimmune or allergic factors that make some persons more susceptible to the bacteria than others. Other disease, such as diabetes or sickle cell anemia, may be present. High blood pressure has been associated with chronic infectious kidney disease, and the importance of malformations or abnormalities in urinary tract structure has received a great deal of attention.

Boys with recurrent urinary tract infections have routinely been referred to the urologists and surgeons for study preliminary to surgery, on the basis that "any factor tending to cause obstruction in the urinary tract may be favorable to the development of infection."[20] One authority said in 1964 that "corrective surgery is indicated" when kidney pathology exists owing to obstruction.[21] However, Stamey, in a recent authoritative book on urinary tract infections, comments on the unnecessary surgery that has been done and says he "feels sorry for" the large number of children who have been operated on when they could have been treated by medication.[22]

Acute pyelonephritis does clear up with treatment, never to return in known form, in many cases. The fact that a child has had one bout does not mean he will have stealthy disease to the point of renal failure. It does mean that a warning has been sounded of possible recurrent kidney disease. Therefore it deserves careful follow-up over a prolonged period, and should not be dismissed as merely an episode.

Malformations or Congenital Anomalies

"There are few instances in all of clinical medicine where early diagnosis and proper treatment are more effective in preventing what may be a fatal diagnosis than in the case of the child with correctable obstructive uropathy."[23] Congenital malformations are relatively common, and many are of little consequence. However, "Collectively, they account for about 45% of cases of chronic renal failure in childhood; they often have a hereditary basis, and are frequently associated with abnormalities in other organ systems."[24] There are many different types of congenital abnormalities, ranging from absence of one or both kidneys to malpositions to malformations of the urinary collecting system, bladder and urethra. The urinary collecting system anomalies are three times more common in boys. Since symptoms are not always evident or clear-cut, they are usually diagnosed by complicated X rays that utilize dye or instruments.[25] Those that create the greatest problems are those leading to chronic infection, those interfering with the flow of urine or the kidney's capacity to function, and from an emotional standpoint those creating abnormalities of the external genitourinary system. "If a child has a demonstrable *significant* anatomical abnormality, that person is at risk of going into chronic renal failure."[26]

The most common abnormalities of the genitourinary system involve the ureters, which are the tubes leading from the kidneys to the bladder. They may hamper passage of urine and lead to gross distortion and dilatation, with eventual loss of vital function of kidneys and bladder. This is the *obstructive uropathy* referred to previously. If the abnormalities are major and do not straighten out as the infant grows, surgery is necessary to prevent serious consequences. Surgery may be simple or it may require removal of an entire kidney and ureter or major reconstruction.

Extrusion of the bladder through the abdominal wall is an uncomfortable malformation with major social implications. The bladder is partially exposed, and often accompanied by other external defects of the genitourinary system. The social and emotional problems are incident to constant odor from seepage of urine and to its unsightly nature. Though the child can live without surgery, medical authorities recommend surgery at three to five years of age.[27] The ureters are transplanted into the intestine and urine is excreted through the rectum. Plastic repair of the external genitalia may also be performed. Surgical treatment may be delayed because of the parents' lack of knowledge, unwillingness, or inability to have the operation performed.

Glomerulonephritis

Acute glomerulonephritis, the most common form of nephritis in children, most frequently occurs in children between three and seven years of age and is more common in boys than in girls.[28] It is usually accompanied by blood in the urine (brown or smoky urine) that the family may have thought due to an accident. The disease, like rheumatic fever, is, in fact, due to an allergic reaction to certain strains of a *beta hemolytic streptococcus*. This reaction may occur suddenly a week or more after a sore throat or scarlet fever. Although the disease may be quickly fatal, most children improve markedly after a week or two, and the underlying kidney disease disappears in several months to a year. Occasionally small amounts of blood or protein persist in the urine for several years. Most children do not seem acutely ill, which makes it difficult for the family to understand the seriousness of the condition.

Treatment in severe cases requires bed rest for the first two or three weeks, limitation of salt intake, and very close medical supervision of the heart and cerebral and urinary output problems that accompany the disease. A high degree of professional competence is required for the medical management of these three major complicating areas, any of which can lead to permanent damage or death. After the child is out of bed, it is still necessary that he be guarded against chilling, overexertion, and infection.[29] Return to school is advocated when return to complete activity does not appear to create any adverse effects (about six to eight weeks); if blood or albumin reappear in the urine, the child should be returned to bed rest.[30]

One source warns against prolonged protein restriction in the diet of a growing child, and also against prolonged activity restriction. The point is emphasized that if the child were kept restricted until all kidney findings were normal, he might be restricted for as much as two years.[31] Another pediatric nephrologist points out that *acute* glomerulonephritis rarely leads to chronic glomerulonephritis.[32]

Chronic proliferative glomerulonephritis is the disease that most often leads to kidney failure, with its awesome choice between death from uremia or prolongation of life on a kidney machine or with a transplanted kidney. Chronic glomerulonephritis begins suddenly in some cases with blood in the urine, generalized swelling or *edema,* or inability to urinate. Unfortunately, however, a stealthy course like that of chronic pyelonephritis is usual, the patient and physician being unaware that anything is amiss until kidney failure and uremia are imminent. "Earlier detection would be an enormously important public health objective, but too little is known of the etiology and pathogenesis of glomerulonephritis and the nephrotic syndrome to achieve these goals."[33]

Frequently glomerulonephritis is discovered by urinalysis during the course of a physical examination, or by its complications, such as high blood pressure, heart trouble, swelling, or anemia. One form of glomerulonephritis does create recurring flare-ups of nephritis, with a gradual loss of kidney function. In this condition, the kidneys suffer further damage with each flare-up. Puberty may create the strain that precipitates complete kidney failure. Most of the time the child is well enough to be up and active, but eventually becomes weak and bedridden, and the crisis arrives of dialysis and transplant versus death. The management of the child by diet is discussed later in relation to *renal failure.*[34]

Nephrosis or Nephrotic Syndrome

Nephrosis is a chronic, relapsing condition characterized by massive losses of body protein through the urine as a result of kidney damage, and by gross swelling of the body in a compensatory physiologic attempt. The disease may be secondary to other conditions including glomerulonephritis and diabetes, but usually is a separate condition in itself, with an unknown cause. Nephrosis has been called "hay fever of the kidney" because of a probable allergic component in causation.[35]

Nephrosis usually begins in children between one and four years of age, and occurs twice as often in boys as in girls. Control of the condition is achieved by steroids and antibiotics in approximately 80 percent of cases. With the advent of current treatment, only 10 percent are now said to progress to renal failure. Children under five who make a rapid response to steroid treatment are said to have a relatively good outlook. However, relapses not only are characteristic but may occur over a very long period, half of the children relapsing up to ten years and 20 percent beyond ten years.[36]

The episodes of acute swelling come on gradually, with puffiness under the eyes, and progress to severe distention of the abdomen, swollen feet, and gross distortion of the swollen eyes. The swelling can become so extreme in some cases that the child's skin splits open. The eyelids may be so swollen they turn inside out. During this period, the child is in great danger from infection. He needs hospitalization for two or three weeks, and is isolated while being treated with steroids, to bring the protein loss and swelling under control. One pediatrician points out the misery of the child and the anxiety of the parents, but emphasizes the need to avoid prolonging the period of isolation, salt-free diet, and steroid treatment. He advocates "constant vigilance against the pitfall of making the treatment worse than the disease."[37] His statement indicates to the lay person the added trauma to the child that treatment itself creates. Steroids have a growth-stunting effect, as pointed out elsewhere. Thus treatment strives to balance lifesaving measures with caution against growth damage. Steroids are now given on an intermittent basis, not daily, after the initial acute attack, in an attempt to minimize the various serious side effects such as cataracts, pathological fractures, and growth retardation.

The ten out of 100 children who do not respond to treatment, and who have severe disease, are now being treated in some centers with chemical drugs used in leukemia such as *cytoxan*. Such drugs have severe side effects, including baldness (*alopecia*) and sterility.[38]

Loss of appetite occurs when wastes are not drained from the system adequately, and the child's refusal to eat becomes a serious problem aggravated by the unpalatability of the salt-free diet. The growing child needs calories and protein, so the absence of food adds to the problems created by the illness and the drugs. The author has seen one young woman of almost model proportions who had childhood nephrosis with relapses every few years until she went into renal failure in late adolescence, but most children seem to be very much undersized. In two instances, mothers told of morning-long efforts to get a child to eat one sandwich. One medical authority says it is impossible to supply sufficient calories for growth to a child whose kidney function has been drastically reduced.[39]

Avoidance of infection is another treatment measure with social implications. Hospital isolation of a very young child, while personnel wear masks and gowns, speaks for itself. A further psychologically harmful but necessary treatment measure is limiting contacts with other children over a prolonged period to avoid contracting colds or childhood diseases.

Chronic Renal Failure

Renal or kidney failure can be acute or chronic. The acute form follows poisoning, burns, shock, or acute glomerulonephritis.[40] The chronic form, which most often concerns social workers, is the end result of progressive glomerulonephritis, pyelonephritis, or other conditions such as cancer or congenital abnormalities. Holliday et al. state that it is fortunately rare in children, occurring most often in adolescents who have chronic glomerulonephritis or untreatable nephrosis. One age peak is at about four to five years, for children with congenital kidney problems, including cancer; and another is at adolescence, for children who have acquired disease, such as glomerulonephritis.[41]

Renal failure means that only a few thousand nephrons out of the original million remain, perhaps 5 percent of the total, depending on the physician's definition of when "failure" has occurred—too few to take care of the water, salt, chemicals, and protein that are taken in. The water is not excreted, but collects in the tissues and creates edema or swelling. In effect, the urine backs up in the blood when the kidneys can no longer purify the wastes and get rid of them. The toxic effect that results is called uremia or uremic poisoning.

Complications

Neurological disorders of two types occur when the kidneys reach a dangerously low level of functioning. The first affects the brain and spinal fluid (the central nervous system) and the other the extremities (in the peripheral nerves), particularly the legs. If water backs up into the brain, or if the normal chemical balance is deranged, mental disturbances result. "In many patients, a tendency to mental fatigue is prominent and is often associated with a slight undercurrent of irritability."[42] Mental dullness, drowsiness, lethargy, and confusion may alternate with periods of normality, but as the condition worsens, muscle spasms, convulsions, and coma develop. Death occurs unless aggressive, modern treatment intervenes.

Muscle weakness "is fairly common,... usually best seen in the large thigh muscles [producing] muscle cramps in the mildly decompensated uremic patient."[43] Some persons develop painful sensations of burning in the feet, or may have such disagreeable aching in the legs that they walk restlessly back and forth in an attempt to get relief. Paralysis of the legs, beginning with the toes and feet, can occur. This is not treatable by diet and dialysis but only by successful transplant, and even then function does not return for several months.[44]

In some instances, the neurological abnormalities are caused by treatment drugs if they build up in the blood of persons whose kidneys are too damaged to excrete them.[45] It is obvious that a child with kidney disease who is showing incipient or actual signs of convulsions or coma needs to be under the care of an expert who is aware of all the possibilities and has the needed facilities at hand.

The kidneys are part of the circulatory system. High blood pressure of any kind is caused by narrowing or constricting of the arterioles, the terminals of the arteries, which act as conduits for the blood being pumped from the heart to the veins, which then return it to the right heart for oxygenation. The kidney excretes *renin*, a substance that constricts the arterioles. In addition, a diseased kidney fails to remove from the blood other substances that cause arteriolar narrowing.[46] Therefore, high blood pressure is a common concomitant of chronic kidney disease, even after such a drastic treatment measure as dialysis has been instituted. The headaches of high blood pressure are one of the several causes of severe discomfort for the child who has chronic renal failure. Unfortunately, not much is known about the treatment of high blood pressure in children,[47] with the result that a specific form of treatment has not been established.

Anemia is a common complication of severe kidney disease, the degree of anemia corresponding roughly to the degree of renal failure. Among the complex causes is a shortened life span of the red blood cells, with greater demand than normal for manufacture of new cells and inability to meet it.[48] Blood transfusions are therefore commonly needed.

One complication of chronic renal failure is bone disease, called *renal osteodystrophy* or *uremic bone disease*. The disease is painful and results in deformities. There are two forms, one in which the bone becomes porous and tends to bend easily or lends itself to incomplete fracture; this is sometimes called *renal rickets*. The other form is *osteitis fibrosa*; as the name implies, the bone becomes filled with a fibrous tissue. One authority, Stanbury, says the bone disease is "eminently amenable to treatment," but that the treatment varies according to the form, and careful diagnosis is necessary. Vitamin D is used in some rachitic cases, and occasionally removal of the parathyroid glands is necessary for osteitis fibrosa.[49] Renal rickets is defined as "dwarfism associated with osteoporosis following prolonged renal insufficiency in early childhood";[50] the importance of its treatment

CHRONIC KIDNEY DISEASES

is self-evident. Bone disease may worsen in patients who are receiving dialysis treatment and is described as extremely disabling. It heals after successful transplant in almost every case.[51]

Diet

Dietary therapy is used where uremia develops slowly and some kidney function remains. Special diet is used when kidney function is materially reduced by any cause. After chronic renal failure, a strict dietary regimen may suffice to keep the child alive or functioning without dialysis for as long as a year,[52] an important advance indeed, in light of the difficulties encountered once dialysis is begun or in some cases a transplanted kidney is received. In an analysis of the University of California Medical Center's experience with the first 53 children dialyzed and/or transplanted, six children were treated by dietary management at first, one for as long as 15 months.[53] Five of the six children were under six years of age.

A major problem in chronic renal disease is poor appetite, contributing to the stunting of growth, characteristic of the condition, because of inadequate nutrition for growth requirements. Loss of appetite as a result of uremia, limited activity due to weakness, immobilization during treatment, and the unpalatability of the diet allowed are some of the reasons for the serious difficulty in getting the child to eat.[54]

Computation of the diet is highly complex. Healthy kidneys, it will be recalled, control the balance of various essential elements such as salt, nitrogen, potassium, and other chemicals. Diseased kidneys lose their ability to excrete excess elements consumed and to conserve the amount needed. Consequently, what is taken in must be regulated with close attention to nitrogen and amino acids, as well as calories needed for muscle tissue (and, in a child, for growth). Diet for children with renal disease is much more difficult to compute than for adults, and it is so unpalatable and restrictive that the University of California Medical Center is experimenting with a "more realistic" approach, permitting the child something he likes, and using deliberate psychology in trying to get him to eat.[55]

The principles involve a "low protein diet of high biological value with sufficient calories for normal metabolism."[56] High biological value requires that the protein contain all the essential amino acids in proper amount and that these carry most of the nitrogen present. "Egg protein has the highest biological value followed by milk, meat, fish and fowl."[57]

The practical problem is that other foods, including vegetables and grains, contain protein also, but of lower biological value. These foods must be excluded, so that the limited protein allowed will all be of high biological value. To achieve a palatable, varied, and nutritious diet capable of providing the calories needed is considered literally impossible. Therefore special dietary foods plus calorie supplements are used to add to weighed amounts of meat and vegetables. Some low-protein wheat starch products that can be made into pancakes, muffins, etc. are Paygel P Baking Mix and Cellu-low Protein Baking Mix. Examples of powders used to add calories are Controlyte and Cal-Powder; these are mixed with water, soft drinks, or juices. Unfortunately, the calorie supplements are described as not very palatable, and the wheat starch products create a sticky, gummy texture.

When patients have edema and high blood pressure, salt must be restricted. Patients with glomerulonephritis are more likely to need salt restriction than those with other kidney conditions including pyelonephritis.[58] Potassium is another element that is usually severely restricted. Fruits and vegetables, such as potatoes and bananas, that contain this element, are excluded.[59]

The carefully constructed diet built around the use of artificial foods is sometimes referred to as the Giovanetti diet, named for the Italian physician who developed it, but modified to accommodate English-American food customs. This diet not only prolongs life and reduces the frequency of dialysis needed, but ameliorates distressing gastrointestinal symptoms and drowsiness. According to a report on two studies, it prevents some particularly distressing feelings of agitation and impending doom for the last week or two before death.[60] In one study of adults on this diet, almost half refused to stay on it because of its unpalatability, but in another group, the relief of symptoms was so pronounced, and the distress so acute following dietary indiscretions, that the sickest patients were motivated to stay on it.

Dialysis

After dietary therapy has been attempted as long as possible, and death is inevitable unless further medical and surgical intervention takes place, certain centers use on children drastic modes of treatment recently established for adults. *Dialysis*, or flushing the kidney wastes by artificial means, may be instituted pending the transplant of a kidney from a live donor or a cadaver. Dialysis is of two kinds: *peritoneal* dialysis, which involves a three-day flushing within the body, and *hemodialysis*, or use of the artificial kidney machine. Peritoneal dialysis is described by those who have had it as very painful; however, some physicians use it as an adjunct to dietary therapy in an effort to prolong life without use of the kidney machine.

Life that is dependent on the kidney machine is not thought of as tolerable indefinitely; too many complications occur medically, and the suffering and financial cost are too great. It is used only during the period awaiting transplant or between unsuccessful transplants. Because transplantation is in itself not a cure but a prolongation, is still experimental especially for children, and has a substantial rate of complications and death in small children, some physicians do not consider dialysis acceptable for children. The family is advised to accept the child's death without subjecting him to the uncertainties and miseries of dialysis and transplantation. However, families who have heard of centers that provide the further treatment, and have the means to get to such a center, may not accept advice to permit the child to die.

Dialysis may be performed at home on adults, if the family has the necessary intellectual, emotional, and physical resources, after a period of training at the center. Young children are not dialyzed at home, since more complications can occur and there is "less margin for error" because of the child's physiology and smaller size. However, if necessary plumbing can be installed to permit use of the machine, and especially if the father is mechanically inclined, this more convenient and less expensive method may be used for adolescents. The youth who otherwise would have to come to the center two or three times a week and remain on the machine seven or eight hours each time, can sometimes sleep while being dialyzed at home at night, and the parent may sleep also, at least sporadically, instead of transporting the child many miles through city traffic and whiling away daytime hours at the bedside or returning later to pick him up.

Hemodialysis, or use of the machine, requires operative preparation of the child's blood vessels to permit the blood from his body to flow via tubes through the machine and back in after the uremic wastes have been extracted. A *shunt* may be prepared in the child's arm vessels or groin, which is large enough to admit the tubing; alternatively, one of his arm veins may be enlarged, or a *fistula* made into which a needle can be admitted. The shunt makes the dialysis procedure easier and less painful, but it limits the child's activity to some extent, because the shunt gradually closes as the arm is exercised. Therefore, fistulas are performed by and for some active children and young persons, especially if their dialysis program is carried on at a center rather than at home. Children who start with shunts have revisions, requiring further minor surgery, or eventually have fistulas created.

Dr. Donald Potter, in charge of treating children at the dialysis center of the University of California Medical Center in San Francisco, sets forth two broad categories of medical problems that disturb the well-being of a child on dialysis.[61] The first is that dialysis does not provide normal kidney function. Children are still subject to problems caused by uremia. They tend to accumulate salt and water, to have episodes of congestive heart failure and high blood pressure, with its accompanying headache. Dialysis does not correct the child's anemia, and as a consequence of the uremia and anemia, the child is lethargic and fatigues easily. Some children develop pericarditis, or infection of the outer lining of the heart, and some develop peripheral neuropathy, the painful neurological complaints earlier described (see pp. 203–4). Sexual impotence occurs, a major problem for adolescent boys. The severe growth retardation mentioned earlier adds to the adolescent's problems. Bone disease creates another common limitation.

The second category of physical problems of the child receiving dialysis pertains to the procedure, which includes shunt revisions at least twice a year. Some children do not feel well while on the machine and for hours after, with symptoms ranging from headache and vomiting to feelings of being, literally, "washed out." Some children have convulsions while being dialyzed. A variety of additional problems arise, including anemia from blood loss in the machine and from continued laboratory blood analyses, necessitating monthly transfusions to replace the loss. Because of the transfusions, and sometimes for other reasons including epidemics in the dialysis center, hepatitis often develops.

Though not frequent, accidents can happen while a child is on dialysis; the shunt can come apart, he can hemorrhage into the brain and sustain paralysis as a result, etc.

The problem that children complain about most is dietary restriction. If, prior to dialysis, they were on the modified Giovanetti diet previously described, the diet is less onerous though different. Dietary restrictions are more severe in children than in adults, because of their small size. This interferes with nutrition, which in turn creates physical problems. Whereas protein is the essential restriction in the diet before dialysis, the salt, fluid, and potassium restrictions become central while on dialysis.[62] Fluid is usually restricted to one quart a day. Constipation is a constant problem.

In commenting on dialysis and transplantation in children, the director of a large center says:[63]

> When extended hemodialysis and homotransplantation are offered to patients in the pediatric age group, there are always a number of children for whom the procedures involved in the treatment program and renal disease itself lead to so much suffering that the question arises whether it would not have been better to desist from treatment altogether. If it could only be predicted which children and which families are those for whom the prolongation of life is justified and which are those for whom rehabilitation will not be successful, decisions about selecting children for the treatment program could be made on a rational basis and with confidence. Unfortunately, so far, no one has the data to predict those families and those children who are good risks for rehabilitation and to identify those who had best be left alone.

Transplantation

The many discussions of transplantation indicate that some criteria have been evolved that guide pediatric nephrologists and surgeons in considering a child for this still rare and drastic procedure, despite some disagreement about details. If the child's disease is believed likely to recur in the new kidney, or if the child is too small, or if he has other widespread disease that has only secondarily destroyed kidney function, he is not generally considered a good candidate. However, because criteria do differ, success rates differ. The centers that are more highly selective have better rates of success. Another factor affecting success rate is the definition of success, and still another, whether the center uses live donors to the extent possible or relies on cadaveric donors. Matters not easily discernible to the outsider also materially affect the outcome, such as the skill of the transplant surgeon and his team, and the degree of coordination among the many specialists and auxiliary staff who participate in the transplanting of a kidney in a child.

Results are said to approximate those achieved in adults.[64] The Tenth Report of the Human Renal Transplant Registry, which provides data from Europe, Australia, and the United States, showed that of nearly 7,000 persons who received kidney transplants and who have been followed up, 62 percent were alive. Three-fourths of this group were surviving with a functioning transplanted kidney, and the others had returned to a life on the kidney machine.[65] Of those transplanted in 1969, 81 percent of those who had received a kidney from an adult sibling (a minor is not permitted to donate) were alive at the end of three years, 71 percent of those who had received kidneys from parents were alive, and 54 percent of those who had received kidneys from cadavers were alive.

The two California centers that provide kidney transplants for children published, in 1970 and 1971, results of treatment of the first sizable groups of children. The 1970 report, from the southern California center, showed that 19 of 23 children ages 2 to 17 years had survived 1 to 32 months with kidney transplants.[66] The report of 53 children treated from 1966 to 1970 at the northern California center showed 42 still alive when the report was prepared in 1971. Fifteen of the 53 had received transplants from living related donors and 16 had received cadaveric kidneys. (The remainder were on dialysis and/or dietary therapy.) Of these 31 children, eight had died, six of the eight in the group that received cadaveric kidneys.[67] Most notable to the lay person was that, of the eight who had died, six were little children weighing less than 65 pounds, although the report points out that cause of death "could be related only indirectly, if at all, to size."

Kidney transplantation is not universally available. Transplants are often repeated, if the body rejects the first kidney received. The person is maintained on dialysis between transplants. Despite the statistical evidence of greater success through use of a sibling or living related donor, the use of cadaveric kidneys is increasing. The reasons seem to relate to social considerations, to be discussed later. One center staff member pointed out the decreasing availability of cadaveric kidneys as more and more transplantations are being performed, or as demand exceeds supply. Another center reported an average wait of three years on dialysis for a cadaveric kidney.[68]

Most children who receive kidney transplants are either adolescents whose kidneys have failed from progressive glomerulonephritis or young children who have congenital abnormalities, nephrosis, or cancer. Preoperative procedures include tissue matching with potential live related donors, or placement on the computerized waiting list for a cadaver kidney with prior tests for the necessary medical data utilized in computer matching, and dialysis just before the operation. In some instances, the child's own useless kidneys are removed prior to the transplant (*nephrectomy*), and in others they are left in. The new kidney is placed in the abdominal cavity, where there is space for an adult kidney, not in the site of the child's old kidneys. The new kidney may be rejected by the body in the first few moments or within the next three months. If after this most critical period it is functioning well, the outlook for retention of the kidney is relatively good, though the body may reject it or complications may occur later. The northern California center's experience with 70 children who received kidney transplants showed that more than half the deaths and kidney rejections occurred in the first six months. The long-term outlook is reported to be good if the transplant holds for as long as two years.[69]

Complications include leakage of urine, gradual chronic rejection, urinary infections, high blood pressure, "transplant lung,"* diabetes, and marked weight gain caused by the effects of the immunosuppressive drugs used to keep the body from rejecting the kidney.[70] One authority states that, in general, surgical complications of transplantation are few and children do very well. The deaths that occur later are largely due to infection.[71] Another, who reported on 106 transplantations in 84 children, said that nine children died and 12 returned to dialysis, but that 80 percent of the total transplants resulted in a functioning new kidney. However, he enumerated 50 children with complications, either infections or problems created by the steroid treatment necessary to keep the kidney from rejecting. The latter included cataracts, diabetes, and ulcers.[72] It should be noted that chicken pox (*varicella*) and shingles (*herpes zoster*), a related virus infection, are very serious for persons taking steroid drugs such as prednisone or cortisone.

Growth failure is a complication of impaired kidney function and of the medication (prednisone) required after transplantation to keep the body from rejecting the kidney. "Growth failure is a complication that seriously affects the quality of life." Experiments are under way varying the dosages of prednisone to determine whether alternate-day administration or low dosage will mitigate its effects yet provide needed suppression of rejection.

* A peculiar syndrome resembling pneumonia, sometimes accompanying threatened rejection of the transplanted kidney or withdrawal of steroid drugs. (Felix T. Rapaport and Jean Dausset, eds., *Human Transplantation* [New York: Grune & Stratton, 1968], pp. 76, 124, 161.)

Thus far, both of the California centers have found that young children show more gains in growth than those who have passed puberty.[73]

PSYCHOSOCIAL IMPLICATIONS

The range and nature of kidney disease, and the variable social situations of the children affected, defeat attempts at categorization. Questions the worker must ask include, first, the kind of kidney disease the child has and, second, its severity and mode of treatment. Obviously, a child with urinary tract infection treated as an outpatient with sulfonamide drugs has a different life framework than a child with relapsing nephrosis treated with steroids, or a child dying with uremia, or a child surviving on dialysis. Gross social variables will come to mind immediately. A boy has a different set of problems than a girl; the child's age is of great importance. Perhaps nowhere is the family's capacity to deal with ambiguities taxed more than when a child is receiving treatment for renal failure; this capacity for understanding abstractions is often related to education, and thus usually to socioeconomic class. The manpower, both institutional and community, and its degree of communication are of equal importance, for skillful, long-term emotional support and help with practical minutiae vie in importance with the nephrologist's skill in outcome of treatment.

There are of course common elements—the pain, intrusive procedures, growth retardation, dependence, body image distortions, diet restriction, and interruptions in school and peer relationships for the child; the anxiety, heavy costs, time burdens, and disrupted relationships for the family. How strongly each of these threads affects the total warp of the family's life varies.

The Young Child

From the foregoing discussion of medical realities in chronic kidney disease, the frequently *early age of onset* stands out as a feature affecting psychosocial considerations. A French psychiatrist at the Children's Hospital in Paris described tersely and well the effect of painful illness and treatment on the development of the young child:[74]

A disease presents itself to the child as an indivisible ensemble made up of physical sensations localized internally, coupled with external aggressions mediated through medical investigations and treatments to which he must submit himself. While the child, during normal development, is constantly attempting to acquire control over the functioning of his body at the same time as he is consolidating ego controls, with the onset of illness he is in many ways dispossessed of his body, which becomes instead a supervised object for others who exercise absolute rights over it, observing it constantly and influencing its responses.... The adults who normally would support his autonomy and self-esteem demonstrate contradictory attitudes in driving him, in the service of his illness, in the direction of submission, dependence and passivity.

Some mothers who have been interviewed seem aware of how damaging and bewildering it would be to the child were they to become part of the group that "punished" him during the many needle injections and catheterizations of supervision and treatment. They have commented on how badly the child behaved during preschool years in screaming and kicking during medical procedures, and how they themselves have refused to help hold him or make him behave. However, the mother is inevitably caught up in the web of adults who "demonstrate contradictory attitudes" in the child's establishment of autonomy, in that she is the person who delivers him into the hands of the medical team and she must give medicines and must force or refuse foods.

The variable reactions children manifest are described in the literature, and have been commented on by staff of special centers. The guilt felt by little children when, during the stage of "magical thinking," they equate pain with punishment for wrongdoing, has been described in several reports. As long ago as 1948, a physician reported, "We have observed several children with hematuria [bloody urine] associated with acute nephritis, who were sure they had caused the damage through masturbation.... Their anxiousness was intense and interfered not only with their adaptation to hospital routines but with their capacity to participate in the therapeutic regimen laid down for them."[75]

The well-known self-blame that little children feel when something bad happens to them is thought by Korsch and Barnett to be aggravated by the feedback that irritable, cranky, miserable, nephrotic children receive. They point out that the negative responses evoked by the child's unpleasant behavior from the mother and others may make the child feel that he is "a very 'bad' child, and that he deserves to be punished."[76] These observers point out the further unfortunate nature of early onset of nephrosis from a developmental standpoint, commenting on the normal need during late infancy and early preschool years for a great amount of physical activity, exploration, and development of skills. The lethargy and malaise of kidney disease and the child's inability to use his body the way he normally would must retard his social development.

That children later repress these anxieties and develop one or more of several defenses including denial has been illustrated in interviews with two adolescents who have described seeing blood in the toilet at four or five years of age as the first warning of kidney disease. One "could not remember much about it," and the other recalled being very frightened but nothing more. One of the defenses the French psychiatrist describes, in addition to repression and denial, is what is termed in psychoanalytic terms "identification with the aggressor" or, in this case, identification with medical staff and becoming, in a sense, their own doctor or nurse.[77] It is a source of discomfort to those who observe and try to help the children become more "normal" that children with chronic renal disease become alienated from their peers through the illness experience, develop a substitute relationship with the medical center staff, and become extremely knowledgeable about the technicalities of their own and other children's medical conditions, using medical terms freely: "I became proteinuric."

Separation from the mother during the vulnerable period of infancy and early preschool age for repeated hospitalizations is another unfortunate aspect of the early onset of illness due to congenital anomalies, nephrosis, or nephritis.

Uncertainty over diagnosis may necessitate two or three brief periods of hospitalization, and, in the case of congenital anomalies, surgery not infrequently requires several more. Mothers interviewed spoke of leaving the child at the hospital so many times they could not remember the exact number, or of six times before the child was age five, or seven between the time he was five and eight, etc. Also typical was the small child's fearfulness of doctors, with crying beginning as soon as he was placed on the examining table and his shirt removed. One child autistically beat his head over and over on his father's shoulder, as he was held after the examination.

A young boy said he could remember the gloom of going to the hospital when he was little, "it was like being in a dark tunnel," but said that after he grew older he looked forward to the hospital because he knew they would make him feel better. The hospital activities were remembered with pleasure by adolescents who spoke retrospectively of their experiences with kidney disease. The kindness of one particular staff member stood out—for example, an X-ray technician who was a ventriloquist, and a head nurse who over the years "was like a mother" to the mother as well as to the child.

Parental anxiety doubtless is conveyed to the child, making the separation more fearful. In each of four cases where Mexican-American parents were interviewed, the parents were afraid to ask the doctor questions, or the one doctor who spoke Spanish had left, and the parents were worried and uncertain about what was happening. In three of these instances the parents had had traumatic experiences during the diagnostic period, with the family physician either downplaying the child's symptoms and their alarm, or not knowing what was wrong, and taking no action until the child became comatose, in convulsions or badly swollen and unable to urinate.

More articulate Anglo mothers spoke feelingly of their worry because of the uncertain outlook, and the fact that there was no end in sight to the child's problem. One mother, however, said the doctor's honesty in this regard had given her great security; that being able to believe him and to know he would tell her as much as he could was a source of great comfort to her. In general, however, the lack of specific information about course and outlook may open the way for parental guilt and aggravate the intense worry.

In a parents' group discussion, Dr. Korsch reports that the parents emphasized "the great need of their children to play out their hospital experiences as a step in mastering them. The parents reported that the children collected urine specimens from their dolls at home, gave injections and transfusions to their Teddy bears and generally inflicted upon their toys and pets all the indignities to which they had been subjected by the medical personnel."[78] The same group brought out "how much the child needs the support of the parents' repeated presence when sick and away from home."

The normal developmental surge for self-control in the young child, which is largely defeated by the adults who drive him, "in the service of his illness, in the direction of submission, dependence and passivity," can and does assert itself in the struggle over food.[79] Carol Levin has pointed out that one way the child can be the master is to refuse to eat—no one can make him swallow, or keep him from spitting up. The critical importance of calories for growth, and of the right amount of the right kind of protein, becomes the focus for "the all-time battle" between mother and child.[80] Two things seem to happen: either the mother gives up and allows the child to control, by eating almost nothing and only those things he likes, or she stays in a state of constant anxiety trying to devise ways to get the child to eat.

The age of the child at onset should provide one guide to the worker in the amount of help she attempts to muster—if the child is young, when stunting will make him a virtual dwarf, the issue is an important one. Not all hospitals or special centers provide individual diet counseling to the mothers, so that the worker's first task is to learn the extent and kind of professional help the mother is getting. A diet list may have been handed to the mother that looks manifestly impossible—"2 oz. of KNa free string beans, 2 oz. of KNa free heavenly hash"—so that she gives up on sight and permits the child to eat a sandwich or chocolate cookie, if this is what appeals to him. A competent, interested dietician, who over a period of time will help the mother incorporate the intricacies of the renal diet, and provide suggestions regarding where to buy, what to buy, and how to make recipes that may tempt and also fit in with the family's food habits and budget, is the first line of defense. The meaning to the child and to the mother of the dietary struggle need not be interpreted to the mother, but the worker needs to be sensitive to the total interplay between the two and to observe how the diet problem fits into the whole. If the struggle for mastery can be switched to other areas, and the intensity of the child's relationship with the mother attenuated through the opportunity for peer relationships, and the child motivated to eat because he sees other children doing so, he may find he can swallow foods and keep them down.

The financial aspect of the renal diet should not be ignored in exploring what the dietary problem consists of. Unlike the diabetic or obesity diet, the renal diet does require purchases from a health food store or the dietetic section of a large grocery; the investment may be difficult or seem unwise if the child is not likely to eat the preparations after they are purchased; in addition, transportation to special stores may be difficult. The calorie supplements, if used as ordered, may cost $100 or more a month, and the family may not have this readily available or may fail to understand the importance of the expenditure. Resources for the supplements should be explored with the special center if this is found to be true. The Kidney Foundation clubs sometimes stock special needs in "co-op" form; private health agencies of broad scope, such as the Tuberculosis and Health Associations in some communities, are willing to provide such tangible health needs.

Latency and Early Adolescence

Scattered through the case reports are those of older children who developed signs of kidney disease suddenly after an infection, or who had no warning of impaired kidney function until a broken leg or routine school examination included a urinalysis that alerted the physician and family to the child's serious kidney disease. In addition, it will be recalled that, although nephrosis may begin during preschool years, it may relapse over a period of ten or more years, and that glomerulonephritis ending in renal failure peaks at adolescence.

Adolescence covers a long period: the child at 12 to 14 is a different person from the young man at 18 or 19. The onset of puberty is most frequently the precipitant of renal failure, and this is also the time of greatest social stress. Entry into junior high school has been shown to be the most stressful period for children in general.[81] When asked why, they mention changing classes and the difference from the sixth grade. Though the lack of support from one teacher and instead having several teachers and changing classes doubtless are important, expectations may cause more of the stress. The American teenager is expected by the public, and therefore by the child, to be unpredictable, peculiar, or lawless; teenage is the beginning of independence; the golden age of childhood is over. For a child who, perforce, must have been dependent because of his physical condition, who has had to rely on his family for social contacts rather than primarily on peers, whose very social development has been interrupted by long-term or relapsing illness, the fantasied demand for independence must be very great indeed. For the child who has not been ill long, the disappointment must be severe.

It is at this time—the onset of puberty, when sexual changes and impulses occur—that the body-image distortions of kidney disease, and the juxtaposition of urinary outlet and sexual anatomy, might be expected to create most severe psychological problems. In a study of normal adolescents, the children were found at early adolescence to have *"greater instability of the self-image,"* lower self-esteem, lower opinions of themselves, and less conviction that others hold favorable opinions of them; they were also more prone to depressive feelings.[82]

Establishing a stable self-image has been described as one of the main "tasks" of adolescence; at this age the child is very body-oriented and the early developer has the greatest advantage. The small child with delayed adolescence has been described as developing the "little-man syndrome," or the "mascot syndrome." Physically normal boys can work off their feelings of aggression acceptably, primarily through sports, and are said to have fewer problems with self-image than girls for this reason. However, the handicapped boy who cannot gravitate to heterosexual interests with his peers is quickly identified as less than masculine, and his parents see him as less than a whole boy.[83]

One of the older boys interviewed used almost the identical words of the academicians in telling the anguished story of his relationship with his parents during adolescence. He was deeply wounded by lack of respect from his father; he said that his father did not think of him as "whole," or in the same terms as he did his younger brother, who could go hunting and fishing with him.

The growth retardation of long-term kidney disease and steroid treatment, and the uncontrollable and unpredictable distortions when the body swells with edema, pain occurs in the head or legs, food nauseates, the urine dries up or is the wrong color, and sleepiness is overwhelming—these manifestations must make the task of "establishing a stable body image" during adolescence a difficult one indeed. And because friends are so important in establishing a satisfactory self-image, the weakness that prevents keeping up with active peers is a further realistic hurdle.

One girl described to me getting through junior high school satisfactorily, because she felt relatively well and her diet was not restricted; this was the time when the others were eating french fries and candy, and she could also. However, she started "getting weak," and in the fall, when she went to high school, she had to drop physical education because she found she could not run around the block as required; she would fall asleep in study hall, and had to fight to stay awake to study. She pushed herself to go to a few football games with friends, but it was difficult. She tried to keep her problems to herself. When she was 14, she entered the hospital, evidently in renal failure, and "took 56 pills a day."

The physical problems that interfere with fulfilling the normal tasks of adolescence may actually heighten the emotional struggle with parents. Ordinarily, teenagers are critical of parents and go out of their way to be different from them, in life-style, hair length, religious or political beliefs, all to accomplish eventual differentiation from family to independent and separate identities. Although no studies have been seen in the literature, observation indicates that teenagers who must remain physically dependent on parents have heightened guilt and conflict about their negative feelings toward the parents. In a few cases they are openly defiant, refusing to take medicine or stay on a diet, or they act irritable and arrogant at home. These seem less unhealthy emotionally than others who seem to have a long-delayed emancipation process and remain childlike and docile.

Adolescents who have the advantage of some creative capacities, good intellect, or special talent, and who receive the necessary recognition, guidance, and instruction, may sublimate their emotional drives into constructive channels. The worker can play an active part in helping the young person discover his talents and receive encouragement and direction through the various resources of the community. It seems sensible to avoid a field of activity in which the parent of the same sex has special competence, to the inevitable discouragement of the child. Encouraging feminine activities in girls and career potentialities in boys helps the child establish his sexual identity.

The adolescent by no means always responds to overtures toward development of interests. Workers often are discouraged when, after investing substantial time and thought in opening channels for a child's activity, the child fails to keep appointments, or fails to continue. The lethargy of kidney disease may be responsible, or the child may be undergoing headache or pain that interferes. Depression may also be the underlying reason the child has little interest in investing himself in anything. Depression in childhood takes many forms, and is not entirely the same as clinical depression in adults.

One authority says that most adolescents express depressive feelings by boredom, restlessness, hypochondriasis, impaired concentration, "acting out," and pursuit of constant stimulation from the radio, television, stereo, drugs, alcohol, poetry, and sexual activity.[84] He states that the depressed adolescent is disorganized and anxious, feels empty, and has poor judgment and perception; that anxiety is the predominant feature, driving the person to seek alternately new thrills and isolation. He postulates that depression is often due to "object loss." This observation closely ties in with experience that loss of sight or mobility creates depression, in contrast to the feelings of young persons who have a congenital defect with which they have grown up. If this proves true over time in respect to adolescents with kidney disease, depression may be more frequent in those whose renal failure develops suddenly late in childhood than in children who have had relapsing nephrosis since early childhood, or whose impaired kidney function follows repeated infections that are due to congenital defect or other congenital kidney disease.

Another psychiatrist who has written about childhood depression makes the helpful point that hopelessness is the critical element in the development of depression. "It is at the point when an individual experiences a sense of helplessness and then begins to give up hope that the feeling of depression occurs. Thus the depressive effect is the result of a helpless position in which the individual gradually gives up hope for relief either through rescue or through his own efforts."[85]

Accordingly, the worker who attempts to help the adolescent with kidney disease develop constructive interests, and to find his identity as a worthwhile human being despite his physical impairment, needs to bear in mind the various possible causes of lack of interest in resources. If failed appointments or other signs of disinterest occur, the worker needs to learn the physical state of the young person, and whether advanced uremia is sufficient cause or whether feelings of hopelessness have dulled his motivation. The hopelessness may be in one of several directions, and can only be dealt with when the problem is understood.

Family relationships cannot be normal when one child has had a serious illness over a long period. The eroding quality of protracted anxiety when a child alternates between feeling well and hanging near death, or of uncertainty whether he is really well this time or will be plunged into even greater danger; the worry when his course is downhill and dotted by new and different complications; the years of sacrificing to try to help him, only to be met by repeated bouts of illness, or his impending death—these experiences demand the utmost in adaptability, and even so take their toll. The child who must stay home much of the time because he lacks energy to be out, and lacks the friends he would have otherwise, is unusually affected by family feelings and activities. Boys are more often affected by the common constellation of family impairment than girls, because of the intensity of their dependence on the mother and the all-too-frequent rejection or seeming indifference of the father to a weakling son. Since this three-way disjunction has been elaborated elsewhere (see the chapters on hemophilia and muscular dystrophy), it is not repeated here. However, as an underlying cause of hopelessness, the family attitudes toward the boy must be kept in mind. Working with the father, or with both parents, may be more important in freeing the child than direct intervention with him.

Dialysis and Transplantation

The decision to prolong life. California centers have found the lower socioeconomic group underrepresented in dialysis and transplant centers. Speculation about cause includes the probability that local physicians screen out children whose families they believe could not cope with the problems involved in dialysis and transplantation. Lack of knowledge of resources may prevent some lower-income families from insisting on the opportunity. Infants and young children of the poor may die of acute disease or complications before coming to chronic renal failure, owing to lack of family capacity to provide recommended medication, diet, and supervision.

A possible reason the poor are underrepresented is that persons who think concretely may have less difficulty in decision making; having less capacity to perceive details, they may see major issues in bolder outline. The capacity to bear ambiguity, of having a child half alive and half dead, may also be less in those who think simplistically. Religious ideas may be a factor, that is, leaving the child's death to God rather than to medical center staff.

Khan et al., who have reported in depth their experience with children treated at the Children's Memorial Hospital in Chicago, state that most parents, confronted with the choice of permitting the child to die from uremia or placing him under a dialysis-transplant program, recoil from letting him die; they have second thoughts primarily because of the pain the child will have to endure, but then decide they must accept the opportunity for extension of his life.[86]

The part that members of the medical profession play in decision making is very great, for much depends on the manner in which they interpret the choices to the family. A few children are ruled out by center physicians because of medical considerations such as other systemic diseases, and the family is given no choice; in other cases, the center staff minimizes the grim possibilities and presents such an optimistic picture that the family can do nothing but consent. One center staff member commented on the difficulty the medical team has in determining how much to tell a family. She said the parents should know enough to have some idea of what to expect, but if they are told too much they may not permit treatment.

Once the child is accepted into the dialysis-transplant program, the medical staff and the family may arrive at different times at the decision to permit death in case treatment is not effective and the child's course is bleak. Parents who visit only in the evenings, or afternoons after most of the "procedures" have been done, may be unaware of how much agony the child is going through; however, there are parents who actually suffer more than the child and, not having his resiliency, may be emotionally overwhelmed. Other family pressures, feelings of grief and loss, may aggravate their emotional burdens, whereas a research-oriented staff may be interested in pursuing further treatment possibilities.

The need for close and continuing communication between family and center staff is clearly an urgent matter. The worker in the community who is aware that parents seldom visit when physicians are on duty, or that the center has either no social worker or one who is not working with the child in question, should take the initiative in attempting to arrange conferences between parents and physicians, the chief resident physician, or chief of staff when possible. If the center has a social worker, this should be arranged through her. Often medical center personnel are unaware of family problems and would welcome a better understanding of the total situation so their decisions could be more soundly based. The worker should be aware that parents may avoid seeing the doctor, either consciously or unconsciously, and may put up barriers to such conferences. In such an instance the worker needs to interview the parents in sufficient depth and length to give opportunity for expression of feelings.

At what age the child himself should be permitted to make the decision about his own death is not known. A few adolescents are reported among the dialysis suicides; they are able to kill themselves by pulling the shunt or overeating and overdrinking. The premature aging that accompanies prolonged suffering in childhood perhaps enables the older adolescent to make a seasoned judgment about whether he wants to live. However, the uremic symptoms of confusion, drowsiness, and occasionally psychotic manifestations, and the labile nature of adolescence, must be taken into account. The literature reports a rational decision by a 16-year-old to discontinue treatment, after prolonged attempts at treatment and a bleak outlook.[87] In one case an 11-year-old boy made the decision to tolerate no more procedures. In confronting his situation, the staff believed he had incorporated his parents' decision, and was, without knowing it, relieving them of the guilt of deciding to take him home to die; they could feel comfortable in the belief they were abiding by his wishes.

Decisions about permitting uremic death versus dialysis and transplant may be expected to increase since financing has become available through Medicare (see p. 221). Waiting periods on dialysis for transplants will become longer as more patients compete for the cadaver kidneys available; and the complications and misery of prolonged dialysis should be kept in mind. Therefore, the decision-making process deserves thought. The worker in the community and the family should be active participants in the decision-making group, and should arrive at their decisions fully informed of the possibilities this particular child faces if treated in the particular center involved. They must not be put off by generalized national statistics, or by evasive answers, or by personal pessimistic tendencies, or yet by excessive solicitude. The whole family's well-being must be taken into account. Respect for the child's life, his right to die with dignity or to have a chance to live, should underlie a shared decision based on full knowledge of knowable facts.

Financial problems and provisions. Dialysis was reported in 1972 by a Midwestern investigator as costing approximately $14,000 a year, home dialysis $10,000 to $12,000 the first year when equipment is purchased, and about $4,000 after that.[88] Current northern California figures are higher, one center reporting about $25,000 for the first year if a youth is dialyzed at home, this amount including $5,000 for the home training sessions and $7,000 for equipment; if, however, the person is dialyzed at the center, the cost is about $15,000 the first year and $2,000 to $5,000 after that.[89] Another major institution reports $30,000 a year for a year's dialysis, at $200 "per run" or session.[90]

In a historic step, the Social Security Administration expanded its Medicare provisions, effective July 1, 1973, to include dialysis and transplant services for wage earners, their dependents, and retirees.[91] A child is eligible if either parent qualifies as a "currently or fully insured wage earner" (or retiree). To be currently insured, the parent must have worked one and a half years out of the last three in Social Security–covered employment; to be fully insured, he must have worked at least six quarters, one quarter for each year that elapses after he reaches 21. Most children will be eligible under these provisions, since the only ones excluded will be those whose parent or parents have never worked, or worked only a short time, under Social Security–covered employment or whose wage-earning parent cannot be located.

Some readjustment of thinking is required to apply Medicare, the provision ordinarily thought of in connection with the aged, to a child. The law places dialysis and transplant treatment under Part B of Medicare, or that part that pertains to outpatient services. This enables the Social Security Administration to pay for physicians' services and laboratory work. However, dialysis may be provided in a hospital or another approved facility or at home. The transplant coverage includes hospital, physician, and other costs for removal of a kidney from a live donor or cadaver, in addition to surgical and hospital care of the patient. At this writing, there is no limitation on the number of transplants that may be paid for if the child's body rejects the transplanted kidney.

Medicare coverage ends 12 months after successful transplant. A kidney that is rejected after that time, requiring the child to have renewed dialysis and eventually another transplant, would be financed according to the original provisions. Limitations on the extent of Medicare payments will mean that the parent must pay part of the costs, or have insurance that does so, or receive Crippled Children's Services or Medicaid. Payment for chronic hemodialysis does not begin until the third month in which dialysis begins, and Medicare pays only 80 percent of "reasonable charges." The deductible feature of other Medicare provisions also applies. Nor are prescription drugs paid for under Medicare, which means that the steroid drugs necessary to keep the body from rejecting the kidney are not included. The many drugs the child may need for complications of chronic kidney failure and treatment such as high blood pressure, cataracts, and bone disease would not be included.

Because the Medicare coverage of dialysis and transplant treatment is so new, the worker may expect revisions in their regulations as the Social Security Administration gains experience. The worker may need to be supportive of the parents when frustration occurs during snarls and red tape, and help them get to appropriate supplementing agencies and also back to the hospital eligibility worker and the District Office of the Social Security Administration. But despite limitations, the new Medicare provisions for dialysis and transplant relieve the parents of the major part of the paralyzing financial burden associated with these life-extending measures. Most gratifying is the release of parents from agency means tests and pay-back provisions that have made other public medical services so burdensome for many families in recent years. The psychological benefits to the child that stem from the parents' release from the heaviest part of financial worries may easily be inferred.

An unknown feature of the Social Security program is the rippling effect it may have on spread of dialysis and transplant services to children of low-income families. Possibly, some children who would not have been referred by the local attending physician to a special center earlier will be, now that the major part of the cost of these services has been removed from the parents. Another effect that cannot be foretold is the shift from home dialysis to that at special centers. Although Medicare may be expected to try to hold the line against such a shift because of the greater expense involved, many patients and families may press for center care. Workers who know the constellation of family feelings and circumstances may have important contributions to make in the decisions about care of individual patients by providing information about them to the center worker or the Social Security office, depending on how Medicare administration crystallizes its procedures for evaluation.

Transportation to the dialysis center two or three times a week, expensive special health foods, costly food supplements, the portion of medical care not covered by Medicare, and the many miscellaneous expenses of illness, including telephone calls, remain to create a financial burden on the family. One young adult who had spent his teen years in renal failure and had had dialysis several years commented perceptively, "One of the most important ways social workers can help is by being up to date about financial measures to relieve the parents. Then they can look on the child as a child, not just a burden. Resources for finances makes it possible for a parent to respect his child, and to think of his other needs, not just how to pay his medical bills."

Fortunately, the drama of dialysis and transplant does open avenues to provide the families with the costly food supplements, or the medical center occasionally prepares and sends home the formulas for young children whose diet must be carefully controlled. One case is reported in the literature of a medical center social worker who secured an automobile for a mother who could not come to the hospital to visit her daughter, seriously ill after transplant rejection.[92] The amount of time and skill necessary to provide for supplemental needs from private sources is well known to all experienced social practitioners, but the enormous investment necessary to treat a child with renal failure may be wasted unless secured by these efforts.

Because transportation to the dialysis center is such a substantial problem, the worker may consider helping the family move near the center. The length of time a child may be expected to be on dialysis may influence the wisdom of uprooting the family. Although no definitive answer can be expected from center physicians, some questions that shed light on duration of dialysis include whether the anticipated transplantation is from a family member or cadaver and, if the latter, the average wait in that community for cadaveric donors. Other questions pertain to the physician's estimate of the child's general condition in respect to success or failure of the anticipated transplant, and his outlook for life. Whereas answers to these questions would be qualified at best—and perhaps there are no answers—in some cases negative factors are known to exist, and might have obvious bearing on the wisdom of a family's move from one community to another. Communication between the worker in the community and the hospital social worker is essential, and a conference between the parents, community social practitioner, and hospital staff may prove helpful.

Diet. As indicated earlier, the size of the child and his chemical balance affect the restrictions in his diet, so that differences exist between diets of different children and change for the same child. The usual dialysis diet is much less restrictive than the diet prescribed while the child was using his damaged or failing kidneys to excrete wastes and maintain chemical balance. Nevertheless, a low-sodium, low-potassium diet and marked fluid restriction are usually necessary during the period of dialysis. One dietician pointed out that palatability depends heavily on the mother's interest in cooking, and her willingness to chop, peel, and mix, rather than relying on TV dinners and other convenience foods in markets.

Low-sodium baking powder is available in the health food stores, so that bread, cake, cookies, etc. can be made at home, as well as pastries that do not require a rising agent. Low-salt peanut butter is relied on heavily for sandwiches, and the child on dialysis can eat regular bread and butter. Protein is not restricted enough to cause a problem. Fruits and vegetables are apt to be high in potassium, especially bananas and potatoes. All canned vegetables have salt except those in dietetic pack. Potato chips and french fried potatoes are probably the snack foods most missed by adolescents; poor families that have relied on frankfurters, pizzas, salami, baloney, and other meats high in salt and preservatives have difficulty finding substitute proteins they can afford.

In practice, children with long-term kidney disease are usually accustomed to low-salt food and do not mind it; their appetites frequently are poor, so that they are not motivated to cheat; and, unfortunately, their peer relationships are usually so meager that they are not in social situations where they are tempted to eat like other teenagers. The problems that do arise stem from the mother's inability to accustom herself to cooking, or her indifference to the child's needs, or to hot-weather trials for the child who is limited to one quart of fluid a day. A constant sense of thirst is said to accompany this severe fluid restriction, and in warm climates or during hot weather the child may drink more colas or Kool-Aid than his body can handle, which results in edema. To some extent the child is "conditioned" not to go beyond the prescribed limits, Carol Levin points out, because if he does he has to be dialyzed to draw off the fluid, and many children dread the period on the machine.[93]

The experience of dialysis. The children's reaction to dialysis also varies. Many have substantial discomfort, from nausea and vomiting, headache or backache, or they have strange sensations that are frightening. The pain of needle or cannula insertion is influenced by whether the shunt is infected. Some children have neurological symptoms, including convulsions. The alarm bell that goes off when any of the mechanical systems goes awry creates nervousness in children who are new to dialysis, as does the sight of the blood flowing around the ropes of glass tubing on the console. However, older children who have grown accustomed to dialysis, physiologically and psychologically, seem to read, study, or perform such craft work as they can. Children with shunts in the groin are virtually immobilized because they must lie still while attached to the machine, but they can use their arms and hands for craft work or holding a book if they feel well enough. Those with shunts in the arm are prevented from any activities, and can only watch bedside TV or take refuge in sleep.

Some children consciously try to drift into sleep or half-sleep to dull the pain and while away time. Other children may cry out, or demand attention for various discomforts. Small children whose mothers remain at the bedside are said to demand more attention and to indicate greater discomfort than those who do not have someone available to sympathize and fetch for them.

Living by means of dialysis unquestionably imposes severe stress on the child, for he lives not only with the three-days-a-week disruption in normal activities at a developmental period when time is most effectively used in learning and socialization, but he lives with some symptoms of uremia—nausea, weakness, and drowsiness—and various pains from bone disease or high blood pressure. The feedback he receives from family and friends must inevitably impose a self-image of a dependent, strange, burdensome person.

The shunt itself is a cause of some problems. This loop of tubing attached from vein to artery, frequently in the inner aspect of the arm above the wrist though variously placed in children who have had several revisions, is wound with bandage. It looks as if the child has had an injury, and therefore is a constant invitation to questions from the curious. "I just tell them about it when they ask," said one adolescent, adding with a smile, "but of course I don't tell them all the details." The shunt must be kept out of water, so that bathing is awkward, and if the shunt is in the groin, the child can have neither tub bath nor shower. The shunt site must be protected from injury—as one mother said, "After all, it is her life line, so she's going to be pretty careful of it." In give-and-take with other children, hitting back is allowed by some parents, "providing they don't hit him below the waist" in case of a groin-placed shunt; in other instances the child may not receive retaliatory blows from siblings or physical punishment, or be permitted active play with other young children.

Preparation of the child. The extent of preparation of the child for the dialysis experience varies in centers according to his medical condition and the medical care provisions. The Toronto Hospital for Sick Children has an integrated service that permits prolonged preparation by skilled staff of those children who have progressive renal failure, for dialysis awaiting transplant. The child visits the dialysis ward, sees the equipment, attends group meetings, etc.[94] However, in cases where the kidney failure is acute, or the child is referred to the center at the last minute by a local physician, or if the center has fragmented service in which the pediatrics, nephrology, and dialysis staffs work separately, the experience may be sudden and frightening. If a worker knows that a child is having a shunt prepared for dialysis, questions should be raised with the parents regarding the preparation they and the child have for the experience. If they are not undergoing psychological preparation, the worker in the community should ask the center worker if plans can be made for it.

Home dialysis. Training of a family to dialyze a child at home seems customarily to require about two months. A mechanically minded, emotionally stable adolescent patient may be one of the team of two needed to participate. However, an unstable adolescent, or one who has an intense relationship with his mother that makes him demanding and irritable with her, may make it impossible for her to manage the procedure. Fear and revulsion may make the mother unable to dialyze the child, or she may show during the training experience insufficient intelligence or general coping ability to make a trustworthy technician. On the other hand, a father who has been virtually excluded and has felt helpless concerning his child may be able to take charge of the dialysis. Because home dialysis is a burden on the parent and greater security exists in the hospital center, pressure to dialyze at a center may be expected as Medicare funds are available. The machine and auxiliary equipment do not take up more space than a kitchen table or a desk, but the presence of medical equipment is a constant physical reminder of machine-dependence. For adolescents who are potential candidates, decisions about home-based versus center dialysis should take into account the family relationships and feelings of siblings, as well as transportation and the plumbing and wiring capacity of the home. A worker who knows the family should make her information available to the center social worker and support the mother or usual caretaker in pressing for a decision based on all the facts.

Home and school relationships under dialysis. Dependency is a central feature of a life that is dependent on artificial measures, be these pacemakers, pills, kidney machines, or other devices. The loss of mastery, and its accompanying fear of death, has to be repressed in order to go about normal activities. Little children, being normally dependent, will not have conflicts in renal failure about general dependency that may be expected later. Adolescents, in the process of breaking the bonds of dependency, might be expected to have extreme conflict. No study is known of adolescents' attitudes toward this aspect of living on dialysis. The youths observed have used massive denial or sublimation to keep themselves in control; though an undertone of sadness is present, they do not talk openly of their feelings of resentment or dependence on parents and the machine. A superficially "good adjustment" by the majority is reported in the studies that have been seen.[95]

Just how disrupting the experience of dialysis is depends on several factors: whether the child is dialyzed four hours or seven, and whether two or three times a week; how far the family must travel to the center, whether 20 minutes or two hours each way; how many months or years the child has been on dialysis; and how flexible the center is with regard to hours of dialysis. In the northern California center, children may be on the machines early or late in order to avoid missing school or to miss as little school as possible; in the southern California center, everyone is dialyzed between 7:00 A.M. and 3:00 P.M.; thus these children miss school three days a week.

Through the use of home teachers and teleteaching aids, and by utilizing special education class facilities at times, most children in the dialysis-transplant program seem to have lost a minimal amount of schooling. The University of California Medical Center at San Francisco analyzes the psychosocial attributes of children treated there; of the first 28 studied, 20 children demonstrated intellectual and academic growth of average or above.[96] Surprisingly, children with long-term renal disease often seem to be only one year behind grade, despite the amount of time they have been drowsy or (when very ill) unable to stay awake, and in spite of the fatigue that sometimes prevents them from going to school. Most remarkable is the ability to remain at about expected grade level when on dialysis, in spite of the discontinuity of schooling. It is possible that the child is promoted to the next grade partly from compassion; his actual knowledge level may be lower than that of his classmates in some cases. The higher-than-average socioeconomic level of children in the dialysis programs may also mean more intellectual stimulation at home than is the norm.

However, a general lack of interest in school activities is a serious indicator of the social disturbance that renal disease creates. Children tend to have solitary interests, to prefer to stay home. Inability to participate in extracurricular activities and to sustain social relationships with schoolmates evidently devitalizes the school experience, giving it less priority than school ordinarily carries for the school-age child.

Korsch presents a bright picture of work with pediatric patients: in an analysis of 84 patients, 55 of whom were one year post-transplant, all but two of the older children were in school or employed and all but two of the younger children were in school. However, this study reported what had been found at the northern California center, that social adaptation had suffered. Dr. Korsch suggested that this could be because the controls "put their best foot forward" in the tests,[97] but Miss Levin finds the children definitely deficient in peer relationships and ability to relate to other children.[98] One bright 16-year-old girl told the author she had at one time wanted to be a nurse, but "now I have second thoughts. I think I would rather just stay home and cook." She denied that a boyfriend had entered the picture. Miss Crittenden, the psychologist member of the team who has interviewed teachers, states that the teachers report the children are "different."[99]

The interruption in relationships created by lying on a bed three days out of seven hooked to a machine, over a long period of time, is self-evident. Only those children who receive a successful transplant relatively quickly and whose medical complications are minimal could be expected to maintain meaningful relationships outside their families unless they have unusual resources. One mother of a seven-year-old boy told of her attempts to keep a young friend coming to the house at least once every two weeks, but "It doesn't work out. Kids that age want to run and wrestle and tumble, and when Kevin can't, the other boy just isn't interested." She felt her child was fortunate in having brothers and sisters, and this appears to be an important factor in the capacity of a chronically ill child to maintain relatively normal social relationships.

The kidney transplant. Children on dialysis look forward, at first, to the wonderful day when they will have a successful new kidney; the transplant is said to be vested with magic. Korsch et al. point out that actual preparation for the transplant by removal of the child's own kidneys (which may or may not be done) is difficult for both child and parents to accept.

"The child himself mourns the loss of part of himself and is troubled by his subsequent complete failure to urinate on his own with the incumbent, apparently even more complete dependence on the machine."[100]

The search for a living related donor may raise problems for families and older children. Siblings are thought to provide the best tissue match, but since minors are not permitted to donate, only children old enough to have an adult sibling have such opportunity. Centers vary in the amount to which medical staff participate in the donor search, but seem usually to leave it up to the family to determine among themselves who will donate. The hypersensitivity felt by the patient in asking someone in the family for a kidney is described by Simmons and Klein,[101] who say that hints are thrown out and direct communication among the group does not ordinarily take place. Mothers most often offer, and small children take it for granted that the mother should give her kidney.[102] The fact has been pointed out that it is easier for a spouse to ask relatives if anyone is willing to donate than for the patient himself to ask; similarly, it is probably easier for a mother to ask in behalf of her child, in case her own tissue proves incompatible.

Donors are actually at infinitesimal risk by virtue of having only one kidney;[103] nevertheless, the pain and risk of any major operation do exist, and potential donors are doubtless aware that their sacrifice may be in vain, that the kidney may be rejected or the life of the patient may not be saved by the donation. However, the literature review of the subject by the Simmons team reports that many donors feel like heroes, achieving deep feelings of inner satisfaction from the sacrifice.[104] That problems lurk for others is evident. Carol Levin states that prior to the transplant the donor receives much praise and publicity, but as soon as the operation is over, the attention turns to the patient, and he is back in obscurity.[105]

Such intense and complicated relationships between donor and donee have been observed that some centers prefer cadaver donors in spite of the greater probability of success if a living related donor gives the kidney. Mother-child relationships cannot be normal when a child has been suffering from renal failure and is brought back from death after great misery, family sacrifice, and the drama attendant on transplant. Guilt and obligation are to be expected on the part of the child, as well as feelings of possession and control on the part of the donor, and depression in both if the kidney is rejected. Bernstein reports the depression of a 16-year-old boy whose body rejected his brother's kidney: "Things became different between Ed and me. It was like one of his good kidneys was thrown in the garbage can. I felt like jumping off the Rand tower."[106]

Simmons and Simmons say that patients evidently accept cadaver kidneys without conflict, but may find it difficult if the donor is not yet dead and the patient must wait an appreciable length of time for him to be declared dead or if, after waiting, the cadaver's kidney is found unusable.[107]

Post-Transplant Adjustment

The complexity and difficulties of a transplant operation are easily apparent. Yet the vital consideration psychologically is its success. The bodies of some children do accept the transplant, and although the children undergo temporary unpleasant aftereffects, they receive new life for an indefinite period. Some persons are known to be alive as long as six years after transplant. One young girl with a successful outcome was attractive, going to college, working weekends, and expecting to be married. But even her story revealed a high price. Her mother was a "nervous wreck," she said; the parents had decided she should be the only child when they found she had kidney disease at age two; her parents' lives had been lived around helping her become a well-adjusted and healthy person; when she was on massive steroids post-transplant, was fat and grew hair on her face, a high school boy had touched her face and said, "You need a shave." This seemed the low point for her, other than two events of physical torture she described, one when she had peritoneal dialysis, and the other when as a little girl she was forcefully held in a university medical center examining room and catheterized at the same time that blood was drawn from her arm.

The University of California psychosocial tests show that some children show an upsurge intellectually after transplant; this is reported elsewhere in the literature. It is as if the new lease on life is total; release from symptoms of uremia and from life on the machine thrusts the person forward socially and intellectually. But unfortunately, the life after transplant is often stormy physically, and therefore filled with apprehensions and periods of depression. Some children reject three or four kidneys, and end the series of surgical traumas by going back on dialysis for an indefinite future. They may have developed painful bone disease, intractable high blood pressure, antibodies against further transplants, side effects of steroids; their lives have become torture.

Even those who have a successful operation have common problems for a year or more. Weight gain is one of the most distressing to teenagers, and difficult for parents. Immediately after the transplant begins to work, the prednisone they take to prevent rejection (and perhaps pre-transplant poor appetite) creates an extraordinary appetite. During hospitalization, they order sandwiches all day, eating and storing four or five more for continuous consumption. They continue to eat as if they are starved after they return home, with the inevitable result. To their own disgust, and that of their parents, they become obese, developing also the "Cushingoid features" of steroid treatment: a puffy face, acne, and in some instances facial hair. Some adolescent girls feel such despair over their appearance that they stop the anti-rejection medicine, with disastrous results.

The pathological hunger wears off when the prednisone is reduced after the first year, but the weight gain can be restricted if the child and mother are helped to realize the cosmetic consequences of overeating and are encouraged to avoid fattening foods and to exercise will power. The worker who is seeing the child and family should work on this problem if the child is a girl and especially if she is of junior high school age, when self-image disturbance is great, or if other factors signal the probability of self-image distress (for example, if the mother is petite and pretty and therefore difficult for the girl to compete with at best).

The growing literature from different centers about children's adaptation to transplantation indicates that extreme behaviors such as suicide and psychosis are the exception. However, reports also indicate that difficult and painful adjustments are the rule.[108] Ambivalent relationships with donors, and various indicators of depression and anxiety, are to be expected. Because most transplanted children are teenagers rather than little children, they understand the hazards of living on immunosuppressive drugs, and they live under the shadow of death just as chronically ill adults do—but without the maturity of adults, and handicapped by the keenness of feelings and lability of adolescence.

Family Reactions to Dialysis and Transplant

The nature and extent of family burden depend on many factors: the child's physical condition and medical center participation, whether the child is dialyzed at the center or at home, whether the center dietician and kitchen send home foods and supplements and give active help with diet preparation, whether an occupational therapist at the center teaches the child handcrafts and provides him with materials to work on at home, how much the center does in arranging school adaptations—home teaching if necessary—how much and how skillfully the center social worker intervenes in a preventive way, and, most important, how available the center medical staff is to the family and how patient and supportive they may be in helping the family understand and tolerate the child's situation.

The geographic location of the home is another important determinant, in respect to the time and exhaustion of the mother in transporting the child for dialysis and her lack of availability two or three days a week to perform the duties required by other children and household maintenance. The financial situation of the family and its practical resources—a second car in good running order, a washer and dryer, a big refrigerator and freezer, etc.—are also obvious factors in the ability of the family to cope with a child receiving dialysis and transplant. A helping grandmother who lives in the same vicinity, or an extended family with aunts and uncles who can substitute for parents and help with siblings, also makes a great difference.

Yet a thread runs through all the conversations with mothers of these seriously ill kidney patients. The wear-and-tear is accepted, whatever its manifestations, from driving mountain roads in old cars to managing care of other sick siblings. This thread is the worry about the child. The constant apprehension and anxiety are the most outstanding feature of mothers' comments and behavior. One exceptionally nervous mother, hovering over her child most of his dialysis time, said, "I'll never have another easy day in my life, even after his transplant, knowing the danger of infection when he is on anti-rejection drugs." One, an exception, refused to talk with me, saying candidly, "It's too painful—I can't put myself through reliving what it has been like. It just isn't worth it."

Observation confirms reports in the literature that some mothers so prepare themselves for the child's death at the time of renal failure that they are slow to accept the prolongation of life via dialysis and transplant. Having been through the anguish of relinquishing him, they dare not let themselves go through it again. Abandonment is detrimental to the child, as has been brought out elsewhere. A psychiatrist, examining the situations of 11 patients out of 48 at one center who died (all adults except for two adolescents), reported, "Eight out of eleven patients who died following renal transplantation had suffered a sense of abandonment by their families or had experienced panic about the outcome of the operation, to a degree not observed among patients who survived."[109] Another report describes the surprising coolness of some of the mothers toward their children during the initial phases of dialysis, and gradual return of normal warmth and concern after the child had been established as a person who was going to live.[110]

One center social worker described a young adult whose mother had devoted her life to his care during the demanding years of his renal disease during infancy and childhood, but who turned her back on him when dialysis was offered as he suffered final, end-stage uremia. She did not want his life prolonged, but because he was old enough to make the decision for himself and wanted a chance to live, he was dialyzed, and was able to return to school on a part-time basis. At another center the staff discussed a five-year-old boy whose mother carefully nursed him through the years when his life hung in the balance, but after dialysis started, she seemed to abandon him to the staff. She dropped him at the center and rushed off every time he was dialyzed, returning in time to take him home. She did only what was required, and felt certain he would die within the year.

A center director states he "is not impressed with the quality of life" of children receiving dialysis and transplant. Two staff members have said they would themselves choose death. Yet the teenagers who have had successful transplants are cautiously glad to be alive, are outwardly composed. It is with those who do not have successful transplants that the worker needs to be concerned, mustering as much support as the human resources of the community can provide. Unfortunately, the community, in which most of the children spend most of their lives and their families spend all of their lives, has not geared itself to provide the support needed. In sociological terms, "Technological advances often outstrip the resources and social organization necessary for their optimal use.... As a major new technology, transplantation may solve important health problems, but in turn it creates unanticipated adjustment problems for the government, the general public, medical organization, and the patient and his family."[111]

Meanwhile, those workers who have contact with families of children undergoing dialysis and/or transplant, or the children themselves, should reach out, both to the families and to the center staffs. Lack of knowledge of potential helpers in the community, and preoccupation with the burdens of each day, prevent the center worker from reaching out to the worker who would be able to help if she knew the unique medical-social needs of the particular client and his family. The depth of pain in child and family is often so great that they exist by use of denial and outward cheerfulness; one contact should not satisfy the worker that no help is needed, but rather a continuing relationship of some sort that the child or family can tap when they are ready to let down their defenses.

The need for enormous amounts of emotional and practical help to these children and their families is a corollary of the technical advances that keep them alive. In the centers observed, the professional staff invests an unusual amount of time and thought and self into the children cared for. The literature reveals that not all centers do so.

CHAPTER EIGHT

Congenital Heart Disease

CONGENITAL HEART DISEASE is the major cause of heart trouble in children. (Rheumatic fever, formerly the major cause, has yielded to control, while surgery and antibiotics have saved children with congenital defects who would have died in infancy 20 years ago. Rheumatic fever is now only about one-tenth as common.)[1] The term refers to abnormalities of the heart or its great vessels, present at birth or occurring immediately thereafter. The seriousness of the condition depends on the kind of defect present and its size and nature, whether it is single or one of several defects, the competence of the physicians to whom the parents have access, and the family's ability to follow treatment recommendation.

The psychosocial ramifications may be long and continuous, repeatedly crisis-centered, or minimal until time for surgery, when the major crisis exists. The condition is usually life-threatening, and often creates medical emergencies that alter social plans. Destructive psychological effects require skillful handling by all who may be concerned with the child and his family. Children of the poor who are not under health supervision may have unrecognized symptoms that the social worker should notice, in order to arrange for early medical examination. Her knowledge of the child's development, behavior, and activities may be very helpful to the physician in making a diagnosis. The social worker may have a key contribution in helping to keep the child alive during the early months and years before he can withstand surgery; throughout this course, she may enhance the quality of family life by helping to alleviate the repeated problems that arise.

THE MEDICAL REALITIES

Approximately six babies of 1,000 live births have congenital heart defects.[2] Many die early, cardiac malformations constituting one of the most common causes of death in infancy.[3] The prevalence of congenital heart disease in this country among school-age children, in different series reported, ranges from almost three to eight per 1,000 children.

A high proportion of children with congenital heart disease have multiple birth defects. These include some with neurological syndromes and chromosomal aberrations. As many as 40 percent of mongoloid children have cardiac defects.[4] The well-known "rubella syndrome" includes cataracts, deafness, and heart defects.[5] In one large New York City study, 22 percent of children with heart abnormalities had more than one heart defect, and 36 had malformations involving other organs, most commonly genitourinary.[6]

The cause of congenital heart disease is unknown, other than in the small percentages of cases where the mother had German measles *(rubella)* during pregnancy or a family tendency exists. Some families have more than one child with a heart defect. Though the hereditary factor is small, the statistical incidence rises from six per 1,000 to between 14 and 22 per 1,000 if the parents already have one child with this condition.[7]

Radiation or drugs during formation of the fetus are also adverse factors, as are very high altitude and maternal pre-diabetes.[8] Mothers between the ages of 40 and 44 are said by one authority, Nadas, to be more likely than younger mothers to give birth to children with one of the most serious combined defects, *tetralogy of Fallot*.[9]

Defects and Their Damage

The heart is a muscular pump that has two parts separated down the middle by a wall of tissue, or *septum*. The right, or smaller side, has a separate function and apparatus from the left. Both sides are structurally similar, to the extent that each has a small upper chamber and a larger lower one, with a valve between the upper and lower chambers. The upper chamber, or *atrium*, in each case is the receptacle for incoming blood, and the lower chamber, or *ventricle*, provides the pumping action. A normal heart has no opening in the septum between the two sides. The right side receives blood that has been circulating around the body giving oxygen to the tissues—blood that is therefore oxygen-depleted—and forces it through a valve to the lungs to receive oxygen, via a great vessel, the pulmonary artery and its tributaries. After this life-renewing passage through the lungs, the blood flows back to the left side of the heart, which pushes it out through another great vessel, the *aorta*, to go around the body again.

A high degree of individualization is essential in understanding the meaning of any one type of defect, or combination of defects, and this can be secured only from the pediatrician. A general background from which to proceed helps in knowing the relevance of his remarks and what questions to ask.

More than three dozen different defects have been identified, but nine or ten types constitute about 90 percent of the whole.[10] Each type of defect has a certain meaning regarding life expectancy, operability, and disability. A wide spectrum exists within any specific defect, so that the type of defect provides only a beginning knowledge of implications. However, the social worker who is helping the family make plans, and needs to understand the child's situation, first must learn what type of defect the child has, and whether it is believed to be single or combined with others.

It is not necessary for a social worker to keep in mind the meaning of all the defects; she should, however, refresh her knowledge of the general meaning of the particular defect of the child she is concerned with. The major defects are described briefly later. The names of the defects are listed here to facilitate the reader's recognition of specific defects in the ensuing remarks about general significance. The most common defects are *ventricular septal defect, atrial septal defect, patent ductus arteriosus, coarctation of the aorta, complete transposition of the great vessels, truncus arteriosus, aortic stenosis,* and *pulmonary stenosis*. These may occur in combined forms, or in a common constellation of defects called *tetralogy of Fallot*.

The physiologic consequences of heart defects have been grouped by Nadas in four ways. They may create insufficient oxygen in the blood, "arterial unsaturation"; overwork on the heart; an inadequate output of blood by the heart; and/or high blood pressure in the blood vessels of the lungs, "pulmonary arterial hypertension."[11]

Insufficient oxygen by and large creates *cyanosis* or a bluish color in the mucous membranes of the mouth and eyes or excessive redness of the lips, cheeks, and fingertips; *clubbing* or widening and thickening of the ends of the toes and fingers; shortness of breath, or *dyspnea*, on exertion; and in severe cases, *anoxic* spells, periods of lack of oxygen to the brain manifested by convulsions, unconsciousness, shortness of breath, and blueness. Nadas says these spells are very serious and may lead to death.[12] In children old enough to walk, a characteristic mannerism of squatting occurs, an instinctive method of improving the amount of oxygen flowing in the blood.

Overwork of the heart, created by an overload of blood in the chambers, may create no symptoms but potentially can so damage the muscles of the heart without warning that sudden death occurs. Or it can lead to congestive failure, a serious condition requiring immediate medical attention, to be described later. *Inadequate output of blood from the heart* creates physical underdevelopment of the child, or stunting of growth. *Pulmonary high blood pressure* is often associated with certain congenital defects. If this is long continued, it leads to damaged blood vessels in later life.[13]

Symptoms and Diagnosis

One of the most serious problems is that "many children who should have surgery are entirely asymptomatic,"[14] so their heart defects are not discovered until a murmur is detected by a physician during a routine examination. Surgery is more hazardous and less likely to effect a complete cure on older persons than in children, and in adolescence than during school age; thus the best chance for cure of a disabling and eventually fatal defect may be missed if diagnosis is not made at an early age.[15]

Symptoms may be so minimal they are not recognized as important, or they may be regarded by the family as behavioral idiosyncrasies. Small size, failure to gain weight, "laziness," crying or whining may be indicative of a variety of conditions and fail to alert the parent (or social worker) to the child's need for a physical examination. Furthermore, some defects produce symptoms only at times of growth spurt or other times of strain. Continuing observation is important. A child who is noted in the case record as active and healthy-looking by a previous worker may not remain so; continuous observation or inquiry should be made.

The general signs and symptoms of congenital heart abnormalities have been listed as follows for infants: choking spells, difficulty with feeding, failure to gain weight, blueness, shortness of breath, rapid pulse, and heart murmurs. The symptoms listed for children are: poor physical development, frequent respiratory infections, squatting, clubbed fingers and toes, poor exercise tolerance, shortness of breath, and heart murmurs. Children cannot articulate symptoms; therefore, adult observation must substitute. Responsibility rests on parents and others who may be helping or caring for them.

Two aspects of diagnosis are of concern to the worker. One pertains to murmurs, and the other to complexity of diagnostic procedures. Murmurs are of special concern if a child is in foster care pending adoption. To prevent unnecessary fright and cardiac crippling by overstating the importance of a murmur, many pediatricians and school physicians tend to label murmurs as meaningless until they are certain they are not. One pediatrician has pointed out that murmurs are not always easy to distinguish. If a baby is crying or other noises distract the physician during examination, he may not be able to hear them clearly. The pediatrician further states that understanding what he hears through the stethoscope is not learned quickly, and that not all doctors have achieved this skill.[16] Nadas says that the murmur of an atrial septal defect is similar to a "functional" or meaningless murmur during the early years of a child's life.[17]

The social worker concerned with a child whose adoption is delayed because of a heart murmur or whose life plans are deeply affected in other ways should discuss securing consultation from a cardiac specialist with the family physician or pediatrician, so that every opportunity can be considered for more definitive diagnosis.

The final determination regarding the nature of heart defects can be made only by *cardiac catheterization*, and in some instances by *angiograms*

(X rays of dye-filled blood vessels). "Cardiac catheterization and angiography are expensive procedures requiring hospitalization. It should be emphasized that there is a small but definite risk to life and limb involved in the performance of these tasks."[18] These tests are made by specialists in pediatric cardiology. "No patient should be denied the opportunity for precise study because he is too small or because death might occur during or after catheterization" in the judgment of one authoritative source.[19]

The *Annual Report of Cardiac Centers* in California reported no deaths in older children during 1970 as a result of diagnostic procedures. The death rate for infants was somewhat less than 2 percent. Complications not resulting in death followed diagnostic procedures in somewhat less than 4 percent of the cases reported by these centers in 1970. Complications associated with catheterization and angiography may be of great gravity, including strokes, followed by permanent paralysis on one or both sides, or brain damage of varying degree.

Nadas, who emphasizes that catheterization is a "major procedure which may terminate in the death of the patient," states that statistics are not valid, for much depends on the skill of the operating team, and on the condition of the person on whom they are working.[20] Fortunately, the fine distinctions requiring catheterization are not always necessary to diagnosis, and where they are, the pediatrician can guide the child through the hazardous early years, if home care is adequate, until complex procedures can be performed with maximum safety.

Surgical Treatment

The constant advance in treatment of congenital heart disease is primarily surgical. Closed-heart surgery, meaning that which does not enter the heart itself but is upon the attached vessels, commenced after World War II with repair of *patent ductus, resection of coarctation of the aorta,* and palliative bypasses or *anastomoses* to relieve *tetralogy of Fallot*. The heart-lung machine, developed in the mid-1950's, made possible techniques to repair defects within the heart itself, and thus gave enormous impetus to surgical treatment.[21]

One consequence of rapid technical advance is the increase of persons operated upon. If a child is not doing well, surgical intervention is usually recommended. Earlier and earlier surgery is performed, and often its ultimate value cannot be assessed because insufficient time has elapsed to accrue adequate follow-up data. A series of operations may be performed and then the procedure abandoned because of the high mortality rate or discovery of late complications. The state of flux attendant upon rapid advance carries dramatic gain—life itself—for some, and death for others.

The *Annual Report of Cardiac Centers* in California for 1970 shows that three-fourths of the more than 5,000 heart operations that year were performed on adults, but that infants, on whom only 6 percent of the operations were performed, sustained 15 percent of the mortality. One pediatric cardiologist commented to me, "For awhile, the largest cause of death in congenital heart disease was surgery—where before children died by inches, they now died swiftly." The most common of the closed operations performed on children in 1970 were repair of patent ductus and correction of coarctation of the aorta; of the open-heart operations, repair of atrial septal defect headed the list.

One pediatric specialist placed the defects in order of amenability to surgical correction, with least surgical risk as follows: patent ductus, simple atrial defect, simple coarctation; with increasing difficulty, tetralogy of Fallot, pulmonary stenosis, aortic stenosis, transposition of the great vessels, total anomalous venous return, and, last, tricuspid atresia.[22]

Until recently, the optimal age for surgery has been thought to be school age, or between six and twelve years. This has been described as the "golden age" for children with congenital heart disease.[23] Some specialists have preferred to operate before age two if absolutely essential or after age four to minimize psychological trauma. In the past, medical experts have preferred to wait as long as possible to perform surgery. Reasons include the larger size of the heart, which makes surgery mechanically easier, the greater strength of the child, and the advantage accrued from surgical experience gained through operations performed earlier.[24] This point of view is still held by more conservative specialists. The younger, more aggressive group believe that the advancement of surgical techniques permits early surgery, and that the earlier the child can be operated on, the less permanent damage his heart will sustain from the abnormal blood flow created by the defect. Four or five years is thought to be the optimal age from this point of view.[25] One cardiac specialist, to whom the author spoke concerning the special psychological vulnerability of children four and five years old, commented on the undoubted psychological gain in repairing the defect (and thus permitting the child maximum vigor) before he begins school.

After surgery, the child is usually in the hospital for ten days to two weeks, spending a variable number of days in the intensive care unit. The immediate postoperative period requires the ultimate in sophisticated nursing and medical skill and elaborate equipment to compensate for the massive assault upon the organism. The psychological aftermath of this experience will be commented upon later.

A recovery period of about six weeks follows cardiac surgery, during which time the child's activity is self-limiting and he is on medication. If the surgery has been successful and the defect completely repaired, the child will need only intermittent medical supervision after this time. In a follow-up study conducted by telephone inquiry by the California Crippled

Children's Services of children operated upon between 1957 and 1961, 75 percent of the children known to have survived surgery (80 percent of those operated on) were located, and of this group 60 percent had been restored to full activity by the operation (the percentages were considerably greater for children operated for ventricular septal defect than tetralogy of Fallot).[26] None were completely disabled. It is to be expected that the figures would be better if a later survey were conducted, owing to the advance in technique since that time.[27]

In a study conducted by the Alabama Vocational Rehabilitation Agency of the outcome of surgery it had financed, one-half of the group of young adults with congenital heart disease were considered entirely rehabilitated, the criteria including return to former status as students, homemakers, or employment.[28] It is to be recalled that surgery on adults is less successful than on children.

The Surgical Risk

The limitations created by congenital heart disease lie across a broad spectrum. Some defects (such as simple patent ductus) lie outside the heart and have been operated on successfully for many years. They create an entirely different picture than other defects that are dangerous in every respect. The differential diagnosis often is difficult, requiring skill and special experience; the decision to operate, when to do so, and what kind of operation require great expertise. Ventricular septal defect, the most common of the heart defects, illustrates these problems, for the opening may be so small that it will close with no intervention, or so large and enmeshed with other defects that its repair is most difficult.

Cardiac surgery is new, in a constant state of flux, and daring operations are devised every decade. Most are too recent to permit evaluation of their long-term results. Open-heart surgery requires a network of complex machines and a team of technical experts. Only those centers with enough patients to keep such a team in constant practice should be entrusted with the critical work that precedes surgery and goes on during the operation and after it. Many children come through the operation with dramatic success; their vigor is greatly improved and they may be capable of normal activity for an indefinite period. Others are left with serious complications, or less than complete alleviation of cardiac limitations.

Much depends on the age of the child when symptoms occur. Many defects do not show up or are not recognized until a routine examination during school age reveals their presence. The most difficult struggles occur when an infant has cardiac symptoms. Early blueness, feeding difficulties, and other signs of respiratory distress may lead to findings of a large or complicated defect. In such cases very careful home management under close medical supervision, with hospital intervals when necessary, may bring the child through the early months until he is large enough in size to have surgery with a greater degree of safety. If he cannot survive without operation, the hazard is substantial. Often early operations are palliative, partial repairs permitting the child to survive until he is large enough for major repair to be attempted, after he is two or three years of age.

But despite dramatic gains made in treating children with congenital heart disease, death remains a significant possibility. Until recently, the increase in number of operations was accompanied by an increase in deaths, according to a statistical evaluation by the California State Department of Public Health.[29] Comments are like the following: "Undoubtedly deaths will continue to be associated with surgical intervention because it is often used in situations that would otherwise be hopeless" and "It is probable that in some cases an operation hastens an inevitable early death, and that in others it adds years to what would have been a short life."[30] The statistics indicate that until the mid-1960's the advent of heart surgery had affected the death rate very little, but that in recent years definite advantages accrued. The *Vital Statistics Records of the California State Department of Public Health* show a decrease in 1970 over 1960 in the death rate from congenital heart disease for all ages up to 40, and a decrease in total number of deaths from this condition.[31]

Individual situations vary so widely that general statistics mean little for a given child, but those of the *Annual Report of Cardiac Centers* in California in 1970 have some significance for the social worker concerned with the cardiac child. The death rate for all heart surgery is shown to be about one in ten, with a somewhat higher risk for those who have open-heart surgery than for those with closed (all closed, death rate of 8.3 percent; all open, 11.8 percent).[32] A great variation occurred by age-group, by type of defect, and by center where the surgery is performed. As indicated earlier, infants under one year have surgery least often, but when they do, they have the highest death rate (surgery would not be performed at this age were they not in serious condition). Of infants who had surgery, 15 percent died, whereas of those between one and four, only 5 percent died, and of those between five and twenty, 8 percent died.[33]

The variable seriousness of different defects must be kept in mind. For example, uncomplicated atrial septal defect had a very low mortality rate, less than 2 percent, whereas tetralogy of Fallot and ventricular septal defect had surgical death rates of around 9 percent, and ventricular septal defect after pulmonary hypertension had developed had 20 percent.[34] In closed-heart surgery, a very low mortality followed surgery for patent ductus arteriosus, about 3 percent, and an extremely high mortality followed banding of the pulmonary artery, almost 25 percent.

Social workers and parents may also wish to know that the cardiac centers in California have different mortality rates. Greatest success has been reported in the centers that have performed neither the highest nor the lowest number of operations.[35] Small centers, where the cardiac teams do not have opportunity for large practice, cannot accumulate the expertise of those at larger centers. Why the largest centers have a proportionately higher death rate may be due to several causes—among them, of course, that they receive the most complicated cases. Large centers are likewise in the forefront of experimental work, forging new paths, with inevitable casualties among the daring successes. The age of patients accepted and other factors at each center also affect the number of deaths.

Medical Management

The goals of medical management are (1) to bring the child through infancy and early childhood safely so that he may have surgery at the optimal time, and (2) to help him live as comfortably as possible within his physical limitations if he is inoperable or has cardiac problems remaining after surgery. The pediatrician focuses on watching the child's weight and on treating or preventing common problems complicating the course of the disease.

Dental care and other semisurgical procedures require penicillin before and after, to prevent possible *bacterial endocarditis*, a dangerous superimposed heart condition to which children with congenital heart disease are particularly susceptible.[36] Carious teeth harbor infection and provide a route to the heart. Prevention of caries through good dental hygiene assumes special importance. *Dental repair that might be thought of as desirable but not essential in a very young child is vital if he has a heart defect. Extensive work may be necessary on baby teeth.*

Prevention of bacterial endocarditis requires prophylactic treatment for kidney examinations and catheterizations, similar to that for dental repair.

Limitation of activity does not pose a disciplinary problem in the preschool child, because fatigue causes him to limit his own play; he comes in from outdoors, or lies down, without reminder. He should be able to rest conveniently and without embarrassment whenever he is tired,[37] a fact to be remembered in nursery school or foster day care of the cardiac child. School age introduces problems. Competition is normal to this phase of development. Boys, especially, may need limitation of the type of play and sports engaged in and should have supervision available to avoid pushing themselves unduly during the excitement of competition.

Some infants and children, those subject to blackouts or fainting spells (*syncope*) and those subject to blue spells due to lack of blood to the brain (*anoxia*), should be prevented from excessive crying or activity that causes breathlessness. Picking up the baby, or distracting the child, is recommended.[38] The child whose blueness is relieved by unusual positions such as squatting should not be discouraged from this, since it makes a real difference in his symptoms.

Upper respiratory infections, including colds and pneumonia, often create complications in cardiac children. Those with defects that cause excessive blood flow to the lungs are subject to repeated bouts of pneumonia, in some cases requiring repeated hospitalization. Such children are treated with antibiotics. Prevention rests on social conditions and good home care.

Other children, those who lack oxygen because of insufficient blood flow to and from the lungs, become anemic. These children may need iron, or blood transfusions.[39]

Heart failure is the most serious medical complication. It requires immediate medical attention, usually hospitalization. As mentioned earlier, young children must be observed by the mother or caretaker because they cannot complain. The outward signs of failure are *sweating* (because of the excessive work of the heart) especially during feeding, *fast breathing* or *tachypnea*, a *worried expression* signifying suffering, and *failure to gain weight* despite adequate food intake. (Failure to thrive may be a sign of serious heart trouble; it is by no means always due to neglect.) A late, grave sign is swelling, or *edema*.[40]

Children who complain of being tired or weak, or who have shortness of breath, *dyspnea*, need immediate medical attention. If they are in heart failure, they are hospitalized for administration of the drug digitalis, in one of its forms as Lanoxin, as an emergency measure. After the correct dosage has been worked out, they may be maintained on digitalis until they are acceptable risks for surgery. Digitalis is dangerous in the incorrect dosage, and can produce toxicity, manifested by diarrhea.[41] Children in failure are also maintained on diuretics, Lasix and Mercuhydrine being medications commonly used now. The latter drug is of concern to those interested in the whole child, since it requires an injection—the "needle" dreaded by all children.

Common Defects and the Outlook for Treatment

By and large, the defects least compatible with survival through infancy, and therefore encountered by family and adoption workers but less frequently in general child-welfare case loads, are *truncus arteriosus, tricuspid atresia, complete transposition of the great vessels*, and some cases of *tetralogy of Fallot* and *coarctation of the aorta*.

Truncus arteriosus is an embryological abnormality in which there is only one large artery leading from the heart, with an accompanying large ventricular septal defect. A highly complicated operation has been devised that will doubtless make this defect less formidable in the future. Tricuspid atresia is another embryological abnormality, in which there is no valve between the two right-sided chambers; the condition also has other accompanying defects. Palliative surgery has been devised, and in a few cases children have survived to four or more years of age.[42]

Complete transposition of the great vessels, as the name implies, is an alteration in the position of the pulmonary artery and the aorta. A recently developed operation permits a much more hopeful outlook for infants affected with this grave condition; the operation has been termed by one pediatric cardiologist "one of the great breakthroughs of the 1960's,"[43] reducing the prognosis for death before the age of six months to an expectation that only one-third will die. Some centers perform an emergency procedure on the baby if he is blue during the first few days of life, and a later major operation at age two. Transposition remains, however, one of the most serious of the heart defects, and not all centers are having success with surgery.

Coarctation of the aorta is of two types: *infantile* or *preductal*, and *postductal*. The former belongs among the group of defects rarely encountered by social workers, other than foster-home placement workers or those who work with families with new babies. Infants afflicted with preductal coarctation frequently have multiple heart defects and present serious symptoms very early. "There were twice as many deaths in the first year of life among children with coarctation as there were in all the children and adults over one year of age during the same interval" in the statistics of the Toronto center.[44]

Postductal coarctation is described as a localized constriction of the aorta, in contrast to the long, diffuse narrowing of the preductal type. Postductal coarctation often causes no symptoms, so that the defect is found only when the child is examined for some other reason. If the child is symptom-free, medical authorities state he should be operated on between eight and twelve years of age to prevent greater surgical risk later when the aorta has become less elastic and before an aneurysm or other condition suddenly and prematurely ends his life.[45]

Operative mortality is described as extremely high in infancy, but substantially less so in childhood. However, surgery for coarctation is always a serious procedure. In a few instances, children have become paraplegic as a consequence of the surgery.[46] The absence of symptoms in a school-age child, with lack of warning to the parents of need for an "elective" operation of this gravity, places coarctation of the aorta in the group of defects frequently accompanied by crisis-centered psychosocial implications.

One measure of the seriousness of the diagnosis of coarctation is the report of a surgeon who followed the surviving patients of his 19 years of experience. He discovered a significant recurrence of the condition in 8.5 percent of those who were located; the majority were children who had been operated on under three years of age. A second operation was necessary on most of them, with a 25 percent mortality during the operative period.[47]

The defects most frequently encountered (because they usually permit life beyond infancy and thus accumulate) are *ventricular septal defect, atrial septal defect, patent ductus arteriosus,* and *tetralogy of Fallot.*

Ventricular septal defect is by far the most common congenital heart defect. Keith et al. say it occurs in combination with other defects in 25 percent of all cases of congenital heart disease, and singly in another 25 percent.[48] The wall between the two sides of the heart normally permits the vigorous pumping action of the left side to function without disturbing the small right side of the heart from its activity in sending venous blood to the lungs for oxygenation. If the hole in the wall is large enough, the high pressure of the left side forces an unusually large amount of blood into the right-sided pulmonary apparatus. This in turn can cause flooding of the lungs with blood, or it can cause the pulmonary arteries to develop a resistance and pulmonary high blood pressure.

Ventricular septal defects vary greatly in size and shape. As earlier indicated some are so small they close themselves without surgery, and others are so large as to be virtually inoperable. Decisions about which cases should be operated and the optimum time for operation require a great degree of skill. Some persons can live to middle age or older without surgery. The risk of surgery is high enough to be a cause of death in itself.[49] The exquisiteness of the decision is sharpened because the children can be well and active despite heart defects, but a significant percentage gradually develop *Eisenmenger's complex* with pulmonary hypertension, which causes death in early adult life and cannot be operated upon with safety in adulthood.[50]

The problem is not always of this nature. Babies with large ventricular defects are short of breath and undernourished, and in advanced conditions may be *cyanotic*; in such instances where threat to life is obvious, the goal is careful supervision and medical management to bring the child through the first year of life, with surgery scheduled in the second or later years according to the child's condition then. *Pulmonary banding*, a surgical procedure frequently attempted as a palliative measure to sustain the child until he is old enough to have the defect patched, has proved to cause later serious problems in those who survive, according to one authority; his center tried complete repair in infants, but gave up after seven out of ten of the babies died as a result of surgery. This specialist advocates surgery prior to the time the child is age four.[51]

One cannot generalize about the significance of ventricular septal defects, for some are insignificant whereas those that are large or complicated by other defects are so serious that this diagnosis has one of the highest mortality rates among all surgical cases.[52]

Atrial septal defects, holes in the walls between upper chambers, uncomplicated by other defects, occur much less frequently. They are in the family of defects that carry a good operative prognosis, providing they are of the "secundum" type, to be differentiated from the "primum" type. After the death in infancy of many children who have combined atrial defects, the remainder often present no sign or symptom until adolescence. The murmur that the doctor thought "functional" when the child was small finally becomes more intense, or the heart enlarges. The optimum age for surgery is said to be between five and ten years of age.[53] When children with atrial septal defects are not known to have a heart problem or are not operated upon, they are said to be thin and have limited endurance, but may survive to 50 years or later without surgical intervention. Under these circumstances, decision about surgery is truly "elective." Not surprisingly, atrial septal defect is said to be the most common congenital defect found among adults.

There is one type of atrial septal defect, designated as an *ostium primum* defect, that is very different in outlook. It is a large defect that involves the mitral and tricuspid valves, and is described by Nadas as a partial *endocardial cushion defect*, which is of special interest to social workers because it is associated with mongolism. These defects, which are in the innermost part of the heart and involve valvular mechanisms as well as the walls, may produce severe heart damage at an early age, with a rapidly downhill course.

The life expectancy of children with ostium primum or partial endocardial cushion defects varies, but they may die in the first few years of life and rarely live to be beyond 30 or 40 years of age, Nadas states.[54] Surgical treatment carries a 10 percent mortality if the endocardial cushion defect is only partial, and 50 percent if complete, in the Boston hospitals with which he is associated. It is recommended between ages five and ten years, or earlier if the child's condition demands intervention.[55]

Patent ductus arteriosus refers to failure of a usual mechanical change from fetal circulation at birth, when the infant must breathe for himself. A muscular structure connecting the left pulmonary artery to the aorta stays open instead of closing as it should. Like simple atrial defect, patent ductus usually is one of the least threatening cardiac defects, if it is not complicated by others. It is the first heart defect for which surgery was performed, because it lies outside the heart and therefore does not require open-heart surgery. Patent ductus is the cardiac defect usually associated with the rubella syndrome.

As described by the medical texts, patent ductus is a common accompaniment of multiple heart defects. In some cases, the open duct compensates for abnormalities in blood flow created by the internal defects. Patent ductus may be associated with coarctation, ventricular septal defects, or valvular abnormalities. When the defect occurs alone, it usually creates no symptoms except that growth is retarded in many children.

In some cases, however, the child has heart failure because of the increased work load on the left heart, and surgery is required as a lifesaving measure. In other cases, the damage, pulmonary hypertension, occurs only slowly, on the right side. Patent ductus needs to be corrected except where it counteracts other defects, or when the situation is too complicated to risk surgery. Before surgery was developed, a 1943 estimate postulated that adolescents with patent ductus arteriosus had half the life expectancy normal for their age.[56] Mortality from surgery in a worldwide survey in 1956 was only 2.3 percent of all children operated on under 14 years of age, according to Keith et al.,[57] and is now lower than this in well-selected cases in skillful hands. Repair of the opening in early life before heart damage has occurred should permit the child to become completely normal, in the opinion of all cardiac experts interviewed by the author.

Tetralogy of Fallot, to the contrary, is a combined cardiac defect with a grave outlook.[58] A baby with this condition is cyanotic in varying degrees and is apt to be short of breath upon feeding and crying, and later when walking. He may have blue spells, or attacks without warning of intense blueness and shortness of breath, which become more frequent and prolonged between nine and 18 months if he survives until then. Such children spontaneously improve after this time. Because the child is tired, as an infant he lies on his side in "fetus position," knees to chest, and as an older child frequently squats, which helps restore the blood flow to the heart. The child is slow to gain weight, or has "failure to thrive." Fatigue is such that some children cannot walk more than a few steps; others with mild defects can walk several blocks.

Keith says children who live through the most hazardous first two years of life tend to get along better until adolescence, when they begin to decline again. Unless surgery is possible, few survive beyond 20 years of age. Early palliative surgery may be performed, a shunt or bypass operation called an *anastomosis* to provide blood to the lungs. Various shunt procedures are used, those commonly seen on medical reports including the Potts shunt and the Blalock-Taussig anastomosis.

One group of physicians, reporting on *total surgical correction* of this condition, says,[59] "In 1955, after 10 years of palliative surgery using various shunt operations, Lillehei accomplished the first successful total correction of the Tetralogy of Fallot. The early mortality was high, often in the range of 40 percent, but today in most centers the operative mortality has been reduced to about 10 percent." In the group of 45 patients they had operated on, 22 percent died either immediately after surgery or later, but they achieved "marked clinical improvement in the surviving 78%." Since the development of the heart-lung machine, total surgical correction is often attempted when the child is between five and ten years of age.

Cautiously tiding the child over until he is old enough to have the best chance of surviving surgery involves close medical supervision and careful home management. Small feedings, particular attention during infections and hot weather, and immediate availability of emergency room or hospital treatment are included, as is "continuous support and encouragement to the family by practitioner and specialist."[60] For those children who can be brought through the critical early years and survive surgery, abnormal heart function remains. Nevertheless, the majority are able to function without major limitations for a number of years. An "important change in psyche and educational drive obtains, with ability to undertake ordinary activity by three months after surgery" according to Keith.[61]

PSYCHOSOCIAL IMPLICATIONS

Heart defects not infrequently are accompanied by other congenital defects. The impact on the child and family, and the influence of the other abnormalities on the treatment of the heart defect, create further variables in this most variable medical problem. That the psychosocial ramifications spread over a wide range need hardly be stated.

The meaning of congenital heart disease to child and family depends primarily on the nature and degree of the physical problem. Whether the heart defect is quickly correctable, severely disabling, or fatal obviously carries greatest significance. Other important determinants of meaning are the child's constitutional vulnerability to experience, his age, the age of the parents, their sociocultural and economic status, the kind of medical care to which they have access, their prior experiences especially with loss, sibling and parent relationships, and the way different aspects of the constellation affect each other. Clues the practitioner can follow in learning individual meaning are revealed by ways congenital heart disease often affects the children and their families.

As earlier stated, many children with heart defects die within the first few days or weeks of life, others have few or no symptoms, and some live beyond middle age with no knowledge of their congenital abnormality. Social agencies are likely to know most of those remaining, because few families can withstand the staggering costs without aid. Financial assistance may in fact be the only help the family needs beyond that given by a compassionate pediatrician. Problems abound, but some families have unusual strengths. They are able to cope with the anxiety related to all heart ailments, the parental guilt constantly encountered in congenital defects, the great demands in caring for symptomatic infants or small children prior to surgery, the intense emotion inherent in submitting the child to an operation of great risk, some psychological crippling in the child, and the strain on family relationships. However, other families need help if the experience is to be weathered with minimum trauma. Most of the children are young, in the life-shaping age and vulnerable to family attitudes. Thus the family experience leaves a permanent imprint on the child. One-parent families, those who are educationally or culturally deprived, and those who have other problems may be in special need of practical aid, emotional support through periods of crisis, and constructive teamwork by the several professional persons or groups involved in the child's care. Whatever the financial or educational status of the family, they can and do have problems during the period a child is in physical jeopardy. Support should be available to them.

Financial Problems

Some infants and toddlers need extensive diagnostic procedures, or have frequent bouts of pneumonia or other respiratory disease or episodes of congestive failure. These necessitate recurrent brief hospitalizations that cost several hundred dollars. Heart surgery recommended for most children who survive the neonatal period costs around $10,000 at the time of this writing. In California, however, the dramatic cost of hospital care is less burdensome for many families than some less expensive items. Most wage earners' group insurance policies cover hospital care for dependents. Programs of the Crippled Children's Services include heart defects among medically eligible conditions, and supplement insurance payments for hospital care where these are insufficient, providing that the family meets eligibility standards. Medicaid provides hospital care in California and other states for families receiving assistance and a dwindling number of other poor.

However, tax-supported sources of medical assistance have become highly restrictive, increasing the number of families who can neither pay nor qualify for aid. Pay-back provisions, or "liability" requirements, may be so high that the family cannot afford to take advantage of technically available public provisions, or if they are able to, they cannot afford the less obvious but equally important expenses incidental to cardiac disease, or meet the needs of their other children. In California, the amount of time and energy required to establish eligibility for Medicaid is a substantial addition to the burden of care for the child. Attempts to discourage use of public funds through erection of formidable procedures create severe hardship for parents of ill children.

Dental care, discussed in relation to prevention of bacterial endocarditis, may be costly if baby teeth must be capped, or if a general anesthetic is required and hospitalization necessary. If the family is financially eligible, Crippled Children's Services or Medicaid (in California) will include dental treatment of a child with heart disease, usually upon special authorization. Some insurance policies cover dental treatment when it is a part of medical care.

Creative effort is most needed in helping the low-income family maintain *general measures to prevent infection.* Nutritious food, warm housing in winter, separate beds and enough bedrooms to reduce transmission of colds from other children, warm clothing, sweaters and rubbers create difficult financial problems. Public housing projects, including federal subsidy to private landlords, have improved the housing of some families hitherto living in drafty shacks with dirt floors or in tenement houses. Private agency resources, though drying up from overuse, still offer potential sources of aid. The Heart Association and Easter Seal Society and other private health agencies, such as the Tuberculosis and Respiratory Disease Association, are among potential sources for extra beds, bedding, or special clothing needs in some communities.

Transportation

Transportation for emergency medical care and for regular office visits or clinic supervision and trips to a distant cardiac specialist often pose special difficulty. Moving a family from one community to another is a drastic measure. However, if an infant or toddler is in frequent cardiac crisis, and the family lives in a community with no resources and the family has none of its own, a move may be necessary. Many families do have extended family, faithful neighbors, or church friends whose automobiles are available at night or on weekends when agencies are closed, although the agency may have to provide money for gasoline. The worker may need to participate in prior arrangements.

In considering the need for help in getting emergency transportation as a factor in the total social plan, workers should keep in mind that infants are most subject to life-threatening emergencies requiring immediate medical care. The vulnerability to frequent emergencies of any cardiac child should be discussed with the pediatrician.

Transportation permitting clinic attendance for regular supervision poses one of the most widespread problems in California. The importance of "weight-watching" of the child by the physician has been described as a means of measuring adequate cardiac function vs. a failing heart and need for early surgery. Changes in the child's appearance or behavior that the mother may have failed to notice may be apparent immediately to the skilled professional; the change may indicate need for immediate action. Yet two large cardiac centers in different parts of the state report an excessive rate of failed appointments (50 percent in one of these).

Cardiac centers draw patients from wide urban areas and surrounding counties; the lack of adequate public transportation systems creates almost insuperable difficulties for low-income families. One hospital social worker in a large city reported that some families have a three-hour bus ride each way, often waiting at transfer points without benches. When they arrive at the clinic, they must wait up to three hours for completion of the electrocardiograms or X rays, for a medical student or resident conference with cardiac specialists, etc. Nine hours for the clinic visit is more than can be expected for the mother who brings a sickly, crying child and often other small children.

Excessive mobility of the very poor, a modern urban problem stemming from rent defaults and evictions, results in failure to receive appointment cards. These reminders may mean little to the family unless the child is in sufficiently obvious distress to take precedence in the mother's mind over the other pressures of poverty.

An additional problem occurs for families who may not be subjected to the pressures of ghetto residents. This is the wide spacing of follow-up appointments for children who are doing well. Six months or yearly intervals between appointments often exist. Under these circumstances, the family may have moved, the weather may be poor, or the mother considers the appointment relatively unimportant if it was couched in terms of "see me in a year."

The worker in the community should intervene actively in helping parents solve problems impeding clinic supervision. The cardiac center may permit the child to be examined during intermediate intervals by a neighborhood pediatrician or health department clinic. If this is not possible, automobile transportation with gasoline paid by the agency, or transportation of the mother and child to the clinic by a volunteer or case aide may be arranged. Occasional chauffeuring by the social worker pays dividends in opportunity to ask questions of the physician and to hear his instructions to the mother and to observe the physician-child-mother relationships. An understanding of what the child is undergoing and how he is reacting is heightened by such occasions.

In discussion of transportation, the worker may want to discuss the clinic experience with the mother and learn her attitudes. She may find the mother does not consider the clinic visits worth while. The child may be in a period of relative well-being, with few overt symptoms. Or the mother may report that she sees a different doctor every time, who repeats the questions she has been asked many times before. When frank criticism of the clinic exists, or lack of understanding of the importance of supervision, this information should be discussed with the clinic to learn whether any modifications are possible.

The Working Mother

Families dependent on income from the mother's work to maintain their standard of living pose a common problem. Some mothers who are under heavy psychological pressure prefer an office job and can rationalize their desire to exchange the crisis-ridden, lonely, and frightening task of caring for a small child with a heart defect for work in an ordered and socially interesting environment. In addition, the life-style of many intellectuals and others includes a concept of self-realization through employment, which is seriously disturbed by the needs of a chronically ill child. They may have good housekeepers, or a grandmother may live in the home and function as a mother substitute. However, during periods when the child is subject to attacks and is in precarious condition, his real insecurity and the need for close attention to changes in behavior and appearance usually contraindicate the mother's employment. When two or more children in the family have cardiac defects, or when a child has multiple handicaps, the mother cannot work outside the home unless an unusually good source of help is readily available or the mother so deeply rejects the child or children that attempts at alleviation are not worth while and placement of the children is necessary.

A most serious consequence of the mother's employment outside the home is her lack of availability for close hospital visitation during periods the child is hospitalized. As brought out elsewhere, the small child's deepest anxiety arises from maternal separation. Especially while he is undergoing terrifying experiences, *the mother needs to be at the hospital* as long and frequently as possible. Hospital visiting hours usually end early in the evening, so that the mother who works during the day can see the child only briefly and infrequently. The child's piteous wails or screaming when she leaves often result in her rationalization that "he is better off when I don't disturb him."

Mothers of one-parent families are caught between inflationary prices and fear of losing a job during a time of high unemployment, especially when creditors press or the rent is behind. However, some mothers are not really in impossible financial situations but lack understanding of the urgency of being with their children during hospitalization. The drag of inertia may keep them working instead of changing quickly to meet the child's needs. Fathers may lack understanding and either reinforce the mother's resistance to stopping work or may actually oppose her doing so.

When a child is hospitalized at a distant heart center, as frequently occurs for diagnostic procedures or heart surgery, money is needed for the mother's board and room and transportation. Additional expenses include those for a homemaker or domestic if the mother has other small children and the sick child is in the precarious first few years of life. The toddler who is too young to understand why he should not strip off his clothing and play in the water when he feels hot and feverish and who is alternately hyperactive and lethargic or whining may be harder to care for than an infant. Preventive attention to the mother's health and to the family's stability and to the siblings' normal needs is warranted from the standpoint alone of preventing greater expense from family disorganization.

The financial implications, then, of cardiac disability in children extend much beyond the obvious costs of medical care for the child. They warrant a careful review of family resources and expenses in light of the total social situation and probable medical need. Understanding of priorities must be ensured to enable the parents to consider possible modifications. Employers are often sympathetic to problems posed by dramatically ill children if the mothers bring their needs to attention. Neighbors and relatives can be imposed upon occasionally but not repeatedly, and should not be considered a basic resource except where close relationships with immediate family exist. Public welfare and public health agency resources for transportation and homemaker service may be tapped, as well as private agencies for small amounts such as may be needed for a mother's hospital stay during a child's catheterization or surgery. The latter expense has an appeal that more mundane needs do not and has the advantage to a private agency of being limited and specific.

Cardiac problems are not static; the child tends to shift from periods of crisis to those of well-being and back again, unless the course is progressively downhill or is interrupted by surgery. Thus the financial situation needs review, and at the beginning the family should be informed of their need to be ready to change financial plans as the medical situation changes. Eligibility workers should anticipate the need for frequent review and potential budgetary changes.

Family Adjustment

The child with minimal symptoms may afford the family few health worries and problems. Families of infants and small children who have abnormalities with marked symptoms often stay in turmoil because of the frequent respiratory infections the child incurs or because he has "anoxic spells" or goes into congestive failure. Children who become acutely ill call forth fear of death. This fear can result in premature psychological separation, or deep and constant anguish.

The age of the parents and the stage of the family life cycle affect their reaction to recurring crises. The mother of a first child tends to be anxious because she lacks experience in differentiating between the normal and the abnormal. Workers usually know some indifferent young mothers whose need for personal fulfillment takes precedence over concern for a child. However, any parent may panic in caring for a child who becomes suddenly limp and turns blue, or an infant who refuses to eat, and lies awake crying. The mother may be impatient with a toddler who whines to be held and wants to be picked up and carried because he is tired or his legs hurt. As in the family of the toddler with juvenile arthritis, the young father may resent the child's competition for his wife's energies and love. His need for rest at home is defeated by an unhappy, crying, insomniac child. Immature young parents with strong self needs may not be able to tolerate the marital strain created.

What it means to have a cardiac infant was described by one young mother who said the baby never slept the night through; customarily he wakes and cries four times every night. Since his birth, the family has never had one night of uninterrupted sleep. Instead of napping during the day two hours at a time, he naps in two sessions, being wakeful and crying in between. As he is unable to take a feeding in one session, or to eat solid foods at the same session in which he takes a bottle, he must be fed a few ounces frequently. His schedule is one of almost constant demand. If he is allowed to cry, he vomits and coughs; thus the mother must keep him from crying by picking him up and distracting him, giving him toys, standing him on her lap, letting him look out of the window, etc. The mother said the hardest part for her has been inability to go anywhere because she could not take him among crowds, even to the grocery store, until recently. Now when she takes him to the store, he is fatigued from the two-block ride in the stroller. He has picked up an infection now, and cries because of earache.

Older mothers, who have a larger proportion of babies with congenital defects, also have special problems. Older parents anticipate the "afterthought baby," or the last of a large family, with varying mixtures of joy, resentment, anxiety, shame, and pride. "Just so he is normal," the universal anxious prayer, meets defeat.

Having lost the resilience of youth, these parents are less able to withstand sleepless nights and continual drain on patience and strength. Their normal needs to settle down are upset. Mothers of children with cardiac defects frequently seem to have health problems such as diabetes, hypertension, or kidney disease. Fathers may be worrying over impending loss of job or insecurity as new young managers take the place of a long-accustomed boss. Teenage or adult siblings frequently provide great help if they are not expected to sacrifice too much of their energies and plans. Exploitation tends to bring out the rage many teenagers feel during the turmoil of adolescence.

Older parents whose cardiac child is among the last of many children not infrequently are ethnic Catholics. *Culturally determined attitudes* are prevalent in those who are first- or second-generation Americans. The extended family add their opinions and experiences with medical care to those of the parents. If recently emigrated from areas where hospital facilities are primitive, they may entertain great fear of what happens in hospitals. They may have attitudes set by childhood memories of hospitals in the old country. Docile and respectful toward the physician, they save his face but do not return to see him or they become suddenly difficult to locate. Unusually complex social situations often are revealed when an understanding social worker, nurse, or aide communicates with them. These may range from simple religious faith that if God has willed that they care for a sickly, small child, they will do so and not interfere in His course, to primitive feelings that the family has been hexed or is being punished for sin. In one instance where the mother had had three children with cardiac defects, two had died, one of them in surgery. She and her husband were not willing to trust a frail little girl whom they loved deeply to the same experience. In another instance, the mother expected a miracle to happen on the child's eighth birthday as a result of prayers and a vision. Great preparations were made for the eighth birthday including a feast to celebrate God's goodness. When the miracle did not occur, complete confusion took place; through the long-sustained effort of a public health nurse, this child was finally trusted to the physicians and fortunately survived the operation.

Because the priest is a central authority among those in whom religion is part of cultural attitudes, he may prove the most helpful ally in interpreting need for care and in providing emotional support. Local workers or aides who speak the language of the family also may be of assistance. If they are part of the extended family or the community group that is embroiled in the situation, they may or may not be supportive of the professional's point of view. It is well to know the aide's feelings and any relationships with the family, especially if the worker does not understand the language.

Reaction to surgery varies over time. Its distance away and the symptoms of the child influence feelings. The hope offered by surgery may relieve the doom of incurability. While the child is frighteningly ill, and surgery remains as a distant goal, the attitude is positive. However, when surgery nears, parents and child are described universally as undergoing deep anxiety. Reactions will be affected by the manner in which the physicians have interpreted the operation, the degree of support given, the cultural background of the parents, their own experience with heart surgery, their experience with loss, and the child's own feelings about the operation.

I and other medical social workers have often observed a regrettable lack of detail in the interpretation of surgery provided to families by some cardiac specialists. Specialists not infrequently gloss over the risks and virtually take over the decision that should be made by the parents. Possibly the high plane of intensity on which they live, feelings of futility about explaining a complex subject, and fear of rousing parental doubts if risks are fully grasped contribute to the paucity of information provided. If the hospital has a social worker, she can be asked to secure more information or arrange for further conferences between physician and parents.

Some physicians do give the families a good deal of information. They may diagram the heart, point out the defect, tell what surgery is planned, and give a rough estimate of prognosis for success of the operation. However, even in these instances, parents may fail to "hear" or to understand;

they often need repeated explanations and several chances to ask questions as their fears surface later or doubts recur about the wisdom of an operation.[62] Unless the parents fully understand the issue and decide that surgery is necessary, their guilt is magnified when they see the suffering of the child postoperatively. If the child dies, they are open to lifelong self-blame, or to blame by the spouse, and distrust of physicians.

When possible, the worker should encourage a relationship with a local pediatrician. A physician to whom they relate and on whom they rely for care of the child before the operation is able to provide a supportive relationship and to interpret the data of the specialist. The parents can discuss with him the child's chances with and without an operation. He can reinforce their courage to accept the child's risk and pain. Those who have worked with hospitalized children point out the need for as much emotional support to the family as possible from all sources during the pre- and postoperative period.[63]

Parents' feelings about subjecting their frightened child to surgery may be extrapolated from an observer's comments about adults who make this decision for themselves: "The challenge to each patient remains the same: to dare to undergo what is ironically at the same time a life threatening, life saving, and usually elective operation, and to agree to incur almost inconceivable amounts of acute anxiety and physical and chemical assault upon the organism."[64] He describes the "exotic equipment [and] eerie science fiction atmosphere" of the intensive care unit. Another seasoned hospital social worker, in discussing parents' anxieties about cardiac surgery on children, describes the "agitated, restless and highly vocal" behavior of other patients in a cardiac surgical ward, and the frequent crises when someone undergoes cardiac arrest or internal bleeding.[65]

The large scar on the child's chest is often not anticipated. One foster mother said she "almost fainted" when she saw the huge red scar on the child she had been caring for and felt at first that she could not possibly take him home. This same feeling of shock to the point of fainting has been described by another mother on first seeing the ugly wound.

Prior experiences, in addition to those undergone at the time of the child's surgery and intensive care, affect parental attitudes. If other children in the immediate or extended family have died of heart defects or after heart surgery, fears about this child may be overwhelming. Partially resolved feelings about the earlier death of a loved one from other causes, or loss through desertion or divorce, may trigger a great reservoir of anxiety about the possible loss of the child. Seemingly "irrational" amounts of fear flood up from the past and focus on the anticipated danger to the child.

In one extreme case, a mother had lost one family member in an automobile accident, another in a heart attack, and her husband had deserted shortly before the time the surgeons suggested operating on her little boy's heart defect. It was impossible for her to agree. Had someone who knew the family situation and her feelings interpreted this mother's "lack of cooperation" to the surgeon, he might have suggested postponing a decision. The worker might have given the mother enough chance to talk that she would have gained some insight into her feelings; she might have reconsidered her decision.

Though the example cited is extreme, practitioners with all age-groups have observed how even the loss of a pet can trigger feelings about earlier losses, and the accumulated emotion can prevent rational thinking unless opportunity for catharsis is provided. In light of the high proportion of one-parent families with whom social workers are involved and the number of parents who are themselves from broken homes, a mother's loss of her husband should be kept in mind, in addition to her earlier life experiences, when heart surgery for the child is under consideration.

A final earlier experience that often affects decisions is that with doctors and other authority figures. Many persons are encountered who have received discourtesy or hasty service from medical practitioners because they are welfare recipients, or because they attended clinics staffed by a changing group of inexperienced interns and residents. Other clients, who have received the most courteous and understanding medical care, may have a generalized mistrust of authority figures owing to maltreatment by their own parents, or to a generalized group hatred of "the establishment." Whereas the latter group can sometimes be reached by understanding workers, those whose attitudes are distorted by early childhood pain and hate are least responsive to intervention of any kind; they can only respond at their own pace and with a great deal of support.

What is the worker's responsibility in persuading parents to permit surgery on a child with congenital heart disease? *Do not persuade anyone to have surgery.* This is a decision that must be made by the patient or, in the case of children, by the parents alone. Remove obstacles, provide clarification, give support, but do not persuade.

The helping person nevertheless may be crucial in permitting parents to arrive at the decision to permit surgery on their child. Listening to the parents' ideas, their anguished pros and cons, their apprehensions, permits not only catharsis but an understanding of how they comprehend the advantages and risks. As often happens in an interview, the client may express outward or superficial issues in detail and only reveal the real problem when the worker starts to leave, sometimes as a half-joke, or as if incidentally. If the underlying problem that prevents permission for surgery is an irrational one, arrangements should be made to discuss this problem when there is time for its serious exploration. If it reveals lack of confidence in the recommendations, arrangements for an independent consultation with another specialist may be indicated. If it reveals need for more accurate understanding, arrangements should be made for a conference with the pediatrician or the specialist. If it reveals discord between marital partners, a joint conference or review of joint interviews with them may be indicated, or a family conference with the appropriate doctor. Care to avoid easy reassurance is important, as is direct influence upon the decision.

Discipline

Inability to discipline a young child with heart disease is a prevalent problem of parents. The aftereffects are serious. One pediatric cardiologist says, "I always tell mothers there is a long distance from the bottom to the heart, and much padding in between,"[66] but spanking or otherwise effectively disciplining a child with a heart defect presents many obstacles. A child who is small and frail and is often observed to be miserable provides an unlikely target for punishment, especially if he is one whose crying may bring on anoxic spells and whose very life has been sustained only by extreme effort. Even though the child may have few if any symptoms, anxiety may prevent objectivity. Parental guilt over any congenital defect is well known, and overprotection is a classic manifestation of guilt feelings. In one study of 150 families of children with congenital heart disease, 50 percent reported difficulty in disciplining the child.[67] Other studies have confirmed the prevalence of the problem.[68] One in-depth study that has been made of 25 families showed the problem of training and discipline to exist in all but one.[69]

"Spoiling" during the early socialization period deprives the young child of opportunity to build inner controls. The child develops serious psychological disturbance when he receives "punishment," not for disobedience, but unpredictably and magically (from his standpoint) from his body and its medical care for fantasized wrongdoing; when he is closely attached to an anxious mother who has given him reason to think he is special in some way;[70] when he is justifiably anxious and has received repeated pain from adults who tried to make him trust them; and finally when he is deprived of inner controls against impulses.[71]

The problem can be observed in the early-school-age child who is fussy and irritable, a tyrant in the house, and in the adolescent who is impulse-ridden. The mother mentioned earlier, who had not permitted surgery in her teenager's childhood, said she sometimes thinks it would have been better for him to have died in surgery than to have grown into a person dangerously hostile and devoid of controls. When he was reexamined in adolescence, the physicians recommended an end to physical restriction. His response had been to say to his mother, "Now I know you'll kill me. You didn't dare lay hands on me before, but you'll make up for it now."

After treatment, as in some cases described from successful surgery on tetralogy of Fallot, a dramatic change in color and alertness provides visual testimony that the child is indeed a different being, who can be treated differently. In many other cases, the child's small, frail stature remains (as a result of growth retardation); he is still behind in school and social development; he is dependent and "spoiled," and the part he feeds into the mother-child interaction tends to hold back a change in parental attitude and treatment.

One source reports that in a series of 12 cases operated, of which eight had good or excellent results, and an additional 13 awaiting surgery, "most of the mothers interviewed were primarily concerned not with how to enforce prescribed restrictions of activity, but rather how to permit the degree of freedom of activity authorized by the physician."[72] Fear, including that of the child's sudden death, guilt due to the congenital nature of the problem, and long-accustomed strain and protection to keep the child alive, in addition to grief over what they have seen the child go through, are not suddenly thrown off.

Social workers encounter some of the occasional cases in which not indulgence but scapegoating of the cardiac child occurs. The puny child at times is scapegoated because of something in the parents' background that creates an abnormal drive for normality. One case reported in the literature describes in a cardiac child what we have seen in the undersized multihandicapped: "We didn't understand him because, constantly, he had to sit on someone's lap. He had a terrible disposition and we would get so tired out, and you worry until you get a little carried away, and we'd spank him a lot of times and treat him a little rougher than we should have . . . he was pale and skinny . . . I wanted all my children to look healthy and strong."[73]

Social workers and other counselors need to lend themselves seriously to helping parents with appropriate discipline of young children. Whether it is dangerous for the child to cry should be checked out with the physician. How much frustration he can tolerate and whether spanking is dangerous also need to be talked over. Fear of sudden death, a common maternal reaction, usually is not realistic. It should be brought out in the open and the possibility discussed with the physician. A child who is in a growth spurt, with increased metabolic demands upon his heart, may not be able to tolerate the frustrations he can withstand later. A rule of thumb at one stage in his development does not hold at another. Furthermore, that which is appropriate for one child with a cardiac defect is not applicable to another child with a different make-up and different defect.

A harassed mother, who has many problems in addition to caring for her sickly cardiac child and who is pulled in many directions, is not always rational or able to control her own temper. She may be afraid of her temper—of letting go. Relieving the mother of some of the pressures on her may be more helpful in enabling her to carry out what she knows to be desirable than teaching or advising her.

The Effects of Long-Term Disability

Personality strands woven by *constitutional sensitivity to experience* and those created by the experience itself cannot be separated. In one case of three-year-old twins with ventricular defects the mother said, "Louise begins to cry as soon as she sees we are going in the car, and cries for a full day and a half after the [very painful] injections there, but Louis doesn't cry until he sees the nurse get the needle ready." One cannot separate the physical and psychological causes of this difference in behavior. True, the little girl has a larger defect, her growth is more severely retarded, her veins are smaller and thus the technician more often repeatedly sticks her, the child has less "padding" or muscle tissue so that intramuscular injections are more painful. However, the mother is more anxious about the little girl, for the physician thinks the boy may be able to get along without surgery, whereas it is inevitable for the girl. Does the mother's anxiety reinforce the child's fear of pain inflicted by treatment? Is the child also more sensitive to experience than her twin?

Unfortunately, the formative years of infancy and preschool are those in which most congenital heart disease creates its greatest physiological problems. Surgery in the late preschool or early school years may overcome the major physical problem, but the psychological impact of the defect and its treatment will remain.

Behavior is the speech of the young child. Infants who have symptomatic cardiac defects are usually described as "sickly and unhappy." They express fright, pain, and insecurity by crying, whining, wanting to be held, eating and sleeping poorly, and looking miserable. One pediatrician said to his nursing staff, "Use your eyes, kids don't verbalize." He remarked on the worried look on an infant's face which signifies pain or discomfort.[74] Another pediatrician has pointed out the tendency for some mothers to mistake cardiac distress for spoiled behavior in infants because they stop crying as soon as they are picked up, the change in position permitting them to breathe more easily.

The small child's psychology of living in the present makes cardiac children seem happy at home and school when they are not ill or in pain or threatened with separation or pain, unless they have suffered long and repeated periods of chronic illness. However, one does not forget the look of terror on the face of a child whose heart is pumping wildly and who is expecting death. The shy, withdrawn behavior of children who have been repeatedly seriously ill is difficult to penetrate. According to one study, "The nonspecific effects of long-standing illness were extremely disabling, particularly for the children who were unable to participate in the physical activities which are of such importance to motor development and the channeled discharge of energy, and to the establishment of healthy peer relationships." The authors of the article describe the morbid feelings of two children about "holes in their heart," one referring to a "broken heart."[75]

The Surgical Experience

Roberta Peay, who has worked with many cardiac children and their parents at the Clinical Center of the National Institutes of Health in Bethesda, Maryland, says that fears prior to surgery range from "what we consider minimal to near panic; these emotions can also vary in terms of the situation at a given time."[76] She discusses the acute distress of the child after surgery, and the need to help the parent understand in advance that he may be angry at them for permitting him to undergo such a shocking experience. The surgical experience is affected by the age of the child, the preparation he has had, the ability of the mother to stay with him before and after surgery, the amount of pain and complications he suffers, and what happens in the intensive care unit while the child is there.

A popular conception is that infants and young children suffer less pain from surgery than older persons. Having less awareness, they presumably have less anxiety, and anxiety is known to affect the degree of pain felt. However, the baby and toddler are not spared the most fundamental anxiety, that of separation from the mother. Furthermore, the immobilization inherent in the postoperative period runs counter to instinctual drives toward activity. Nurses have observed despair develop as a result of repeatedly painful procedures and new forms of pain as treatment progresses.[77]

An illustration of psychic scarring from cardiac surgery was described with bewilderment by the mother of an eight-year-old girl who cringed and cried when undressed at a clinic. She said the child's heart surgery at age ten months had been uneventful and the baby had evidenced no outward distress that she was aware of. However, when the child had her tonsils removed at age six, she suffered total psychological collapse, remaining in a near-coma for several days. Her fear of doctors remained so deep that she still cried when prepared for a physical examination.

Age-related fantasies and realistic fears about pain, mutilation, and death are well documented in the psychiatric and child development literature.[78] The mother of an eight-year-old child was presented to a psychiatric seminar because of the boy's aggressive behavior after open-heart surgery with prolonged complications. She said, "Help him with his fears. For some strange reason, he's scared to death of everything—pesticides, bugs, anything." The teacher had worried because he drew tombstones on which he printed the names of children who he felt tormented him.

In an exceptionally delicate piece of work with a withdrawn eight-year-old boy, a doctoral social work student has described the fantasies the child revealed after a relationship slowly permitted their expression in stories.[79] "Once upon a time there was a big dinosaur who thought he was going to die, and he said to himself, 'I am going to die, I know it, I'm going to die.' He walked through the forest and all the other animals were happy but he was the only one who was sad because he was sick." The child told other stories that revealed helplessness and fear. Eventually he cried and talked about his heart operation. It was fear about the knife that had given him nightmares. "He drew, hesitantly, a picture of a large curved knife with a sharp tooth edge....When I asked how long he thought it was, he held his hands about two feet apart." Regarding other frightening things, "he looked at the floor and asked if the blood clots he coughed up were pieces of his heart."

The management of the surgical experience greatly affects the psychological trauma. One mother, a teacher, telephoned the hospital for help in preparing her four-year-old child for heart surgery. A student nurse assigned to the project took the child through the pediatric ward, and showed her the door to the intensive care unit and operating room; she secured pictures of doctors and nurses, and pamphlets for children about hospitals; the child was told about the tubes that would be attached to her body and why, when she came to in the recovery room, and what the intensive care unit would look like. The success of the carefully contrived preparation was beyond expectations. Another child of the same age in the intensive care unit at the same time provided an unfortunate "control." This child's terror and anxiety were much greater than that of the prepared child.

The attitude of the parents is of paramount importance in the nonverbal preparation of the child for surgery. The National Institutes of Health cardiac service in Bethesda not only prepares the parents with intellectual explanations but explores their fears and provides emotional support and practical help throughout their stay. Pamphlets have been prepared for the parents and for the children.

The size, management, and staffing of the intensive care units affect the child's experience. Wide differences exist; sophisticated child-oriented pediatric units provide for maximum continuity of supportive nursing staff, plan ahead for the parents to visit the child five minutes every hour, and shield the child insofar as possible from the terrifying sounds and sights of other patients in the unit at the same time. Many hospital personnel feel strongly that children should not be removed from pediatrics to adult surgical management and facilities at the time of most critical need for child-oriented measures, but even in facilities of excellent standards children are placed in intensive care units with adults who may be groaning or hemorrhaging, and under care of doctors and nurses they have never seen before and who have not specialized in child care.

Intensive care means a place where critically ill persons are monitored and treated; some die or have major crises. One pediatric cardiac specialist said of the psychological effects on children in his own high-standard facility, "We don't know if it [the intensive care unit experience] makes a scratch, a dent, or a hole in the child's personality. Certainly we can tell by the dilated pupils and rapid pulse that children are in a state of chronic fear while there. They may see other children die, or mysterious things happen that look as if someone is dying."[80]

The worker in the community may have minimal opportunity to influence the choice of medical center and to know whether the child will have the best or worst of experiences associated with surgery. In some instances, however, she may be able to see that options are available, and help the parents consider the relative merits of a local versus a distant center. She may want to make inquiry about the amount of work done in a local heart center and, if it is minimal, ask the pediatrician to help guide the parents toward the best available care for the child.

The worker can make an important contribution to alleviating surgical trauma by helping with the practical problems that will enable the mother to remain with the child, by securing help in psychological preparation of the child for the hospital experience, and by allowing opportunity for sustained psychological support to parents and child before and after the crisis that heart surgery creates.

Growth Retardation

Stunting and its effect upon social relationships will be commented on in respect to children with juvenile arthritis; obviously, the problem is more severe psychologically for boys than for girls. Unfortunately growth retardation commonly results from heart defects. "Failure to thrive" in an infant should trigger in the worker not an automatic response that the child is neglected but a question whether he has had a thorough physical examination by a physician who is skilled in the use of the stethoscope on infants.

The physical growth and intellectual development of children with congenital heart disease have been studied in several series. In one study of 317 Caucasian children without defects other than cardiac, they were significantly smaller than normal, both preoperatively and postoperatively, the surgery having been only slightly beneficial in helping them catch up in size.[81] In another series of 463 children, severe growth failure occurred among children with all types of cardiac defects, the severity of the growth retardation generally correlating with the severity of the cardiac defect.[82]

However, in this study the authors noted improvement in growth within months of surgery, except in palliative procedures for tetralogy of Fallot.

Sibling Relationships

Siblings of the disabled cardiac child cannot receive an equal share of the parents' attention. Indeed, older children may be pressed into service by the harassed mother. To a five-year-old sister of a three-year-old, one mother said during an interview, "Run out and see if Lucy's playing in the water; go upstairs and get Lucy a clean pair of pants; now go outdoors and play—can't you see I'm busy?" This sibling needed attention so badly that in kindergarten she distracted the other children with constant bids for attention, so much so that she was not permitted to continue to attend.

Another mother of a chronically ill cardiac child said that the other children were not permitted to go among crowds for fear of bringing home infections. "They don't like to miss out on the movies and picnics and swimming and all, but they know they've got to, for awhile anyway." Nor do siblings dare to express resentment against the ill child in the usual brother-sister fashion of hitting, kicking, or slapping. They are deprived of the normal outlet for childhood anger if they internalize and share the parents' prohibitions.

Guilt feelings over hostile wishes enlarge fears for themselves. The fears to which siblings are prone have been described in a report of a series of 150 families previously cited. Some children express fears that they too may have holes in their hearts, or that they are defective in some manner. Some take on parental fears over possible death of the cardiac child, which may be inevitable where the family income, plans, recreation, housing, and relationships are all focused around the recurring crises or frailty and fatigability of the child with a heart defect.

School Adjustment and Social Relationships

Children with heart defects rarely attend special schools for the physically handicapped, but may do so if no other school will admit them or if bus transportation is available there but not elsewhere. Many who have had surgery do well, and their capacity for vigor gives joy to those who have known them previously. No activity limitation is placed upon them and the physician emphasizes the child's ability to limit his own activity according to his fatigue.

However, as with asthmatic and diabetic children, cardiac children do not have the advantage of teachers oriented to special physical needs. Thus they may occasionally be excluded from class because of the teacher's unwarranted fears or, to the contrary, meet with less consideration than needed because of a stereotyped response that handicapped children should be forced to be independent.

Cardiac children often attend special classes for educationally handicapped children. Studies of intellectual development show there is nothing incompatible with normal intellect in a cardiac defect, but it is true that many children with heart disease do not measure normal on standardized tests. In an English study of 43 children, all of whom had severe cardiac defects of varied nature and most of whom were between four and ten years of age, a wide scatter of intellectual capacity appeared on psychological tests. The authors concluded that the mean scores and the scatter showed normal intellectual development.[83] Some of the children were precocious because of constant association with adults and preoccupation with books and quiet pursuits; 13 of the 43 children had IQ scores of 110 or above. However, more than the normal number of children had IQ's under 90, with nine below 70. The lack of opportunity for schooling and physical fatigue, with slow reaction and manipulation of objects, and emotional disturbance or anxiety, were believed responsible. "The more intelligent child, deprived of school teaching, may be reading on his own, [and] improve his performance on a verbal scale such as the Stanford Binet, whereas the dull child, who cannot utilize his time in this way, falls yet further behind."[84] This observation has particular applicability to the culturally deprived child.

Of special note in this small study was the marked effect of fatigue. One-fourth of the children were too tired to lift blocks or handle pencils with ordinary speed or tired very early in the interviews. Fatigue this great may easily be mistaken for mental dullness.

A French study of 114 children between five and 14 years of age who were hospitalized for cardiac surgery used psychometric tests and interviews to determine intellectual and social development. The study reported "a deficiency in perceptual and motor functioning particularly in the cyanotic cases, the conspicuous disturbances tending to corroborate the hypothesis of an organic susceptibility produced by an inadequate blood flow." Yet the investigators questioned whether the large percentage of low IQ's found were due to true intellectual retardation or resulted from irregular school attendance and lack of stimuli that "eventually reduces the child to a state of passive withdrawal thereby further diminishing his interests and motivations."[85]

In a recent massive study by Johns Hopkins Hospital staff of over a thousand children who had severe heart defects and were operated on in the early years of palliative surgery for tetralogy of Fallot, 64 percent of those who had left the hospital were still alive, and provided elementary data about themselves at the beginning of the fifteenth postoperative year.[86] However, out of this group, less than a third gave information about their life adjustment. Those who did included over fifty persons who had achieved professional status as doctors, lawyers, teachers, and the like. The

CONGENITAL HEART DISEASE

great proportion who failed to answer the questions about occupation and schooling creates speculation that many had either done poorly, were disappointed in themselves, or were psychologically or physically disabled. A significant number, particularly persons who had had surgery in the preschool years, had had to have second operations, and some even third and fourth operations; from this fact, as well as from the deaths that had occurred from brain abscess or bacterial endocarditis, one can imagine the school interruptions and social deprivations they had undergone.

Interruption of class attendance by illness may put the cardiac child further behind. If he does attend classes for the educationally handicapped, he may be with slow learners and the curriculum may be geared to mental dullness. He may not secure the stimulation from peers that would normally take place. Lack of discipline and internalized expectations of less than normal performance may aggravate problems of learning.

Relationships with peers can be normal for those children who have few symptoms or who have had entirely successful surgery early in life; others are handicapped by small size, immature social development, lack of self-confidence, and lack of acceptance by others. The study of French children found that the younger ones were very insecure and in need of reassurance. The children over eight years old had strong feelings of being different from others, with feelings of anxiety expressed in either excitation or withdrawal. A body image of disjointedness and incapacity appeared. The authors point out the inhibiting effect on the child's social development of a close relationship with an anxious, overprotective mother. Unfortunately, this perceptive study was carried out at a time and place (during hospitalization for cardiac surgery) that could not but have affected the content of the children's revelations about their feelings and reactions.[87]

"He never learned how to play with others" has been mentioned several times by mothers whose children are physically well during school age as a result of surgery but were disabled as infants and young children. A maturational lag in social development takes place when a child is too tired to play outdoors long at a time and must come in and rest, or when he can never keep up with the other children and thus learns not to compete but instead expects always to fail. One mother described her son, possessed with newfound vigor after surgery, as rushing up and shaking other children. "He wants to play, but he doesn't know how," so the other children dislike him.

The Multihandicapped Child

Heart defects combine frequently with other congenital malformations. A wide range of physical combinations exists, and there is an entire gamut of psychosocial ramifications. The two most frequent physical combinations are those occasioned by the rubella syndrome, which includes blindness, deafness, and patent ductus arteriosus, and by mongolism, which is often accompanied by an endocardial cushion defect (see discussion of atrial septal defect, primum type, p. 245). These two illustrate the high degree of individualization necessary in medical and social planning, and they bring out the issues frequently encountered.

Many stable families in every socioeconomic class take care of multihandicapped children with minimal help. Social workers tend to know those who arrive at a point where they can no longer carry on and ask for institutional placement of the child. The worker who is helping unwed mothers or who works in a protective agency may be concerned with a multihandicapped newborn. The social worker's responsibility varies from that *in loco parentis* to that of counseling anguished families. Whatever her responsibility, she should be clear about the cardiac defect and its place in the spectrum of problems.

The blind, deaf child with patent ductus arteriosus may well have a heart defect that creates few, if any, symptoms in early life. Recalling the discussion in the Medical Realities section of this chapter, the worker needs to keep in mind that this defect does not require open-heart surgery (providing it is not one of a combination of heart defects) and has been operated upon for the longest period with the greatest success. The defect will, however, shorten the child's life if not repaired, and will be much more difficult to repair safely as he grows older.

The blind and deaf child presents urgent medical problems that sap the energies of the mother or foster mother and command the worker's attention. The many visits to an ophthalmologist for treatment of his eyes and an aggressive speech-and-hearing program mean numerous trips to other physicians, securing reports from counselors and therapists, fitting glasses and hearing aids, etc. The heart problem that causes no overt symptoms is pushed into the background. Worker turnover and large case loads sometimes result in the new workers' complete lack of knowledge that a heart problem exists. They may look at the last recordings, see nothing except notes about eye examinations or speech-and-hearing examinations, and fail to note the existence of patent ductus—or, finding it, not know what the term implies.

The worker's first responsibility is to arrive at a decision with those concerned with the child regarding advisability of heart surgery. Questions arise about his mentality and the probabilities of prolonging his life: How much of his retardation is due to lying in a crib in an institutional setting, devoid of tactile, emotional, or aural stimuli? How much from being deprived of the essentials of normal psychological growth owing to the admittedly inadequate care he very likely receives? From lack of mothering? From deprivation of learning opportunities? Is the child autistic or retarded, or both, as well as blind and deaf? Does his mother want him, or could she be helped to want him if she had less stress to cope with and more love to give? Is her current situation known, or has she been all but frozen out by the foster mother and not "bothered" by the agency? For what purpose shall he be put through the unquestioned pain and terror of repair of his heart defect? Will his life, if saved and prolonged, hold any happiness or merely stretch into an infinitude of bleakness?

The same fundamental questions must be answered for the child with mongolism, or Down's syndrome, but here different physical factors influence the decision. If the child has an endocardial cushion defect, partial or complete, the defect may cause death in early infancy before he is large enough to be a good surgical risk. The defect he has is one of the most complex and difficult, requiring open-heart surgery and carrying a high mortality risk. His mental limits, though not known with certainty, can be guessed, for the majority of children with his condition do not develop capacity for abstract thinking and frequently are found in the "moderately" retarded classification, which from a practical standpoint means those with severe mental limitations. Postponing surgery until the child has survived the most hazardous years of early life and is at optimum childhood strength and resiliency is not neglect but common sense. Thus, a sharp point of difference exists between the issues for him and his multihandicapped brother with patent ductus, who is blind and deaf.

But the underlying questions remain. Shall an attempt be made to salvage this child's life? "Who Shall Live"* is the ultimate in philosophical problems.

As technology continues to outstrip value formulations and brings vital issues into conflict with each other, a new area, that of bioethics, has developed. Legal, theological, medical, social work, and philosophical experts have begun to grapple with questions such as those posed by the advisability of cardiac surgery on the multihandicapped child. Some comments on the subject have been made in Chapter 2.

Unfortunately, this most difficult issue is decided by the physician alone in some cases, or unwittingly by the social worker alone, without consultation or full exploration of the child's total situation. The worker usually raises no question when the physician notes on the medical record that surgery "is not indicated because of other problems." She may silently agree that obstacles to this child's achievement of a satisfying life are so multiple and serious that putting him through the pain and trauma of surgery is not warranted. Or she may not dare question the surgeon's judgment, failing to realize that he is as human and vulnerable to subjective responses as she. In some cases, the worker alone determines that a child's

* *Who Shall Live? Man's Control over Birth and Death*, A Report Prepared for the American Friends Service Committee (New York: Hill and Wang, 1970), deals with the moral and theological questions that arise.

life is not worth saving. She does this, not by conscious decision, but by placing the child susceptible to infection and without the cardiac reserve to withstand infection, in a nursery with a number of other children—or in other words, in a setting where recurrent infection is inevitable.

Desirably, no person alone should make the decision regarding the possibility of saving the child's life and the risks that should be taken to save it. Moral and philosophical positions vary. Bias in one direction may correct itself when a group of persons discuss the problem. Some consensus should be reached, on the basis of all the information available. Participants should, of course, include the parent or parents if they are available and have technical custody, and in some cases grandparents or other relatives who have remained concerned about the child. They should include the foster mother and, if relevant, nursery staff who provide the child with physical care. These persons have observed the child's reaction to stimuli, his response to pain and fear, and can help in arriving at some estimate of the child's probable degree of retardation. In some instances their love is invested in his welfare. All those who care, and have knowledge to pool, can help make life-and-death decisions in the child's behalf.

An overriding practical issue is finding placement for the multihandicapped child with a cardiac defect when the parents will not or cannot care for him at home. In some counties, foster-home funding is adequate for the need. In other counties, the only bonuses available are for foster homes that accept the retarded or emotionally disturbed. Special funding is critical, in that no foster parent can afford to accept a child with 24-hour care needs unless the board rate provides for domestic help or regular relief. If the county does not make such provision, the child must be placed in institutional-type care where, as earlier brought out, cross-infections will guarantee the shortening of life. In such instances, it is the worker's obligation to let her superiors know the institutional responsibility the agency is taking. A card file of cases may be kept that can be used as ammunition by the supervisor or director in presenting to the authorities the needs for special payments to foster mothers who can care for physically handicapped children only if they have paid assistants.

CHAPTER NINE

Cystic Fibrosis

THE FULL, formal name of cystic fibrosis, cystic fibrosis of the pancreas, is a curious misnomer, for chronic lung impairment is usually the most critical feature. Sometimes called *mucoviscidosis*, or *fibrocystic disease*, the condition is a generalized, hereditary disorder wherein the mucus-secreting and sweat glands are abnormal, and in which unusually thick and sticky mucus interferes with the functioning of the lungs and digestive system. It is a grave disease, for no cure has been discovered at the time of this writing.

Cystic fibrosis was not identified until 1936. For lack of formulation of effective treatment, children usually died within the first one or two years of life. The number of children with the disease has grown greatly, possibly because of a real increase and also because earlier diagnosis and improved treatment have increased the life expectancy, with consequent increase in living children. It is now one of the most common chronic diseases of childhood and is the most serious lung condition among children.[1]

Cystic fibrosis seems to be almost entirely a disease of Caucasians, with Negro children seldom affected and Oriental children almost never affected.[2] Sex distribution is equal. Geographical distribution in the United States apparently is greater in the Northeast and North-central states, the prevalence possibly affected by congregation of families around several major treatment centers. The case rate is estimated at about one in 1,000 to 1,500 live births.[3] The deaths account for 2 to 4 percent of all deaths in childhood.

Cystic fibrosis is of special concern to social workers because of the massive social implications for the families affected. In perhaps no other disease is successful medical treatment, and therefore the life of the child, so dependent upon alteration in normal family life. The demands upon the family are formidable and spectacular; these become apparent as the disease and its treatment are understood. The disease creates almost irreparable problems for adolescents. Those concerned with counseling affected children and their families need as much understanding as possible of the meaning of cystic fibrosis.

THE MEDICAL REALITIES

The one fortunate aspect of cystic fibrosis is its hereditary pattern. The gene is recessive, thus requiring both parents to carry it and eliminating the destructive tendency of the parents to "climb each other's family tree," as in cases where birth defects are inherited from one side of the family alone. In cystic fibrosis, the statistically average chances are that in a family of four children whose parents carry the gene, one child will be normal, one will have cystic fibrosis, and two will be carriers. In actual practice, many affected families have more than one child with the disease, the incidence of two or more in the same family being estimated at 24 percent.[4]

Nature and Symptoms

According to foremost medical authorities, a feature in approximately 85 percent of persons with cystic fibrosis is pancreatic insufficiency leading to the absence of enzymes needed for the absorption of food.[5] The pancreatic ducts are plugged by mucus, preventing the pancreatic enzymes from reaching the intestine to help break down fat and protein into an absorbable form. Approximately half of the fat eaten is not absorbed. This may result in a voracious appetite and an inadequate weight gain. A related problem is evacuation of very foul, bulky, greasy stools. The sweat glands have a salt concentration markedly greater than that of normal persons. A notable use of this peculiarity of cystic fibrosis is sweat analysis to diagnose the disease with the so-called "sweat test." In hot weather, massive salt loss through sweat can lead to shock and even death.

Problems of the liver are relatively uncommon, but in some cases they lead to severe complications that create serious manifestations of the disease.[6] *Portal hypertension* resulting from thick mucus in the bile ducts may cause liver damage and enlargement. It may also result in varicose veins of the esophagus, which may suddenly break with severe bleeding. Another consequence of portal hypertension may be enlargement of the spleen with trapping of blood elements, which may lead to increased ease of bleeding or anemia.

Babies may incur *meconium ileus,* or thick, molasses-like stools that create obstruction of the bowel, necessitating surgery usually in the first few days of life. Children who survive the surgery may develop serious gastrointestinal and respiratory symptoms later.[7]

But by far the most widespread difficulty is lung involvement.[8] The infant or child develops a dry hacking cough, and after an upper respiratory infection, or especially after measles or whooping cough, he develops bronchial obstruction and secondary infection. This is usually brought under control with antibiotics, but it recurs, and as the pattern is repeated over and over the child eventually succumbs.

The process should be understood, for much rests on it.[9] The bronchi are lined with fine hairs called *cilia*, which under ordinary circumstances waft bacteria and air pollutants up from the lungs in systematic waves, coated in a fluid bath of thin, slippery mucus. The infectious material is swallowed or coughed out. In cystic fibrosis, where the secreted mucus is too thick to be brought up, one of the body's systems of getting rid of bacteria is destroyed. The most critical feature of treatment is to remove the mucus and bacteria. If this is not achieved, infection of the bronchial tubes and trapping of the air in the lungs result. More and more areas of the lungs lose their function. As the air becomes trapped, the gaseous exchange is impaired, with resulting shortness of breath from lack of oxygen and excessive carbon dioxide in the bloodstream and body tissues. Recurrent infections lead to more mucus, which plugs the airways and creates more damage to the bronchial walls and the lungs. Bronchial pneumonia recurs and, though temporarily and partially subject to control with antibiotics, eventually overcomes the child. The most usual infectious agents reported are *staphylococcus* and *pseudomonas*, though others may be found. Unfortunately, the bacteria are those that frequently become resistant to antibiotics.

Not all children with cystic fibrosis are affected in the same way, and the disease differs in severity so that not all children have the same symptoms. Symptoms may appear in early infancy or not until the child is older. In general, it is said that the earlier the disease appears, the more serious it will be. The disease is characterized by ups and downs, with long periods of stability between spells of illness; although the disease itself is always present, the child appears to be relatively well much of the time until late in the course of the illness. Early symptoms in general usually include exceptionally foul bulky stools, protruding abdomen, hacking cough, and chronic chest disease leading to recurrent chest infections. Retarded physical development is usually apparent, though notable variation is observed even in children in the same family. Children with cystic fibrosis often "fail to thrive" as infants, and later they look several years younger than they are and are small for their age. Most are thin, showing the effects of incapacity to gain, no matter how good the diet.

When generalized bronchial obstruction occurs, the child has hyperinflated lungs and shares some of the appearance of the *emphysematous* adult. He develops a *barrel chest*, may be obviously short of breath even on speaking or mild exertion, and have big fingertips with rounded nails. The medical report may indicate that the physician hears *rales* in the child's chest, and the X-ray report may describe a *honeycomb* or *snowflake appearance*.

Coughing is one of the most significant outward signs of illness in the child with cystic fibrosis. The cough is frequent, and usually though not always loose. The absence of cough may simply mean that the child cannot bring up the secretions—a poor sign—but more usually it shows that the disease is under control and is to be welcomed.

Treatment

Except for occasional periods of hospitalization during episodes of acute worsening of the lung disease, treatment is conducted in the home.* The regime is often established in the hospital over a two- or three-week period, when the physical therapist may teach the postural drainage exercises to the parents and the inhalation therapist may help them with the ordering and establishment of equipment in the home. Medical care or its direction should be conducted by a specialist who has a treatment team to help him, first because it is so grave, and second because treatment is so complex. Treatment measures have two general purposes: first is to keep the lungs clear of obstructive secretions and thus to prevent or reduce infection and damage to the bronchial walls; second is to compensate by diet for loss of nutriments to the stools.

Frequent feedings may be necessary, with every effort made to satisfy the child's hunger. The diet is of high-caloric, low-fat content with pancreatic extracts. The extracts are from animal pancreas and replace some of the missing enzymes to help digestion of fat and protein. Degree of involvement of the pancreas varies from one child to another. Some children are said to need little dietary restriction, whereas others need restriction of fatty foods such as whole milk, peanut butter, butter, potato chips, fat meat, and pastry. The child's growth and the character of the stools influence the physician's determination of dietary needs. High-calorie snacks are recommended between meals and at bedtime.

Extra salt is encouraged, especially in hot weather, when the physician may prescribe heavy amounts of added salt every day. This is necessary because of the increased loss of salt in the sweat in this disease.

Treatment of the lungs, in addition to use of antibiotics, is sometimes referred to as the "pulmonary toilet." The aim is to clean out stagnant secretions, which invite infection and impair the cleansing action of the cilia. This is done by reducing the stickiness of the mucus and improving drainage, through the use of (1) aerosol administration of drugs that constrict blood vessels and dilate bronchial tubes, (2) postural drainage, with percussion and vibration of the chest, and (3) physical activity. Aerosol

---

* The account of treatment is that provided under Dr. Harvey's direction at the Children's Hospital at Stanford, as well as treatment described by Di Sant'Agnese (notes 5, 8); by Doershuk and Mathews (note 2) at the School of Medicine, Western Reserve University; and by L. W. Mathews et al. at the Department of Pediatrics at Western Reserve, in "A Therapeutic Regimen for Patients with Cystic Fibrosis," the report of an investigation supported by the Cystic Fibrosis Foundation (note 12).

treatment, followed by percussion and drainage, usually takes place two to four times a day, usually before meals and at bedtime. *These treatments must be carried out daily for the entire duration of life.*

Postural drainage treatments immediately follow the aerosol treatment. The child is placed on the parent's lap or a table in various prescribed positions that permit gravity to assist, and the therapist or parent claps his cupped hands on the child's chest. This is followed by a finer vibratory movement. Older children can be taught to clap some of the chest areas themselves. The purpose is to jar the secretions loose and let them drain out. Some families use electrically driven mechanical percussors and vibrators. Each percussion and drainage treatment requires approximately 30–60 minutes and substantial physical vigor. Some major cystic fibrosis centers teach parents of infants and toddlers to suction the secretions until the children are old enough to cough on command, after the percussion of each lobar area. The suction procedure is uncomfortable for the child and may cause him to cry.

Breathing exercises to improve the efficiency of respiration and posture may be beneficial; the child lies or sits and breathes in and out slowly as taught. Usual knee bends, push-ups, etc. are used. Children are encouraged to learn to play wind instruments, and to run and play actively, as aids to deep breathing. Small children or severely ill patients need to have their position changed frequently.

Adequate treatment requires equipment. The "nebulization therapy," or aerosol and mist-tent treatments, are designed to deposit medication directly on the mucus coating in the recesses of the bronchial system, and to wet and thin down the secretions. A nebulizer with face mask or mouthpiece is necessary. At night the child may sleep in a mist tent in order to breathe the wet medicated air all night. Compressed air, not oxygen, is used, with medications blown into the tent. If he sleeps in a tent, the mist should be so dense an observer can barely see the child. As is apparent, this keeps the bedclothes and mattress wet. The tent is not only expensive, but the motor, like any that keeps an appliance going eight to ten hours a day, frequently needs repair and return to the factory for maintenance work. Access to substitute equipment is necessary while the tent or motor is out of order. Arguments about responsibility for repair between the local vendor and the factory seem not infrequent.

During the past five years or so, some studies have thrown considerable doubt on the efficacy of mist-tent therapy.[10] At the Children's Hospital at Stanford and its outpatient service, children who have been sleeping in mist tents are, for the most part, continued in them, but at this writing mist-tent therapy is not begun in newly diagnosed children.[11] If further studies fail to confirm the value of this treatment, families will be relieved of many problems in the home care of their children because tents have been a constant source of work, expense, contention, and potential infection.

In certain children who do not respond to the aerosol and percussion and drainage treatments, or who cannot cooperate in them because of weakness or pain, *intermittent positive pressure breathing* (IPPB) of oxygen or air, from a specially designed machine, is administered. Some parents have these machines at home. Whether prolonged use is helpful or harmful evidently is debatable.

Antihistamine therapy and desensitization therapy are used to treat respiratory tract allergies. Chronic sinusitis is common and can be a constant source of infection for the whole respiratory tract and is therefore treated. Measles and influenza are particularly serious for patients, so that all children need measles vaccine at one year of age and should have yearly influenza vaccine injections. Pediatricians who specialize in treatment of cystic fibrosis believe that the underlying principle of the treatment program is not only to treat the disease process but to use good preventive medicine—to attempt to avoid or prevent infections and to keep the child in as good physical and psychological health as possible. Prevention of measles and influenza by vaccination and immunization is urged because of the complications that exist. Normal school attendance and usual childhood activity insofar as possible are recommended.

The psychologic attitudes and problems of the patients are closely followed and every effort is made to help the individual adjust to life with a chronic disease. Information and instruction are provided as the child becomes capable of accepting and understanding the material.... Every effort is made to keep both the patient and his family enthusiastic, hopeful, and secure in their approach to life. Our success with this program permits us to share this attitude with them.[12]

Outlook

The life expectancy of children with cystic fibrosis is continuously revised upward. Whereas older materials showed the majority of living children to be under five years of age, and later under ten, the statistical average age of death has risen to approximately age 14.[13] The mean age of 53 patients of the Children's Hospital Medical Center in Boston who died during 1968 and 1969 was 15 years.[14] A number of children are living to be young adults, some of them marrying and having families.

Increased sophistication in treatment techniques, advances in chemotherapy, increased communication among physicians, and the growth of parents' organizations to promote availability of drugs and needed equipment must be credited with the rapid advances. Despite the gains, cystic fibrosis remains a fatal disease. Publicity accompanying fund-raising campaigns makes this fact known to parents and children alike. Literature designed for their consumption underplays the outlook, but they do not escape sharing the general awareness of the community. Fortunately, no child's fate can be determined by the average, or general, considerations. A wide range of probabilities exists. The most important factor, as has been stated, is whether the disease is diagnosed and effectively treated before extensive irreversible damage occurs in the bronchial walls. Because the "effective treatment" is a matter first of medical competence and second of parental ability to exert a lifetime of daily effort in the child's behalf, the crux of the prognosis is social—e.g. the family's ability to secure competent medical care early, and the ability to carry out the medical recommendations.

PSYCHOSOCIAL IMPLICATIONS
Family Adjustment

The characteristics of the disease and the extraordinary nature of treatment shape the social implications of cystic fibrosis, as does the gravity of outlook. Under present treatment methods, the child's life depends on nothing less than the family's ability to put him first so long as he lives. Unlike the family of a child with cancer, they cannot expect a relatively defined period of disequilibrium; unlike the family of a severely retarded child, they have no subterranean assurance that an institution will take him if the needs of other family members become overriding.

The guilty knowledge that the child with cystic fibrosis will die if the family tries to accommodate his needs to theirs confronts them as relapses follow the slighting of his treatment program. Medical advice that they should maintain a normal family life sometimes places the mother in an impossible situation, between a husband who is not willing to accommodate his demands and the child who cannot do so. One experienced observer says of the grave outlook:

Death may come in one month or in twenty years. The suspense and uncertainty keep the parents in a turmoil and prevent them from reaching a stable adjustment. ... Especially damaging to a parent's self-esteem may be his death wishes for the child as a way of ending the uncertainty. Such wishes are often compensated for by overprotection or by avoidance of involvement with the child—the latter is especially seen in many fathers of our patients with cystic fibrosis.[15]

The parents face not role change but role intensification, which may lead to chronic family disequilibrium, or if the parents are strong enough and circumstances fortunate, it may lead to an unusual knitting of family life. The upward-striving characteristic of young middle- and upper-lower-class families in our culture is defeated as child-care burdens prevent the mother from adding to the family income and material comforts by working outside the home. The breadwinner is not aided by his wife but, to the contrary, he must share her responsibility for the child's treatment and support her emotionally, in addition to earning and perhaps borrowing enough for the treatment program.

Problems of open communication between family members regarding deprivations the child's illness creates are mentioned by various observers. One study reported that "we found finances leading the list" of difficult things to discuss with the spouse.[16] Deprivations not only of money but of time for the parents to be alone together, of energy for sexual relationships, of outside social activities and stimulation, and of vacations inevitably arise from the illness and treatment demands. Depending upon the parents' personal characteristics, the strength of the marriage, and other tensions they are under, the deprivations can lead to feelings of isolation and lack of emotional support.

In a major study of the effect of cystic fibrosis on family life, McCollum and Gibson of the Yale New Haven Hospital outlined what they have observed about the disease and its diagnosis and treatment at different stages of the child's development.[17] They emphasize the anxiety and frustration parents feel over the infant's voracious appetite, failure to gain, and frequent foul stools during the long period that often elapses before diagnosis is made, and the anger they often project on others after the diagnosis, as a result of their grief, guilt, and anxiety. Toilet training is particularly difficult, because of the revolting smell and irregularity of the child's massive stools.

Postural drainage treatments, always a potential cause of contention, are especially difficult when the child goes through the "negative stage" of emerging need for autonomy and motor activity. The child's sleep interruption, often accompanied by enuresis, and consequently the parents' broken sleep, add to the problems. Other tensions include concern for the child's siblings, and management of their problems including those related and unrelated to the sick child. Parents worry that their other children must forgo activities and relinquish or defer their own desires.[18] Normal siblings face an emotional dilemma, for they dare not hate a brother or sister with a fatal illness, but they are deprived of their fair share of family income and parental attention and cannot escape resentment. Siblings with cystic fibrosis may, according to their age, face the terror of watching a sister or brother with the same diagnosis progress downward and die.

The social worker's task is of heroic proportions, for it is to help the child and family in this framework to live as normally as they can and with the best cheer possible, while ensuring that the child's treatment needs are met. From the worker's viewpoint there are two broad groups of families, those who have the financial and emotional resources to adapt to the child's needs without destruction of themselves and those who cannot give the child the care he needs—who may have other serious health problems or too limited ability to rise to the heights demanded. With the former group, services will be minimal; with the latter group, the worker should be prepared to invest very heavily over a long period of time, to utilize a wide variety of resources, and to adapt her efforts to the needs of the family as a whole.

As with all persons, the individual child is impinged on by the psychological interplay between family members, and impinges upon it. The treatment regimen, and therefore his life, may be more effectively aided by indirect than direct means. If the mother does not provide the daily treatment regimen necessary, it may be because she is too burdened by the problems of another child or her husband, or by her own health problems. She may deny the importance of the child's care or shut off the significance of neglect, because she is not capable of tolerating one more demand. Efforts directed toward relief of the most immediate pressing demand she feels may be the route toward helping her give the needed care and attention to the child with cystic fibrosis.

Financial Problems

Financial problems and housing are among the first concerns to be brought to the social worker's attention. Periodic outlays for hospitalization and equipment require large sums. Costs vary by locality, by treatment used, and by the relative activity or stability of the disease during the year. Facts presented at a northern California conference in 1972 showed average medical costs for children at one center to be over $4,000 per year for vitamin supplements, enzymes, and medications; $770 for a mist tent and nebulizer expected to last 18 months; and in the care of one child described, $135 per day for hospitalization that totaled 88 days during the year. The total was $16,650 for the year for all costs.[19] California medical care costs are higher than in some states, but I have seen references to costs elsewhere of approximately $10,000 per year during earlier years when medical care was less expensive.

Many state crippled children's services now include cystic fibrosis as an eligible diagnosis, and provide an excellent resource for large items. Major medical insurance of the breadwinner that includes dependents is another common resource, but its use for equipment depends on the interpretation of the particular insurance company. When major medical insurance does provide good coverage for the needs of a child with this expensive disease, the parent may feel that he cannot afford to dissociate himself from the company's policy. There may be a feeling of entrapment in employment—the inability to leave an undesirable job or to accept a better job because of uncertainty about insurance benefits.

Medicaid payments are available for children who qualify for disability benefits and, in some states, for families who can be linked to, or can qualify for, public assistance and who can meet the liability requirements. Military families can be helped through military Medicare, although this resource frequently involves long delays because of the intricacy of the procedural requirements. The Easter Seal Society and other private agencies and service clubs may help with expensive equipment and its repair, the purchase of equipment especially lending itself to the philanthropic aims and customs of service clubs and private health organizations.

The continuing cost of drugs and food supplements is more difficult to arrange unless the family lives in the area of a Cystic Fibrosis Foundation chapter that sponsors a drug bank. The reduced (wholesale) costs materially relieve the middle class; the poor, however, will find even these too high but may be able to get the medicines free through the drug bank, depending on local Foundation policies. In some instances major medical insurance covers drug costs.

"Hidden costs" include the large supply of high-protein, low-fat foods that are urged on the child in generous amounts in order that he may gain weight or at least hold his weight if at all possible. For children still receiving mist-tent treatment, costs also include the extra bedding necessary in order to replace mattresses, blankets, sheets, and pillows that mildew or rot from the nightly damp of the mist tent, and necessary for substitute use when bedding hung out to dry in the morning does not dry before nightfall in humid weather. Heavy plastic sheeting under the bedsheets and folded on top of the blankets is an additional expense. Although the diet, like the medicine, does not lend itself well to gifts from service clubs or agencies, bedding supplies can often be secured from church or lodge groups that make small tangible gifts to disabled individuals.

Housing

Housing constitutes one of the most difficult financial problems for large families or for those receiving public assistance in flat-grant form. Children who sleep in mist tents and need special equipment in the bedroom and who cough a good deal in the night and early morning should have rooms of their own. Bedrooms of these children should be on the ground floor to prevent need for the mother to go up and down stairs daily with the wet bedding. Laundry facilities are imperative, including a dryer in localities subject to long periods of rain or snow.

A location accessible to a cystic fibrosis clinic is one of the most important elements in the child's life and creates one of the few justifications for moving to another geographical area. Since such centers are in large cities where medical schools are located, suburban housing is most often chosen. Accessibility of reliable transportation to the clinic is essential.

All these requisites add to the cost of housing for the one-income and public assistance families. Some form of supplementation for AFDC families is a necessity. If a flat grant permits no leeway, special permission from the administration should be sought because of the relationship of the child's longevity to the adequacy of his care at home.

Household Assistance and Foster Care

One of the most urgent common needs is for physical help to the mother with the housework or with the percussion and drainage treatments. Unless the father, relatives, or teenage siblings take an active part in child care and domestic chores, a home health aide or some form of domestic service is imperative if there are several children or the mother is not very vigorous. The poverty programs may be able to assist with household aide service through their career training programs. Relatives may be able to help, although their own circumstances may require adjustments.

The normal need for respite from the responsibilities of day-to-day care is magnified enormously in parents of children with cystic fibrosis. Unfortunately, it is seldom adequately met. Baby-sitters may prefer not to care for a chronically ill child, and some parents are too anxious to entrust their children to anyone but close relatives. Family vacations must not involve plane flights or high altitude. Electricity must be available to run equipment. Medical attention must be readily available. All these limitations often make vacations seem too much trouble, so the family just does not get away as most middle-class families do. This is hard not only on the parents but on the normal siblings and the affected child.

The needs for foster care or day care constitute other reasons parents of children with cystic fibrosis come to the attention of workers in the community. One-parent families are not uncommon. Men may leave who are not mature enough to rise to the extraordinary demands on family life that this disease creates; marriages break up that are subject to other stresses if the partners do not have unusual strengths and ties; neurotic conflicts receive reinforcement by guilt components in the situation, and some mothers become mentally ill.

The extraordinary capacity required of a foster home is obvious. Few can tolerate the physical burden and emotional strain of a child with this disease. The foster mother need not be a nurse, although a nursing background may make learning the treatments seem less formidable to her. Visiting nurse services on a daily basis may sometimes be feasible, as may employment of a high school student or other person to come in and give one or more of the percussion and drainage treatments daily. The pressure for placement may create the temptation to try any home that seems remotely suitable. In the care of the very young child, the risk may be justified if the alternative is prolonged hospitalization. However, the prospect of several replacements is a negative one to be avoided for a child who already carries the emotional consequences of cystic fibrosis.

Adequate day care is less difficult to secure because the parents will retain major responsibility for percussion and drainage and for care of the mist tent and bedding if the tent is used. However, the physical capacity of a mother to work and carry on the other responsibilities may be short-lived. Thus, homemaker or more health aide service would seem preferable to day care outside the home under most circumstances.

The Parents' Anxiety

Since relatively normal living and hopeful attitudes are goals that may be thwarted by unvoiced fear, the worker would like to be of help to the parents in relief of anxiety. As one therapist said of the parents, "They come here smiling on the outside but they are crying inside." The worker may be baffled by the inability of the parents to discuss their feelings. In their long engagement with anxiety they must defend themselves from dread thoughts; only at time of crisis may they be able to talk about their inmost worries unless strong relationships have been established. Because these outward defenses may well be essential to the parents' equilibrium, they should not be disturbed unless they are obviously destructive, and then only by workers who are prepared to deal with the responses that are substituted for the defenses.

Tacit understanding and indirect support are usual means of helping. The knowledge that a burden is shared with a reliable person who understands and cares is a fundamental source of help. The indirect nature of the helping process does not devalue its usefulness. One-parent families may have relatives or long-time friends who meet these needs, or pastors or church friends. These meaningful contacts should be not only encouraged but actively facilitated. The most basic relationship is with the physician, if over a period of time the child is under care of one doctor who is interested in his patients and their families. Next to a deep religious faith, complete trust in the doctor is the most important source of help a family can have in undergoing the downward progression of a sick child. When a change of location is considered because of some change in social circumstance, the importance of remaining accessible to the trusted physician merits major consideration.

During crisis periods when the parents want or need to talk about the child's condition and its meaning to them, false reassurance must be avoided despite the natural desire to relieve the worker's own pain as well as that of the parents. Positive aspects that permit hope should be brought out, but only those aspects that in fact exist. Otherwise the mother will receive the message that the worker does not understand or does not want her to talk. Anger is a natural and inevitable part of pain, often projected on a safe object instead of the real one, and should be permitted. The selfish need of the mother or father to consider himself is also a part of the

The Child's Anxiety

Unless a child is very young or too ill, he is fearful of signs of deterioration. Children quickly read or hear such phrases as "CF is the number one killer of children." Hospitalized or clinic children watch with wide eyes and sober expressions the physical signs that are bad omens and absorb the expressions and phrases of their parents and physicians. The child's fears may be projected on minor complications or procedures or felt as anger toward the world or nearby persons. Although the child's questions should be answered, hope and the best possible cheer should be maintained. Serious attacks upon the condition or situation on which the child has projected concern are also important, for these efforts symbolize attacks on the enemy.

A child who is very ill receives more security from the mother's presence than from any other source. Often the worker can be of very significant service to the hospitalized child by creating ways for the mother to spend a good deal of time at the hospital. Transportation and board costs usually can be secured from a service club, church, or special fund without difficulty if the family budget does not permit her frequent visiting.

Fortunately, most of the time the child is relatively stable or getting better. During these periods the worker engages with the child around the activities, events, or problems that are of concern to normal children but colored by his disease—school, diet, clothing, living arrangements, relationships with siblings and peers, recreational opportunities—as well as around physical needs incident to his disease, such as repair of equipment and transportation to the clinic.

A problem unique to cystic fibrosis is the feeling of shame common to the school-age and adolescent child.[20] Although feelings of being different are common among children with major chronic illnesses, no other group known has the peculiar difficulty that arises from the pervasive odor of foul stools and flatulence or gas. The bad odor of undigested fat in the stools is difficult for others to tolerate. The offender is embarrassed among his siblings and schoolmates. One may postulate, in addition to such obvious problems, that the mother's revulsion during the child's toilet-training period—especially if it had been a protracted and stormy one—is ingrained in the child's psyche. Shame is used by mothers as a weapon in toilet training; "bad child, stink," are connected in the child's mind.

Not only does the child stink up the environment but he has an unpleasantly loose cough and the need to spit phlegm, similar to that of the adult with bronchiectasis. Some children with cystic fibrosis try to avoid coughing, and instead develop an annoying throat-clearing habit, which jars the nerves of their schoolmates and teachers.[21]

A direct discussion of shame with the child would seem to be indicated only after work toward eradicating its cause. Dietary fat affects the amount of foul-smelling undigested fat that will be passed. A child who eats peanut butter sandwiches, fried tortillas, fried potatoes, fat-filled hamburgers and frankfurters, or beans and french fries has bowel problems that may be difficult to correct if they are financially and/or culturally induced or come about from lack of parental supervision or from the child's rebellion against dietary restriction. Since ignorance or lack of clarity about diet may exist, however, help may be sought first from physician and dietician, and other areas may be attacked as exploration indicates their relevance. If the diet of the entire family is modified to include less fat, tensions are less.

Enzyme medication, to aid digestion of fats, and adequate postural drainage and antibiotics, for cough, are other practical measures to reduce causes for shame. The worker's first efforts therefore should be to try to see that the child has competent medical care, and that the family is able to follow through with purchase of prescribed medicines and is providing the postural drainage treatments and the recommended diet.

Special Problems of Adolescents

At adolescence, problems become extreme. Obvious conflict results from prolonged physical dependence on the parents for treatments during a time when normal development brings ambivalent needs for dependency with strong surges of independence and hostility. The intensity of the relationship between mother and child is fostered by the physical contact inherent in the treatment method. Older children should be taught to give themselves their own percussion and drainage treatments to the extent possible, in order to avoid the situation where a parent beats on his chest and where dependence is symbolized.

The adolescent boy who is undersize and who is looked down on as a "pee-wee" or who feels unable to compete with his peers may be more in despair over his social situation than his physical condition. His foul-smelling stools, his cough, his inability to compete in athletics may make him a social misfit—or feel that he is. He may know that almost all adult males with cystic fibrosis are sterile,[22] and this fact further damages his self-esteem. To sleep in a mist tent may seem unendurable humiliation if other boys know about it.

If the youth leaves home for college, as happens occasionally, he may be eligible at age 18 for attendant-care services under the Social Security disability program, or if under 18 under the crippled children's program, for help in financing the daily percussion and drainage he cannot administer to himself. Other students, house mothers, or church associates may sometimes be engaged to help.

Cystic fibrosis is not incompatible with adult life, or with independence, employment, and successful social relationships and marriage. A study reported in 1965 of 65 young adults (over 17 years of age) who had been treated at the Children's Hospital Medical Center in Boston showed that four had completed college and were working and seven had married — one of whom had been married for five years. One man had survived to the age of 33. Some of these young persons had had mild disease, and two-thirds were male, although the sex incidence is equal in infancy and childhood.[23] Despite the qualifications inherent in these facts, the constant slow increase in longevity of children with cystic fibrosis means that a larger number increasingly may be expected to attain relatively normal social experience.

Realistically, however, most children with cystic fibrosis currently under care will not live to become adults. This seems especially true for girls, and for all children with severe disease in early life. Focus on preparation for independence and on a vocational future is denial of reality. The worker who pretends something that parents and child know to be improbable cannot expect wholehearted participation or an honest and meaningful relationship. Without denying hope, the worker can instead help them focus on limited goals that will be of value whatever the future.

The achievement of identity as a separate person is generally accepted as the adolescent's major developmental task. Erikson, the father of this concept, writes at length of the importance of ideals and philosophy in establishing identity.[24] The adolescent's interest in religion, whether in traditional form or Eastern, occult or bizarre, is testimony to the universality of his need to find a philosophical base. Knowledge of foreseeable death heightens the urgency of achieving philosophical identity. This aspect of the normal adolescent task therefore is appropriate to encourage in the young person with cystic fibrosis. Whether he lives or dies, philosophy, psychology, and religion will afford avenues for learning, stimulation, growth, and escape.

Life enrichment studies and activities provide outlet for escape from grim thoughts and for self-expression in the present. At the same time they may develop talents or skills for later vocational use if this is to be pertinent. Since many adolescents will lose physical strength as they grow older, learning to enjoy and become proficient in endeavors that can be performed at home, sitting or reclining, carries obvious advantage. Vulnerability to infection and interruptions for acute illness and hospitalization are part of the dismal reality. Ignoring the disease in social planning merely leads to repeated disappointment and apathy.

Difficulty in maintaining fruitful social relationships, depression, and preoccupation with death are probably the most serious obstacles to worthwhile living, depending on the severity of the disease and the temperament and family circumstances of the adolescent. One young woman on a panel of young adults with cystic fibrosis said openly that she had held herself aloof from social relationships because she feared rejection.

Some authorities have said it is important for the adolescent to seek an identity as a lovable person rather than as a cystic fibrosis patient.[25] This is a realistic goal for some, if cause for shame has been kept to a minimum and parents have been steadfast and loving. The attitude of the worker can be a strong healing force. Because individuals incorporate others' ideas about themselves and build self-esteem accordingly, the adolescent whom the worker likes and respects will absorb some of the worker's feelings. Teachers are also a potential source of help, particularly for bright children. "The teacher, more than anybody else, represents the reality of the outside world, and his acceptance, encouragement and respect for the child may tilt the balance toward a favorable adjustment even when the home situation is less than adequate."[26] In the large impersonal high school, the worker may need to make a substantial effort to find the best teacher or a counselor who will show special interest in the child. To some extent, the lovable-person identity goal is workable.

However, the peer group is most important to the adolescent. Whether young persons with diseases carrying a fatal outlook should be encouraged to form patient clubs seems questionable. McCollum points out the limitations in parent group discussions in depth, "since exposure of the deep fears of one member can readily threaten the defenses of the others."[27] This is applicable to groups of patients in whom the death of one reinforces the fears of the others. Relationships with other, "normal" peers obviously are preferable, to the extent that they can be fostered.

Young people's groups in churches would appear to offer a compassionate atmosphere for socialization and opportunity for possible identification with a counselor or chaplain in lieu of the athletic coach so often of vital importance in a boy's maturation. One young man on the panel previously mentioned said that jobs in small organizations also offer a chance for social relationships; he felt that large organizations are too impersonal to provide the same opportunity. Interest groups seem to provide the most natural opportunity to form friendships.

Preoccupation with death was found to be almost universal in one small study reported from Canada.[28] Popular literature had exerted a negative effect. Some parents have felt that too much is said about diagnosis and prognosis by medical staff in front of the child.[29] The adverse effects of fund-raising events on television are commonly reported. Difficulty in communication in the family about the subject of death is common. One study states that children whose parents tried to conceal the diagnosis and avoided discussion were most apt to be ashamed of their disease and uncooperative in treatment.[30] The study by McCollum, referred to earlier, states:[31]

Parents able to master the grief, guilt and anxiety stimulated by such questions [raised by their children about the future and whether they were going to die] characteristically responded with a statement such as "None of us knows when we're going to die. That's something God decides. But it's up to us to do everything possible to live as long as we can, and that's why you must sleep in your tent."

A girl with cystic fibrosis on the panel mentioned earlier said that the subject is like sex—the less openly it is discussed the more intriguing it becomes and the more urgent for the child to investigate. The McCollum study showed that about a third of the families, who were largely middle-class, avoided giving information to the child about his illness.

Because the child's need to communicate honestly about his fears has been discussed elsewhere (see chapters on leukemia and muscular dystrophy), it need not be elaborated here. However, the worker should bear in mind that the manner of dying is one of the aspects of death that can be most terrifying to the fatally ill and their families. The Foundation of Thanatology has supported a collection of papers, issued in book form as *The Psychological Aspects of Cystic Fibrosis*, from 26 cystic fibrosis centers, in which the main emphasis is upon physicians' observations of the terminal stage.[32] It is clear from these papers as well as from my own research that medical management varies widely and the role of the social worker will vary accordingly. It will depend, in some measure, on what point in the illness the physician makes the decision to withhold extraordinary life support measures and let the child die. That there is no uniformity in this is illustrated by some descriptions of death as prolonged, tormented, and suffering,[33] whereas other physicians can assure parents and the child who is able to ask "How will I die?" that death will usually come during gradually deepening coma, with no awareness or feeling when it actually occurs.[34]

Whether death is peaceful or difficult, some parents will not be able to bear to be with their child during the last hours. Social workers from the Montreal Children's Hospital point out that physicians and social workers should give support to parents in whatever they feel able to do, and for those who cannot stay, a substitute should be found.[35] Readers may note the similarity here with the position of experienced social workers on leukemia services.

The community social worker's responsibility during this period stands out through a revelation made in this same collection of papers. In a survey of 135 centers, of which fewer than half responded, only 34 reported employing a social worker. Obviously, the community helping person cannot count on the hospital to have staff with primary responsibility for family and personal problems; the worker who knows the family and is involved with them must keep in touch, relegating the responsibility to the hospital worker if there is one functioning on the cystic fibrosis ward with the child in question, but otherwise doing what must be done herself.

It is unfortunately true that at this stage of medical science, prolongation of life has postponed death from cystic fibrosis to an age that, in general, permits neither the ignorance of early childhood nor the maturity of adulthood. Because teenagers and young adults and their parents and siblings have a tragic and overwhelming task in coping with what they face, a wide range of attack has been mounted from Orange County, California, to Cincinnati, Philadelphia, and Boston; these attacks vary from studies to learn more specifically what the problems are, to day camps, parent groups, and programs on genetics for teenagers and siblings. Helping persons in the community can investigate what resources may exist in the community, and if the population is large enough to contain several or a number of children with cystic fibrosis, they can cooperate in or stimulate group effort to help parents and children meet their problems with the most suitable resources available.

Pediatricians, hospital social workers, clergymen, psychologists, school and vocational counselors, parents, and representatives of the patient group are among those who can pool their ideas. The National Cystic Fibrosis Foundation is available to provide literature and advice.

CHAPTER TEN

Head Injury

ACCIDENTS KILL more children than the three most common diseases of childhood combined, and about a quarter of these violent deaths are due to head injuries. Unlike most diseases this waste of young lives is on a steady incline and is truly a modern dilemma, in large part a product of the automotive age."[1]

An estimated 200,000 children are hospitalized annually for head injury; 10,000 to 20,000 have prolonged impairment or significant aftereffects; over 3,000 children die annually from its effects.[2] Social work is concerned not only with the children who die needlessly but with those who survive as multi-handicapped persons. Permanent neurological defects have been ascribed to varying proportions of head-injured children in different studies, varying from less than 1 percent to almost 6 percent.[3]

The majority of head injuries are said to occur in cities and are due to automobile accidents.[4] Children between the ages of 3 and 7 are most frequently involved—"an alarming number of toddlers are injured when running between parked cars and playing in the street." A significant number of adolescents also sustain head injuries while riding in automobiles or on motorcycles.

The age of the children involved and their stage of development need to be borne in mind with respect to the psychosocial implications for child and family. A study in Los Angeles charted the ages of 237 injured children in a shape like an inverted bell. By far the largest number of children were either 4 to 6 years or 16 to 18 years old, with numbers descending from each of the high ends of the graph, and lowest in the 8-to-10 year bracket. (When more children were added to this study, the peak age occurred at 4–5 years.)[5]

Although the general discussion here focuses on the group most commonly encountered, those injured in automobile accidents, the social worker in practice is concerned with individual cases, including those of children injured by battering. One physician divided young head-injured children into groups according to whether the accident resulted from their being struck (battered) or dropped, from falling, etc. He stated that "children who were in the struck group were clearly disadvantaged. They were predominantly non-white and came from low socioeconomic status, broken families in which the mother had little education and few supportive resources available to her." In addition, he stated, "frequency of pregnancy within the previous year was significantly high among the struck-group mothers. We feel that this is a major source of stress associated with the occurrence of physical abuse."[6] Other social features are known to be of importance also, such as illegitimacy, financial stress, and immaturity. Whatever the cause of the injury, the child and his family constitute a challenging problem for social workers.

THE MEDICAL REALITIES

The Brain and Its Functions

"The central nervous system is more complex and more mysterious in the way it works than all the man-developed computers and other man-made informational systems put together."[7] An increasing amount of information is being gathered about the way the brain works, but much remains unknown.

Some readily understood ideas about the function of the brain are, however, worth bearing in mind.[8] The brain consists of the *cerebrum*, two hemispheres covered by a "bark," or *cortex*; the brain stem, which includes the *thalamus* and the *hypothalamus*; the *pons*; the *medulla*; and the *cerebellum*. The cortex or outer layer of the cerebrum is of particular concern in understanding the behavior of head-injured or brain-damaged children. It is composed of four lobes, the *frontal, temporal, occipital,* and *parietal.* The lobes are located as their names indicate, the frontal in the front, the temporal on the sides or temples, the parietal in the middle or on top, and the occipital in the back.

The brain functions as a whole, so that damage to one area inevitably affects to some extent the total functioning of the person. However, each area also has its special tasks. The frontal lobe is involved with the patterns of motor association. Thoughts, words, sentences, etc., are fed into this part of the cortex, from which impulses are sent to the different muscles of the body allowing for appropriate muscular response. ("Stop!" and the person draws back from what he is doing.)

The temporal lobes at the sides of the head are concerned with time, memory, auditory stimulation, and the capacity to recognize or perceive sounds and produce speech. The occipital lobes in the back of the head have a close relationship with the visual area, so that damage to this part of the brain may result in decreased visual acuity. The parietal or top lobes relate to sensory matters such as touch and position sense.

Deep in the brain are the areas that control the autonomic nervous system. This system controls the physiological functions and structures that control sleeping and waking, eating, sexual activities, respiration, heartbeat, and other vital functions. This brain-stem area also includes the thalamus, which has control over emotions and the affective qualities of different sensations. The thalamus is said also to play a role in controlling muscle movement.

The brain has a central coordinating and integrating mechanism that is thought to lie in the thalamus deep in the base of the brain. The system that affects the activity of most of the other parts of the brain, the so-called *centroencephalic* system, is not fully understood.

One other part of the brain that frequently comes in for attention is the meninges, the protective covering of the cerebral cortex. The meninges can become infected through the blood stream, resulting in meningitis. Infection of the brain itself is called encephalitis.

Of interest in understanding intellectual and behavioral impairments in a head-injured child is the fact that the central nervous system is not fully developed when the child is born. The brain and nerves receive their last fatty layer of myelin at different times, beginning at the top of the head and going down the spinal cord. Most maturation has occurred by the age of 4, but complete development does not occur until the beginning of puberty.

Experts disagree on the effect of the child's age on the outlook. Since the brain is in a formative stage, flexibility of function should permit greater capacity for compensatory activity. However, the child who has not learned prior to the accident does not have the base of information and behavioral habits to return to after recovery, nor has he mastered the language and reading skills so essential to later learning. If an injured brain impairs his learning during the critical preschool years, he is deprived of an essential period of development. The younger child has a high incidence of retardation after a head injury.

*Nature and Course of Recovery**

The highly variable nature of the outcome of a head injury is related to the variable effect of the accident upon the brain. Skull fractures occur in some instances, but in others the child receives a concussion accom-

---

* I am indebted to the professional staff at the Rancho Los Amigos Hospital at Downey, Calif., for sharing their observations and extensive experience regarding the nature of the impairment after severe head injury in children. They include Joyce D. Brink, M.D., Chief, Pediatric Service; Martha Carol, R.N., Head Nurse, Pediatrics; Marilyn Lister, R.P.P., Supervisor, Pediatrics Physical Therapy; Charles Koontz, Principal, RLA School; Chris Hagen, Ph.D., Chief, Communication Disorders; Steve Heck, Coordinator for Vocational Rehabilitation Services; Laura L. Edwards, M.S.W., Medical Social Worker, Pediatrics; and Anna Hanson, Teacher Title VI, Bay Center for Cerebral Palsied Children.

panied by bruising and swelling of brain tissue and sometimes by hemorrhage. A fracture is not necessarily more serious than a concussion. Concussion technically is not a mild occurrence as commonly understood, but rather refers to a "syndrome due to a sudden mechanical head injury characterized by a transient loss of consciousness *and impairment of related neural functions* with subsequent amnesia for the actual traumatic incident. The disturbance of consciousness and memory evoked by the trauma usually varies in duration from a few moments to an hour or so, but occasionally [lasts] a much longer period."[9] The coma or traumatic stupor may last many weeks. The nerve involvement frequently causes paralysis and spasticity of the limbs, with resultant contractured deformities, unless preventive measures are instituted.

Neurosurgeons can estimate something of what is going on in the brain according to the symptoms when a child is in coma. However, whether the child will recover or how long it will take cannot be told. When a child remains comatose over 24 hours, the outlook for permanent impairment is serious.[10] He is fed by a nasogastric tube if coma lasts a week or more. In some instances the child's breathing is so jeopardized that a *tracheotomy* (an opening in the throat) must be performed. The opening allows an airway and also permits removal of secretions. The child is incontinent, not because of a physical loss of bowel and bladder control but because of lack of awareness. The child may require skilled and sometimes hazardous diagnostic procedures such as an *angiogram* (X rays of the blood vessels) and *pneumoencephalograms* (X rays of the ventricles of the brain) and may require burr holes (removal of a bony portion of the skull to reduce the pressure caused by swelling or hemorrhage). Skilled nursing care and highly specialized medical care obviously are essential during the early period.

Consciousness may return with a sudden capacity to speak, or the return may be gradual and speech may be greatly delayed. Headaches, dizziness, irritability, confusion, and distractability occur. If the coma is prolonged, some authorities believe it desirable to bombard a child with a variety of visual and auditory stimuli and stimulant drugs. The family may be asked to come to the hospital and speak to the child so he will hear familiar voices. Tape recordings may be helpful.

Although an occasional parent takes a child home before consciousness is fully regained and while he still needs extensive care, the family is advised to leave the child in the hospital or nursing home during the months of his helplessness and need for intensive, complicated nursing care. He will probably need to remain in the hospital for at least three to six months; a heavy financial burden is therefore implicit.

Children who survive severe head injuries with a week or more of coma usually need extensive rehabilitation. Many are left with spasticity and an ataxic gait, or suffer from severe incoordination; some have double vision or other visual disturbances; some are partially or entirely deaf; some have seizures; many have speech defects; defects in mental activity and emotional control are very frequent (about two-thirds of children are so affected).[11] Speech therapy, special school, orthopedic treatment of the spastic muscles—which may include surgery or bracing—and careful structuring of the environment are frequent concomitants of medical care.

During the early stages the child has orthopedic problems that not only necessitate preventive treatment through splinting and bracing but may require corrective surgery if deformities have resulted from spasticity. A child may also develop bedsores, sometimes requiring surgery, if he has not had close attention during the time he was comatose and/or paralyzed. Because the accident that injured his head may also have fractured ribs, ruptured spleen, or broken legs, the child may have any variety and combination of physical problems coincident with those due to the neurologic impairment resulting from the injury to the brain.

Aftereffects

The outlook remains uncertain for several months, and children may improve for up to three years after the injury, although the greatest return takes place during the first year.[12]

The variety of locations of brain injuries and the specialized functions of different parts of the brain would lead one to expect different behavioral aftereffects in different children. They do differ in attributes caused by neurological impairment such as impairments of speech, vision, and motor ability, and degree of mental retardation. However, professional persons who work with head-injured children categorize their behavior as having an essential core of similarity, depending upon age.

They agree that older children seem to be left with a curious and unfortunate lack of judgment, lowered impulse control, impairment in perception of social cues, and an inability to adapt. These attributes exist independently of scores made on intelligence tests. Depression and emotional disturbance caused by worry over separation from family and what is going on at home, and frustration over physical handicaps, are interlaced with personality problems occasioned by the organic brain injury. In younger children temper tantrums, distractability, hyperactivity, aggressive behavior, and impulsiveness are common.[13]

A study made of 247 severely injured children, of whom 89 percent had been in a coma for more than a week and some of whom were still comatose for more than a year, showed that 75 percent recovered physically to the point where they could get around by themselves and were independent in self-care, although some required braces and crutches. Only 13 percent were normal neurologically. The more pervasive and serious effects related to mental retardation and personality change. Of the 15 older children who had intelligence tests before the injury and who were available for comparison, all showed a decrease of at least 10 IQ points. A third of the children were assessed to be within the normal IQ range, but only 16 percent were able to attend regular classes in public school. Most of the younger children attended schools for the physically handicapped.

Analysis of an unselected series of 105 consecutive cases treated at the Johns Hopkins Hospital included a majority of children in coma an hour or less—in other words, a group with less severe head injury than those discussed in this chapter. The majority of the children made complete recoveries after a year, but over a third developed substantial behavioral problems similar in nature to those described here.[14]

PSYCHOSOCIAL IMPLICATIONS

A child's serious injury and its aftereffects constitute only one problem in the family's constellation of concerns. How they can meet his needs, and how he is affected in turn, will depend on other things that are happening. A review of 37 case records of head-injured children at Rancho Los Amigos Hospital showed that 28 of the families were in the midst of serious problems when the accident occurred. (Owing to the brevity of the records, the proportion may have been higher.) Problems included the mother's serious physical or mental illness, the death of one or both parents, family break-up or parental imprisonment, severe financial deprivation in one-parent families with a large number of minor children, etc. Marital discord, foster-home placement, older siblings with behavior problems, divorce, alcoholism, child neglect, asthma, ulcers, and other indications of disturbance were common in the records.

The importance of the mother's "coping ability" has been described in relation to her central role in controlling the safety of the young child's environment.[15] Coping ability was defined as including such personal traits as accuracy, risk-taking, planning, and emotional disturbance. The types of control failures on the part of the mother that resulted in the child's injury were grouped as follows: (1) the mother was in an incompetent state and failed to appoint a competent caretaker; (2) the mother placed the child in an unsafe position or inappropriately used baby equipment; (3) the mother failed to protect the child from dangerous objects; (4) the mother failed to control the behavior of other persons potentially dangerous to the child; and (5) the mother failed to control her own behavior.

In a study of traffic accidents involving young children, Dr. John Read commented that "studies of family characteristics show the children tend to come from families in which there is illness, maternal preoccupation and less opportunities for protected play."[16] It is therefore not unexpected that brain-injured children themselves are characterized by those who work with them as having been "accident-prone" or "highly motoric" (active) or "emotionally disturbed" before the accident occurred.

The multiple stress of the parents is undoubtedly important in reducing their capacity both to cope with the child's needs prior to the accident and to rise to his greatly heightened needs afterward. If the mother is working outside the home, additional negative factors exist. Not only may she rightly feel guilty about leaving a small child with a less-than-adequate baby-sitter or an adolescent without supervision, but she is torn between the child's need of her and her need to keep on working for financial reasons. With little psychic or physical energy, and in the face of multiple demands and great emotional stress, she may act in what seems to be an irrational or irresponsible manner.

The Early Stage

Early and late stages of the child's injury bring separate ordeals for the family. Other problems must be pushed aside, no matter how serious, during the first critical phase while the child lies unconscious in the hospital. Other children must shift for themselves; jobs must be left, transportation borrowed, debts incurred. The child's unseeing eyes, pale face, the tubes hanging from his body evoke terror in the parent racked by uncertainty over his life. The hospital may add greatly to the *parents' burden* or may ease it, depending on the institution. Getting information from an ever-shifting staff in a large public hospital may be very difficult for the parent. In the admitting office, unrealistic financial demands may be made by clerks working under rules framed by collection- and tax-minded superiors. In other hospitals or in other wards, however, the family's experience may be entirely different, with heartwarming, compassionate family-minded staff and consideration throughout.

During the later phase, when the parent's irrationality may add many obstacles to the worker's attempts to help the child and family, the early experience of the parent during the child's first few day or weeks in the hospital should be kept in mind. Not only the pre-accident family picture but the early accident phase will influence the circumstances of the case and the outlooks of the people involved at the time the social worker enters the picture.

Some early trauma can be alleviated. While medical and nursing staff concentrate on the child, the social workers can support the parents (often a mother alone) with physical measures and psychological help. Elaboration of the physicians' comments in lay terms and at times when the parents express concern is an important adjunct to the often technical explanations the parent has received. An experienced social worker has said that the phrase "expected intellectual deficits and poor impulse control" needs to be interpreted as "acting like a three-year-old."

Through coordination of the social workers of the hospital, the welfare department, and any private agencies involved, information may be provided about the best times to telephone, which doctors to see and when, maximum financial aid, and child-care resources for the children at home. However, coordination generally is honored more in the breach than in the observance. It takes time and patience to try to reach busy people by phone. Which worker is to take responsibility for what services should be clarified.

In some hospitals the social worker becomes the one hospital staff member in the family's life who does not rotate or leave, and who can be counted on to get information about the child's condition or to coordinate efforts. Under urban traffic conditions, and especially with working mothers, the social worker's maximum use of the telephone, to make sure that referrals are appropriate and that the mother's trips will yield results, is essential in helping arrange for financial, home-making, or transportation resources. Follow-through on referrals is essential. Volunteers from church or service club can often be secured to help because the need is dramatic and obvious.

A parent's regressive behavior, or a heightened need to lean, dependency, and even demanding behavior need not be thought of as pathological or lasting. Encouraging relatives and clerics to help relieves the social worker and hospital staff. Parent groups led by social workers have also proved therapeutic as parents are given an opportunity to share experiences, feelings, and uncertainties and to receive emotional support from each other. As a mother receives support and the child's crisis abates, her needs also will usually abate for the time being.

While the child is in coma, his life in peril, *the siblings* are shoved aside—to stay with grandma perhaps, or to get along by themselves while the mother arranges hospital payments, works with lawyers to sue the driver who ran over the child, sits by the bed, or waits to see someone about his care. Resentful brothers and sisters may be waiting, therefore, when he comes home from the hospital. The child's poor impulse control and generally maladaptive behavior and long, regressive experience, coupled with the feelings of his siblings, can be expected to create rivalries and retaliations that not infrequently are physical. The older brother who beats the poorly behaved convalescent child, or the sister who slaps and pushes him, may create real hazards for a child whose balance is poor or who cannot defend himself while wearing braces or splints or who has an arm or leg in a cast.

Thus, if only from the negative standpoint of prevention of later physical problems, the needs of the siblings should be recognized from the start. In some instances, they have been drivers of the car in which the child was injured, or were left in charge of him, or have some justified or fancied guilt over his accident. Adequate plans for their care while the mother is at the hospital, their participation in plans, and recognition of their efforts and sacrifices can result in strengthening rather than diminishing family relationships. In some case illustrations of families who have weathered the problem exceptionally well, a helpful older sibling has proved a great ally to both the child and his parents.

What of the child himself? The bewilderment and fear he must feel as he wakes are not easy to comprehend, with amnesia concerning the accident itself and memories of home, parents, siblings, etc., that are at complete odds with his hospital surroundings. The discontinuity must extend to weirdness when even his body is strange—if, in searching for words, none or wrong words come; if in reaching, his wrist droops and his fingers fail to open, or his arm fails to respond at all.

In the *very young child,* who needs the reassurance of his mother's presence for even a small bump, the panic proportions of his abandonment and distress in a hospital ward conceivably may aggravate the brain-damaged quality of his behavior. One wonders if the restless hyperactivity, repetitive and odd postures and actions may be in part a child's expression of an adult's agitated depression. If his parents are focusing their own disharmonies on disagreements about his care, blaming each other for the accident, or if they are alternately failing to visit, then showering him with attention, how much greater is his psychological need.

The child who has become overnight an orthopedic and neurological cripple requires that an infinite amount be done to him, for him, and about him. If he as a person is overlooked in the process, this is easy to understand. Yet how he feels must inevitably influence his behavior, and this becomes the major problem of the late stage.

Each age-group of children has different problems, in addition to their individual neurological impairments in speech, vision, or gait and balance. The young child who has no previously learned patterns and knowledge to fall back upon must learn fundamentals while hindered by the learning difficulties of cortical damage.

The Later Stage

A common characteristic of a head-injured child is an inability to sort out stimuli. In other words, he responds indiscriminately to everything that goes on, including background noises and peripheral sights.[17] He therefore needs to be protected from them in order to concentrate on such tasks as dressing himself, bathing, eating, and speaking properly. The home environment, with the television on, other children coming in and out, the mother needing to give attention to meals, the telephone, laundry, and the usual daily tasks, is far from conducive to the structuring and limiting that these children need.

Unfortunately, many parents think they can "make" the child learn if he will just try hard enough, because they find themselves unable to accept the finality and sometimes the maddening strangeness of brain-injured behavior. The fine line between spoiling the child and unrealistic expectation that he "should be treated like everyone else" is hard to find at best. When the parent feels guilty and torn and is under many strains, the "fine line" is hidden under other considerations.

Young brain-injured persons usually need to be placed in special classes at school. These classes, if well taught, give the child an opportunity to progress at an individualized pace, and perhaps more important, they place him under the care of persons who, having had experience with the mentally retarded or neurologically handicapped, have adapted to their own frustration and have learned how to help the slow-learning child. It is unfortunately true that the self-image of the brain-injured child may suffer from being grouped with retarded children when his memory of himself is that of a normal person.* If he can accept the necessity for attending a special class until he "catches up" after his accident, some of his depression and confusion about role may perhaps be alleviated.

Schools that refuse to permit physically handicapped children to attend regular classes or even to attend school at all do so out of concern that the child on crutches or a child wearing a brace may be hurt by other children. This concern may be justified in some schools; however, in others the restriction arises from unwarranted fear and rigidity and should be questioned.

The school placement and the location of the home in a school district best suited to the child's needs take serious consideration, because of the importance of school not only in the difficult and important task of learning but in the contribution it makes to the self-image. In considering housing, rent budgets, and transportation, the social worker needs to take into account the particular importance of the school for the head-injured child.

Special Problems of Adolescents

The older child has serious problems of schooling, vocational preparation, and emancipation from parental control. Learning difficulties that affect the older child's adaptive capacity stem from lack of memory for recent events and lack of capacity for retention. The person who cannot hold anything new in mind long enough to learn it must fall back on previously established knowledge and patterns. Lacking an understanding of the present, he applies the past in a way that is inappropriate. Lack of capacity for social adaptation is the mark of mental retardation.

* Sheldon R. Rappaport (editor, "Childhood Aphasia and Brain Damage," Pathway School publication, Livingston Publishing Co., Narberth, Pa., p. 43) states that the advantages of placement in a good special school (versus a regular school) outweigh the disadvantages for the child: "It is a relief for him to be in an environment where his difficulties are not awesome or terrible.... In this haven of security he no longer has to cope alone with his frustrating skill deficiencies and inadequate controls. He no longer feels different and rejected."

Parents of a brain-injured adolescent find great difficulty in incorporating the changed behavior of the child. He may have recovered physically to the point where they are led to believe he is almost well. He seems to be a disciplinary problem rather than a medical problem. They cannot realize that the injury in some fashion wiped out the socializing experiences of his childhood; that he is unable organically to control his impulses and that poor judgment was inflicted on him indefinitely by the accident. The great change in his behavior is not perceived immediately. It is too different and too dismaying to grasp. The parents need long-continued support and reinterpretation over a period of time and help in coping with the daily problems his behavior creates. Owing to the intense frustration and depression felt by the adolescent and by those working with him, aggressive acting-out behavior may be expected. The physical vigor of youth combined with poor judgment and the anger that accompanies frustration make an extraordinarily difficult combination. The boy who is constantly in fights, who forgets what he started to do, who loses interest quickly, and who "acts like a three-year-old" is rejected by peers and finally by parents who cannot take any more. The seriously damaged adolescent is sometimes imprisoned or taken to a state mental hospital by police. The discouragement and frustration of the professional workers involved add their own input of negative forces.

At this stage of knowledge we do not know why a head-injured child manifests more severe behavior problems than the cerebral palsied, but it seems possible that the discontinuity of experience of both the child and his family creates a disharmony that adds to the emotional burdens. The bewilderment and lack of understanding seem to be contributing factors.

The *vocational future* of an adolescent with a severe head injury realistically is a dark one. Bizarre or highly unrealistic goals are not uncommon in boys who retain old dreams but who may be incapable of elementary school work. Unreality creates lack of motivation for the mundane tasks they may be capable of and frustration in reaching goals that are not feasible.

A common vocational problem involves learning to drive. The boy not only assumes he is capable of driving in common with his peers, but he needs to learn to drive to work or to a workshop. When he is aggressive, lacking in impulse control, and subject to poor judgment, and particularly when his emotional and intellectual problems are compounded by lack of coordination, visual difficulties, or other physical impediments to safe driving, the social workers and others involved need to be firm in helping the boy realize that, however inconvenient, driving must be postponed until later. It is conceivable that in five or ten years he may have matured enough to drive, whereas it is not possible at the time other young men are taking driver education courses and applying for licenses.

Structured living during a long period of relearning social behavior is needed by the adolescent head-injured boy. Some aggressive, uncontrolled youths need institutional care during late adolescence and early adult life. They may "calm down" as physical vigor ebbs and as some self-acceptance and maturity emerge. Unfortunately, mental hospitals at the time of this writing tend to release the brain-injured youths as soon as organic injury has been diagnosed, and prisons are poor places for the kind of care they need.

Police intervention and mental hospital admission, occasioned by intense conflict at home, may sometimes be avoided by limited goals and compromises, even though they represent in themselves inadequate solutions. Boarding-home living or sharing an apartment with other youths can occasionally give some respite to the family and an outlet for the urge to independence of the young adult. An active, sustaining relationship may sufficiently alleviate the family's anger and despair over the adolescent's behavior to prevent culmination in final rejection.

Development of Needed Resources

The development of needed community resources is an urgent challenge to social work. These include clinic services where parents of the head-injured can be seen regularly and may obtain help with the management of their own feelings and the behavior of the child. A specialized staff would appear to be necessary to accumulate enough experience to differentiate between what is appropriate for the young, organically damaged person and for a child with functional behavior disorders. Community needs also include halfway houses where the necessary structured existence and resocialization opportunities can be provided in an atmosphere freed of the intensity of home conflicts.

Counseling with the youths may be expected to yield less helpful results than environmental manipulation. Although the brain-injured often acts like a sociopath, he is not. The use of techniques that benefit certain groups and that utilize deliberate provocation of anxiety and strong measures of "reality" is not suitable for persons whose inhibitory mechanisms have been impaired and who cannot hold new facts in mind long enough to integrate them. The temptation to use aggressive and sometimes harsh techniques is strong when the counselor is frustrated and angry, or when he has not differentiated between the organically and the functionally impaired person. Insufficient experience has been accumulated with the head-injured or other organically impaired youth to know what, if any, techniques may be devised that will be fruitful. Dr. Rappaport, psychologist at the Pathway School, utilizes measures to enhance self-concept and helps the person recognize feelings of rejection and loss of control.[18] Behavior modification techniques with rewards for correct responses are reported to have been successful. In coping with violence, social workers will need to experiment with ways to help the brain-injured, without themselves becoming victims of frustration.

Meanwhile, some hope is offered by measures designed to reduce frustration, depression, aggression, anxiety, and insecurity, and by measures designed to impart knowledge and support slowly and repetitively and with a minimum of excitement. Borrowing from what we have learned in working with the mentally retarded, we find that verbal cues from the nonarticulate, slow client can be counted on less by the counselor than behavioral cues. Response to feeling is imperative. Flexibility on the part of the counselor, rather than by the client, is paramount; and a slow patient tempo is the only feasible one. Fortunately, feeling is transmitted from one person to another without intellectual or verbal means. The counselor who can maintain empathy with the brain-injured holds the key to success with him as with others.

CHAPTER ELEVEN

Hemophilia

HEMOPHILIA is a "hemorrhagic disease resulting from a congenital deficiency of certain blood coagulation factors."[1] The common type is due to a deficiency of coagulation "factor 8," and is called Hemophilia A; an uncommon form is due to a deficiency of "factor 9," and is called Hemophilia B or Christmas disease. They have the same effects but are treated differently. The following discussion confines itself to children with the common type of hemophilia, or "factor 8" disease.

The disease is highly individualistic, with a wide range of clotting deficiencies. As a consequence, some persons with hemophilia incur little disability throughout life, whereas others are so seriously affected they have little chance of survival. Because of phenomenal advances in medical treatment and organization that make possible rapid transfusion, life expectancy has increased greatly for children who live near urban treatment centers. Whereas only 25 percent were expected to survive to 16 years of age 25 years ago, almost all children to whom good medical care is available are now expected to reach adult life.[2] As in diabetes, the emotional ramifications are shifting from those related to fatality to those related to long-term, though dangerous, illness.

Contrary to the stereotype of this disease as a killer, its most common long-term effect is crippling. Now that life-saving treatment is generally available for small children, the long-term orthopedic problems that occur from bleeding into the joints, called *hemarthrosis*, are the major manifestations of hemophilia in older children and adults.

As hemophilia becomes less of a rarity (estimated to occur in one in 10,000 of the male population),[3] owing to the prolongation of life of those it affects, its importance for human services workers increases. Out-patient treatment in lieu of long hospitalizations places more responsibility and opportunity for services on workers in the community and less on hospital staff. The disease is of special interest to those concerned with family relationships because, like Duchenne's muscular dystrophy, it highlights and intensifies a psychological problem often found in the families of chronically ill children, the tendency for the father to separate himself from a weak or defective child. The problem is more marked with boys, and hemophilia usually occurs only in boys. A further reason for special concern among social workers is that children from the lower socioeconomic classes are underrepresented in programs that offer specialized services for children with hemophilia (in California, and doubtless in other geographic areas). What happens to children of the poor is not known—do they die early and undiagnosed, or are they scattered throughout the communities without benefit of the special medical and auxiliary resources they need?

THE MEDICAL REALITIES

Pattern of Inheritance

Hemophilia is transmitted from the mother to her male progeny according to a recessive genetic pattern. Both types of hemophilia are inherited as follows: (1) all daughters of a man with hemophilia are carriers; (2) all sons of a man with hemophilia are normal; (3) approximately half of the sisters of a boy with hemophilia are carriers; (4) approximately half of the daughters of a carrier will be carriers; and (5) approximately half of the sons of the carrier will have hemophilia.[4]

In other words, if a man with hemophilia marries a noncarrier, none of the sons will be born with hemophilia but all the daughters will be carriers. If a carrier marries a man who does not have hemophilia, each son has a fifty-fifty chance of being a victim and each daughter has a fifty-fifty chance of being a carrier. No one can predict whether or not a given child will be affected.[5]

Although about 60 percent of the known cases have a family history of hemophilia, the remainder are "new" cases that arise from hidden inheritance or from a genetic mutation. There has been no way of detecting female carriers by laboratory tests until recently.[6]

Course of the Disease

Hemophilia may show up at circumcision, but babyhood is usually uneventful until the child begins to walk and fall, at which time excessive nosebleeds or bleeding of the mouth may follow a bump or other hemorrhages may occur.[7] Toddlers are subject to many injuries as they explore, fall, and learn.

Internal bleeding is more common and more of a hazard than bleeding from cuts. Twisting, jumping, or seemingly even excessive excitement may cause inner bleeding.[8] Spontaneous, unpredictable bleeding is one of the major characteristics of the disease, and one that holds obviously great potential for disruption and justification for anxiety. Bleeding is painful when the accumulation into the tissues causes swelling and pressure on nerves. Sometimes nerve pressure causes paralysis. Flexion deformities may occur while the child holds his limb in a flexed position to avoid pain. Repeated bleeding into the same joint irritates the joint lining, and can cause the same type of pathology and disability as arthritis. Death may occur from bleeding into the brain or throat. Head injuries are most dangerous and call for immediate medical attention, as does a sore throat, for though it may be inconsequential, it may mean that bleeding into the throat has begun.

Until the child is old enough to understand the relationship between a fall or bump and the painful hemorrhages he incurs, the parents almost inevitably must be overprotective to shield him from experiences that are physically dangerous though essential for normal emotional growth. As children reach better understanding and the ability to assume responsibility in hazardous experiences, and as they develop stronger musculature that protects the organs and joints, most are said to get along better. Some children apparently do better than others, for no objective reason. The course of the disease is characterized by cycles, with periods when one hemorrhage seems to lead to another, in part because the abnormal body position used to avoid pain creates more abnormalities.[9]

Great differences exist not only in variation in disease severity but between children who have access to comprehensive medical care in large treatment centers and those who do not. The former have a better chance to survive, and with less emotional damage as a result of the supportive guidance given to parents and the precautions used in treatment. Further, they have a better chance of avoiding the contractures of knees and hips and elbows common in children who have sat in wheelchairs for long periods or who have suffered repeated episodes of prolonged bleeding into the same joint.

Treatment

Recent advances in medical care have revolutionized the lives of children with hemophilia and their families. Children born since the advent of the new treatment may look forward to much less crippling, danger, and disruption.[10] The antihemophilic, or clotting, factor "AHF" has been identified and drying methods devised for storing it. Clotting factor 8 has been prepared in two forms, either as a concentrate or as a frozen plasma derivative called "cryoprecipitate." Concentrate (available for either factor 8 or factor 9 deficiency) is made by commercial drug companies, and comes in convenient-sized small bottles that may be stored in the refrigerator at home; a recent advance has also produced a concentrate that can be kept without refrigeration for a short period and thus permits travel, a great boon to child and family. Cryoprecipitate, often referred to as "cryo," is a blood bank product available only to persons with the common form of hemophilia, factor 8 deficiency disease. Its advantage is that it is less expensive than the concentrate and can be replaced by blood credit at the blood bank rather than cash. Blood banks may exchange three bags of "cryo" for one pint of blood, thereby lowering the number of donors. The disadvantage is that it must be kept frozen in a reliable freezer.

The great advantage of these concentrated blood-clotting materials is that they can infuse large amounts of the needed substance into the body quickly without the accompanying fluid of plasma. They therefore replace the massive transfusions of ordinary plasma that had to be limited by the amount of fluid the body could safely incorporate. Transfusions have to be given in the hospital, whereas the concentrated forms can be given by injection in an emergency room, the doctor's office, or at home, if the parent and child have been trained through a home-care program. This may save the child's life or prevent such a serious consequence as paralysis. By preventing large hemorrhages into the joints, it prevents destruction of joint tissue with subsequent crippling; by acting in a hurry, it shortens or prevents long periods of bed rest and hospital supervision and reduces pain. The new treatment makes dental work and even major surgery possible that could not have been performed before. Greater daily risks in activity can be taken. The child's life and that of his family become more normal.

Modern treatment includes supervised gradual exercise designed to strengthen muscles and encouragement of recreation that also increases vigor. Some braces are used to protect vulnerable joints, but the old method of extensive bracing and rest has advanced to more adventurous risk-taking measures, with the knowledge that if bleeding results it can be controlled with cryoprecipitate or concentrate.

Hospitalization, formerly frequent and prolonged, is now reserved for life-threatening bleeds or for surgical procedures. However, arrangement ahead of time is essential for emergency hospitalization, and for emergency room or office treatment on a 24-hour-a-day, 365-day basis. Families need to make sure that a physician is available at all times who knows the child's condition.

The home-care program provided through some specialized centers requires training of parent and child in background information and resources, in observation of their capacities, and in instruction about equipment, as well as further technical training of the child to administer his own cryoprecipitate. Dr. Jack Lazerson commented: "It occurred to us shortly after starting our program that in many cases there was no need for a doctor or nurse to administer cryoprecipitate. Young patients with diabetes learn to inject themselves with insulin, and young dope addicts become adept at intravenous infusion."[11] The Children's Hospital at Stanford, which administers a home-care program, started with teaching a 13-year-old boy but has now trained boys as young as 6 or 7.

Equipment needed at home includes a freezer that maintains a constant temperature if the cryoprecipitate is used, otherwise a refrigerator for storage of concentrate. Children who administer their own cryoprecipitate must have the necessary vials, tourniquets, tubing, needle, and syringes, and a "tempscribe" recording device to make certain of the freezer's constant temperature. Some children need plastic ice bags for cold compresses, and the small child may need a padded crib and playpen, knee pads, and helmet to avoid trauma from falling or bumps. (This is a controversial measure, not advised by some physicians; the severity of the disease and the intelligence of supervision provided are factors of importance.) Specially designed casts, splints, and braces have been created for treatment of deformed joints, which provide support and yet allow supervised exercise of affected parts. Children need wheelchairs and crutches during periods of joint crippling.

Dental Care

A major problem for both the child and those caring for him has been dental care. Bleeding in the mouth is hard to control. The injection of a local anesthetic can create severe bleeding. In the past, no local anesthetic was used for filling teeth and a general anesthetic had to be used when teeth were pulled. Older hemophiliacs therefore have tended to avoid dental care, missing appointments or finding excuses after having had experiences in which weeks or months of hospitalization followed a tooth extraction. Delay in securing needed dental care is serious in a child with hemophilia because of the later problems it ensures. Cryoprecipitate now makes possible dental care on an outpatient basis, in contrast to the former need for hospitalization. A child may receive an injection of cryoprecipitate, go to the dentist, go back to the physician for another injection following the dental work (or if he is trained for home care, give himself another injection), and get along well. In addition, an oral drug, Amicar, is used four times a day for ten days when dental work is done.

PSYCHOSOCIAL IMPLICATIONS

As in every condition, the meaning to any individual child and family arises from the total constellation of medical, psychological, and social circumstances. There are some recurring features in hemophilia, however, that will be discussed as a springboard for understanding a particular child and family.

Family Problems

Financial burdens.* The financial burden of hemophilia is staggering. Hospitalization and medical care are costly, but transfusions are much more so. Estimates of costs per year vary, and can only reflect statistics. The Orthopedic Hospital in Los Angeles estimated the annual cost per child for medical care at $5,000 in 1970.[12] Some children need more transfusions than others; as body size increases with growth, each hemorrhage requires a greater volume of blood replacement.

Blood bank policies vary in the credits they will accept, and commercial blood banks differ from the American Red Cross Blood Banks. Unfortunately, by no means do all blood banks fractionate blood in such a way as to extract the antihemophilic factor, or cryoprecipitate. (By 1973, all 59 regional American Red Cross Blood Banks were separating cryoprecipitate.[13]) Families that live in those areas where they must use the commercially bottled concentrate must pay more. At the time of this writing, one bag of precipitate costs $10 and four to five bags may be used for one hemorrhage. The child may have another hemorrhage in a few days and may have several over a period. In California, the Crippled Children's Services will pay for cryoprecipitate for persons under 21 years of age, providing the family meets eligibility requirements, is able to meet the pay-back provisions, and the program has funds. In California and in some other states as well, Medicaid provisions are available for children of indigent families.

Insurance is a frequent bulwark if the child is covered under a group policy that includes blood (many insurance policies do not include blood products). Insurance provisions for employees often determine the father's choice of employment, and his ability to change jobs. Large organizations often have blood pool arrangements with the Red Cross or commercial blood bank, and provide primary resources for recruitment of donors. Replacing the units of blood used not only reduces costs but ordinarily is required, whatever resource pays for processing the blood.

Blood replacement. Instances are known where a post office or fire department staff will "adopt" a child with hemophilia and donate the blood he needs; a recent Associated Press dispatch described a fraternity that has taken responsibility for donating blood for one boy for 12 years. "Each year, Timmy is inherited by a new wave of students.... Since they first began in 1961, University students have donated 2,400 pints of blood to the boy most of them will never see. Timothy needs at least 100 pints a year."[14] However, not all blood banks will permit this type of group credit for an individual child.

* See note at end of chapter, p. 319.

Many parents feel defeated by the impossible task of securing replacement for all the blood the child needs; they acknowledge the debt, do what they can to meet it sporadically as a resource becomes known to them, but have given up hope of replacing enough blood to meet the child's demands. Others resort to desperate measures. "Her Deal: Booze for Blood" was a front-page headline of an Associated Press dispatch in October 1973 newspapers, describing a mother's attempt to solicit Skid Row alcoholics to act as blood donors in return for a drink.[15]

The ultimate success of the home-care program in preventing crippling and promoting normal activity would appear to rest on the ability of parents to secure cryoprecipitate in sufficient quantities and on the progress blood banks make in fractionating the antihemophilic factor from plasma. When blood banks do this, the rest of the blood can be used for other patients; this is why they can afford to exchange several units of cryoprecipitate for one pint of blood donated. The child who is using cryoprecipitate at home to permit normal activity uses a great quantity. For example, one boy seen was about to go on a three-day bicycle trip; he planned to give himself an infusion just before leaving, and another when he returned. He receives many bumps and hemorrhages from his bicycling, but nonchalantly administers precipitate to take care of them. The amount of cryoprecipitate required for such a way of life obviously is very great over a period of time, in addition to that needed for physical therapy (with an infusion before and after each treatment), elective surgical procedures and dental care, and accidental hemorrhages. In the not unusual families that have more than one boy with hemophilia, and the communities in which families settle to take advantage of special medical care resources, the demands are enormous.

The shift from hospital care during hemorrhages to outpatient or home infusions of cryoprecipitate transfers the burden for financial support from hospital fund raisers and collection officers to parents, welfare departments, local blood banks, and other community sources. Home and community costs rise while institutional costs decrease for care of these children. Unless a child is on home care, immediate transportation to a hospital emergency room or doctor's office must always be available. This means having a second car in good running order at home, or the father's using a car pool or public transportation.

The mother's employment. The burden of the catastrophic financial problem on the marriage, for which the mother feels responsible, may be eased if she contributes money. If she goes to work for a large organization that has a group insurance policy, she can feel that her insurance underwrites the father's insurance, in case the latter cannot finance more blood. Unfortunately, when the boy or boys are preschool age and most subject to falls, the mother is most needed at home. Repeated decisions must be made in the boy's behalf—should he be allowed to play with a certain toy, should an ice pack be applied, should a doctor be called, how should the child's tantrums be handled? Since these decisions can have life-and-death meaning—especially if the child is not under a home-care program, as most are not—and are vital emotionally and financially, the mother is caught between two conflicting needs. Sitters and even grandmothers should not have to make the decisions and provide the care. Agencies working with the family should help parents weigh those alternatives that will be of greatest value to the child in the long run, and try to hold in abeyance agency policy that encourages all mothers to work. When the child is of school age, the mother's part-time employment during school hours may be possible, especially if the school system has a school nurse or teacher or principal who has evidenced capacity to act during emergencies without penalizing the child.

Family location. Hemophilia affects the family's location, for not only does the father need to work for a company with a broad group health insurance policy, but accessibility to a special treatment center and to cryoprecipitate may well determine the child's life and future. The school is important also; schools vary greatly in the understanding shown by principals and teachers for chronically ill children. Many cautions must be exercised in counseling a family to move. Thorough exploration of the projected new site is necessary and warranted because the needs of the child with hemophilia are unique and of such import.

Attitudes and relationships. Family relationships deserve very close attention to individual differences. The relative dominance that hemophilia assumes in family life depends not only on its severity but upon the values, personalities, and social circumstances of the family. The constellations seem to have more than the usual complexity. First, the family frequently includes extended family members. Maternal grandparents who have reared sons with hemophilia, or whose sons have died, may maintain a close relationship with carrier daughters who are repeating their family's tragedy, though in a different way because of the variations in each nuclear family. Adult maternal uncles with hemophilia may remain an important part of the total family picture, as models, mentors, warnings, authorities, or loved persons. Those who have died may also remain in family memories, conversations, and fears.

The paternal grandparents may also be a continuing strand in the web. In-law tensions are easily heightened when the daughter-in-law is considered "to blame" for a beloved grandchild's pain and crippling. If the grandparents knew of her heritage, they may have disapproved of the marriage and attempted to prevent it. The child's father may be caught between loyalty to his wife and son or sons and loyalty to his parents. If no one knew of hemophilia in the mother's family, the paternal grandparents may suspect her of hiding guilty family secrets. The infinite ways in which they may react to the child include both overprotection and masked rejection with favoritism to siblings; how actively they fuel the tension between father and son requires delicate exploration.

A second reason for the intensity of family relationships is the dampening effect a child with hemophilia often has on socialization, and thus on the attenuation of family interaction. Most parents cannot participate actively in club, church, or other group activities during the periods they are tied down by the unpredictability of emergencies and by caring for the child. Some parents are isolated from peers other than relatives and long-time neighbors.

The overprotective mother is the classical stereotype in hemophilia; frequent corollaries to that stereotype are the intense dependence of the child upon the mother and the emotional distance of both from the father. By and large, the mother can be assumed to be harboring feelings of guilt, feelings that vary from one mother to the next and in their effects on the child and the marriage. An overlay of defiance and denial may cover the guilt feelings, or they may be manifested in severe, undisguised anxiety. The word "guilt" is also a generalized term that serves to insulate the worker from the mother's pain. But the depth of a mother's fear, worry, self-blame, and despair is not difficult for the worker to comprehend after hearing the stories of onset, and remembering what the sight of blood does to many people. One mother told with anguish of her shock when the child's tooth was knocked out in a fall, and the bleeding would not stop. He was finally hospitalized, and when she went back to see him at evening visiting hours, his head was lying in a pool of blood.

Education about caring for the child is important, but probably less so than the mother's personality and the availability of understanding and long-term, steady support in dealing with continuing crises. The advent of cryoprecipitate lessens the reality of her stress. Knowing that critical episodes can be brought under control provides the possibility of mastery.

It is in fact the rare mother who can provide a normally supportive relationship: normal discipline is difficult to administer, and oversolicitude is "normal," or at least inevitable, when a child's head injury may cause death and a bump may cause pain and crippling; and ensuing medical treatment always carries the pain of needles and, frequently, immobilization. Medical authorities have emphasized for years the importance of permitting the child normal activity, despite the bumps, in order to strengthen his muscles and to prevent emotional crippling. The mother who identifies herself with a medical role in treating the child can take on some of this attitude.

The degree to which a mother may be expected to be "sensible" will depend on her early experiences with her brother's and her child's hemophilia, what happened at onset, her husband's support, her health, her temperament, and other stresses she is under. Depending on her personality and the degree to which she permits expression of aggressive feelings, she may protect herself from victimization or she may yield to it. An aggressive mother who habitually projects her anger on others (and is thus more difficult for persons in helping roles) may be more firm with her child and less prone to baby him. The "more civilized" mother, who cannot permit herself to feel anger openly, seems to blame herself more, be more understanding, suffer more with the child, and yield to his and other family pressures; she finds it harder to discipline her son or to permit him to take risks, and therefore does overprotect.

Charles Hurt, the social worker of the Regional Hemophilia Center at the Los Angeles Children's Hospital who has had extensive experience with parents of boys with hemophilia, says that fathers of hemophiliacs have often become bystanders by the time a child is school-age; that the mother's feelings of responsibility for her boy's condition reinforce the usual maternal caretaking role. She has brought the child to the doctor and learned all the facts, whereas the father may be frightened that the child will bleed to death, may be anxious and feel left out. Mr. Hurt has found that middle-class fathers, who can often take time off from work to come to the clinic if asked, frequently respond very well—they want to be involved and to play their normal role as parent, and they respond to casework or therapeutic efforts. Men of lower socioeconomic levels, who tend to be less verbal and less accustomed to talking about their feelings, may respond less well, and realistically cannot get off work during the day when the doctors are available for conferences. If there is no intervention, the normal course of events plays itself out, the mother-child relationship becomes intense, and the father removes himself physically or psychologically, as much as possible.

Situations observed confirm the literature that fathers, by and large, separate themselves from the hemophiliac child and his care as much as is decently possible, and the boy is reared primarily by his mother. The father's capacity for understanding the mother's feeling, and for loving her compassionately, probably affects the degree to which he is willing to share what seems to be her burden, the rearing of the child. One mother said, "Lots of fathers resent sons with hemophilia," because they cannot participate in sports and physically arduous activities. She said that since her brother had hemophilia, "I was my father's son." She added that she knew enough "not to marry a sports freak." Her remark highlighted the fact that ability to obtain satisfactions as a parent from a child affects the relationship. A father whose values center on intellectual or creative achievement takes pride in an intelligent, creative son, whereas a father whose values equate athletic ability with masculinity is disappointed in a physically weak son.

The effects of absence of the father in a boy's life are unusually well delineated by Tess Forest in "The Paternal Roots of Male Character Development."[16] "The sensation of father's strength and responsive experience of his own strength is the infant's first intimation of the exciting pleasure of nonprotective but stimulating and evocative physical contact. It is also his first knowledge that father's strength is available when his own fails." The father is the "first stranger" and, as such, represents the outside world, widening the infant's relationship from that with his mother alone and signifying pleasure from other than mother. He dilutes the symbiotic relationship with the mother. "The lack of physical exchange with father deprives the child of the sense of his own survival power and strength relative to father's. He is left feeling fragile and vulnerable to any touch but mother's protective caress." Dr. Forest also develops the way in which absence of the father deprives the child of example, companionship, and concepts required to enjoy his surroundings, leaving him confused, without male standards, and increasingly dependent on the mother. She says the child "hungers for father's acknowledgment, rages at his abandonment, and clings to mother in humiliation, despair, and defiance."[17]

The child's age at the time the parents become aware of his hemophilia should be kept in mind in considering the effect of the father on the child's personality. An early definitive study[18] showed that 8 of 35 boys, or nearly a fourth, made a notably poor adjustment; the rest got along well, at least outwardly. It would be helpful to know whether one factor contributing to this difference could have been age at time of diagnosis. Certainly the withdrawal of the father from the boy at any age is harmful, but by the time the child is old enough to have relationships with others than the mother and father and stimulation from a wide assortment of objects, one could predicate less severe psychic damage. (Though most children with hemophilia are found to have the condition when they first begin to explore and fall, it is not discovered in others until teeth are pulled, and still others are known to have the condition from birth or during the early months.)

The study referred to points out that fathers of the boys who were poorly adjusted had left the home, or left all decisions and care to their wives, whereas the children who were well adjusted had fathers who took an active part in the children's care.[19]

The siblings in a hemophilic family pose another range of problems. Sibling relationships cannot be "normal" in an abnormal reality. Unaffected children cannot receive their fair share of the mother's attention. They are left alone or with their father or shifted to the care of relatives or neighbors when emergencies demand that the mother take the boy to the emergency room or stay at the hospital. The drama created by the brother's "bleeds" and the attention focused on him hold potential for deep resentment; in addition, feelings of anger toward the brother can be complicated by sympathy, and guilt that they do feel resentful. Doubtless, the boy's behavior has much to do with their reactions to him; an infantilized tyrant cannot but create more sibling hostility than a matter-of-fact child.

Relationships between hemophilic brothers are more complex. The advent of cryoprecipitate has come earlier in the lives of the younger boys with hemophilia; they have been spared the numerous separations for hospitalization; they have a greater feeling of mastery; they have not had the school interruptions; they have experienced less intensity of maternal anxiety; they have had a chance for more normal personality development. Other reasons for difference in personalities exist. Each child has his own genetic background and constitutional vulnerability to experience; each has varying degrees of clotting factor—all manner of differences exist, so that the sons with hemophilia cannot be thought of as having the same capacities and experiences. It seems probable that the brother with the least physical difficulty will be caught in the middle: he does not receive the excess attention given to his more severely affected brother, and he lacks the physical security of his physically normal siblings. In other words, this boy may be in the worst position and in need of especially careful evaluation.

Girl siblings, of course, suffer under an entirely different set of burdens. They know they have a fifty-fifty chance of being carriers. Some evidently do feel inferior and labor under conflict about marriage. However, denial seems to operate often when a girl falls in love and marriage becomes a specific possibility. Katz's recent study of adults with hemophilia showed that only 30 percent of those who married were childless.[20] The girl can always rationalize that she may not be a carrier, that her children may not be boys, that she and her husband could adopt a child, etc. There is often a "conspiracy of silence" in a family about unpleasant matters pertaining to illness. Unless opportunities are made for private, meaningful conversation, the girls may bury their worries and carry a burden of ill-formulated resentments and anxieties.

What hemophilia in one or more children means to the whole family was summed up tersely in one mother's comment about the value of "cryo" infusions at home, *"Now we no longer have to live life with an IF."* She elaborated: before home infusions, commitments for family outings, etc., were made with a silent qualification, "We can do this—IF no one is in the hospital." Mr. Hurt states that hemorrhages always seem to occur at the most inconvenient times. For example, a child may injure his knee and start hemorrhaging in the joint, contain his pain because he knows his mother is giving a dinner party, but find the pain too great to bear just before the guests arrive. He then has to be taken to the emergency room for an infusion, or hospitalized depending on the availability of concentrate or precipitate, and "always at the wrong moment." Thus the family's feelings toward the child cannot but be contaminated to some degree by resentment.[21] The fortunate children who have been trained to give their own infusions avoid this negative constellation of feelings.

The Child's Adjustment

Mr. Hurt has pointed out that as the child with hemophilia grows older he is made well aware of the conflicting feelings his disease arouses and the inconvenience it produces; the mother's guilt and father's resentment may be poorly concealed. Their anger and irritation over the inconvenience of his bleeds are quickly felt—"he is aware from early on that he is a pain in the neck." Though the preceding pages have dealt with the family's attitudes and adjustments, the powerful impact of these on the child's *own* adjustment should be apparent throughout.

School experience. Home relationships seem more important than usual to boys with hemophilia because the disease diminishes the amount of satisfaction the child receives from school. School interlocks with home relationships in the socialization of the boy.

The Katz study of adults with hemophilia showed that 34 percent did not finish high school, and 6 percent had had no school at all other than through private tutoring or home teaching. The school achievement of the total group was "significantly lower than the general United States average."[22] The school experience had been "marked by attendance gaps and inconsistencies in programming," and teachers were not "adequately prepared to cope with or even accept comfortably the youngster with hemophilia."[23]

Discontinuity stands out as a special feature in the school life of these children. Access to cryoprecipitate and home training will prevent much of the problem, but without these advantages the boy with hemophilia is a part-time cripple, an unpredictable cripple. Repeated bleeds into the knee or hip joints put him on crutches or into a wheelchair for an indeterminate period. He may then recover, with treatment, and become outwardly healthy again. Then, with more hemorrhages, he again has an orthopedic problem, with suffering and impaired gait and appearance. Some years, he goes to regular school; in others, he has a home teacher for six months; and in still others, he is in special classes, or in a special school for the handicapped. No wonder then that, as one boy put it, "school isn't all that important to me." The peer identifications, school loyalties, the recognition and competition, and the extracurricular activities through which social life takes place cannot proceed in a natural fashion. The intelligent child from a culturally stimulating home may surpass his peers in some fields if his time is spent reading and in pursuit of hobbies, especially if he has a natural bent for mathematics, music, art, electronics, etc. But the fun, and the growth experience, as well as the natural progression of education, are spoiled.

HEMOPHILIA

The not infrequent inability of teachers to "accept comfortably the youngster with hemophilia" is illustrated in one mother's account of the damage done to her child by a rejecting teacher. She said the boy had begun to feel inferior, and "different," and to dislike school for the first time. He had been a good student before, interested in his studies, but now he made various excuses to avoid attending school and doing homework. At her conference with the teacher at the beginning of the school year, she had failed to detect what became clearly evident in later conferences. The teacher felt "put upon" to have a child in class whose physical condition might create a problem. She already felt burdened by the size of the class, and most important, she was afraid that the child might bleed and cause some terrible, unsightly incident that she could not cope with. The mother blamed herself for not picking up this attitude in the teacher at the beginning of the year, and said she would have put the boy in a private school, or had him moved, if she had known.

Fear of the student with hemophilia, because of misunderstanding about external bleeding or fatal accident, is not uncommon, and the concern that many overburdened teachers feel about one more problem is not unusual. Children should not be refused the privilege of regular school attendance because of misapprehension. The social worker can make an important contribution to the child's socialization process and his education by helping the family to intervene if the school refuses to accept the child, or the child suffers from a teacher's rejection.

These unfortunate aspects of hemophilia do not hold true in all cases or at all times. Some children do not have severe medical problems, as mentioned earlier. Those who have access to "cryo" and intelligent supervision may go through the school years with little interference with normal life. Other children, who have uncontrolled problems, may have the good fortune to have exceptionally interested and innovative school teachers. In one case three children with hemophilia from different families are attending one elementary school, in part because the first family who moved into the neighborhood found the principal and teacher so helpful. This school adapts itself to their needs. An entire class has been moved from one floor to another to eliminate stairs. Extra sets of books are provided, so the boys can have books at home and not carry them (recommended by authorities for all children with hemophilia). The boys are kept in regular classes, provided with home teachers when they cannot attend, and treated with normal expectations.

During elementary school, a certain degree of social continuity is maintained if the child remains in the same school, for most families know each other, and the teachers know about children with special problems in earlier grades before they themselves are involved; the rough edges of fear get worn off among all concerned; neither the child with hemophilia nor his peers or teachers feel the discomfort of newness. However, entry into junior high school, or high school, precipitates numerous problems. The change of classes, the lack of acquaintance, the steps, and the jostling arrive at the very time the child is most self-conscious and emotionally labile.

Two special problems have been noted that are due to this unfortunate confluence. The first is that home teachers may be very hard to secure, for the person who can teach mathematics may not be able to teach Spanish, and the child needs help in several subjects. Owing to the scarcity of home teachers, the school may have a policy of not placing a request for a home teacher until a certain time has elapsed, and then only when a doctor's certificate guarantees that the child will have to remain home for a certain length of time—two weeks, or a month. Such a policy, justifiable from a school administration viewpoint, is entirely incompatible with the needs of the boy with hemophilia. He very often is absent for a few days only; he can return to class when his bleed has been controlled. Thus, he misses lessons entirely; if he has many bleeds, he may miss lessons repeatedly.

A related problem pertains to the personal adjustment of the boy. When school has become a miserable experience—he knows no one, feels different, cannot keep up—it is very easy for him to say that his knee (hip, elbow, stomach) is sore, or in other words, a bleed has begun. No one can say it has not. The degree to which he fakes his bleeds is a serious problem in some boys. One boy told the author he often did so; the mother of another said that her son used his disease to get out of all kinds of disagreeable situations, including school, home chores, and responsibilities to siblings. In another situation, a boy said that he does not fake his bleeds but that schoolmates in junior high school accused him of doing so. In elementary school, his peers knew him, but in junior high school, no one knew anyone else very well.

Many parents dislike their children attending special classes for the handicapped. A substantial number of the child's classmates there have mental or emotional problems that interfere with learning, in addition to orthopedic problems; thus the curriculum is generally adapted to slow learners. One adolescent, in discussing special school experience, said, "If everybody thinks of you as a weirdo, you'd come up thinking you were one—it would be terrible." The stigma, and the arts and crafts emphasis in the curriculum, had poisoned him against special school.

One advantage of special schools should not be overlooked, however, for the child in a wheelchair. Their bus system, calling for the child and helping him in and out, may make the difference between his being able to attend school or having a home teacher. The latter is not always the worst choice; some home teachers are exceptional in their interest in the child and do much to help him develop special talents or academic interests. Children who have brothers and sisters, or an extended family with various people to relate to who come in and out of the home, or who live in a neighborhood of friendly children who come to play, may be better off with a home teacher (if one is readily available) than going to a special school. The merits of the choices must be weighed after the total situation is studied, including the family relationships and curriculum and makeup of the student body at the special school.

Recreation. Recreation, so closely related to the school experience for most children, has several major values, and thus deserves the worker's thought and ingenuity. Boys with hemophilia should be encouraged to engage in noncompetitive forms of physical activity—swimming, fishing, hiking, 4-H club, and sometimes Boy Scout or church group activities, and bicycling if the physician approves. Boys who have home training in the use of precipitate and access to an amount permitting prophylactic use can now take part in almost every activity except body sports. Gradual development of muscle strength safeguards inner organs, keeps the boy's weight down, which is important, and gives him self-confidence. Since he can be part of a peer group, the damaging emotional effects of the disease are lessened. However, development of sedentary interests and solitary pursuits is essential for the periods when he is disabled, and prevents constant absorption in television. Small children can enjoy costumes for dressing up to play Indian, fireman, etc., and enjoy blackboards and coloring. Older children may enjoy aquariums, electronics, playing pool, table games, and making models. Recreational activities are especially valuable in helping the handicapped adolescent secure a sense of identity and self-worth; they have further value in pointing toward possible careers.

Vocational preparation. Vocational choice is affected by self-discovery—experiences that demonstrate the pleasure of mastery in one or more areas. Budding vocational choice during adolescence is part of the usual high school experience. The Katz study of men with hemophilia showed that the majority were employed, at a wide range of occupations clustered predominantly around white-collar technical and clerical jobs.[24] However, a significant percentage, largely those who had severe physical handicaps, were unemployed or had not worked, and many who were employed wished they were in some other job (not unlike the attitude of many average healthy workers). Though the adult with hemophilia may engage in a wide range of occupations, very early vocational counseling is emphasized by persons experienced in working with children who have the disease. Technological development has lessened vocational problems because of the machinery that has lightened office and factory work. However, certain types of occupations have to be excluded, such as those that are hazardous, that involve heavy lifting, that put strain on certain groups of joints or muscles, or positions that are "one of a kind" in an office or factory. The latter are unsuitable because the entire firm will be disrupted when the man with hemophilia is off work unpredictably with a hemorrhage.[25] Consequently, the adolescent needs to think of a career early. He should have aptitude tests and beginning vocational counseling in junior high school, and an opportunity to attend career days, exhibits, college open houses, etc. Guidance staff should keep in mind that he may be crippled further as he gets older.

Sex and marriage. Regarding sex and marriage, genetic problems may be of greater immediate concern to the adolescent boy's carrier sisters than to him, for although his daughters will be carriers (and his possible grandsons victims), his sons will be normal. As indicated, a "conspiracy of silence" sometimes prevails, and girls do not share their worries with their families. Technically, transmission of the gene need not be a concern during an era that has seen the rapid advance in birth control methods and of acceptance of selective abortions unless religious considerations exist. However, adolescents who have a physical abnormality sometimes seem particularly anxious to have children to prove themselves physically normal.

When adolescent boys or girls from a family with hemophilia indicate conflict about sexual alliances and marriage, the worker should be clear in her own mind that she does not need to be neutral, and to know how she stands. Often people become so closely identified with a person with a potentially transmissible defect that their values become blurred. The laissez-faire attitude of some families, and the frequent use of denial, are not abnormal in families involved, or in girls in love. However, the social worker expects to be objective. Prevention of a defect that has such disastrous effects upon a child and his family seems to warrant a clear stand that the boy with hemophilia or the carrier girl should plan a marriage that includes use of reliable birth control.

Attitude toward illness. The final factor determining the boy's personal adjustment is his attitude toward his illness. Common sense is confirmed by the Katz study, which showed "success" in life to be closely related to severity of the disease.[26] Employment was used as the criterion, with linked variables such as schooling, need for financial aid, marriage, and activity. Despite the truisms about (and the sometimes overstated emphasis on) emotional factors such as motivation, the severity of an illness determines the restrictions it imposes, the preoccupation with pain and malaise required of the human organism, and consequently the opportunities the person has for self-development. A child who frequently hemorrhages with no apparent cause, or who has hemorrhaged into the brain and is partially paralyzed or brain-damaged, obviously must have a different attitude toward his handicap than one who is only mildly affected.

Yet it is also true that "feelings are facts," and that these stem from constitutional vulnerability to experience or a general sensitivity, from human experiences, and from the feedback of others. Feelings of difference from others seem to begin as soon as the child's cognitive capacity can comprehend abstract ideas, and as soon as school exposes him to his peers and to adults outside the family. One mother commented that her boy began to notice he was "different" and to indicate concern about this at age seven. One nine-year-old boy had been told by his mother that the worker wanted to know what it was actually like to have hemophilia, and he said bluntly, "It feels like you're bruised all over, and like it's not very nice to be a hemophiliac." Not until later was it learned that not he, but his healthy brother, was subject to constant bruises. As a cover-up for having revealed himself, this boy launched into all the good things that happen if you have hemophilia, describing a wonderful special camp experience so vividly that it sounded current, whereas it had actually happened several years previously.

Feelings of precariousness, of never knowing whether one can count on one's body to perform functionally or whether it will painfully disrupt present or future plans, must create anxiety; the psychological effect of sudden changes in body image, from an active, upright person to a bedfast, wheelchair-bound or crutch-limited person, can readily be understood. No studies are known that show a correlation between episodes of bleeding with critical ages of development; it can be assumed that bleeding cycles at puberty and at the early age of beginning autonomy would be most destructive personally unless active intervention occurs.

One of the greatest values of home training in the use of cryoprecipitate reveals itself in the attitude boys have toward self-determination about injections, with ability to control the pain of the needle. A common complaint of families and children is having to "sit around" a hospital emergency room or clinic waiting for someone else, interns or other physicians, to decide whether to transfuse; by the time the transportation and the waiting have combined, bleeding has begun in earnest. Thus more severe pain, more disability, more blood replacement, and slower recovery occur. A boy who knows that he can make his own decision when he first feels soreness or stiffness in a joint, and can transfuse himself, has realistic reasons to incorporate less resentment about his disease. Resentment against interns for fumbling attempts to find a vein ("they shouldn't allow interns to learn on little kids") and resentment against all physicians ("they don't know as much as we do about when we are having a bleed") would appear to be in part projection of anger against the pain, inconvenience, and danger of hemophilia, in part realistic, and in part an expression of frustration over the dependence on others that such a disease creates.

Despite the realistic reasons for poor personal adjustment that hemophilia poses, both the study of 35 boys previously mentioned[27] and the Katz study show a surprisingly large percentage who achieve better adjustment than would be expected. Only 20 or 25 percent had gross measurable indications of a "spoiled identity," or severe personal or social problems (withdrawal or depression or lack of ability to seek or hold a job, etc.). Since these persons did not have the advantage of advances in treatment including precipitate, future children may expect a still better outlook, statistically.

The Worker's Role in the Community

Social workers and other practitioners in the community are likely to be involved with those children who have manifest problems, or to be working with families in prevention of problems among those who are struggling with crises. Areas where meaningful help can be offered have been brought out in the foregoing. Locating resources for skilled medical care, or helping to develop access to a home-training program and cryoprecipitate, is the single most important job a worker can perform if the family is not enrolled in such a program. The current emphasis in social work on "advocacy" and "reaching out," in contrast to "therapy," is advantageous in reinforcing the worker's awareness of the dignity of what may be an arduous task. Group endeavor through a local hemophilia association or informal group of parents may be an appropriate method.

Working with the father, so that he is not excluded but, to the contrary, fulfills his various essential roles in the development of the male child, may also be one of the most important contributions the social worker can make. Evening visits, or waiting for a reluctant father to get out of bed and join the interview, may be necessary. With the many families in which there is no father, or an indifferent stepfather, finding a male substitute may be possible. Male social workers are themselves potential good models providing they do not abruptly leave the agency, unwittingly reinforcing the child's feelings of abandonment. Because social workers are migratory, by and large, and subject to case-load changes, they may need to locate persons who have greater likelihood of becoming a stable male figure in the child's life. The athletic coach who performs such an important function in the usual teenage boy's life is not feasible for the boy with hemophilia, but a male teacher, minister, policeman, or volunteer may act in this capacity. Identification with medical care personnel is natural and, if not involving an intern or resident (who is transient by nature of his position), may also be fruitful.

Special Problems in Adoption

Should the social worker encourage a couple to adopt a child known to have hemophilia? Or encourage a couple to keep a child who was not known to be a bleeder at time of placement? The first reality factor to be explored is the severity of the bleeding difficulty. A detailed report from a physician is necessary in understanding the particular child's problem. Other constitutional characteristics need to be considered also. Some boys are said to be remarkably "healthy" and cheerful, resilient in spite of the hemophilia, whereas others, possibly more sensitive and frail, have great difficulty coping with the physical affliction. The age at which bleeding becomes apparent and the child's response over a period of time give some clue to the individualized nature of his condition.

A special problem in finding suitable adoptive parents for the child with hemophilia is the financial cost and the burden of finding blood donors and of paying for blood; and this problem increases as the child grows larger. Unless government funding becomes available, the prospective adoptive family needs to have unusual financial resources or unusual capacity to locate and sustain, over the years, a supply of donors. The unpredictability of bleeds means that the family also needs to be flexible, able to rearrange plans quickly without undue upset. The prospective father merits special scrutiny and understanding, for he will need to participate in child-care decisions and responsibilities, and also not be disappointed in a child who cannot become an athlete. The foster mother should be a person capable of administering the injections until the child is old enough to do it himself, if they live near a center that provides a home-care program.

If the child is to be placed, the geographic area of the adoptive parents is a vital factor in their selection. As pointed out earlier, proximity to a special medical center and access to a blood bank that fractionates cryoprecipitate have a life-and-death bearing on the child's condition and the family burden. Foster parents to whom home training is available, and who have the emotional stability to help the boy learn to administer his own infusions, would appear to be critical in the success of the placement.

NOTE: Since this chapter was written, Congress passed legislation authorizing over two billion dollars for special health measures, including one that "authorizes the Secretary [of HEW] to make grants to and enter into contracts with public and nonprofit private entities for projects for the establishment of comprehensive hemophilia diagnostic and treatment centers. Authorizes to be appropriated for such grants and contracts $3,000,000 for fiscal year 1976 and $4,000,000 for fiscal year 1977. Authorizes the Secretary to make grants to and enter into contracts with public and nonprofit private entities for projects to develop and expand existing blood separation centers. Authorizes to be appropriated for such grants and contracts $4,000,000 for fiscal year 1976 and $5,000,000 for fiscal year 1977." (Title VI of HR 4925, reconciled with provisions of SB 66, the Special Health Revenue Sharing Act of 1975, passed over the President's veto on July 26, 1975.) If the funds are appropriated as authorized, and the programs implemented, the legislation will constitute an opening gun in the battle against the financial catastrophe of blood costs to parents of children with hemophilia. (From House Bills, p. E499, Democratic Study Group Report for the week of July 28, 1975.)

CHAPTER TWELVE

Juvenile Rheumatoid Arthritis

GRASPING THE MEANING of juvenile rheumatoid arthritis presents many pitfalls. Much about the disease is unknown; its onset is variable and its course "capricious." The range of medical and social disability is so wide as to defy generalization. Stereotyping juvenile rheumatoid arthritis as a relentless, progressive crippler, as in the severe adult form, is a mistake. Juvenile rheumatoid arthritis differs from adult arthritis in several ways, most remarkably in prognosis. Up to two-thirds of the children with this disease eventually recover. Some are left with deformities and some may develop arthritis again as adults, but the active arthritis of childhood disappears. A study of 46 arthritic adults with arthritis in childhood showed 35 able to work and maintain a relatively normal family life.[1]

Generalized statistics, however, do not describe individual cases, and may in fact be misleading. Children of the poor are more likely to suffer severe crippling, since home care and skilled medical supervision during the early critical phases often alter the outlook for functional improvement. The adoption worker who learns that a child awaiting placement in her agency's charge is arthritic may be able to predict a different possible outcome than the worker in Aid to Families with Dependent Children. Intelligent use of guidance and continuing care by a skilled pediatrician and other specialists available to adoption agencies, and the good nutrition provided in most foster homes, frequently are not available to families receiving public assistance. Home, not hospital, is the major setting for care of the child with this long-term disease. Prevention of severe crippling of the child may rest on the efforts of a helping person in mustering resources and in coordinating family, child, specialists, and community activity over a long period of time.

Although accurate data regarding prevalence cannot be obtained, one authority estimates about 175,000 cases in the United States, which would make juvenile arthritis the major chronic crippling disease of childhood.[2]

THE MEDICAL REALITIES

Juvenile rheumatoid arthritis is a puzzling disease that is better described than defined. An acknowledged authority on the disease, John Calabro, says its "variable modes of onset are accompanied by a myriad of signs, symptoms and manifestations and are followed by an apparently unpredictable course."[3] Patterns have been identified, however, that follow several modes of onset, and these will be presented as described in the literature.

The cause is unknown, though infection or trauma frequently precedes the onset.[4] Psychological factors, so widely considered a cause of adult rheumatoid arthritis, are not sufficiently notable to have been observed and recorded by social workers involved with a group of the families whose records were studied by University of Chicago students.[5] Although the "role played by psychological factors in juvenile rheumatoid arthritis has received relatively little attention in the literature,"[6] the studies that have been done, not surprisingly, fail to agree on or establish any significant elements. The human personality is, after all, essentially in constant movement, interacting with and acting on many facets of itself and the environment, hence unable to "stand still" for a picture of any one of its parts; because control of all significant variables is virtually impossible, many statistical research efforts involving personality have proved sterile or disappointing. Personality attributes of arthritic children are discussed later.

Onset and Symptoms

JRA, or *juvenile rheumatoid arthritis*, strikes very young children and more girls than boys. It may begin as early as six months, but the peak incidence occurs between two and four years, and between 8 and 11 years.[7] These peaks have significance in relation to the difference in stages of development of the child's personality and, frequently, in the stage of the family life cycle.

The modes of onset are three, and each has meaning for the future. *Still's Disease*, or the acute systemic (body-wide effects) type, affects about one-fourth of the children. *Oligoarticular arthritis*, or arthritis of less than four joints (sometimes referred to as *monoarticular* because it first begins in one joint), affects roughly another fourth. *Polyarticular arthritis*, or arthritis of many joints, affects about half the children with this disease. (The polyarticular form, generally called "polyarthritis," is the most likely to lead to crippling.[8])

As discussed by the authorities cited, the oligoarticular type of JRA has the best outlook, except for one feature of special note. The disease is sometimes accompanied by inflammation in the eyes that may lead to blindness. This complication is discussed later. The term "oligoarticular" on a medical report should alert the worker to the need to ensure eye examinations to prevent the possibility of irreversible impairment of vision.

Still's disease presents difficulty in diagnosis. It begins as a "fever of unknown origin." There are few joint symptoms and the symptoms that do occur are present in many other conditions. These are intermittent fever, evanescent rash, lethargy, and irritability. The child is very ill, and delay in diagnosis has many ramifications for cost, energy, patience, and most of all initiation of appropriate treatment for the sick child.

Polyarthritis has less severe systemic or body-wide manifestations than the Still's disease form, and is characterized by swelling and tenderness of joints. The child is moderately ill. Though there are remissions (periods of freedom from symptoms), his chance of developing progressive arthritis is greater than that of children with the other forms of the disease. He is more apt to become severely crippled.

During the unpredictable flare-ups, or periods of exacerbation, children with JRA have pain and stiffness in the involved joints, especially at night and after periods of inactivity. Some wake at night and cry, several times every night. Home care may require turning the child or giving him a hot bath during the night. All children with JRA, at some stage in their disease, are stiff on waking in the morning, and may need a hot bath to relieve the stiffness. Although children with arthritis are thought to have less pain than adults, pain is a significant factor.[9]

Involvement of various joints obviously creates particular problems of function. Ankle involvement is described as creating a ducklike, flat-footed gait; if the feet are affected, there is a *cavus* (inward-turning) deformity with a cock-up toe. Brewer states that rheumatoid involvement of the wrist creates one of the most troublesome and restricting problems in children. Stiffness and muscular weakness occur and—ultimately, when the disease process stops—destructive changes in bone that create deformity. Involved hands lose muscle strength, grip, and mobility. The cervical spine, or neck, commonly affected, becomes stiff so that the child moves head, neck, and shoulders as a unit. Hip involvement creates pain down the thigh to the knee. If pain is severe and lasting, hip involvement is one of the most disabling of the functional impairments. Limping, muscle atrophy, and, in severe cases, *osteoporosis*, or fragile bones, occur. Shoulders are also commonly affected, causing serious limitation of motion. In some severe cases, the jaw joints are affected, resulting in difficulty in chewing and loss of growth of the mandible, causing an "angular pinched expression."[10]

Course and Prognosis

Calabro states that there is no way of forecasting what will happen to any individual child in the early stages of JRA.[11] In the study previously cited, of adults with arthritis known to have developed it in childhood, "there was no demonstrable correlation between the functional outcome and the age of disease onset, duration of disease, sex, ... or types of drug therapy used."[12] Calabro states that the disease process stops in about two-thirds of the children by the end of ten years. About one-half can expect disease activity for an average of three years; the remainder have an unknown and unpredictable duration. A tabulation by Brewer, with results of nine studies pertaining to crippling, shows that complete functional recovery occurred in about one-third, minimal or moderate crippling in about one-third, and severe crippling in the others, in the series of cases reported. Death is reported to occur from the disease or its treatment in 4 percent or more of the cases in the series. It is most apt to take place during the early stage of severe illness, or later among children who have severe, relentless disease.[13]

Brewer says, "Patients with monoarticular [oligoarticular] arthritis who have clinical remission with less than three years activity probably have the best chance to avoid recurrence. When the disease lasts longer than three years the chances of remission in less than ten years are remote. Duration is based on severity of the polyarthritis and whether or not progressive erosive arthritis occurs."

Differences in prognosis reported by various works are due in part to the very recent development of studies on juvenile arthritis covering a period of time, and in part to the delays in diagnosis, which obscure the length of time the child has had the disease. The more current optimistic outlook arises from the recent ability to include mild cases in totals studied. The statistical averages differ from those obtained when only patients with easily identifiable disease with severe symptoms were counted.

The disease process cannot be cured but it can be controlled. Arthritis flares up, dies down, flares, and finally ends for no reason understood at this time.[14] Nevertheless, active treatment from the beginning is very important to prevent destructive changes and crippling.

Complications

Ocular complications, especially in connection with oligoarticular disease, as pointed out earlier, are highly dangerous because they may not be detected in early stages, when treatment is most effective, except by slit-lamp examination by an ophthalmologist. Children who complain that light hurts their eyes, or who rub their eyes, or whose eyes are red should have an eye examination without delay. Because the eye disorders can occur at any time, whether the disease is active in the joints or not, it is essential to have continued, regular examinations by a medical eye specialist. Rheumatologists' recommendations regarding frequency of needed eye examinations vary from every three months to once a year.[15] The eye disorder may be in one or both eyes, and may consist of a simple inflammation of the iris, *iritis*, or may progress to *iridocyclitis*, a spreading involvement leading at times to a fibrosis of the cornea called *band keratopathy*. Eye complications may lead to glaucoma or cataracts, or both. The eyes are easily treated by steroid medication in the early stage, but if the disease is permitted to progress, severe visual impairment results, including blindness.

Miller states that *heart complications* are unusual and ordinarily mild but may be lethal.[16] In their moderately severe form they create substantial pain, and in very severe cases, pain and a murmur. Abrupt heart failure can occur. Either *pericarditis* or *myocarditis* can develop.[17] The social worker whose caseload includes a child with JRA who has developed heart complications should anticipate the possible need for hospital care.

Children with severe JRA are subject to *growth disturbance* for a variety of reasons. These include poor nutrition, retardation of bone growth, and the steroid treatment often required if other measures fail to control dangerous or painful symptoms. Growth stunting of the jaw is called *micrognathia*. It is one of the unfortunate results of childhood arthritis that last into adult life, though Brewer states that some children catch up, at least in part, when the disease process ends.[18]

Treatment

Drug therapy. Aspirin is the basic element in treatment. Its common use and its pain reducing characteristics mislead parents and relatives. They tend to downgrade its importance, or think it is for pain, and thus to disregard its regular continuing use after pain subsides. Aspirin, acetylsalicylic acid, is in fact a specific for reduction of inflammation, and thus for the ill effects of JRA, an inflammatory process.[19]

Ordinarily, large doses are prescribed, to be taken four times a day. The large doses create undesirable side effects in some instances. Stomach pain is frequent. The ill-informed parent, or the adolescent who is expected to take his medication without supervision, may discontinue or decrease the dose to avoid the pain. Fortunately, this pain can be prevented by use of milk or other food taken with the aspirin.[20] The family that has been educated about the problem and receives sufficient medical supervision should not have continued difficulty unless psychological or relationship problems complicate the giving of medication. Aspirin toxicity can occur, creating ringing of the ears, or *tinnitus*, fever, shortness of breath, and in severe instances, lethargy. When any of these symptoms occur, the physician should be notified so that he can secure laboratory tests and, if necessary, decrease the dosage.

If six months of aspirin therapy has not controlled symptoms, the Children's Hospital at Stanford considers the use of gold. Gold therapy, which has been in and out of favor over a period of years, should be administered only by physicians who are experienced in its use.[21] Gold is administered by injection once a week for approximately three months at the Children's Hospital at Stanford.

Other medications sometimes used include certain dangerous drugs. Indocin, commonly used for adults, is rarely used for children.[22] Certain other drugs for adults are contraindicated for children. Steroid drugs, such as cortisone and prednisone, hailed at their discovery as the remedy for rheumatoid arthritis, now are known to have such serious side effects that they are used only in emergencies and as moderately and for as short a time as possible. They are only indicated when heart failure or blindness threatens.[23] A child known to be receiving steroid drugs should be under close and skilled medical supervision.

The injection of steroids directly into affected joints is not as dangerous as their systemic use, though specialist care is needed. This treatment is used in some cases where one or two joints are seriously affected.[24]

Physical therapy is, like aspirin, a staple of treatment, though not all children receive continued, professionally directed exercise. Designed to prevent or rectify deformities, physical therapy consists of the use of exercise provided with adequate attention to protection and rest of affected muscles and joints. Because hospitalization and clinic attendance form only minute intervals in the long treatment of JRA, the foundation of the physical therapy program takes place in the community and at home. Applications of hot paraffin are sometimes used for heat preceding exercise. However, the most practical means of providing moist heat at home is by warm tub baths. One bath on awakening, to reduce morning stiffness, and one before bedtime are sometimes recommended.[25]

Prevention of deformity requires proper positioning of the child in bed, chair, or (while watching TV) on the floor. There is a natural tendency to favor a painful joint by keeping the limb in a flexed position. The position becomes fixed and deformity may result. Exercises, often performed by the child himself through a "range of motion" (ROM), are used to counteract this tendency and to keep the involved parts supple. The amount and type of exercise depend on the state of the particular joint being treated and the purpose of the exercise. Different exercise programs may be conducted on different joints in the same child, and at different times.

Moving an inflamed joint is painful; stretching after the inflammation has ceased is less so. Correction and prevention of deformity in quiescent joints require stretching, sometimes beyond the point of pain. Because parents cannot and should not be relied upon to inflict painful treatments, professional physical therapists should perform these exercises. In some areas schools for handicapped children provide physical therapy services for children for whom physical therapy is recommended. Those who do not have this advantage must be taken to a clinic or office frequently and regularly over extended periods. Ordinarily, parent and child perform daily exercises they can do at home, to supplement those provided by a professional therapist.

Damage to joints or fracture of weakened bones constitutes a danger if exercise is too enthusiastic or incorrectly performed. Rest is as necessary as exercise. The popular myth that arthritics should "keep active" may lead uninformed parents and teachers to minimize the essential nature of rest. Children need a balanced program. The little child at home will control his own activities. However, the school-age child in whom peer competition is psychologically inherent may push himself to keep up or win. Permanent destruction of joint space cartilage and bone can occur if the child's play is excessively active or unsupervised.

Play as exercise needs careful prescription. A written medical recommendation specifying what sports and play are permissible should be used at school. By and large, swimming is the most beneficial sport, with bicycle riding also recommended. During the acute stages of arthritis, all jarring, twisting activities are prohibited (jumping rope, other jumping up and down, roller skating, trampoline, wrestling, etc.). Competitive activities are prohibited because the child will not feel able to stop when fatigued or in pain. Contact sports are also prohibited because of the possible trauma to the joints.[26]

Orthopedic measures including surgery. Skilled orthopedic care is an integral part of the treatment of protracted and severe arthritis. Braces and splints to correct deformity are occasionally used. They are said to do more harm than good if improperly applied. A child's limbs are growing and supple, making him more vulnerable to harmful effects than an adult.[27] Corrective devices must be modified as the deformity straightens or as the child grows. Night braces and splints are used in some cases. These are heavy and impede the child's turning at night, increasing his irritability and the family's loss of sleep. These aspects of orthopedic treatment make obvious the need for skilled medical supervision.

Surgery is used in relatively few cases, in comparison with the total number treated by medication and physical therapy. In recent years, surgery has been employed directly on the actively inflamed joint in an operation called a *synovectomy*, or removal of the *synovium*, the joint lining. This operation is performed only after conservative measures have failed to prevent continued joint destruction and when surgery seems essential to save the cartilage from destruction. It is used primarily when only one or two joints are involved, usually a knee or hand.[28] Synovectomies are considered to be successful in achieving temporary goals. The condition may recur in the same joint, so that repeated operations may be necessary. Scarring, with permanent substantial loss of joint motion, follows surgery.[29]

Other operations performed on children with JRA include *flexion contracture release*, a measure to improve the function of a rigid deformed joint that has not yielded to physical therapy and devices. *Osteotomy*, or change in position of the bone, is performed on children over 11 years of age if serious deformity of wrist or knee seems to require this procedure. *Arthrodesis*, or joint fusion, is rarely used in children. This procedure results in a permanent position of the limb or part affected, usually the hip or wrist. Other orthopedic operative procedures include manipulation of joints under anesthesia, and sometimes surgical equalization of length of the lower extremities if one leg is longer than the other.[30] The development of artificial joints promises benefits in the future.

The usual length of hospitalization for surgical procedures ranges from weeks to months. In order to reduce hospital costs, the child is often sent home for a convalescent period, and returned to the hospital for intense physical therapy, a very painful period, for several weeks.

PSYCHOSOCIAL IMPLICATIONS

A striking range of psychosocial problems exists, in variety and intensity. Their nature arises from the interplay among the various factors of current age and personality of the child and age of onset of the disease; the family structure, physical circumstances, attitudes, and relationships; the severity and nature of each child's disease and medical treatment. No two configurations can be the same. Some common threads occur, however, that provide clues of value in deriving understanding of the individual. The salient characteristics of the disease that interweave with social aspects are the frequently early age of onset, its long duration and unpredictable character, treatment requirements, pain, limitations of activity, and cosmetic deformities, including stunting of growth.

Family Adjustment

Experience strikes most deeply when the organism is young and in a period of rapid growth (see Chapter 2). Because arthritis is a long-term illness that sometimes begins as early as six months of age, it must leave an imprint on personality even after the disease process has disappeared. A small child who cannot respond freely to the drive for activity inherent in his stage of development and whose explorational activities are inhibited sustains a maturational setback. If the child must be carried because walking is too painful, and the mother often holds and lifts him during prolonged illness, dependency is increased. The child with mild, oligoarticular disease may be only slightly affected, but the child with severe polyarthritis is profoundly affected.

Long duration guarantees many family changes. Siblings are born to usurp the child's place with the mother. Fathers may disappear and stepfathers emerge. Other children may become ill, claiming the mother's attention. Unemployment, alcoholism, or other disruptive changes may occur. Mothers often go to work in order to bring in more funds. Older siblings or indifferent sitters may take the place of the formerly hovering mother.

Young children often have young parents who are in the vulnerable early years of marriage. Parents who have not themselves reached complete emotional maturity, and whose normal expectations include good times and self-fulfillment, are most open to disappointing home life if painful illness keeps a child crying at night and exhausting the mother from lack of sleep. One Eastern center describes its use of special measures to enlist the participation and interest of the father in caring for the young child, after discovering that over half the fathers of arthritic patients over 16 had separated from their families, had died, or "were trapped in irreversible medical and social problems."[31]

Long duration of any stress wears away the capacity to cope with it. "She's angry," one mother said of an outwardly placid child at the clinic. "She's tired of coming to clinic and going to therapy and having to stay home from school and all the pain and everything." The mother was tired of it too. Her grim voice revealed her frustration.

The child's attitude changes abruptly when the symptoms disappear. "He's a different child—I can hardly believe it." The formerly listless, withdrawn little boy has become a happy, active youngster. The parents of such children can now believe the physician's optimistic comments that two-thirds of the children finally get well. They express hope that a cure has taken place, that they are through with arthritis. The parents renew their strength, and the child cautiously or aggressively begins to take part in the play of his peers. Not infrequently, the mother discontinues aspirin or exercises prematurely, with variable results.

The flu, a tumble, or nothing at all occurs, and another joint or joints swell, stiffness and pain recur—the disease is active again. (Some children have flare-ups as often as three times a year; others may go for years with no symptoms.) The child is again depressed, and the parents frustrated. "It's a discouraging disease," one mother said heavily. The severity of the recurrence, the family's finances, and human resources influence such decisions as whether the mother should quit work and how the child is to be cared for. Father and mother may react differently, the father sometimes angry and the mother resigned or overprotective. The potential for marital discord is always present.

One parent voiced the difficulty in disciplining a child who is alternately sick and well. "I noticed that even when she was well she expected me to pick up her toys for her. Spoiling is the greatest temptation—I am so thankful my husband agrees with me that she must be treated just like any other child when she is not sick."

Children who have been hospitalized often seem spoiled to parents or foster parents, and have difficulty with their siblings when they go home. The child has learned a pattern wherein caretaking adults withhold discipline and wait upon him while he is in pain and distress. Failing to distinguish appropriate behaviors when he recovers, he continues to expect special consideration.

Confusion of another nature also rises from the remitting, exacerbating character of juvenile arthritis. Home care demands that the mother take responsibility for many daily decisions about the child's play, rest, medication, exercise, and utilization of medical resources. Severe exacerbations or treatment procedures necessitating hospitalization require that parents relinquish responsibility to the hospital staff. Just how much responsibility the mother should continue often confuses her. If she participates too actively, asking questions or making suggestions, she may be made to feel a meddler, or too anxious; if she welcomes the rest and relinquishes entirely, she may be thought of as an abandoning parent.

Financial Problems

Arthritis is an expensive disease. Children who require neither hospitalization nor appliances nevertheless have many physician's visits, X rays, an abundance of laboratory work, drugs, and, frequently, physical therapy treatments. The cost of an office or private clinic visit on the West Coast may range up to $90 or more, depending upon the amount of laboratory work performed in connection with the physician's evaluation, and whether X rays are taken, and how many. Physical therapy currently costs about $15 per session in California. (All costs quoted necessarily are those in effect at the time of this writing and in the author's locality, northern California.) If hospital care is necessary, the current cost in this state is at least $100 per day because of the physical therapy treatments, laboratory work, and drugs that are added to the cost of board and room, which may range from $60 to $80 a day at this writing. A two-week hospital stay for intensive therapy and diagnostic studies may cost around $1,500.

If surgery is necessary, and appliances, these greatly add to the expense. An operation costs an average of $1,500. Braces currently cost approximately $300, and a folding, nonmotorized wheelchair, if essential, about $500 if several attachments are included.

Miscellaneous expenses are small for middle-class families but difficult for the poor. An electric blanket may be useful in lessening the arthritic child's pain at night. Fortunately, such an item may be secured from a service club if the family is unable to provide it.

The cost of drugs is not a major item unless gold is used. Weekly gold injections may be approximately $5 each, but are accompanied by laboratory analyses that extend the cost of each to around $15. Steroid drugs can also become a major expense if a number of tablets are prescribed daily over a long period of time, but this is not the general rule except in severe cases.

Juvenile rheumatoid arthritis is among the diseases for which Crippled Children's Services will assist with payment, providing a family is eligible. A child with JRA should also qualify for Social Security disability benefits, if the family is financially eligible. However, the remitting characteristic of the disease, combined with the administrative problems pertaining to standardized adjudication of disability during early stages of a new program, indicates that some families will have difficulty securing these benefits. They may need aid in presenting further evidence of disability. The worker who knows the family and the extent of the child's physical problems may be able to help them formulate substantiating materials. (See p. 82.)

In California, Medicaid provisions include payment for hospital care, laboratory work, X rays, and drugs for children of parents receiving public assistance or disability benefits. Insurance of employed parents, especially if it includes major medical provisions, is a frequent resource not only for hospital costs but for X rays and laboratory work, and in some instances braces or other appliances, and it may include drugs.

The variety of resources, therefore, aids most families of middle income or lowest income. Most serious financial problems occur among families who are medically indigent but who have incomes above the stringent AFDC standards, or who have more income than the Crippled Children's Services or Social Security provisions allow.

Housing and Transportation

The value of hot tub baths in the home care of arthritic children makes essential a dwelling with an accessible bathtub, and with an adequate hot water heater. Families in substandard rural or tenement dwellings, or forced by low income and large families to rent substandard houses, often must be helped to move. Major reconstruction or moving is also necessary for families of badly crippled children who cannot get wheelchairs through narrow doorways or up steps, or who need lifts or standing tables for which no room exists. Flat grants in public assistance make such individualized consideration very difficult, especially since allowance for rent, although an item included in the budget, is at an unrealistically low figure or is utilized for necessary items not included in the budget. Sums secured from private sources to supplement rent may be deducted from the grant, and therefore can be used only if top-level supervisory advice has been secured from the public assistance agency. Supervisors who are experienced in the use of regulations to help clients, and who are thoroughly familiar with agency resources, often can find ways around seemingly impossible obstacles in public assistance, and their aid therefore should be enlisted. If public housing is available in the community but a waiting list prevents access to its limited facilities, conference with the manager and public assistance supervisor is sometimes helpful.

The other major financial problem is for transportation for long-term, frequent physical therapy treatments and for clinic or hospital visits. Those children who attend special schools for the handicapped may receive physical therapy treatments there, and receive free bus transportation. Those who attend regular school or are not in school often must go by automobile to physical therapy sessions in another town or across the city three times a week indefinitely. A second car may be necessary if the father's work is so located that he too must drive. Car pools are sometimes feasible alternatives, or the mother may be able to drive the father back and forth to work or in certain communities to a train to work. Volunteers secured by the American Red Cross or other private agencies sometimes are helpful if the therapist's availability and the child's school hours can be fitted to the volunteer's available time. In some areas the Elks Club provides a traveling physical therapy unit; doubtless other private resources exist in various counties.

Like housing, transportation may be one of the most time-consuming and difficult social problems to solve, but its tangible and prosaic nature should not obscure the priority it deserves when physical therapy treatments are necessary to prevent crippling. When cost alone is the obstacle, private resources usually can be utilized without jeopardy to the public assistance budget, if the family receives public assistance, although supervisory confirmation may be important in preventing later deductions for "overpayments."

Problems with Treatment

The least expensive aspirin is as effective as any buffered or highly advertised product,[32] but constant advertising of time-release, buffered, or other expensive forms tempts the family to needless expense. The cheapest aspirin in bottles of 1,000 tablets is recommended.[33]

The simplicity of aspirin as a major tool of treatment introduces problems, as has been pointed out. The mother may understand the physician's explanation of its specificity in reducing joint inflammation if she has a physician who has taken the time to talk with her and whom she trusts, but her husband, mother-in-law, or other intimates may dispute, arguing for something less mundane, when the child continues to cry with pain and the disease is seemingly endless.

Equally troublesome in aspirin therapy is the gastric distress that has been described. Taking the medicine with milk or meals seems a simple solution, but in repeated instances the mother either does not know of this remedy or the child's irregular eating habits or refusal to eat interferes. Adolescents who try to deny their disease, or have conflict about their identity as a sick person, sometimes extend their conflicts to the regular swallowing of pills. One mother explained that her adolescent son's enuresis cleared up immediately when she told him to stop taking his aspirin. The physician later commented that aspirin could not physiologically affect bed-wetting. Less extreme instances manifest themselves in the adolescents who "forget" to take medicine.

Gold treatment must be administered by intramuscular injection at the physician's office. Frequent analysis of blood samples accompanies the treatment, to avoid dangers from toxicity. Weekly visits to an office that may be many miles away create self-evident problems for the mother in arranging child care for other small children, and in finding the time, energy, and money. School or home teaching schedules may need to be rearranged during the three-month period that the gold is being administered.

The gold injection is said to be only moderately painful, creating a stinging sensation similar to that following a penicillin injection. The needling that goes with drawing blood for analysis, however, is greatly feared by some children. The variety in response of different children appears related to the skill of the technician and the sharpness of the needle, to age, to the size of blood vessels, and to the relative ease or difficulty the physician or technician has in getting into the vein. The child's previous experiences with needling and pain also influence his reaction, as does his psychological response to bodily intrusion. By and large, all children hate intrusive measures, and some have symbolic fears that magnify their distress.

Physical therapy. Inflicting pain upon the child is inherent in physical therapy,* especially during the acute phases of disease when moving an inflamed joint may be very painful. If a child has fever, feels sick, or is subject to other painful procedures, his physical therapy sessions may be dreaded in the extreme.

Much rests upon the qualities of the therapist. A therapist who may be competent in working with cerebral palsied or other children may not be

---

* Miss Margarite Dilley, RPT, Children's Hospital at Stanford, provided valuable insights into the therapist's problems in working with arthritic children, and shared with the writer her experience with children and their families.

able to work well with arthritic children, because of the complexities in attitude and technique that the child's pain introduces. If the child is to be as relaxed as possible so that he can cooperate, he must trust the therapist to stop when he tells her he can stand no more. The forceful therapist, accustomed to stretching spastic muscles, or the therapist who cannot resist pushing just a little beyond the point where the child has called a halt, loses the child's confidence. If he resists, the exercises hurt worse, and "bulldozing ahead" becomes a battle, not treatment. Thus a therapist who is wise in the ways of relating to children and who can cope with her own emotions about inflicting pain, in addition to mastering the techniques required, is a vital person in the success of treatment for arthritis. Unfortunately, by no means all therapists combine these unique qualities, and as a result, physical therapy may be intermittent or unsatisfactory or traumatizing to the child.

One mother vividly described the difference in therapists in her community. The sacrifices she and the child had to make to get to the therapy office miles away three times a week, "rain or shine," had not seemed worth it when the therapist had reacted to his difficult task by being late, lackadaisical, and seemingly uninterested in the child. Now a new therapist had arrived in the community. She worked with unusual dedication, skill, and concern. Both mother and child responded by working as hard as possible with exercises at home and never missed an office session, to take advantage of the new therapist's help.

The length of time a child must go to physical therapy varies, some needing nothing more than an annual muscle-and-joint or "range of motion" evaluation. When physical therapy is indicated, however, months or years, not days or weeks, must be planned for. A usual routine of three times a week after school interferes with the extracurricular activities that are prevalent among older children. They may be left out of orchestra, marching band, 4-H club, or similar activities because they have to go to "PT." The mother's work schedule must be adjusted to physical therapy visits. One mother commented that the entire life of the family was dominated by the need for physical therapy sessions, since in her child's case the treatment continued week in and week out all year round, during illness or health, vacations or work.

Daily exercises at home are part of the usual physical therapy program. Some parents can handle the problem of working to the point of pain, and others cannot. Some parents expect too much of little children; an understanding of age-level competence is needed, as well as discipline and compassion. A regular time of day and conscientious adherence to the schedule are important, else the exercises will be pushed aside for lack of a suitable time to perform them. Orderly families, able to develop routines for other things, can fit in an exercise schedule; disorganized families may need a great deal of help in doing so. The writer recalls a child she knew who was dismissed from a clinic as "uncooperative"; investigation revealed that the child's mother was dead and the father had told an older sibling to conduct the exercises. The high school-age sibling resented the burden of care for her younger sister and performed the exercises only fitfully.

The contrast in family capacity is pointed up by one mother who has little difficulty with the exercise routine. She has chosen a time when the baby naps and when the arthritic child can watch television while mother and child do the exercises. In another family, where there are eight children and the rural family migrates with the crops, the arthritic child is retarded and the parents are preoccupied with securing food and shelter; there is no physical therapy beyond that provided once a week when volunteers take the child to a therapist's office.

If a child is in urgent need of concentrated physical therapy that cannot be provided on an outpatient basis, hospitalization for two or three weeks may be recommended. A child who has been through such an experience previously and knows the pain involved may need a good deal of emotional support to accept such a recommendation.

Many exercises can be learned, and performed, by the child if there is some supervision. Mildly involved children or those in remission may receive sufficient exercise from play, and have no exercises prescribed. The child who has a bicycle, or the toddler whose drive to explore keeps him moving, may secure all the exercise needed. The older child whose school gymnasium provides a swimming pool, or who has access to neighborhood pools, may also gain sufficient exercise if length and regularity of the sessions are planned and supervised. A thorough knowledge of the child's regular activity and discussion with the physician are preliminary to reconsideration of physical therapy that has become an excessive burden or is exceptionally difficult to arrange.

Orthopedic measures and surgery. Heavy casts or splints interrupt or prevent sleep. Some parents, unable to bear the child's distress or their own need for sleep, remove the offending appliances. Children who have been crippled to the point of need for stretching under anesthesia, casting, or surgery are those who have been neglected during the early stages of disease, or whose disease is so severe that it does not respond to drug treatment and physical therapy. In either instance, they are prone to need more extensive social planning, discussed later.

Surgery on the knees leaves half-moon scars—"smiles" that create a major cosmetic problem to girls—and leaves enough scar tissue to prevent full extension of the knees, creating ungainliness and awkwardness of use. An evaluation of personality is considered a prerequisite to surgery from a therapeutic standpoint, since intensive physical therapy involving severe, prolonged pain is necessary to make surgery successful. The hoped-for results in relieving pain from arthritis or saving cartilage from destruction should be evaluated against the temporary nature of the remedy and the cost in terms of money and postoperative pain.

Pain

Long-continued pain distinguishes arthritis from other childhood illnesses. The hemophiliac who is bleeding into the joints, the child with sickle cell anemia in a sickling crisis, the leukemic child receiving chemotherapy, and the cardiac recovering from surgery, all have severe pain as a substantial part of their illness experience. Unfortunately, all hospitalized children, in this age of biochemical medicine, are victims of many needlings. However, continuous recurrent pain over a period of many months—or in some cases, years—seems unique to juvenile arthritis.

Experience indicates a wide range of reactions to pain among young children. Many will not cry out, so that only by watching for grimaces can the parent or treatment staff tell when the point of pain has been reached in examination or therapy. Some latency-age children seem to become unusually thoughtful, sober, and mature for their years out of their experience with illness and pain. Also found are fearful, apprehensive children who whimper when a white-coated figure appears, struggle and scream when blood is drawn, or scream during the whole of physical therapy sessions. A few seem overly sensitized to pain. In one extreme instance the mother of a five-year-old girl said the child screamed in terror when she saw table legs sawed off and when a purse fell on the floor. She ascribed the child's overreaction to an experience during infancy when a new intern tried for an hour and a half to get a needle into the child's vein. This kind of overreaction at a later age, stemming from an early experience with pain, has been seen in other cases.

A physiologist who approachs pain in organic terms has written, "Pain is no more a simple perception of a sensory experience than insult is a simple perception of sound."[34] He elaborates that there are "multifarious associations for pain," relays and circuits that have been laid down in the cerebral cortex in the course of past experiences.

Two social psychologists published a study showing that in their subjects, who were stimulated with electric shocks, group identification increased the ability to tolerate pain: "The greater the strength of identification, the greater the increase in pain tolerance."[35] They explained that if one has pride in a group, one wants to defend it against attack, takes pride in its accomplishments, and therefore holds out longer against pain to avoid shaming the group by appearing a weakling. The mechanism of group identification seems to be exploited unconsciously by parents and also by treatment personnel. With boys, "You want to be a man" identifies the boy with his father, the doctor, and other males he looks up to. With boys or girls, the pride in being a member of a brave group that does not cry out, that tolerates therapy, is played upon by the staff.

Younger children are said to feel less pain than older persons. They have not had as much experience, and therefore anxiety, laid down in the cerebral pathways. Pain from within and pain inflicted from without are considered to be indistinguishable to the young child, and any pain is a frightening experience. Before children have the cognitive capacity for rational thinking, and are in the "magical" stage of thinking, pain is perceived as punishment for imagined wrongdoing. Psychiatric observations identify the oedipal period, from around four to six years of age, as one especially vulnerable to adverse long-term effect because of the unconscious sexual fantasies of this period.

A child analyst, Anna Freud, has written about the remarkable differences in children's reactions to pain, and ascribes the difference to the psychic meaning of the pain. She states that the child feels pain as maltreatment, harm, punishment, persecution, threat of annihilation, but if the anxiety is minimal, he bears pain well and forgets it easily; if pain "is augmented by anxiety it represents a major event in the child's life and is remembered a long time afterward."[36] She further comments that "in the first year of life, the threshold of resistance against stimulation is low and painful sensations assume quickly the dignity of traumatic events.... The *actual response* of the infant, *whether it occurs instantaneously,* or after a time lag of varying length, *or remains invisible altogether,* is *no reliable guide* to an assessment of the shock caused by pain [italics added]."[37]

Observation indicates that the onslaught of pain from arthritis is poorly endured during early adolescence: just when the childhood organism is coming under the stress of disorganizing in order to incorporate the changes necessary for adulthood, and therefore is in turmoil, the physical stress of illness adds to the emotional burdens. Feelings about being ill and different heighten the anxiety, which adds to the psychic meaning of pain. The heightened capacity for awareness of stimuli of all kinds may also add to the degree of pain felt.

It is among arthritic teenagers that one can observe the lasting imprint of earlier painful experience, although it is impossible to sort out the effect of this from other regressive features of long-term illness. Saul's dictum that "anger is to pain as heat is to friction"[38] not infrequently appears in sarcasm and hostile behavior. One gifted adolescent vented her spleen in a clever essay, intended to be humorous, in which she neatly pilloried the weaknesses of all the staff who treated her. The physical therapist appeared as the "physical torturist," the occupational therapist as the "other torturist," etc. Direct anger is the most healthy expression of angry feelings and therefore to be welcomed in social treatment, but it complicates the living situations of older children struggling with normal adolescent rebellion and the effects of their illness. Separation from the family sometimes becomes the only apparent solution. If the young person qualifies for Social Security benefits or has access to other funds, some form of group or independent living arrangements may prove desirable. Foster home placement seems less prone to success than group living. In one case known, a private boarding school has proved the solution to a difficult medical-social problem.

At any age, pain is accompanied by depression. Even a severe toothache blots out interest in the outside world. The depressed, listless, withdrawn child who is in an active phase of disease should be considered normal, not abnormal. Literature that imputes psychiatric problems to arthritic children because of their depression seems singularly out of touch with reality, as do staff efforts to "treat" withdrawal in a sick child. The organism must use its energy in coping with distress; this is necessary to healing.

Limitation of Activity

Activity limitation among arthritic children varies at different times in the same child, and varies among children. Frequently the limitation extends only to competitive sports, to activities that use one joint such as piano practice or typing, and to jarring or twisting play. At the other end of the spectrum is the need of some severely crippled children to be lifted, carried, or fed, or to undergo temporary immobilization of a body part.

In those instances where immobilization of one or more parts of the body takes place, either from pain or orthopedic treatment, Anna Freud points out the hardship to the child: "Children defend their freedom of movement to the utmost wherever they are not defeated by the type or intensity of the illness itself. It is well known that children with minor indispositions cannot be kept in bed at home. Young toddlers are known to stand up stubbornly in their beds (in hospitals) for the whole course even of severe illness until exhaustion forces them to adopt the lying position."[39]

She later says, "The punitive character of these restrictive measures has always been known to parents and has been exploited by them. To send a child to bed, confine him in his room, deprive him of certain dishes, have been used as punishment over the ages." She also comments on the work of other analysts, notably Bergmann,[40] who observed children in an orthopedic ward for three years and described the mechanisms children used in order to bear the restraint—increased docility but rages and tantrums when the restraint was partially, not wholly, lifted, or when chance deprivations outside the expected medical procedure were added to it unexpectedly. Bergmann emphasized a relationship between the immobilized limb and the other parts of the body, commenting that restraint might extend to other parts of the body, create tics elsewhere, or that certain ego skills might be speeded up as a compensation.[41]

Prohibition of certain forms of play (in contrast to complete immobilization) has meaning according to the age of the child, how long he has been ill, and the available resources that can be substituted for creative endeavor. Play is the channel for discharge of surplus energy, for learning, for release of anxieties, for socialization, and for testing reality. Small children who can run around at home and who are not tempted into excessive activity are denied few of the functions of play if they have at least moderate supervision. The unsupervised child whose companions are jumping up and down, tumbling, climbing, and wrestling either cannot keep up with them and drops back defeated or, in the excitement of the group, disregards his painful joints and jeopardizes his physical condition. The arrangements that working mothers may make for neighbors or older children to act as sitters or for day care in low-standard facilities are not suitable for the preschool arthritic child. He needs attentive watchfulness, if he is to receive the essential benefits of play without playing too long and tiring himself or indulging in harmful forms of play.

Successful competition with peers is a major psychological need of the elementary school child. Arthritis strikes at a fundamental psychological growth task during latency. The child is building his future self-image, his self-confidence, during this period, according to the way he compares with his peers. If a boy cannot engage in a Little League type of after-school sports or participate in the informal rough-and-tumble at recess or in the neighborhood, he must find other ways to be superior or to secure recognition if he is to build self-confidence for the future. A YMCA membership that permits development of expertise in swimming, the enlistment of a Big Brother, the provision of a bicycle may have important bearing on his personality development. In all instances, the understanding and ingenuity of principal, teacher, physical education teacher, school nurse, and visiting teacher are necessary in maximizing opportunities for him to achieve competence in relation to his schoolmates.

Latency-age girls are often less disadvantaged by play restrictions than boys, if their competitive endeavors tend to be scholastic or artistic. Nevertheless, membership in the Camp Fire Girls, with its emphasis upon symbolism and crafts, access to a library and the assistance of the librarian in helping to develop reading satisfactions, or other measures that are suitable to the child's situation, such as help in the Sunday school, should be considered.

The minority-group child, if he is also poor and ashamed of his clothes and lack of lunch money, is in special need of services that build toward self-respect. These may be focused on clothing or other items not related to the physical handicap but nevertheless important in relieving stress upon a specially painful or vulnerable psychological area.

Despite the particular problems of young children, this group has some advantages over the child whose arthritis occurs at adolescence. Many school-age children seem to have incorporated a quiet way of life. They have gradually learned to play alone, to enjoy television programs, solitary games, record players, dolls, making cookies with mother, etc. They seem to accept their difference, at least outwardly, and do not expect to participate with their peers.

Adolescents who have been healthy hitherto find most bitter the loss of friends when they can no longer do the same things the others do. To be like everyone else of the age-group seems imperative at this age; to be dropped is tragedy. The mother of one boy who had been an outstanding athlete described the manner in which attentions had been showered on him the first two weeks he was sick. Then the calls dwindled and stopped altogether. "Active young people have active friends," she said. If one cannot keep up, one loses out.

The length of time the child is away from school, the frequency of flare-ups, the response the child makes to medication, whether other joints become involved, the extent of permanent crippling, if any, are among the unpredictable factors that determine the permanence and severity of the psychosocial problem. Help in becoming a camera buff or a chemistry expert, learning to play the guitar, or developing other interests and skills that permit a reordered group life helps the young arthritic find a few new companions and new satisfactions. The assistance of church leaders, deans of students, or relatives supplements the supportive efforts of parents, siblings, and social workers in helping the arthritic teenager make the transition to modified activity.

Children who have severe functional limitations from permanent stiffening, contractures, or deformities, or who are immobilized in casts or cylinders or heavy braces over substantial periods of time, have problems of much greater importance. These may be temporary or permanent, and pertain both to reality and to psychological reactions.

Temporary major activity restriction occurs in relation to acute flare-ups of several joints and to orthopedic treatment. The special equipment and staff that long-term hospital care formerly provided to ease the burdens of incapacity during these periods rarely is available, because of the exorbitant cost of institutional medical care. The child is sent home soon after surgery or manipulation of joints, often in a cast, cylinders, or braces. Inept family and home furnishings must make do. Social needs are massive and complex if the family is poor and uneducated. Rapid prior planning is essential in order that recommendations may be received for equipment, measurements made, financial resources secured, equipment borrowed or rented, etc. Plans that predicate supervision and care by siblings usually fail, as do those in which the mother works at night and is at home during the day, without regard to her need for sleep.

Localities that provide adequate public health nursing service or make visiting nurse service available and that have home health aides, homemaker service, or traveling physical therapists may be able to relieve pressing physical needs except those for medical supervision and advice. The public health nurse may secure medical advice through the hospital's liaison nurse or through the medical consultant of the Crippled Children's Services, or the specialist in a clinic may become available by telephone. Hospitals that have medical social workers provide a resource for liaison to the physician. If, however, the community's resources and the child's needs and family situation are too far apart, a move into a nursing home may be an improvement even though none suitable for children exists. Pressure on medical agencies to authorize extensions of hospital care usually should be made through the child's specialist, who has most influence and frequently is most aware of the damage done by inadequate home care.

School Attendance Problems

It is indeed fortunate that only a small proportion of arthritic children have serious crippling. Except during exacerbation of illness, most attend regular classes. A surprising number keep up to grade through the use of home teachers during periods at home and through temporary use of special classes for the handicapped. In attending regular classes, children may suffer considerable fatigue and joint pain, especially in grades where classroom changes require long walks at a pace faster than they feel able to go. They may need to leave one class early to get to the next in time. Schools for normal children vary in the grade levels where class changing begins. Class changing, especially when stair climbing is necessary, limits the crippled child's ability to attend regular school. Unlike the paraplegic with strong arms and hands, the arthritic may have deformed hands and weak wrists and shoulders. Severely impaired children usually attend special schools or classes for the handicapped. The bus drivers to aid in lifting, the trained teachers and auxiliary personnel, and the specially designed physical facilities not only minimize the child's feelings of dependence and difference from others but afford the family a much needed opportunity to keep the schedules of others.

No solid evidence exists to prove the advantages of special classes over regular classes. The auxiliary services offered by some special schools, particularly in physical therapy, may not be available in any other manner, and thus force the child to attend a special school. Some parents strenuously object, thinking that the education offered is inferior, consisting largely of arts and crafts in lieu of solid subjects, or designed primarily for persons with mental retardation in addition to physical handicap: "My daughter couldn't possibly go to a school for the handicapped—she's a gifted child." A child who attends a school for the crippled tends to think of himself as crippled. Many arthritic children will get well, or will have only minor permanent crippling. Arthritis damages the self-image of a child at best, so that negative reinforcement should be avoided. However, constant inability to achieve success in competition with schoolmates, especially during elementary school age, should be weighed against the disadvantages of attending special classes for the handicapped.

Busing creates special problems for the arthritic child, who needs to be able to get up and walk around every 15 minutes or half-hour to keep from getting stiff. Long bus rides may undo the good that has been done by physical therapy at school. The worker should become involved in this uniquely complex problem of modern urban life, to make certain the arthritic child attends the school nearest home or avoids long self-defeating bus rides for the sake of short periods of physical therapy.

The coordination of changing medical recommendations, potential school adaptations, transportation, special equipment, helpers for toileting and class changing, finances, parental wishes, and—most important— the interests of the child requires teamwork by many persons. Recruiting the team and keeping the members together are often the job of the social worker. The child's willingness to study, and to take advantage of opportunities, is requisite to the continued efforts of his many helpers. Emotional support and practical help during recurring crises are essential to the child's ability to keep going.

Personality

Very few personality studies of the arthritic child have been reported. An early analysis of 28 hospitalized children described them as profoundly depressed and typically withdrawn and apathetic. "The children resembled the picture of anaclitic depression described by Rene Spitz"[42] (virtually autistic behavior). The mother-child relationship was described as one of unusual intensity. However, this study did not encompass a follow-up of the children after their disease remitted; the description is one that might be expected of sick children in pain, subjected to painful treatment and separated from their mothers. A later study of outpatients, which by its nature would include those in remission and those with only mild symptoms, reports, "There does not seem to be any uniformity among the arthritic children."[43] This study, which used psychological tests, and therefore would exclude parents and children unable or unwilling to take them, found that the mothers remembered their children as having been more active than usual before the disease began and the investigators rated the children high in perceptual-motor skills. A number of mothers commented on the stoicism of the child in respect to bearing pain.

The lack of any distinguishing personality characteristics other than depression when in pain is concordant with both experience and general knowledge of personality. The varying interacting influences—constitutional, familial, age-related, medical, and experiential—would seem to rule out the possibility that arthritic children would resemble each other. Those who have experienced long severe pain and anxiety during psychologically vulnerable periods must, however, show in some way, directly or indirectly, the anger and insecurity their lives have created.

Understanding of physiological mechanisms involved in stress states is ever more sophisticated. It is conceivable that tools will emerge that permit refinements in study not now in existence, and that future investigators will determine some of the psychological concomitants in the cause and effects of juvenile arthritis. A study of young adults who have had JRA since various stages of development would lend exactitude to knowledge of the permanent impact of pain and activity limitations. Meanwhile, helping persons will seek to understand each child with whom they are involved, and to aid the community and medical teams in alleviating or overcoming the particular problems of that child and the family.

CHAPTER THIRTEEN

Juvenile Diabetes

JUVENILE DIABETES differs from the adult form. A minor difference in physiology and the fact of childhood create major changes. Knowledge of the meaning to an elderly person fails to equip the social worker or other counselor to help the diabetic child.

Childhood diabetes is not statistically significant in the general population. Diabetes is the seventh-leading cause of death, affecting several million persons and occurring in every social class and race. Its incidence increases with age:[1] only about 1 percent of children have diabetes, whereas over 5 percent of the elderly are diabetic.[2] However, diabetes runs in families and strikes the population unevenly. When a child does have diabetes, every aspect of his life and his family's life is affected. The social implications are so pervasive that helping persons should understand and take into account the changes in family life that the disease causes.

Furthermore, diabetes leads to serious medical complications with special reference to kidney disease and blindness; it also shortens life and handicaps personality development, vocational outlook, and marriage potential. And of special interest to social workers and other counselors is the recently documented, long-suspected role of the emotions in precipitating flare-ups and handicapping maintenance of control.

A popularized explanation of diabetes, addressed to diabetics themselves, asks in headline, "Do You Know How Lucky You Are?" This unfortunate hypocrisy reflects only the great gains made in life saving. Luckily, the use of insulin, discovered by F. G. Banting in 1921, is now so well incorporated into medical practice that nearly everyone knows diabetes can be controlled; what the client may not understand is that he must take insulin (or, if he has the adult form, control his diet and weight) regularly the rest of his life. He will live by the clock, ruled by time to eat and time to take insulin, not spontaneously as he has done before. But it is true that the diabetic has cause for gratification that he lives in the latter part of the twentieth century. Not only do means of control exist, but the possibility of finding an eventual cure is seriously considered.[3]

THE MEDICAL REALITIES

Diabetes mellitus is a metabolic disease of unknown origin in which lack of insulin production prevents utilization of carbohydrates for energy; instead, the major food intended for fuel, sugar, bypasses normal routes and spills into the blood and from there into the urine, being lost for strength and energy.[4] The lack of insulin or impairment in the insulin mechanism may be due to several biochemical or structural defects. "An underlying genetic defect is generally assumed."[5] Juvenile diabetes is a form that develops before age 15, and is sometimes called *pre-maturity onset diabetes*. In juvenile diabetes the pancreas manufactures no insulin at all; in *maturity onset diabetes*, some is made but is insufficient for need. Juvenile diabetes is almost always severe and is due to the complete absence of insulin. This contrasts with the adult form, which may be of any degree of severity.

An associated degenerative disorder of the blood vessels exists that accounts for most of the deaths and complications in long-standing diabetes. In the past, a cause-and-effect relationship was presumed, that the diabetes caused the atherosclerotic disorders. However, at present the relationship is under question. Some authorities believe that the conditions coexist but do not believe the diabetes causes the vascular disorder.[6] Ramifications of the current uncertainty create divergences in medical practice, and are discussed later.

Diabetes is inherited through a recessive gene, or more probably through several genes (*multifactorial inheritance*), and develops through a combination of constitutional and environmental factors.[7] Both parents must carry the gene for a child to develop diabetes. An authoritative source indicates that when both parents are diabetics the chances of the child's developing diabetes are 50 percent.[8] Close relatives of diabetics run a risk of developing diabetes three times greater than the normal population. Some persons object to camps for diabetic children and to group meetings for diabetics, on the grounds that acquaintance with other diabetics of the opposite sex encourages romance and ipso facto offspring. In point of fact, the fertility rate is low when two diabetics marry, and current permissiveness regarding contraception lessens the hazard of further "contamination of the human gene pool" through this means.

Onset, Symptoms, and Course

Childhood diabetes usually develops abruptly and severely, after the child has been feeling run-down or fatigued for a period of time. An infection sometimes precipitates the overt diabetes. Although children may develop diabetes at any age, including infancy, the peak incidence is during the prepubertal growth spurt, at an average of 11 years of age. The classical symptoms of diabetes are intense thirst, *polydypsia*; frequent urination, *polyuria*; severe hunger, *polyphagia*; and weight loss. These symptoms, as well as sudden development of enuresis, stimulate the mother to take the child to a doctor. The child often is critically ill. He must be hospitalized to establish the diabetic regimen and educate the child and family in the changes they must make in his diet and way of life. Length of hospitalization varies from one to three weeks, depending on local practice, the severity of the illness, and how rapidly a regime and the accompanying education can be established.[9]

During the acute onset, the child may have severe abdominal pain, and may go into coma, or *ketoacidosis*. (The absence of body fuel from carbohydrates, or sugar, that has been spilled directly into the blood requires the body to utilize fat for fuel, releasing *ketone bodies* or fat products. Brain symptoms result—in this case, coma.) The child has accompanying *hyperglycemia*, or sugar spilling into the blood. He must have close medical and nursing care during this stage. Soon after proper treatment has been established, the child's health responds, so well for a few months that parents and child may find it difficult to accept that he has a serious condition. He needs less insulin during the early recovery period.[10] But his insulin need will increase again, often breeding discouragement in parents and child.

The differences in childhood diabetes from adult-type diabetes include not only the body's complete lack of insulin but absence of obesity as a general problem. The opposite is true: children with diabetes usually are undernourished. Their nutritional requirements are greater and are constantly changing because they are in a period of relatively sudden spurts of growth. The suddenness and severity of the onset, with accompanying *ketosis*, or *ketoacidosis*, are additional differentiating characteristics of juvenile diabetes. When diabetes begins at puberty, the emotional concomitants are severe, as would be expected, and they greatly aggravate the management of the disease.

Diabetics' blood vessels age prematurely. This is particularly true of the small vessels. *Microangiopathy* is the medical term used. Juvenile diabetics are prone to cataracts also, especially those who have not adhered to the required regime and have been out of control for substantial periods of time. This serious consequence is the one documented argument for control of the blood sugar.[11]

Although the lay literature emphasizes the normal life attainable if a reasonable regime is followed, the adverse effects on adult health and longevity are universally acknowledged in the professional literature. Death and disability occur primarily as a result of blood-vessel problems.

A study of patients at the famed Joslin Clinic in Boston, of over 4,000 juvenile diabetics, showed that fewer than five hundred had survived between 30 and 46 years.[12] Another study reports that of 162 persons whose diabetes began before age 16, one-fourth were dead 15 years later. One-fifth of the living were partially or totally disabled, but the other four-fifths were "entirely functional."[13] Age at death is related to age of onset. Most juvenile diabetics live approximately 30 years after onset.[14] The gloomy outlook for length of life, however restrictive a regimen, has stirred concern to enhance quality of life. This spurs emphasis on normal living, in contrast to rigid adherence to regimen.

Treatment Goals

Understanding what the child and family are confronted with, and the effects on family life, requires some comprehension of the special treatment of emergency conditions and of the lifelong, everyday treatment: insulin injection, nutrition, control of energy expenditure, care during impending coma, care during insulin reaction (the functional opposite of coma), and skin care.

The broad-gauge goals of treatment are to help the diabetic child live as healthily, happily, and long as possible; that is, within the restrictions imposed by lack of bodily insulin, to grow normally, feel comfortable, and achieve adequate personality development and relationships, while avoiding unnecessarily early disability or death.

The specific goal is to achieve a relative equilibrium among food, energy expenditure, and insulin. Blood sugar in the normal person rises and falls in relation to food intake. Insulin is secreted "on demand" by the pancreas to the extent necessary to convert the sugar consumed into energy, or to store the excess in the liver and body fat.[15] However, the person who has no natural insulin must receive it by injection in some set amount at a set time. Until the insulin dosage can be changed, the food consumed and the energy expended must be adjusted to the amount of insulin that has been injected. If the child eats less than anticipated, the physician can decrease the prescription for insulin, if he is informed of the change. When special stress occurs, as happens during an infection or surgery or period of emotional strain, extra insulin may be needed. The optimal relationship between insulin, food, and energy must be tailored individually by the physician for the patient, and altered as necessary according to the experiences of the particular patient.

Social workers justifiably may be confused by the difference in treatment approach of various physicians of equal stature. So much has been learned in recent years that old dogmas regarding treatment are challenged:[16]

Current practice in this country ranges from one extreme to the other. Some physicians advocate complete normalization of carbohydrate metabolism with normal blood sugar values and the total absence of *glycosuria* (sugar showing in the urine), precise dietary prescriptions, frequent evaluation of urinary and blood glucose levels, and what one must consider relatively rigid control of daily activity. At the other extreme is disregard of carbohydrate metabolism and dietary intake, with provision of enough insulin to prevent ketosis and acidosis (release of fat-produced substances in the blood stream) and to provide adequate growth.

The reason why treatment approaches differ is because ideas are changing about the relationship of vascular complications to the degree of diabetic control. The older, orthodox treatment method, that of attempting rigid control through rigid means, presumes that heart disease, kidney breakdown, other circulation disorders, and blindness—or, in other words, the vascular complications of diabetes—can be prevented or delayed by maintaining precise balance between insulin, food, and energy expenditures. In recent years, studies have shown no relationship, except for the advent of cataracts, to *precision* of control. Thus physicians oriented to recent studies, and indoctrinated with appreciation of emotional problems of diabetic children and their families, allow more leeway in the diet to permit more nearly normal living, and are less concerned about some spilling of sugar into the urine than are physicians trained in the orthodox older way.[17]

The newer, more relaxed approach to treatment is of course relative. Less concern about degree of control does not mean the child is permitted to go into near-coma, or its opposite, *insulin reaction* (the common term for *hypoglycemia*, or seriously low blood sugar). The goals of treatment outlined at the American Academy of Pediatrics Conference on diabetes in July 1971 were (1) normal growth, (2) absence of *ketoacidosis* (toxic effects of fat products accompanying spillage of sugar), (3) absence of *hypoglycemic* episodes (the opposite of item 2), (4) absence of *polyuria* (excessive urination), and (5) absence of *ketonuria* (fat products being spilled into the urine). These were described as the modern criteria of control of diabetes in children.[18]

Insulin Injections

Insulin injections are essential for every child with diabetes. Children cannot be treated with oral substitutes. This is due to the total absence of bodily insulin (the oral compounds merely magnify the effects of insulin already present; they do not serve as insulin itself). It will be recalled that the essential difference in juvenile and maturity onset diabetes is that juvenile diabetics manufacture no insulin at all, after the diabetes is truly established.[19]

Insulin usually comes in two strengths, called U40 and U80; the latter is twice as powerful as the former. U40 carries a red label and U80 a green. Syringes, which ordinarily hold 1 cc of insulin, are usually made for either U40 or U80 with matching red or green markings; if a child welfare worker, foster mother, or other person is purchasing the insulin and syringes, it is essential to know what strength has been ordered and to make sure the appropriate strength is secured. Persons who take over about 30 units per day will usually use U80 to avoid injecting themselves twice, unless injections at different times of the day have been ordered; the markings on the syringes for more concentrated insulin are closer together and harder to see, which should be kept in mind if the child who is giving his own insulin has blurred vision or is otherwise handicapped.

Insulin of different kinds acts at various rates. Its administration is geared to match the rise and fall of blood-sugar levels from food as well as possible. "Regular" or crystalline insulin is fast-acting but lasts only a few hours. It is used to cover immediate need for insulin. Most children receive one shot of intermediate-acting insulin (named NPH or Lente) per day once their regimes have been established. The injection ordinarily is given before breakfast. Sometimes the intermediate-acting insulin is mixed with regular insulin for a quick boost over breakfast. Children who are newly diagnosed and in the difficult periods of adjustment, or who remain difficult to treat or are undergoing special stress, receive as many as four injections a day of regular insulin. Some children require two injections of intermediate-acting insulin, the second shot just before the evening meal.[20]

Other things a helping person may need to know about insulin are that regular insulin is clear, and intermediate and long-lasting insulin are cloudy. It need not be refrigerated, though it is best kept in the refrigerator; excessive heat and excessive cold cause it to spoil. Whether pork or beef insulin is used is of no importance.[21]

Rotation of places injected is essential to avoid tissue breakdown, with development of unsightly lumps, a cosmetic problem of particular concern to girls. Thighs, buttocks, lower abdomen, and arms are the sites used. Young children can be taught to inject themselves, taking responsibility first for injections in the spots that are easy to reach, while parents alternate with the child for the hard-to-reach spots. Difference of opinion exists regarding the age at which children should be taught to accept responsibility for their own injections. The traditional view has been "the earlier the better." Some professionals question why children, who normally rely on their parents for other types of medication and care, should be prematurely burdened with self-responsibility for injections. Agreement does exist that the child should learn to inject himself before adolescence. Otherwise, the normal adolescent struggle for independence and resentment of parental domination or touching or intrusion become entwined with the insulin administration, greatly complicating management.

Insulin injections are the most hated part of the diabetic regime. They hurt.

Testing Urine

If injections are the most hated, because painful, testing is the most embarrassing to the child, and particularly to the adolescent. However, it is the foundation stone for medical supervision; without knowledge of the extent of sugar spillage, the physician cannot tell whether his dosage of insulin is matching the child's food intake and energy output. Family supervision of daily fluctuations is essential to adequate professional supervision. The family member must know whether balance is satisfactory, take responsibility for minor adjustments, and notify the doctor if alarming signs occur.

The number of urine tests needed each day decreases after the child's condition stabilizes and while he is in periods of good health. At first, or during exacerbations, they may be required four or more times a day. Ordinarily, the second voided urine in the morning (before breakfast) and one at four in the afternoon or before the evening meal are necessary.[22] This means the child must get up, or be roused, a half-hour early to void, and then void again and test, during the before-breakfast, before-school flurry. Although the test is in itself simple, involving two test tubes, a clear vial or glass, and a product such as a Clinitest tablet and two clean eye-droppers, one for urine and one for water, it requires privacy to minimize embarrassment. Occasionally the more convenient "testape" can be used, but it is not as reliable as the use of tablets.

The time of testing is determined by its purpose, that is, to measure the amount of sugar spillage before the blood-sugar level is stimulated by eating, in order that accuracy can be estimated. *Urine tests should not be negative all day.* If they are, the blood-sugar level may be dangerously low, forewarning a dangerous insulin reaction. Ideally, tests should show "one-plus" or "two-plus" sugar; if, however, at the top of the scale they consistently show four-plus sugar spillage, they indicate that the amount of insulin and energy output (exercise has the same effect as added insulin) is too low for the food intake. An additional phase of testing must be added if the reactions are four-plus. Urine acetone, or ketones (fat breakdown products), may be present. A drop of urine from the eye dropper is placed on an Acetest tablet and the results read by chart. A less satisfactory product (similar to the Clinistix called Ketostix) can be substituted when the child is away from home. The *presence of acetone is the danger signal* signifying the need for more insulin to avoid coma.[23]

Charting of daily test results is the final aspect of urine testing. Children can write down the results themselves if normally intelligent, responsible, and willing to be truthful. The chart shows the child, parent, and physician how well the diabetes is in control and when it went out of control, with clues to why. A chart that consistently shows "one-plus" sugar despite known dietary departures obviously has not been kept truthfully; temptation exists to make the chart look good.

Nutrition

Most helpful in the necessary treatment of juvenile diabetes is the satisfying amount of food allowed. In contrast to adult diabetics, who by and large are deprived and depressed, with their oral needs unfulfilled, the juvenile diabetic, frequently underweight or undersized, is encouraged to eat. He is deprived of candy bars and other carbohydrates that burn immediately, but can have slowly digesting sweets such as ice cream. Since he is allowed enough food to satisfy his hunger, he is much less apt to sneak sweets and subsequently to feel guilty. Many professionals emphasize the dangers of cholesterol because of the vascular damage that awaits the diabetic.

The flexibility suggested in the diets of juvenile diabetics can be misleading. A "free" diet is by no means free. The "exchange system" ordinarily used for adult diabetics is used for children. Dieticians say it should and can be based on the family's cultural food patterns, and as nearly like that of the rest of the family as possible. The exchange system is a division of all foods into six lists, in which the amount of calories and the grams of carbohydrates, protein, and fat have been computed and are the same as other foods on the list. For example, on the bread exchange list, one slice of bread equals three-fourths cup of dry cereal. Manuals for diabetics listing the grams of carbohydrates, fat, and protein in common foods are readily available.[24] Expanded lists of gourmet and foreign foods also may be obtained.

The most obvious problem is that common foods include "exchanges" of more than one kind. Though one slice of bread is merely one bread exchange, as is one small potato, and one small apple is one fruit exchange, most items are made up of more than one major component. Thus one finds that three ounces of ice cream is one bread exchange and two fat exchanges. Almost every other common item is a similar compound of two or more kinds of exchanges. Some exchanges have no readily apparent rationale, and must be memorized by rote, such as that one cola drink equals two fruit exchanges. Although it is true, as some Diabetes Association literature states, that generally speaking, there is no food a diabetic cannot include in his diet *provided that he knows and takes into account its food value,* a diabetic has written, only half in jest, that "a diabetic ... even just to be a bit free wheeling in the selection of his meals, has to be a walking table of food logarithms."[25] It's not easy. She also comments, "Here's the hitch: in order to get the proper balance of calories, carbohydrates, proteins and fats, we had to work out as many complex calculations as it would take to figure a moon shot."

Weighing food is recommended by physicians who believe in the rigid method of treatment. Weighing each portion is often recommended to mothers of new diabetics and used at camp where children are taught nutrition, as a means of teaching how to estimate portion size. One meat exchange is, for example, one ounce of meat, and few lay persons can estimate the size of one ounce of meat accurately until they have had special instruction or practice.

Constancy is the most restrictive aspect of the juvenile diabetic's diet. He need not eat the same thing every day at exactly the same time, but he must eat the same food values, and always at the same time. His insulin dosage has been worked out to take into account blood-sugar levels at various times of day; thus the blood sugar must be kept at these levels or he will have too much or too little insulin.[26] Even though the rest of the family may sleep late on Sundays, the diabetic child may not do so, for he must eat his breakfast at the same time as he always does. In many instances his mother also must get up, to give his insulin shot and prepare his breakfast. The other members of the family may have a big meal late Sunday afternoon and no supper, but the diabetic child must eat lunch and dinner at the same time as he does the rest of the week.

Insulin Reaction and Coma

Though the stereotype of a diabetic's greatest hazard is coma, the opposite may be the danger. The insulin-dependent, juvenile diabetic's *greatest hazard is insulin reaction* or hypoglycemia—not enough food, or burning food too rapidly by exercise, to balance the amount of insulin earlier injected. *Insulin reaction* is especially dangerous because it comes suddenly, in contrast to coma, which provides a longer warning period; dangerous because the convulsions and unconsciousness created can *cause permanent mental retardation* through brain damage if untreated. Even a short period of brain impairment can be dangerous by causing accidents.[27]

Insulin reaction carries warning signals, varying from one person to another, but frequently consisting of trembling, sweating, shakiness, dizziness, sleepiness, vomiting, or emotional outbursts. Older children, who can identify their own particular warning signals, can avert full-blown reactions by quickly drinking a sweetened soft drink or orange juice, or eating a sugar cube, a small piece of chocolate, a few lifesavers, a small box of raisins—some quickly burning sugar.[28]

Once the reaction becomes severe, the child frequently becomes stubborn and perverse, refusing to cooperate in consuming the quick sugar that will avert convulsions. For this reason, others need to be informed of his problem and, if they cannot get him to eat, to secure help quickly. It is easier to make him swallow orange juice or a soft drink than to get him to chew sugar or chocolate, but if he is unconscious one must not pour liquids down his throat for fear of strangling him. The parent, foster mother, or school nurse may give an intramuscular shot of *glucagon*, which comes in two bottles, the contents of which are mixed and administered with the insulin syringe. If the child does not become normal within a few minutes and is not able to eat a meal, he must be rushed to the hospital for emergency treatment. Dr. Christiansen states, "Normally, I tell parents that, if they think the reaction is severe enough to require glucagon, they should start to the hospital without giving the glucagon. It is no shame to arrive at the hospital with the child alert."[29]

Prevention of insulin reaction is vital. The first essential is eating meals *on schedule*, and eating the full amount of the meal. Another is eating a snack before unusual exercise, including play, athletics, or yard work. Snacks before bedtime and after school are a usual feature of the diabetic regime, the former because insulin reaction not infrequently occurs in the night because of length of time since the evening meal. Identifying the time that insulin reactions repeatedly occur in a particular child, and correcting the dietary regime and insulin accordingly, is another means of preventing emergencies. Reactions in the night are a special hazard, for though the child frequently wakes others by screaming or thrashing about, others do not always hear him.[30] A completely negative urine test first thing in the morning is less desirable than one showing that the child has been spilling a little sugar or, in other words, had enough in his body to spare.

Child welfare workers who take children on outings, helping persons who transport children to distant clinics, foster parents whose charges attend school by bus, and social workers responsible for family budgets and counseling need to keep in mind (1) that a diabetic child's meals cannot be delayed, and (2) that traffic jams, snowstorms, or other unforeseen causes of delay in meals are a part of life. Therefore, sweets or soft drinks must be carried by or on behalf of the diabetic. The schoolteacher, school bus driver, and counselor should also keep sugar cubes or small chocolate bars in the office or bus when working with a diabetic child. Orange juice or Cokes should be kept in the refrigerator at home or, if other family members drink them when accessible, should be hidden for emergency use.

One physician says, "If a diabetic feels poorly in any way or behaves strangely, he should be treated for insulin reaction immediately—even if the symptoms are doubtful or do not follow a regular pattern. Relatives, friends, and others who are close to the diabetic should be ready to act the instant he shows any deviation from normal behavior."[31]

Ketoacidosis, coma, or the consequence of too much sugar for the amount of insulin, is the Scylla to insulin reaction's Charybdis—the opposite hazard the diabetic must avoid. In the absence of enough insulin to utilize the carbohydrate, the body utilizes its fat, releasing toxic ketone bodies. The forerunner of coma is copious urination, thirst, hunger, weakness and drowsiness, vomiting, and finally unconsciousness.[32]

The child old enough to recognize symptoms usually knows when he is "out of control," for he does not feel well, and is usually aware his feelings are the result of eating forbidden candy or overindulging in pizzas or potato chips or syrup on pancakes. He can ask for or give himself extra insulin. However, the irritable, drowsy, flushed child may be too apathetic to do so, or rebel against calling attention to his condition.

A common cause of ketoacidosis is infection or decrease in physical activity. When children sleep longer, read more or play less, catch cold, or when girls menstruate, they need more insulin. Unless the dosage is adjusted upward, the urine tests will show four-plus sugar and possibly ketone bodies, testifying to the need for action in increasing the insulin or decreasing carbohydrate intake.

Coma is more of a problem in girls than boys, because of menstruation and because they tend to be less athletic and spend more time in quiet pursuits. Coma is more rapid in onset in children than in adults. One pediatric diabetician said that about 10 percent of his clinic patients are frequently in trouble with ketoacidosis, and that he can see no difference in their organic problems from the 90 percent who are well controlled. He attributes their repeated difficulties to social and emotional causes.[33] Long-suspected sugar spillage due to psychological stress now has been documented by studies demonstrating rise in blood-glucose levels after artificially induced stress experiences.[34]

Coma is fatal if untreated in time. Until recent years brought greater alertness and better treatment, coma was a major cause of death in diabetics. A comatose child must be taken to a hospital emergency room immediately. As in its opposite hazard, insulin reaction, prevention is vital. Prevention is achieved by adequate regimen and by ready accessibility to and use of a physician's advice when a cold, toothache, or unusual physical stress occurs.

"Brittle" or "labile" diabetes seems to exist in some children—that is, they swing from insufficient insulin to too much insulin at the slightest provocation, and are extremely difficult to keep under medical control. What may seem to be a peculiarly difficult physiological problem, however, may be improper administration of insulin, with the child suffering accordingly.[35] Hospitalization, with consultation from a pediatrician who specializes in diabetes, is indicated when a child has been labeled "brittle."

Long-Term Complications

Diabetes for ten or more years is accompanied by disease of the small blood vessels of the eyes and kidneys, muscles, nerves, and skin. *Retinopathy*, or disease of the retina of the eyes, appears in some cases and may finally progress to blindness. Retinitis becomes a serious problem in reducing vision among those juvenile diabetics who have survived over 20 years since the onset of the disease.[36] However, one authority states that only 5 percent of juvenile diabetics become totally blind, even after many years of the disease.

More serious for a large number of juvenile diabetics is diabetic *nephropathy*, a kidney condition that becomes manifest a few years after problems in the retina have begun. A Joslin Clinic study shows that in half of the patients whose diabetes began before age 15, the chief cause of death was chronic renal (kidney) disease.[37] When and if kidney complications reach a defined degree of kind and severity, they are referred to as *Kimmelsteil-Wilson* or *K-W* syndrome.[38] A poor prognosis for life is associated. Chronic, severe kidney disease is less hopeless since the advent of dialysis and transplants, but few families are able to secure the advantages of these advanced and expensive forms of treatment, especially when the child has underlying systemic disease and other complications.

Disease of the peripheral blood vessels of the extremities (primarily the legs), or *diabetic neuropathy*, is also associated with long-term diabetes. Numbness and uncomfortable sensations and, not infrequently, severe pain develop. Gangrene is a specter. The person whose impaired circulation keeps him from feeling pressure, pain, or heat readily must make special effort to prevent common accidents from blisters, burns, and cuts. Well-fitting shoes, daily foot washing, clean stockings or socks without holes, clean shorts, etc. are essential. Lack of a good supply of blood to an injured part impedes healing. Pressure sores and gangrene, requiring amputation, arise from neglect of precautions.

The three complications of retinopathy, nephropathy, and neuropathy cast an obvious pall over the vocational future of the diabetic child.

PSYCHOSOCIAL IMPLICATIONS

The physician cannot live with the family, recommending insulin changes for every change in the child's life; thus the major responsibility for daily supervision rests on the mother or caretaker. Ramifications of diabetes are so pervasive and complex that the disease has been called a "way of life." In some families, and during the periods of good adjustment, the child's diabetic management seems easily incorporated and causes few outward signs of disturbance. At the other extreme are families that break up or where constant turmoil is the rule. Factors that affect the meaning of diabetes to the particular child and his family are the interaction and characteristics of medical management, the marital situation of the parents, socioeconomic class, and the age and other personal attributes of the child and his parents.

The management of juvenile diabetes is a team function. At home it is a "two-man job." The two may be a mother and a competent, stable child, or a mother and father or older sibling, or mother and extended family members, or some other duo. The need for two persons is especially acute during the first year. This is the time the family is learning the truly complicated diet, how to distinguish the danger signals of insulin reaction and coma from each other and from behavior problems, and how to incorporate into the family routines the daily urine testing and insulin administration. The child who is prone to insulin reactions continues to need a protective friend, sibling, neighbor, teacher, or constellation of persons. During the periods of ill health, stressful adjustments, or complications of the disease, all diabetic children need someone close by who recognizes danger signals and knows how to help.

The goal of a "normal life" under these circumstances is elusive. Unusual good fortune must exist or exceptionally skillful management, or both.

Clues useful in knowing when help is needed by the family, and where, may emerge from examination of recurring psychosocial issues. These are finances and material needs, medical care, parental adjustment, personal adjustment, adjustment away from home, sex and marriage, and availability of special resources for the child and his family.

Financial Problems

The initial hospitalization in diabetes lasts from one to three weeks; depending on the existence of insurance or Medicaid eligibility, and the hospital's policy of billing indigent families, the initial financial burden may be small, oppressive, or catastrophic. At current rates, the cost of board and care, laboratory work, and medical care will range from $1,000 to $3,000 in California, and many county hospitals will bill and indebt indigent families or impose an indefinite "liability" upon them.

Additional emergency-room visits or continued brief hospital periods for treatment of coma or insulin reaction may be expected during the first year and during infections, tooth extractions, fractures, and the onset of menstruation in girls. Costs are unpredictable but loom as a financial strain, depriving all but the well insured or wealthy of security and planned vacations, clothes, appliances, etc.

The diabetic child's diet need not be more expensive than that for other nutritiously fed children. Diabetic desserts, fruit, and candy do help and do cost more than ordinary foods, but the total cost is not substantial. The major financial burden of the diet arises from inability to take advantage of sales and to rely on cost-cutting casseroles, hunger-satisfying high-carbohydrate meals of macaroni, grits, peanut butter sandwiches, or tortillas, as the case may be. Families receiving Aid to Families with Dependent Children allowances who must use food budgets for rent, and those who are supplied with surplus commodities in lieu of cash, find that the "normal, nutritious" diet recommended for a growing child is a "special diet," and a very expensive one indeed. Therefore the worker will need to assist such families to secure recommendations for a "special diet" from a physician who understands the difference between "normal" in his terms and in welfare department terms. In addition, help may be provided by protection of the food budget for food, through assistance with other allowable items from outside agencies or resources. Where flat grants are used by the welfare department and no special needs allowed, "adoption" of the diabetic child may be secured by a club that can be guided to help in a way that safeguards the child's self-esteem.

Families on marginal incomes are known to go without food frequently toward the end of the grant period.[39] The worker should ascertain the usual family practice of existence until the next grant arrives, and make certain that the diabetic child has sufficient food to balance his insulin during this period.

Special food for the diabetic child is practical only if he eats separately. If his schedule varies from older or younger children, or if he is an only child or special circumstances exist, some separation can be made to seem natural; breakfasts and lunches are eaten separately in many families. However, excluding the child from the evening meal if all the others eat together defeats the larger purpose. Special money for his special diet may be used to fortify his breakfast, lunch, and snacks.

Costs of insulin, syringes, and urine-testing equipment are higher if disposable syringes are used. These avoid the necessity for sterilization equipment and routine, and therefore meet the need in households where an unsupervised child must give his own injections or where household equipment and management are so scanty that one cannot count on clean utensils for sterilization. If regular syringes are used, and a clean pan is available and used only for sterilizing the needle, the cost of test tubes, tablets, insulin, and swabs varies from about $10 to $15 a month in California at the time of this writing. Thus, if a special grant is secured for extra food and supplies for a diabetic child, the request may be approximately $20 to $25 a month. The amount obviously varies over time and in different localities and according to inflation.

Extra glasses may be needed by the diabetic child whose vision is being affected. However, blurring vision may indicate that the diabetes is out of control, and may disappear when better management of the disease has been obtained. New glasses should not be purchased until it is determined whether the visual difficulty is transient. The most important action is securing medical evaluation of the diabetes and helping with necessary adjustments in regimen.

A "Medic Alert" bracelet or locket is worn by many diabetic children. The locket, worn under the clothing, is less conspicuous and is preferred by boys. The child needs some form of identification worn at all times. The mother feels less anxious about possible accidents to the child when he is away from home, and security is greatly increased. A free identification card and tiny lapel pin supplied by a pharmaceutical company may be secured from the local Diabetes Association. The card is not as satisfactory as a locket because it may not be on the person when needed. The drug age has heightened the need for identification for children whose skin bears marks of needle puncture. "I act like I'm stoned" one adolescent said of his beginning insulin reactions. If an uninformed police officer were to pick up such a child, catastrophe could occur. Medic Alert bracelets and lockets, secured from the Medical Alert Foundation at Turlock, California, cost approximately $10.

A final item of cost may be for literature on management and diet. Many pamphlets are free, and available from the local diabetes or heart association. Books on diabetic management are also available from the public library. However, many families will want and profit from a manual they can keep and use as a reference. The manual should be one recommended by the physician.

Medical Care

The diabetic child's family needs one physician on whom to lean for advice. In other words, continuity of care is essential, especially during the first year and during periods of special difficulty. The family needs someone they can call during the night and on weekends, not merely during clinic hours. However, they also need a pediatrician who understands and wants to treat diabetic children—not all physicians feel able to carry this kind of responsibility.

A county hospital clinic, with turnover in residents and interns, may be especially unsatisfactory in this regard, as may be a teaching hospital. However, some hospitals have special diabetes clinics where a specialist in charge remains over a continuous period, and may participate actively and make special arrangements for availability through the emergency room outside of clinic hours. In some county hospitals a medical social worker or liaison nurse participates actively in the diabetes clinic, is available for questions, and can arrange medical care in emergencies.

The ideal is a well-informed local pediatrician available to the family at all times, who utilizes consultation from specialists when indicated. This can be arranged for children in foster care by many agencies, for insured families known to family counseling agencies, and for those receiving public assistance or benefits in which Medicaid pays for private care.

Continuity of care is especially needed for the diabetic child because of the variation in medical approach previously described. Mother and child are badly confused when one physician prescribes close adherence to regime and another loose control. The confusion is often used by the child against the mother: "Dr. Smith said I could eat candy bars." The mother, anxious over diet computation and other problems, with memories of critical episodes of coma or insulin reaction, usually tries to enforce the scheme proposed by the more rigid physician.

The Child's Adjustment

The child's feelings about having diabetes greatly influence the degree of responsibility he assumes for staying on the diet, testing urine, and injecting himself with insulin. They affect the kind of person he grows to be, and often adversely affect his sense of identity and self-esteem. His feelings depend upon his age, his previously established security, his family's reactions to the disease, and the members' basic patterns and relationships. They are affected by the physician's philosophy and treatment, and the severity of his medical condition.

Unfortunately, attitude is always influenced by initial experience, and the onset period is the time when parents' anxiety is usually highest, carbohydrate restriction is most severe, weighing of food recommended so portion size can be mastered, and the frightening experiences of insulin reaction and coma or near-coma often encountered.

The small child's main problems not infrequently are his hatred of the shots and his view of his mother as the punishing person who administers them. She may also be the depriving person who does not let him have the kind of food he wants. Since image of "mother" is inextricably bound up with food-giving, a faulty child-parent relationship is likely to develop. The mother of a toddler is faced with obtaining a urine sample from a wriggling child, and providing a diet he does not understand, in addition to catching and holding a screaming child while she forces herself to shoot a needle into him. Because he cannot understand and tell her of feelings that warn of insulin reaction, her scrutiny of his behavior must be more constant.

The panic, continual anxiety, and sense of harassment of such a mother are inevitable unless she has a strong ally in her husband, who shares in the job of caring for the child, and who understands and sustains her. In the absence of a husband, some other continuing ally is essential. The feelings of the child about himself and his mother and his diabetes can hardly be "normal." A realistic goal is to secure an optimal situation until the child becomes old enough to conceptualize and to learn how to give his own injections, at least part of the time, to report physical responses, and to develop some capacity for restraint. Respite for the mother, with efforts to decrease her other concurrent pressures, may be the social worker's major contribution.

The age of the child is usually a potent factor in personal adjustment. The latency-age child who cheerfully and matter of factly sits down to eat his "snack" at ten and three o'clock, is in marked contrast to the restless, moody teenager who wants no one to know he is a diabetic and broods by himself. Diabetic children are in fact sometimes characterized as being "loners" who have difficulty socializing. Teenagers report that although they are not openly teased, their peers show curiosity. "Are you eating your sugar now?" they ask if he eats a snack in front of them.

Low self-esteem seems a common problem among diabetic teenagers. The feeling of being different is an inevitable consequence of a condition that does indeed make life different from that of other children. The suffering of being different from peers during adolescence is well known. One young girl recalled with an expression of distaste that she associated diabetes with "being a grandmother." A report of the fantasies of five diabetic teenagers revealed that they all felt seriously damaged by their disease. Despite adequate intellectual understanding of diabetes, they had distorted images of themselves and their bodies.[40]

Eating with others is an integral part of normal social life. Food obviously has values that transcend nutrition. Someone has said that a birthday party is a serious event in the life of a diabetic child. In reality, an event of this nature that can be planned ahead is less difficult to manage than the spontaneous, irregular eating that usual adolescent social life entails. Thoughtful mothers can arrange birthday celebrations that involve going out for pizza for dinner, instead of ice cream and cake in the middle of the afternoon, or a movie timed to precede the usual evening or afternoon snack. Furthermore, occasional breaks from routine can be tolerated, providing the break is truly occasional (not frequent). The serious barrier to normal social life is the habit of stopping for a milkshake, french fries, or sundae when the peer group is bored or a leader feels hungry. If the food intake occurs every day at the same time, even if it is a doughnut every morning on the way to school, it can be incorporated into the insulin-food-exercise regimen, and subtracted from a meal. Nevertheless, it is the exceptionally mature and intelligent child, or the indifferent one, who does not find the dietary restrictions of diabetes a serious handicap to normal peer relationships.

An agony of embarrassment accompanies any mention of urine testing. One mother says that all she has to do to get her boy in to dinner on schedule is to call, "It's time for your ——," and even the possibility that she might use the word "test" is enough to bring him running. Urine tests in the middle of the day are impractical during the school year unless the child goes home for lunch. The 24-hour collection of urine for special tests conducted several times a year may require the child to stay home from school. However, the school nurse's cooperation can be enlisted if the issue presents a serious problem—in schools that have a nurse.

The rebellious child or adolescent can use a variety of ways to show his anger. Rebellion takes the form of "sneaking" sweets or of refusing to eat the meals the mother has laboriously calculated and prepared, an especially dangerous way of acting out. Another common way is to insist on testing and charting urine without supervision and altering the findings, or not testing at all and charting regularly "one-pluses" (implying that his diabetes is in perfect control and that he never breaks over his diet).

Denial is a common form of defense against the pain of feeling defective and different. Teenage boys frequently use it if their conditions have stabilized sufficiently that they can avoid serious immediate effect even though staying in poor control. Exercise helps them avoid coma by utilizing some of their excess carbohydrates, and a continuously high carbohydrate level prevents insulin reaction. Even though diet colas are in the vending machine, they deliberately choose high-sugar regular colas, saying the diet cola "tastes funny"; they refuse to carry sugar or candy bars even when exercising strenuously, as if to demonstrate that the danger they have been warned against is untrue, or that they are "supermen."

Girls seem less able to utilize the denial mechanism effectively, because they have vaginal itching due to sugar in the urine, which is very uncomfortable, and they are more apt to be ill because of the physiological swings of the menstrual cycle.[41] Hostility against the mother may be heightened as the girl feels the scales loaded against her in unconscious rivalry with the mother. The timid, shy girl who stays home because she feels defective and different is particularly vulnerable to an intense relationship with the mother.

As in any chronic illness, the diabetic child, especially a bright one, may use illness to get what he wants, or to get the upper hand over the mother. He may do so directly, feigning sleepiness or reporting feelings of shakiness in order to get a sweet, or indirectly by persisting in dangerous behavior. Often parent-child or sibling-child animosities preexist, but may not be overt or intense. The diabetic condition with its manifold requirements reinforces the underlying difficulties. Quarreling or stubbornness over the diabetic regime may merely mask deeper problems. However, the worker needs to be aware that a child's irritability or apathy may in fact be due to hypoglycemia, and to make certain that he is receiving continuing medical evaluation.

The physician and his philosophy become part of the child-family struggle. Some pediatricians who are not convinced that rigid control reduces later complications, and having learned not to expect honest reporting of urine tests from most adolescents, advocate "loose control" with a view to providing less for the child to fight over or resent. However, the mother loses her ally in enforcing dietary restrictions and may even find an adversary. She must possess greater sophistication and intelligence in dietary planning than is needed in adhering to a simple, repetitious diet, and must be mature enough to withstand a greater degree of anxiety. All involved need awareness that the physician takes for granted certain limitations and boundaries. However, the child may focus, not on the limitations, but rather on the freedom and normality that have been emphasized.

Family Adjustment

In a large study in which social psychologists administered four standardized psychological tests, the data supported the hypothesis of the investigators that diabetes in a child adversely affects the parents' marriage.[42] A nurse-sociologist whose doctoral dissertation was written from a study of nine diabetic children and their families, all of whom were middle or working class and attended an outstanding clinic, said that four of the nine families lived in a state of recurring crisis.[43] The child's unwillingness to cooperate in one of more aspects of care was an important cause of extreme discord.

Another form of family adjustment, the one that is possibly most common in the lower-class family with a number of children, is seeming indifference. The absence of anxiety over the diabetic child may give the impression of good adjustment to diabetes. In contrast to the worried middle-class mother with her innumerable questions and harassed look, the unconcerned mother may seem a welcome contrast. If she has learned the rudiments of carbohydrate computation, uses low-cost substitutes for meat proteins such as peanut butter and beans, and has adapted the general family diet to include more protein and juice and very occasional cookies and candy, she may indeed have made the best possible adjustment and provided the child with a healthy, matter-of-fact attitude toward his disease.

Lower socioeconomic class carries so many pressing worries about subsistence, marital cohesion, transportation, toothaches and earaches, drug problems, etc. that the needs of the diabetic child are only one more pressure, less urgent than how to pay the rent. When one uneducated but intelligent mother was interviewed, she said, "Oh, I didn't know diabetes was a chronic illness," but she had learned and adhered to rudimentary diet measures and gave insulin injections on schedule. Another mother said she cried a great deal, but it was not about the diabetic child; it was how to feed the whole family when her husband was out of work.

Low socioeconomic status must always be considered a risk factor in juvenile diabetes, but not simply because of lack of money for the plentiful nutritious food needed by the child. Dr. Marian Metz, Chief of Social Service at the University of California Medical Center, has pointed out that to be a "good diabetic" one needs typical middle-class values—postponement of gratification, and the hope that one's efforts will be rewarded.[44] Sociologists have pointed out that these are lacking in the most deprived, who have learned to take their pleasures where they find them and have found that hopes do not materialize. Experience indicates the difficulty of constancy, the sine qua non of good diabetic control, in those severely deprived families whose way of life is one of disorganization and who respond only to the most painful or urgent needs.

The diabetic child's problem of low self-esteem, or a poor self-image, is reinforced by poverty. In addition to being physically different, he must dress shabbily, cannot participate in the many school activities that require money, and is often subject to contempt from peers and teachers because of coming from a welfare family. Tensions within the family are heightened by the child's resentment over his parents' inability to give him what other children have. Lack of privacy in crowded housing for urine testing and insulin injections, and lack of sterile equipment, add to the problems poverty imposes.

The manner in which dietary and other instructions are provided during the child's initial hospitalization influences the reactions and capacity of the mother to follow the regimen when the child comes home. Management of the disease may not seem too formidable if only elementary information is presented, the details being added gradually after the initial shock has been absorbed. An overwhelming amount of detail is sometimes presented, however, so that feelings of defeat or rejection of the child and his needs may occur. One small child, readmitted to a county teaching hospital in near-coma, displayed great distress because her angry mother said she intended to give her away; that she could not cope with all the special diet and insulin requirements on top of everything else she had to do. Many mothers feel similar anger, and no doubt transmit it to the child, though not necessarily in words.

Another problem in dietary instruction is insufficient repetition and explanation. Working mothers, or those dependent on working husbands or neighbors for transportation to the hospital, may not be able to visit during the hours the staff is available to educate the mother. Workers who know the family during the period of onset may need to see that special arrangements are made for the mother's daily instruction in diet, insulin, and urine testing, either through some adaptation of time by hospital staff or daytime visits by the mother.

The single parent's great need for outside help is apparent, as is her need to quit work, if working outside the home, for the several months or year required for establishment of predictable insulin-food response. However, women with husbands may be as alone, or in even greater difficulty. The diet, different physicians' ideas about it, and the child's fear and disturbance over injections provide ready fuel for arguments if the two parents have different attitudes toward the child, toward physicians and illness, or if they have other sources of tension between them.

When family relationships have been strained, the prolonged stress of a poorly adjusted or labile diabetic child can be the proverbial straw. Inability to travel for vacations, to have normal recreation, to give each other needed love and attention obviously tips the scales against marital adjustment. One mother whose child was prone to insulin-reaction convulsions at night said: "The parents of a diabetic child can never close the bedroom door at night." Less concerned parents, or those whose children are spilling sugar continuously rather than maintaining a marginal sugar, do not have this problem. One mother of a very ill child who had many critical episodes due to diabetic complications said she simply had to explain to her younger children that "their turn would come" to have her attention, but now Bud simply had to have it all. She added, with some doubt in her voice, that she thought they understood.

Two common threads are seen among the poorly adjusted families. One is abdication by one parent, usually the father, of any responsibility for the child. He frequently takes a second job, which gives him a reason to be away from home at night and on weekends. The family's need for extra money frees him from guilt or family blame. Or, if the father is at home, he does not involve himself in the child's problems or his wife's problems in management. The cause of a mother's excessive anxiety may sometimes be revealed by acquaintance with an abdicating father.

Another relatively common problem is the presence of diabetes in a parent who provides a poor model for the child. He may ignore dietary restrictions or denigrate medical recommendations. Because of the hereditary factor, two persons with diabetes are not infrequently found in the same family. Since the maturity onset form (which can occur in late adolescence or early adult life) does differ in its requirements, the child with serious juvenile diabetes may be misled, even though an older sibling or parent does actually remain in relatively good control despite considerable latitude in regime.

Perhaps most difficult is the problem occasioned when one or both parents are self-centered or immature, and are unwilling to make sacrifices themselves in behalf of the child. Parents who eat candy in front of the diabetic child, or set out cookies or doughnuts for the rest of the family and expect the child to abstain, lay the basis for trouble. He either breaks his routine, unable to avoid temptation, or feels angry and deprived. Whether such parents are in reality punitive, scapegoating the diabetic, or merely immature can only be ascertained by evaluating their other attitudes and behavior.

Managing Away from Home

School, bus travel, and, for the middle-class child, vacations, visiting relatives, slumber parties, and going to camp are parts of normal life that need advance planning when a child is diabetic. While children are too young to inject themselves with insulin and eat and play without supervision, the schoolteacher, school nurse, and bus driver must be educated and able to participate in diabetic management. As welfare department regulations increase their emphasis upon mothers' working, day care facilities must be equipped with similar knowledge and equipment. Neighbors, relatives, and church members frequently also are involved in subsidiary care of a diabetic child. They may need opportunity to air their anxieties and get answers to questions if they are to act responsibly without embarrassing the child or showing undue anxiety. They need at minimum to understand the simple principles of insulin-food-exercise balance and of quickly available sugar, in orange juice, Coke, chocolate bars, or sugar cubes; further, they need the physician's name and telephone number if the mother or foster mother cannot be reached.

Children who look "normal" and attend regular schools do not have the advantage that orthopedically handicapped children have in a teacher who has had special training in work with the exceptional child. The teacher, who represents adult authority, is a potential friend or enemy in the child's emotional adjustment and should be brought into planning for a diabetic child who is having difficulty staying in control. She should know that psychological stress raises blood-sugar levels, and help to minimize it during the child's school attendance.

Ordinarily, children too young to give their own insulin injections do not stay away from home overnight unless near enough for the mother to go and give the child's injection. Urine testing can be omitted (and when the child is in good control, it often is omitted for several days in a row). In case of children removed from home suddenly because of need for protection or a mother's hospitalization, the child welfare worker will need to utilize the help of a foster mother with a nursing background or previous experience with diabetes, or take the child to a hospital for injections, which he cannot go without. Conference with the physician is essential in emergency cases.

Airlines will provide diabetic meals if asked in advance, in case travel to a distant point is necessary. By using disposable syringes and urine-testing kits, travel is not impossible for the responsible and educated adolescent diabetic. Obviously, a Medic Alert locket or bracelet is important, as are sufficient funds to purchase food if delays in schedule occur, and a handbag or briefcase large enough that emergency supplies can be carried by the child (not stored away in a baggage compartment).

Diabetic camps offer children many advantages. They appear to be utilized primarily by the middle class; the extra effort necessary to secure a "campership" (a sort of scholarship or financial grant), transportation, and required clothing changes should be made in behalf of children from families on assistance. Camp is a painful experience for many children during the first several days. Not only does the customary homesickness occur, but camp food is not tailored to the child's likes. He is required to eat everything served, including vegetables he is not made to eat at home. Children by and large do not seem to enjoy meals at camp. However, they enjoy the games, crafts, and social life, and they learn a great deal about management of their disease that can be of immeasurable help later. Children from single-parent homes, or from culturally deprived homes, particularly need these advantages. Learning that they are not alone, not as "different" as they thought, and making friendships with other diabetic young people are a significant part of the camp experience.

Marriage, Sex, and Pregnancy

As earlier pointed out, girls have more trouble living with diabetes than boys. One study of the emotional adjustment of 26 selected diabetic children showed that nine of the ten who manifested significant emotional maladjustment were girls.[45] Whether girls are more upset emotionally because they are more often ill, or vice versa, is difficult to know, but physical discomfort and physiological irritability would affect emotional stability. Girls often are more concerned than boys with interpersonal relationships, attractiveness to the opposite sex, and chances for marriage. These areas are indeed adversely affected by diabetes. Adolescents are highly sensitive, and those with diabetes are not unaware of the shadows on their future.

A study of illegitimate pregnancies among adolescent girls with heart disease, referred to earlier, postulated that girls who feel defective physically try harder to prove their normalcy as females by becoming pregnant.[46] No information is available about illegitimate pregnancies among diabetic girls. Fortunately, in some respects (genetically and socially) the fertility rate among juvenile diabetics is not high, and the pregnancies that do occur have a higher rate of termination in miscarriages or stillbirths than normal.[47]

Pregnancy requires close medical supervision, and diabetic control is difficult, especially if morning sickness and vomiting occur. Late in pregnancy, there is a hazard that the baby will die in utero if the mother's diabetes does go out of control. Hospitalization is essential when emergencies exist.

Reproduction is a precious human privilege, but in light of the serious problems for the diabetic young woman, her infant, and society, birth control must be considered when a juvenile diabetic girl begins a sexual relationship, in or out of marriage. The method of birth control requires careful medical evaluation, for "the pill" is controversial for diabetics, and a gynecological consultation is needed with regard to methods, including sterilization.[48] The probability that the young mother of a surviving infant will become blind, disabled by kidney or heart disease, and that her life expectancy is materially shortened, weighs on the side of prevention of pregnancy. (See pp. 138–39, 146, 151.)

Resources for Diabetic Children

Because of the rising costs of hospital care, fewer specialized facilities exist than formerly for the care of the chronically ill child; consequently, those persons who help the parent care for the child at home carry greater responsibility. Resources for home care become increasingly more important.

Rural children or those living in small towns have few special resources unless medical consultation has been arranged in a city whose special facilities may be tapped. Some connection with a specialized clinic that offers consultation to the local physician and provides periodic examinations for the child provides opportunity to secure the advantage of auxiliary services. A liaison relationship with such a clinic can frequently ensure special class instruction for parents and the child, consultation with dieticians, and help from a hospital social worker. Nutrition counselors of the 4-H and Grange organizations, and public health nurses affiliated with the county or state health department, can be queried regarding direct service or their availability for consultation.

The American Diabetes Association has branches in most large and moderate-sized cities. These may be manned by volunteers, so that more initiative may be required to take advantage of the society's services than in the case of larger health organizations staffed by professional workers. The organization has free literature in English and Spanish for parents and children regarding diet and insulin administration, lists of specialists interested in diabetes, information regarding group meetings, and news bulletins for parents and physicians, and can provide information about camps. A cooperative arrangement may exist with the local branch of the Heart Association whereby the dietician there will give advice to diabetic persons. The local Tuberculosis and Health Association or the Heart Association may provide educational materials and information on activities regarding diabetes if no branch of the Diabetes Association exists in the community.

Parent groups and youth groups are forming, after the pattern of groups related to cerebral palsy, mental retardation, etc. Because ignorance and feelings of isolation are common enemies of the diabetic, group membership is usually beneficial. Middle-class, two-parent families that have readily available transportation tend to dominate parent groups. The single-parent, minority members or welfare recipients may need emotional support or help with transportation in order to attend.

CHAPTER FOURTEEN

Leukemia

LEUKEMIA HAS BEEN a uniformly fatal illness, the term so fraught with dread that a family crisis occurs with its diagnosis. Recent dramatic gains in treatment now permit hope of five-year survival and even of ultimate cure of some children. Treatment remains in a state of change, and thus the meaning of the disease is changing. What is true today may not be true tomorrow. Nevertheless, leukemia still creates mental and physical anguish, and still terminates in death for most children who have the disease. The social worker should understand leukemia as well as possible, and know the ways she can alleviate some of the suffering it inflicts.

The number of children with leukemia is relatively small. Many more elderly persons are afflicted. Yet cancer is the highest cause of death, next to accidents, among children ages 1–14; and acute leukemia is the most frequent type of cancer in children.[1] Furthermore, its incidence is increasing.[2] Leukemia is a prominent disease because of the extensive research mounted throughout the nation. Progress has caused excitement. The progress has been in extending disease-free intervals. The children "in remission" are, for all practical purposes, well. Many children who receive the new forms of treatment do not have the old problem of prolonged dying but a new problem. They must learn to live under a shadow, but with the hope they will be among those who are spared.

Workers in the community therefore have increasing reason to become involved with leukemic children and their families. The child is in the hospital for shorter periods, at home and at school for longer periods.

THE MEDICAL REALITIES

The Disease, Its Cause and Distribution

Leukemia is a malignancy of the blood-forming organs. Abnormal blood cells accumulate in the blood and bone marrow.[3] Leukemia cannot be prevented from spreading by early diagnosis and treatment, because it is disseminated throughout the body.

The cause is still unknown. "It seems likely that several factors, perhaps some as yet unknown, may have to act together."[4] The Hiroshima experience proved that radiation can be one of the causes. Genetic factors are implicated also by the unusually high incidence of leukemia in children with *Down's syndrome*, or *mongolism*, a group with an abnormal number of chromosomes.[5] Leukemia is not familial or inherited, nor is it catching, although the possibility of virus causation is widely discussed. There is no justifiable reason for parents to feel or project guilt, looking for blame. However, mothers often feel that they have been responsible in some way.

More boys than girls have cancer, and more Whites than non-Whites. Nearly one-half of childhood cancer (46.6 percent) is leukemia. The age-group most affected is children under ten, with a decline in incidence after five years of age and a still greater decline among the age-group 10–14.[6] The peak incidence for the most frequent form, *acute lymphoblastic* or *lymphocytic leukemia* (abbreviated ALL) occurs between the ages of three and four years.[7] Mauer, a leading authority, states that about 2,300 children die each year in this country as a result of acute leukemia.[8] How many are living with it is not known.

To understand what leukemia is, and what it does, one needs some comprehension of the work of the blood cells. A pamphlet for parents, "Childhood Leukemia," prepared by the U.S. Department of Health, Education, and Welfare, explains in substance that blood cells are formed in the bone marrow and consist of red cells, which carry oxygen to the tissues; *platelets*, which prevent abnormal bleeding; and white cells, which defend against infection. The white cells are called *leukocytes* and are of two kinds, *neutrophils* and *lymphocytes*. They both defend against foreign substances, such as invading bacteria, but do so by different mechanisms.

In leukemia, abnormal white cells replace normal bone marrow and then appear in the blood and subsequently in other tissues. When the abnormality occurs in the cells that normally become lymphocytes, the disease is called *lymphoblastic* or *lymphocytic* leukemia. A less common form with unfavorable prognosis is acute *myelocytic* leukemia. A few children have chronic myelocytic leukemia. The chronic form of lymphocytic leukemia occurs in adults. The rapidly growing number of abnormal white cells in acute disease crowd out and inhibit production of normal white cells, red cells, and platelets. The resulting lack of normal cells creates the symptoms of this disease.

Course and Outlook

Because of the decrease in red cells, the child is anemic. Therefore he is pale and tired. He is lethargic and cannot perform his usual activities, and may be completely prostrated by fatigue. Because of the decrease in platelets, the child bleeds and bruises excessively or without apparent cause. He may have heavy nosebleeds, or bleed from the rectum or have tiny red spots on the skin, called *petechiae*. Because the normal white cells are reduced, he picks up infections easily, and often is unable to throw them off. Many children have bone pain.[9]

The child's pain and discomforts, and the time and manner of death, are closely related to treatment employed. Mauer states that the course and complications are "related to the consequences of marrow replacement, the invasion of leukemia cells into other organs, and the side effects of therapy."[10] A digression regarding changes in treatment throws light on the physical experience of children who receive older and newer forms of therapy.

Untreated, acute lymphocytic leukemia is fatal in about six months; only 5 percent of affected children are said to survive for a year.[11] Acute myelocytic leukemia responds to treatment briefly, but remains an essentially fatal disease with much worse prognosis than acute lymphocytic leukemia.[12] More than 20 years ago, acute lymphocytic leukemia showed response to drug therapy. Various drugs were administered separately until resistance developed; then a different drug was given. Each produced short disease-free intervals. Two drugs used together proved more effective (prednisone and vincristine) in killing leukemia cells and therefore in creating cessation of symptoms. Still another drug, methotrexate, prolonged the disease-free period. The usual mode of treatment eventually became that of an intensive "induction" period of about two months, followed by "consolidation" and "maintenance" of remission, or the disease-free interval. In more recent years, with increasingly aggressive and sophisticated drug administration, supplemented by countermeasures to sustain the child during the heavy drug assault, the period of first remission became as long as a year and a half in many cases.

But then came relapse. Relapse was a "bad sign."[13] Further inductions were administered, but each was increasingly painful for the child and followed by a shorter period of remission, until finally remissions and relapses blurred into a long and often terrible period of dying, unless raging infection, stroke, or other accident quickly terminated the child's life. Mauer, writing in 1969, gave the median survival time as 17 months, and calculated that 25 percent of the children survived 28 months. In one center using a massive drug-assault program much like those used today in advanced centers, a median survival time of 33 months had been reported in 1967.[14] Leading research physicians have reported that in December 1971 55 percent of the children under their management achieved a three-and-one-half-year survival rate.[15] Thus it may be seen that over the 20 years of drug therapy enormous gains were made in prolonging life for some children, but for most the prolongation was relatively brief.

An institution that concentrates on research-oriented treatment of children with leukemia, St. Jude's Research Hospital in Memphis, Tennessee, released reports in 1972 and 1973 of studies supported by the National Cancer Institute that showed dramatic gains. They have used a very heavy multiple-drug assault, coupled with radiation of the child's head and spinal cord, followed by maintenance doses of multiple drugs for a three-year period. They call their program "total therapy," and state that "results of recent studies indicate that acute lymphocytic leukemia can no longer be considered an incurable disease.... Total therapy has resulted in a 17% seven-year leukemia-free survival rate for children admitted for treatment studies at St. Jude's Hospital in 1962 to 1965. Patients admitted to the 1967 to 1968 study have a 51% four-year leukemia-free survival rate."[16]

In 1955 the National Cancer Institute had launched a comprehensive cancer chemotherapy research program. The program continues to provide funds and direction to develop drugs, and to evaluate them on animals and then on human beings.[17] Twenty-six research centers and 80 medical schools scattered throughout the United States—or, in effect, all the major treatment centers—have become part of the national research network. Chemotherapy, the cutting edge of progress in cancer treatment, is more effective with disseminated cancer than with solid tumors; hence children with leukemia are the subject of widespread interest in cancer research circles in providing inspiration and possible clues to progress in treating other forms of cancer.[18]

The Pains and Limitations of Treatment

With death as the adversary, the research-oriented physician "pushes the child to the brink of death" to kill the leukemic cells.[19] The drugs used are chemical poisons that damage or kill cells undergoing growth and multiplication.[20] Those in common use are prednisone, vincristine, 6-mercaptopurine, methotrexate, and cytoxan. Others are being tested, and are in limited use. The first two remain the cornerstones of induction. The other drugs are used for maintenance.[21] Since the drugs do not single out malignant cells alone but damage normal cells as well, their side effects are life-threatening and highly distressing. They kill the cells of the hair follicles, causing baldness (*alopecia*); they kill the cells of the mucous membranes of the mouth and gastrointestinal tract, causing ulcers and diarrhea, nausea and vomiting, and malnutrition. They cause kidney damage, producing bloody urine, kidney infection, etc., and cause double vision, headache, and other symptoms.[22]

The drugs aggravate, temporarily, the very hazards of the disease itself by lowering the body's defenses against infection (the effect known as immunosuppression) and damaging the clotting capacity of the blood through platelet suppression. Prolonged upper respiratory infections, with pneumonitis or pneumonia, are also dangerous. Moreover, germs always present within the gastrointestinal tract may enter the child's bloodstream (septicemia) from drug-induced ulcerations. Altogether, the most vulnerable period is during a time of intense treatment, either at the beginning or when an exacerbation has occurred. Infection now accounts for 70 percent of deaths of leukemic children.[23] One St. Jude's study reported that 10 percent of the children died of infection during complete remission, in addition to those who died before remission had been achieved.[24]

Authorities state that medical capacity to achieve longer remissions has come about because of "supportive measures"[25] that permit the child to survive the trauma of the drug assault. "Support" leans heavily on transfusions of platelets. These have had dramatic effect in reducing death from hemorrhage resulting from platelet deficiency. A child may need twice-weekly transfusions for as long as three months—or, during hemorrhage, much more frequently.[26] Modern blood-bank techniques, available to some but not all special centers, permit extraction of platelets from the donor's blood and return of the blood to him, thus enabling him to give platelets as often as twice a week. A small pool of donors known to the family, ideally including the parents themselves, reduces the possibility of giving the child blood contaminated by hepatitis.[27]

As mentioned, part of "total therapy" during the initial intensive treatment phase is prophylaxis against a common complication, leukemia of the central nervous system. The brain, kidneys, and testicles are hiding places where drugs cannot penetrate to completely destroy leukemic cells. In the past, from one-fourth to one-half of children with acute leukemia have developed *meningeal disease* (in the outer covering of brain and cord), and almost half of them develop some form of nerve involvement.[28] It is now believed that two-thirds of children will develop central-nervous-system disease if they have a significant remission.[29] Because those who will develop nervous-system leukemia cannot be distinguished from those who will not, all children in some centers now receive radiation to the head by use of cobalt or linear accelerator equipment during the initial phase of treatment.

As described by Dr. Probert of the Faculty of Radiology at the Stanford University Medical Center, the brain and spinal cord are irradiated one area at a time for two or three minutes each day, five days a week, for three or four weeks. He said the treatment is too recent to permit evaluation of any possible long-term side effects, and that adverse mental effect (retardation) has not been observed thus far where small doses of radiation have been used by specialists sophisticated in this method of treatment. Immediate side effects include loss of hair and in some cases nausea and vomiting. A lumbar puncture and bone marrow biopsy must be performed before initiation of radiation. Dr. Probert emphasized that X-ray therapy is a two-edged sword, a valuable treatment form but one dangerous in unskilled hands and advisable only in centers where physicists work out the dosage and professional staff have sufficient number of leukemia patients to maintain proficiency.[30] Many centers are now using radiation to the head alone and direct injections of methotrexate into the spinal cord for all children during induction as insurance against central-nervous-system leukemia; the use of radiation and/or intrathecal methotrexate is obviously costly and frightening, and since loss of hair occurs, it has major psychological connotations.

During the period of remission, when all symptoms have disappeared, maintenance drugs must be continued with absolute regularity.[31] As mentioned earlier, the St. Jude's "protocol" continues drugs for three years. Children may take eight to ten pills daily. Reports from mothers vary in regard to children's reactions. Some children have no difficulty swallowing the pills; others complain of the size or bad taste. Treatment regimens requiring the child to take methotrexate and cytoxan on a once-a-week basis may cause nausea and malaise so severe as to limit school attendance the next day.

Testing of blood, bone marrow, and spinal fluid at regular intervals continues during remission. Weekly blood tests may be performed by a local physician. The remission period requires watchfulness at home and school for any signals of recurrence or need for preventive measures. Fever, cough, earache, abdominal pain, diarrhea, abscesses, massive nosebleeds, blood in the stools or urine, or petechiae, all require immediate medical attention.[32] If the platelet count has dropped and the disease has become resistant to the drugs that have been used for maintenance, a reinduction may be attempted with the original induction drugs or with a different combination.

When the disease increases in severity, the child is again especially vulnerable to infection and hemorrhage. Exposure to infection in hospitals is so general that home care is preferred whenever possible. However, the child may be hospitalized for transfusions, drug administration, and treatment of toxicity problems. Rigid measures to prevent exposure to infection, including isolation, may be used.

Two common complications—several kinds of kidney pathology (including uremia) and enlargement of the testicles—require expert medical scrutiny to determine whether treatment should be initiated, and if so, what type of therapy. The drug allipurinol has been found effective for uremia; testicular enlargement may be treated by surgical removal of the testicles or by radiation or drugs, or may be left alone.

Children who have been started on older methods cannot be switched to the new "total therapy" regimen. Institutions vary in the treatment regimens employed; not all physicians have the same philosophy about research and about treatment. However, the goal of all is a long first remission. This is the period when child and family can enjoy a relatively normal life. The length of first remission is directly related to length of life.³³ Relapse from "total therapy" leaves the physician without other tested drugs to use on the child because their effectiveness has been completely exhausted simultaneously during initial induction and heavy maintenance. Thus these children may die quickly from an infection that is especially hazardous for them, or from uncontrolled bleeding. Children on older, less-aggressive treatment programs are placed on additional drugs, and short periods of remission may be achieved. Thus they may die slowly, over a gradual downhill period.

The splendid news of seven-year survival for 17 percent of one series of children at St. Jude's, and the general hope for a 50 percent survival for newly diagnosed children treated with "total therapy," are tempered by awareness that 83 percent of children receiving the most modern treatment did die before seven years, and 50 percent before five years after onset. Leukemia is still a grim disease. Investigational chemotherapy essential for prolongation of life and for the possible eventual cure of leukemia adds to the trauma for many children and their families. The price all leukemic children pay in suffering so that some may live longer today, and still more tomorrow, is very high. The psychosocial effects on today's children are yet to be measured. The next section describes what we know from yesterday and believe will remain valid.

PSYCHOSOCIAL IMPLICATIONS

The meaning of leukemia to the child and his family changes with the course of the disease and is a highly variable experience. Onset—with early symptoms, diagnosis, first awareness of meaning, hospitalization, and massive treatment—constitutes a family crisis. When remission occurs, and the child looks and feels well again, the medication, his hair loss, and the clinic visits keep alive memories of the early period. If the first remission becomes a long one, as now may be expected for many, the early trauma fades into a shadow over an essentially well child. In the majority of cases, relapse occurs, sooner or later, bringing the beginning of the terminal stage. The child may die quickly, or he may suffer more relapses, shorter periods of remission, complications, hemorrhages, pneumonia, other infections, nausea, pain; he may undergo repeated hospitalizations, drastic treatment and misery, transfusions and needles. For these children and their families, hope wanes and anxiety increases. Living with leukemia merges into the experience of dying and death for the child and mourning for the family. Thus "leukemia" means a sequence of several different experiences.

The length and variations of the experience vary greatly, depending on the course and complications of the disease process, the medical care received, the child's age and temperament, what he means to his parents, and the family constellation and circumstance. The uniqueness of each child and what happens to him combines with the changing outlook in leukemia to make generalizations questionable. Yet some experience has been amassed that can be synthesized. It offers clues regarding what the individual child and family may be going through, and provides the worker with ideas about how to help.

Leukemia in children has been synonymous with dying until so recently that almost no literature exists on living with it. Foreknowledge of impending doom is so frightening to associates of the person who is to die that a barrier rises to impede communication. Social work literature gives the impression that the profession has avoided relating to the dying child by concentrating on the mourning family. One article cautions that "it is prudent to avoid interaction with the child" in order to avoid being overwhelmed by needs of both family and child.[34] Recently, dying has become the subject of intense interest, possibly as part of the general anxiety over violence. A few experts have emerged who are working to break down the communication barriers.

Case records, interviews, and observation do provide a picture of some of the determinants in living with leukemia. Major determinants are medical care and the effect of leukemia on family life, for the child is most affected by the adults in charge at home and in the hospital. Though the child's personal problems are intertwined with his family's, an attempt has been made to separate them for the sake of clarity in presentation; they are elaborated in a later section of this chapter.

The Family and the Medical Team

Since the treatment of leukemia is difficult and highly specialized, the family doctor or pediatrician will usually send the child to a specialized center, frequently at a distance. The extent to which center specialists utilize the local physician for interim care varies; the local pediatrician can remain the key figure for parent and child, or one of the physicians at the center may become the most important doctor. In life-threatening illness, "God and the doctor" are the patient's only hope, and the doctor frequently functions as the representative of God. Faith in the doctor is the most important single mainstay, until the child's last breath, except in the dwindling number of families who place their main reliance on God Himself.

Because the relationship is so important, problems that can interfere with optimum patient-doctor relationships are significant. Repeatedly, physicians who first impart overwhelmingly bad news are blamed. They are thought of as cruel, brusque, indifferent, and may be deeply disliked and distrusted, in a response that has been compared to that of the early Greeks who put to death the messengers of bad tidings in battle. Nor is the family response always unwarranted. Physicians are not devoid of emotion, and vary in their mechanisms of control. To tell parents that a child has leukemia, aware of the horror this illness often brings, must call forth all needed unconscious mechanisms, including those of distance. Other negative realities in medical care include the number and turnover of medical staff in research or teaching centers. Some chiefs, who determine the medical protocol or regime to be used, remain aloof from the treatment of individual children. They are spared the sights and sounds of suffering that result from investigational methods. Interns, residents, and medical students who flow through teaching centers striving for experience and knowledge may be inept in needling techniques and in the management of difficult relationships and their own feelings. Teaching centers sometimes utilize a bewildering array of young physicians, each of whom may ask the same questions every time the child comes to the clinics, and subject him to painful injections and frightening experiences. When these things happen, the child and his family are deprived of the one most important relationship during critical illness, that with their doctor.

Small wonder then that some middle-class families destroy themselves financially and travel far from home when they find a physician they trust. Or that the child places his faith sometimes in a resident or intern who is compassionate and gentle. One physician to provide continuity of care, who is available on weekends and nights in emergencies and whom the family trusts, is essential to the psychological well-being of child and family. Such a person is not easily found and not necessarily in the largest centers with the most outstanding reputations. The family may feel a need for some medical shopping at first. They may need help with travel or involved family and financial arrangements. Helping them find a local pediatrician on whom the family can rely and who extends the care of the special center may be the single most important contribution to the child and family the worker can make.

The worker and parents should be aware of the treatment philosophy in the center to which the child is sent, because great differences exist, and these have major impact on the child's experience. Some centers emphasize preparation for fatality, and others, hope for cure. Some center chiefs distinguish between prolonging life and prolonging death in the care they order lower-level staff to provide; some physicians believe in keeping the patient comfortable and not fighting the inevitable after a second or third relapse, others attempt repeated inductions and more danger in every attempt to prolong survival. Some are flexible according to family wishes and capacities; others adhere to rigid research protocols. Parents of children who have died vary in their opinions about research-oriented treatment. Most whose comments have been noted feel it is a comfort to know every latest method to prolong life has been tried; others think the price in suffering that the child paid was too high when in the end it was "for nothing."

Parent participation in the care of their children during hospitalization is permitted in varying degrees at some centers.[35] Of great social significance is the practice of requiring the mother or a substitute relative to remain in the hospital during the child's stay. At the leukemia center in the Children's Hospital at Stanford, mothers sleep on cots near the child's bed. The mother feeds and bathes the child, and some mothers who are able are taught to give intravenous medication through an established needle (one put in position by a doctor and fixed to remain there until he or a nurse removes it). The child is provided with the greatest source of emotional security, his mother, at the time of greatest need. He may be able to leave the hospital earlier if the mother has learned to administer chemotherapy under outpatient supervision. Furthermore, "the child needs an advocate," says Miss Dutcher, the assistant to Dr. J. R. Wilbur at Stanford, someone who will raise questions if the "whole child" seems to get lost in the fragmented complexities of specialized care. A study made of the parent-participation program at the City of Hope in southern California points out that the quality of parent participation, not the quantity, was the essential element in determining its effectiveness there.[36]

The influence of the medical care facility on the child's experience with leukemia extends beyond medical competence to the attitudes and skills of paramedical staff. "The doctors and the nurses are so nice, Stanford seems like a second home," one mother said of the Pediatrics Department at Stanford Medical Center. Children seem better able to tolerate painful treatment when they like and trust the staff, who have been taught the nuances of children's needs and their own interactions with them. Awareness of the trauma for staff in treating fatally ill children has brought psychiatric, social work, and chaplain participants into the teams of many specialized cancer facilities. They help medical staff and each other, in addition to the patients and families. Hospital social workers who do involve themselves directly with leukemic children lift great burdens from mothers and provide direct and indirect support to the children. They are the link with the outside world, an excellent resource for the worker in the community who needs information in her plans pertaining to continuing concerns in the home. Many hospitals have liaison nurses who act as a link with public health nurses in home communities.

Some centers that use the team approach now pay special attention to the first conference with the family when the physicians inform parents of the diagnosis. Dr. C. M. Binger, who acts as psychiatric consultant to the Pediatrics Department of the University of California Medical Center, says families "loosen up" during onset and diagnosis, as is to be expected during crisis, and are thereby accessible to help. Staff at that time can implant knowledge that they will be available to help when later problems arise.[37] This accessibility to help, and the importance of capitalizing on it during the diagnostic period, should be borne in mind by the agency worker, who otherwise might think it better to wait until matters are more settled before telephoning or making a home visit.

The Crisis of Diagnosis

The social worker is concerned with family adjustment to the child's leukemia for at least three reasons. Dr. David Kaplan points out that the family "mediates stress" for the child, the way shock absorbers cushion the impact of bumps on the road.[38] Second, severe behavioral and emotional maladjustment among family members has been observed as a late manifestation of the prolonged severe stress on the family. Dr. Binger states that, in evaluating patients with psychiatric problems at the Langley Porter Psychiatric Institute, he is struck with the frequent incidence of an earlier death in the family.[39] Third, and of critical importance to the child's well-being, is the danger that a family's "grief work" or mourning will begin when they first accept the diagnosis. This can result in premature emotional separation from the child, resulting in his actual or emotional abandonment.

In addition to these reasons for concern is the impact of leukemia on the community. The financing agencies, including unions and public coffers, face enormous bills after family resources have been depleted. Massive chemotherapy necessitates repeated expensive bone punctures for monitoring purposes and extensive transfusions to combat hemorrhages. Bankrupt and/or disrupted families produce a financially crippling effect in their human surroundings, so that relatives, fellow employees, lodge members, taxpayers, and philanthropists are all affected by a disease in which exorbitantly costly treatment is involved.

Case records reveal a wide range of parental behaviors during the period of diagnosis. Parents have been through a period when the child screams behind closed doors while his blood and spinal fluid are drawn, and when the young child may continue to sob with fright and bewilderment long afterward or fall into exhausted sleep. The hospital admission forms have required them to rummage for insurance papers, Social Security numbers, and data on expenditures and sources of income. Hasty arrangements for work and care of other children have been made. The physicians have been serious or remote and busy. The nurses and other parents have looked sad and commiserating. The anxiety, feelings of harassment and bewilderment culminate in the shock of hearing the diagnosis. One father said he refused to accept it—he still had not fully accepted it after the child's death. At first he had thought, "Why me, what have I done to deserve this?" Then he felt it was a bad dream and would go away. Then he started "bugging the doctors about the new drugs he read about." Should they go to England? To Dallas? To Boston? It was "just hell."

Parents have been described by some observers as acting "stunned," disbelieving, or so delayed in taking in the information that they may appear uncaring, or unaffected by the news.[40] Perhaps they will be less so when more hope can be imparted. Acute grief reactions are common, however, with weeping, desperate attempts to avoid crying in front of the child, hovering over him, and other reactions of solicitude that unfortunately are sensed as frightening by the child. Rose Grobstein has said that all families go through several stages, that of denial or disbelief, anger often directed at the doctors and nurses, guilt over something they may have done or failed to do, depression, and eventually acceptance, although the latter may come too late to be of help to the child.[41]

Parents' guilt after they hear the diagnosis is easy to understand in light of the behavioral similarity between laziness and fatigue in a child too young to articulate how he feels. The toddler or preschool child who cries to be carried because he is too tired and his legs too painful to walk may well be ignored, shamed, slapped, or whipped by his tired mother or impatient father. Guilt need not last if professional staff give sufficient attention to discussion with the parents and explanation that they did not cause the disease. If the agency worker finds the parents are burdened by guilt, she should arrange further conferences with the physician; if guilt continues, the parents should have opportunity for counseling from the best available source.

Stanford Medical Center social service staff believe they can predict the families who will need help later on, by the manner in which parents cope with the crisis of the diagnostic period. Kaplan et al. theorize that each stage of the experience, including remission, constitutes a crisis, and that each must be worked through successfully if the later crises are to be resolved constructively.[42] (Another possibility is that emotionally mature parents who have a good marriage cope successfully with each stage of the experience, and that clues to immaturity reveal themselves during the crisis of onset.) This attractive theory, backed by their study of 50 cases, does not seem to allow for my own conviction that different breaking points exist for all, and that the course and treatment of the illness and other concurrent stresses are critical variables in determining how much any given family can stand. (See Chapter 2, discussion of stress, pp. 17–20.)

Where both partners are mature and the marriage pattern is one of sharing and communicating, they are able to sustain each other and the child. The Stanford survey showed that only one-fourth of their series of 50 families were able to cope adequately. Inevitably, the heavy stress of this period acts as a polarizing agent. The intensity of emotion pulls some parents together and thrusts others apart. Parents who agree on other matters of child rearing and on how to deal with the leukemic child seem to be drawn together. If they share the information with older siblings, who also react in a mature manner, the family acts as a unit. It is probably strengthened by the terrible experience; no doubt such a family cushions the blows for the child in a way nothing else can.

The agency worker often is concerned with families who are not cohesive.

Divorce may have already occurred, the mother is either alone or remarried, or the marriage is tenuous and subject to various other strains, such as the immaturity of one partner, alcoholism, the illness of a parent or of one or more of the other children, poverty, ignorance, etc. Often women seem to talk and cry out their emotions, whereas many men, struggling for control, become irritated, impatient, or angry over the mother's need to talk and be comforted. The child's leukemia usually is experienced differently by fathers and mothers, causing one aspect of polarization in which the worker can sometimes intervene.

Cynthia Mikkleson of the University of California Medical Center in San Francisco points out that the father's self-concept of responsibility for his family and of fending off harm has suddenly become endangered by a situation in which he is helpless. The mother's nurturing role is heightened. She becomes more and more involved in the situation, watching the child's appearance, talking with the doctors, taking the child to the clinic, sitting with him in the hospital. The father, on the contrary, not only is away from home, working to pay the bills, but usually has difficulty taking time from work to talk with the doctors—they have gone home when he visits in the evening. When the illness progresses, the father may be almost excluded, while mother and child grow closer, more interdependent. She is the authority on medical care and the father knows only what she tells him.[48]

The worker can sometimes help prevent this. She can encourage the father to take the mother and child to the clinic or to relieve the mother at the hospital. She can consult him about what the doctor said and expect him to function as the responsible head of the family.

Parents may disagree on how much to favor the child and how to discipline him. A father may see the mother's tender, compassionate feelings for the threatened child as a shift of love away from himself, and the child is resented. One father was observed to be very stern with the child, creating scenes over small disciplinary matters. He later abandoned the mother and child—with the support of his sensitivity group, which placed an emphasis on his own self-fulfillment. Another father so indulged his leukemic son that the confused and frightened youngster bullied the mother into giving him his way in everything; he became impossible to discipline.

Among the potential differences of opinion between parents is what to tell the child about his diagnosis. One parent may find it intolerable to tell the child, and the other may think it better that the child hear from them rather than run the danger of hearing it inadvertently from neighbors, siblings, peers, or hospital staff.

As has been observed regarding other illness, the position of the child in the family affects the parents' reaction to the child's condition. When parents' satisfactions spread over a number of children and daily demands for parental attention are multiple, catastrophe to one child usually is more bearable because the emotion is less intense. However, it has been observed that some children mean more or less to father or mother irrespective of place or number of other children. A hitherto happy toddler whose progress has brought joy to the family, a beautiful little girl, or a boy whose vigor has been his father's special pride does mean more than an unwanted child, expressing his rejection in whining behavior.

The Phenomenon of Denial

Denial, the first reaction to catastrophe, is an unconscious phenomenon often employed when pain is too great to bear; it prevents psychic collapse and is to this extent a constructive mechanism. Denial of a child's leukemia will depend on the parents' idea of the disease, how the situation is presented, and how ill he becomes. It ranges in degree from optimism that their child will be cured, to a pathological refusal to entertain the diagnosis. After initial treatment, the phenomenon is nourished by the child's renewed vigor. "I have to have hope or I couldn't live," one mother said. Some parents will not call the disease leukemia but use the word "anemia," and take comfort in an inner assurance of heavenly protection or in the hope that their child will be one of the few to receive a cure. One mother said she believed in God and therefore had to believe that her child would be one of the few cured; however, she felt guilty toward the other mothers, for if her child were spared, theirs could not be.

Denial may be easier for the father than the mother. She maintains a continuing relationship with the clinic or physician's office by taking the child to the doctor, and waits nervously for his screaming and then the report of his blood count. She watches him at home for symptoms, gives him his pills. The father may hold two jobs in order to make money toward the enormous expenses, and remains busy, exhausted, and away from home most of the time. The father who does not want to talk with the mother about the child's behavior or illness may increase her burden of loneliness.

Professional opinions differ on how to deal with a parent's denial. Because it prevents open communication and thus sharing and mutual support, some social workers intervene actively to prevent the use of this defense. They feel that realism is essential from the beginning in order that family and child can support each other through the difficult periods and especially the late stage, whenever it comes. Stress, as described in Chapter 2, is more severe if sudden. Dr. Binger tells of one child deprived of both parents' emotional support because each held to a pathological degree of denial; when the child lay dying he finally asked the parents to leave the room so he could die in peace.

However, defenses are generally respected, and no attempt is made to remove them until the person indicates he is ready to do so. Consequently, the person striving to help a family in which one or all members are using denial faces a dilemma. Dr. Binger suggests the worker can be guided by the extent of the denial and its pathology. She need not take part in the pretense but can permit the parent to hope. She should respond to any unrealistic suggestions in terms of understanding why the parents would want to think the way they do.

Informing the Child

At the conclusion of the diagnostic period, parents and professionals wonder *what, how, and when to tell the child.* Awareness of the diagnosis and its implications seems to come to most children of seven or eight years or older, and to many who are younger. In a study of 50 children with cancer, 42 of whom had leukemia, admitted to the City of Hope during the early 1960's, Morrissey reports that only one-third were suspicious of or aware of their prognosis. Two-thirds of the children made a good adjustment, correlated to the level of anxiety, as well as to effective parent participation. The older children were most likely to be aware of their diagnosis and subject to death anxiety. "Actually most or all of these children had considerable anxiety about the entire experience, with the exception of the very young child.... The younger children were primarily oriented to physical comfort and maternal security and support."[44]

The degree of insecurity that is acted out does not seem to vary widely whether the child has been officially told his diagnosis. Older and some young children hospitalized in pediatric or cancer research wards invariably pick up the threat of death to themselves from the outright communication of other children, the death of other children with the same illness, the furtive voices of nurses' aides outside the door, medical lectures at their bedside, the mother's red eyes, strained behavior, or hysterical weeping, the forced jollity of grandparents. It is difficult indeed for the hospitalized child, except the very young, not to know that he has something seriously wrong. When he goes home he sees television marathons on leukemia for fund raising, sees newspaper accounts of leukemic children having early Christmases, and receives presents his siblings do not receive. Some children are prayed for aloud in church or taken to prayer meetings for the laying on of hands.

Dr. Sigler at Johns Hopkins Hospital in Baltimore has advocated that children be told they have a chronic illness, usually called anemia, requiring numerous shots, pills, and possible transfusions, but "they are usually not told the diagnosis or their probable fate. This approach permits them to be realistic about their own limitations but never leads them to hopelessness or despondency."[45] Several persons have said that children's questions should be answered but not elaborated, nor should additional information be given, and that most children do not ask directly what is wrong with them. When a child at the U.C. Medical Center persists in asking the physician his diagnosis and its significance, the matter is discussed at length by the staff, and the decision made thoughtfully according to the individual child's situation. Drs. Solnit and Green, of Yale and Indiana universities, respectively, point out something that should not be taken lightly: "One of the most powerful fears is that which results from the prediction by an authoritative trusted person that one is going to die soon, before he has lived out his potential."[46]

Nonetheless, social workers have urged for many years that persons with cancer, including children, be told their diagnosis. Their reasons have included emotional responses—"He has the right to know; if it were I, I would want to know"—and the pragmatic reason that the patient suspects or will find out anyway and that pretense or deviousness isolates him from communication during the very time he is most in need of opportunity to share. Several instances have been quoted of children who have protected their parents, by pretending not to know, or who have told professional staff of their poignant but frustrated desire to talk with their parents about impending death.

In one case the father of a child who had died said the children should be made aware of the outlook, but gradually and a bit at a time, as warranted by the problem. However, in two cases known, the child pestered the parent, backing him into a corner about his condition until, exasperated and in an angry manner, the father told the child he had leukemia, and yes, he would likely die. In one of these, the child's schoolwork improved quickly. Where he had been a poor student, though intelligent, he now applied himself with great diligence, evidently hoping that he would live if he were a good boy. The long cultural heritage of the Western world equates catastrophe with punishment for wrongdoing. This feeling is very strong in young children.

Sigler points out that emphasizing death in relation to leukemia is not in consonance with its ever-increasing life span and the long interval many children have in complete remission. He believes children should not have a shadow thrown on them during the time they are well. The Children's Hospital at Stanford has a policy of complete sharing of diagnosis with all children, but places its main emphasis upon the need for the children to cooperate with the doctors who are working to help them, and on the "difference" between each child and the other children there who die. This institution does not regard leukemia as an incurable disease and therefore emphasizes hope.

Whether and what a child should be told about a disease that is still predominantly fatal would appear to depend on what seems likely to happen after he has been informed. This usually depends on the family's solidarity and usual pattern of communication. In the many families whose cohesion is tenuous and who are not meeting other stresses with great strength, it would seem preferable to leave the child with some hope that his suspicions are wrong. Families should not be forced into communication that is false to their mode, and the consequences of which they will be unable to handle.

Children with psychotic mothers, or with emotionally disorganized parents seen frequently by social workers, may be helped by substitute parents if this is carefully arranged. Psychiatric interviews or other scheduled opportunities may give the older child a chance to voice his anxieties and to receive support and renewed hope through his ordeals, and to ask questions that concern him most deeply. In the long run, communication of information as highly charged as that about death would seem to need the most careful individualization, with plans well in hand for dealing with the child's feelings after he has been told.

One social worker experienced in working with children with fatal illness says that children in jeopardy want most to know "What is it like to die?" In other words, fear of the dying process haunts children just as it does adults. This may well be due to realistic fears and also to the various pictorial symbolic representations of death. Asked what they think it is like, some children have a surprisingly simple and comforting answer for themselves, such as "I think it is like going to sleep."

Children's concepts of death have been investigated by child psychologists, who have found that they are age-related and linked to the children's evolving concept of life. Since children are incapable of abstract thinking until they are about eight years old, it is not surprising that children under five tend to think of death as reversible, a temporary separation. M. H. Nagy, the authority whose works from the 1940's are usually the basic source, described three stages in the child's ideas of death: the first as described above; the second occurring from about age five to nine. This stage is one in which death is personified: a figure who catches you. Since you may be able to elude him, your own death is remote and not inevitable. After about age nine, the adult conception of death takes shape, and the child understands that death is irreversible and inevitable.[47]

Dr. Binger points out that just because a child's concept of death is partial does not mean his anxiety is less intense.[48] The lengthening survival rate of children with leukemia places more of them in the age-group at death with more accurate concepts of its meaning. This may not mean that more children will suffer greater anxiety, but possibly that there will be a different form of anxiety. In fact, Schowalter says that it is at about age six that the fear of death first occurs, and the child is "horrified, confused, and angered by the discovery." He states, in regard to their questions:[49]

Seldom do they want to know the truth, but they are expressing their realization that they are very sick. Most children are content with an explanation of why they are feeling so bad and with reassurance they will be taken care of. If a child continually returns to his original question, he probably should be told, but what and by whom should first be discussed with his parents. No child should be told more than he asks, and hope must never be totally abolished.

All knowledgeable professionals emphasize the need for the adult to permit the child to ask questions, not to shut him off with false cheeriness or avoidance.

Realistically, the worker should keep in mind that neither she nor most of the professional persons with whom she works are able to bear the death of a child, which Schowalter calls "one of the outrages of nature."[50] A person who is so upset that he finds reason to avoid the child is destructive. Consequently, most agency workers' activity in this area will then be to search for the right person to visit the child regularly who can talk about death with him *if he wishes to talk,* and to sustain the parents so that they will be able to answer questions while assuring the child they will be there. In no instance should the worker inform the child he is going to die and force the issue of talking about it. The recent intense fascination with death shown by some professionals has led to crude, destructive incidents by persons who wanted to help but did not know how.

Financial Problems

Adding to the stress of the period of diagnosis and initial treatment but providing a channel for activity, which in turn helps drain off anxiety, is the need to secure funds for astronomical medical expenses. The board-and-room cost of hospitalization, expensive as it is, pales beside the cost of treatment drugs, spinal taps, and bone marrow punctures, radiation of the child's head, and in many instances blood transfusions. Insurance of the employed father and savings accounts are an immediate bulwark for working parents. In some states leukemia is an eligible diagnosis of the Crippled Children's Service, and when the agency has funds, it supplements family insurance and savings, providing they are financially eligible. Some states such as California provide Medicaid for families receiving public assistance and for a few others, subject to stringent pay-back provisions. The American Cancer Society and the leukemia associations vary according to locality in providing some financial aid for incidental expenses such as parents' board and room near the treatment center and transportation to the clinic.

An increasing phenomenon of the times is the plight of families whose income is too large to qualify them for financial assistance for food and shelter, but is insufficient for expensive medical care. Increasing governmental emphasis on saving taxes and decreasing emphasis on human services combine with the high cost of medical care to place such families in a desperate position. Bankruptcy or declaration of pauperism may become necessary, depending in part on the course of the illness. In cases that involve lengthy drug administration, repeated spinal punctures, complications requiring specialist consultation and/or hospitalization and transfusions, the family must decide on the lengths to which they will go to qualify for public welfare, in order to secure payment for medical care.

The total cost of care is greatly influenced by the cost of blood transfusions. Ordinarily, the need for repeated transfusions arises not in the onset period but late in the child's illness, when the amount of drugs is stepped up to combat the advance of leukemia.[51] However, they are a significant part of the total financial burden. When blood is replaced by donors, the handling costs remain, but are substantially less (at this writing, in this locality, $15 per transfusion as against $65). The family may replace blood by securing a wide pool of donors. Relatives or friends can give blood locally and credit the bank in the area where the child lives. Platelet transfusions may be given twice a week over an extended period by relatives in centers that have equipment permitting return of red cells to the donor. Some children need only a few transfusions; others may need up to 1,000 units of blood (platelets).

Church groups, unions, other employee groups, service clubs are frequently mobilized. If families do not belong to groups, some may choose to advertise their need in the newspapers. Some parents faced with finding a hundred or more donors may do so without help. Others, overwhelmed with the sick child's need and their own anxiety and lack of sleep, the problems of other children at home, and other stresses, may greatly need assistance with the community organizing necessary to secure large numbers of donors. If advertising is resorted to, or service clubs make a project of the child's need for blood, advance thought should be given to preventing photographers and press write-ups from frightening the child and embarrassing the family. (A child who reads in the newspaper that he is soon going to die receives deep and unnecessary trauma.) Letters must be screened if the child's situation has been publicized in the newspapers. He receives letters from strangers, religious pamphlets, and letters from fanatics or disturbed persons that upset him.

The Family and the First Remission

The child who achieves complete remission often comes home from the hospital looking well, and full of vigor. However, one mother told a social worker she felt as if she were bringing home a new baby. She felt she wanted to put her son in a glass cage; she had to stifle the urge to get up twice a night to make sure he was still breathing. The debts, the child's loss of hair, the daily pills, the weekly or biweekly clinic visits for spinal taps, blood and bone marrow tests, remain to remind him and his parents of the storm he has been through. However, "no man can sustain a grand emotion." The intensity of fear gradually attenuates, the pills and clinic trips are incorporated into routine in most cases, and children's fortunate absorption in the present makes the future seem far away and unreal.

During this period of relative relief from acute stress, potential problems remain, depending upon parental temperaments and family circumstances. In the absence of studies, but from interviews, case records, and the experiences of hospital social workers and other staff, parents' recurring problems seem to include the use of denial as a defense, how to discipline the child, excessive gift giving, and sibling and extended family relationships. Anxiety and loneliness may also occur during this period. These problems become more severe if the child has complications or relapses and begins a long downhill course.

Those who work with leukemic children and their parents agree that remission is a period when parents by and large want to escape discussion of the gloomy implications of the disease. Some parents hurry by the hospital offices as if afraid the hospital worker will open the subject, or they are "too busy" to talk, unless about finances or transportation. One experienced social worker said that she takes her cue from the mother's irritability and hostility. If the mother begins to express a number of negative feelings about a variety of subjects, the worker senses that she is worried about the child—that symptoms have begun that are breaking down her defenses. An opening to talk about the child's condition, and how he is getting along, may permit the parent to pour forth her worries, and the defense comes down of itself.

Gift giving seems a universal response to knowledge that a child has a life-threatening illness. Parents need to give to the child, as much as they possibly can, in special recreation and in toys. One father voiced the common reaction, after his child's death. "We just did everything—went to Disneyland, to ball games, to San Francisco to ride the cable cars, went fishing, and Johnny just had a ball. He loved every minute." Parents justifiably want to enrich the quality of the child's life if it likely will be brief. The parent who receives public assistance or who barely survives financially feels special bitterness when his circumstances force him to deprive the child of what he wants to give. One mother on public welfare hated the world because she had not been able to afford a Christmas tree, which the child wanted, the last Christmas of his life. (One wonders where the social worker was.)

This need to give should not be discouraged, but balance is necessary. Receipt of bounteous gifts of toys and baskets of mail confirm to the child that he is ill indeed; he is further set apart, more alone. When the family has other children, the sick child can become spoiled and arrogant, and the other children deprived and resentful. A moderate course consists of special events on weekends and especially generous birthdays and Christmases.

Discipline is a recurring theme in parents' comments about problems in living with leukemia. One mother said, "It's almost impossible to bring myself to punish him." The physician has told the parents, "Treat him normally"; at the same time, he has cautioned the mother to watch for symptoms and bring the child back immediately if he begins to develop bruises, if small red dots show up on any part of his body, if he acts lethargic, if he is not eating properly, if he is not playing as much as usual, if he acts drowsy, if he feels warm and feverish, if he sleeps a lot, etc. As one experienced nurse said, "We put the families in a double bind." No wonder the mother cannot bring herself to punish the child to whom she is administering eight or ten pills a day, and whom she must watch so carefully. Yet the area can be one of disagreement between parents, with the father insisting "The hospital said he must be treated normally," and the mother highly protective.

Nutrition is a related problem. Dr. Pinkel points out that malnutrition is a major problem during drug treatment, predisposing the child to hazards from infection and side effects from the drugs. Yet parents tend to let the child have what pleases him—cookies, soft drinks, potato chips, etc.—instead of insisting on nutritious foods. If malnutrition continues despite dietary counseling and food supplements, the drug dosage must be reduced until appetite improves and better nutrition is established.[52]

As in hemophilia, danger of bleeding from trauma is always present, though less so if the platelet count is known to be good at the time. This complicates methods of punishment, and also management of the fights that are part of small boys' relationships with peers and siblings. The child should not be kicked. Neither should he be belted with a strap, or slapped hard across the face. Parents who treat siblings in this manner, but "let Johnny get away with murder" in the eyes of his brothers and sisters, make him feel special in a frightening way. One mother said that since their child's diagnosis, and later their realization of their unfairness to the other children, she and her husband had compromised on the discipline of all the children. They swatted Johnny like the rest, but eased up on hitting all of them.

Sibling Relationships

The relationships with siblings are especially affected if they feel the parents are unfair, holding them accountable for their misdeeds but not the sick child. One family told of their decision to inform an older sibling of the child's diagnosis because he had grown so resentful of the preferred treatment given the leukemic child. After he knew the reason, he too became protective of his younger brother.

All children know there is something seriously wrong when their parents' eyes are red from crying, when the sick child is treated suddenly with great consideration and tenderness, and when there is a terrible air of constraint in the home. No solid data exist about how to minimize damage to siblings, but children old enough to understand would seem to profit by overt mention that the ill sibling has a serious medical problem, and by willingness to include them in the family tragedy. One seasoned social worker believes that siblings gain assurance that they too will receive special attention if they ever need it, by seeing how the parents respond to the illness of one child in the family.

Very serious personality disturbances have been reported among siblings after a child's death.[53] That they are neglected by the mother is inevitable during the period she is engrossed in anguish, in duties that take her away from home, and in the multiple financial and other practical problems leukemia brings. The ages of siblings obviously influence the effect of separations from their mother, and also the extent to which they appropriately may be included in intellectual understanding of what is happening to the ill child. One father said that as soon as the doctors told him the diagnosis, he asked the priest to come to the house for a family conference in which all children were present: at the time they were told that Johnny had a serious disease from which he might not recover. The mother thought it essential that the other children understand from the beginning what was going on. This family was satisfied they did the right thing. Other parents have said they told the older children but not the younger.

One couple whose child had died called in their teenage boy during conference with me. They had said previously they did not tell him his sister's diagnosis for fear that during a quarrel he would taunt her that she was going to die. His father asked him if he felt this had been the right thing to do. The boy answered in a slow, troubled voice that his parents had done right in protecting him from himself; that he might have yielded to an angry impulse to say something cruel to his little sister. Despite his affirmation, his manner gave the impression that he was burdened by the lack of trust that had been shown in him. In another case the mother said she tried to tell the boy's adolescent sister, but a veil came down over the girl's eyes every time the mother broached the boy's serious illness. The mother concluded the girl did not want to hear. The resentful girl, guilty later over the hate she felt for the intense relationship she saw between her mother and brother, said, "But why didn't you tell me?" The mother said she had tried, but in vain. Sibling rivalries probably had existed before the boy's illness, or the girl filtered what she saw through adolescent hatred for her mother. Now, after the boy's death, this family was more alienated than ever.

Adjustments and Anxieties of the Child

The young child's inability to articulate his feelings, the changing nature of leukemia's course, and professional avoidance of doomed individuals probably account for the paucity of recorded information on the meaning to the child of his experience with leukemia. Studies doubtless will be reported within the next few years of the reactions of children in long remission and those who receive "cures." Meanwhile, experience and observation indicate that the effects on the child depend primarily on the course and medical treatment of the disease, parental capacity to provide emotional support, and the child's age. The uniqueness of any child's experience also depends on his constitutional sensitivity to experience, and the geographic, financial, cultural, and marital status of his parents.

When the hitherto healthy small child becomes very tired and subject to nosebleeds, has difficulty breathing, experiences bone pain and general malaise, he undergoes the additionally frightening experience of painful and intrusive procedures at the hands of professional adults, which take place with his parents' encouragement or acquiescence. He is then separated from the parents, placed in a strange environment, and subjected to further bewilderment and painful treatment. "When the child, during the first three years, becomes sick, he feels anger at the parents for failing to protect him and experiences a fear that he will be abandoned.... Death anxiety and separation anxiety remain juxtaposed at all ages, but their fusion is greatest while the organism is youngest and most dependent," says Schowalter,[54] a psychiatrist whose comments on loss and grief are recommended to all who are interested in children's reactions to serious threat.

The well-known trauma of separation from parents is most terrifying for children under three, but becomes mixed with fantasies of punishment for wrongdoing as he grows older. The child by then is capable of realizing he can be safe under the care of others. Kubler-Ross, a specialist on the dying, quotes child behavior experts as saying that fears of mutilation are especially strong in the older preschool child.[55]

The worker's most helpful contribution to the preschool child is to assist as necessary in making possible the mother's stay at or near the hospital during his hospitalization for diagnosis and beginning treatment. The parents may most need assistance at this time because of their stunned and overwhelmed reactions and the haste with which they have to make arrangements for other children, work responsibilities, etc.

Accounts of the meaning of hospitalization to children point out the frequency of changed behavior after return home.[56] Thus it is not unique to leukemia that the child returns home from diagnostic tests and initial induction changed in some ways. The torment he has been through, mental and physical, and the questions and fear that have been aroused not infrequently leave him quiet, withdrawn, somber, and older than his years. He sometimes is seemingly indifferent to his parents and siblings. One child who had been especially close to a sibling one year older would not speak to him for several days, and never kissed him again, the mother reported, though he had been very affectionate before then. Or the child may be unwilling to let the mother out of his sight for a time. In several instances, mothers have commented that the return clinic visits also leave the child quiet for a few days.

Dr. Burgert of the Mayo Clinic writes that in 23 years of working with leukemic children he has seen them display many different reactions: anger, fear, depression, anxiety, isolation, and also acceptance and hope.[57] Children are also seen to display insecurity and irritability, and some take an unusual interest in the mysteries of science or religion. As time elapses, they continue to seem older than their age; yet as children, they live for the day.

Manifestations of anxiety and insecurity may occur at any time throughout the illness, and are influenced by factors other than the illness, such as parental fighting or separation, the father's loss of employment or alcoholism, sibling hostility, school failure, etc. Though no record exists of children's reactions to the appearance of *petechiae* (the little bright red dots indicating skin hemorrhage), bruises, and resurgence of pain, it is obvious that the mother's frightened response to these indications of recurrence must set off fright in the child; blood and bleeding create revulsion and horror in many persons. Thus the effect of the illness upon the child's personal adjustment becomes more profound if the child has relapses or complications that bring frightening experiences, disruptions in school, and rehospitalizations for nauseous and injected drug induction and transfusions. The premature aging of these children becomes more apparent. "They remind me of little old men," one hospital social worker said of the seriously ill children on the ward, and "They have to grow up fast," commented another.

Night is a time when fear takes hold. At home, between periods of acute illness, the child may hesitate to go to bed, reluctant to face the dark, making excuses to get up, stay up, or to ask a question, or to sit on his father's lap to watch television. Several mothers have told of school-age children unable to sleep who crawl into bed with them. This need for closeness can create a problem when children sleep between father and mother for any protracted period. Yet the need for closeness should be met as much as possible, for protection by the parent and faith in the doctor are the only strength the child has when he fears that death may be near.

Leukemic children have been observed to have abnormal concern for other persons or pets who are under threat. Seeing the Apollo astronauts safely down and rescued from the water was so imperative to one child that he refused to go to school until he saw the rescue completed on television. Similar intensity of interest in the astronauts' safety was expressed by another school-age leukemic child. Deep concern for other children in the hospital, and for their own pets, has been observed or reported from several sources.

Two mothers have said that their leukemic children experienced terrible anxiety over the death of a pet. One said that her boy, like many children, placed his entire hope in the physician. When the kitten lay dying, the child frantically urged calling the veterinary. He ran for his piggy bank and said, "Take my money and pay the vet to save the kitty." Although the kitten manifestly was already dead or *in extremis*, this wise mother took the cat, dead on arrival, to the veterinary. A ritual is surely called for in mourning for a pet.

Anxiety can be channeled into constructive activity if strong support is given and outlets secured. Excerpts follow from a newspaper account of how one adolescent was helped to sustain a full life during remission and into the terminal period:[58]

> Glen Berendes died Monday of leukemia, one badge short of his Eagle rank. He was confined to a wheelchair and finally a hospital bed but still continued to study and pass the merit badge tests. Only last week he completed work on his coin badge and changed his last requirement from fishing to fingerprinting because he was no longer able to leave Children's Hospital at Stanford.
>
> Berendes served Troop 600 as senior patrol leader. During his periods of hospital confinement, the youth began to help his sickroom companions. He led a neighborhood toy gathering and repair effort and hauled a truckload of toys to his hospital friends. He climbed out of bed to direct 16 fellow Scouts in planting 30,000 square feet of ice plant at the hospital.
>
> "He set the most unbelievable standard of courage I've seen in years of Scouting," said Rollen Avey, a troop committee member who often helped the youth in his projects.

The help of the "troop committee member," played down in the account, obviously was great. The projects described required substantial time and organization, in addition to encouragement. That the help was given by a volunteer highlights the potential services that can be performed.

School entrance and adolescence are the times when loss of hair from irradiation or medication seems most catastrophic to the child, since he is most vulnerable to peer acceptance at these times. Hair comes out suddenly in clumps, an outward and inescapable sign that something abnormal is going on. Though the hair grows back in, it does so slowly, unevenly, and with a different texture. The schoolchild sees himself in the mirror as a strange child, someone others will tease. He has been set apart as different. He may wear a wig, or one of an assortment of happy-looking hats or visored caps, but as he sits in school with his hat on, or in his wig, he knows other children may try to grab it off to see what he really looks like and that they will ask questions. The child who can say, "I had radiation when I was sick," and who can show a friend or two what he looks like without his cap, has overcome the worst of the hurdles about hair. The teacher or the principal probably knows what peers are usual troublemakers, and may talk with them privately, if asked to help. But even when hair problems at school have been overcome, the sensitive child sees his baldness as a continuing reminder of the illness that hangs over him. One mother described her children's happy shouts when grandparents drove in from a distance. The other children ran out to greet them; the leukemic child started with the others, stopped, ran back for his hat, put it on, started again, but then fled to the bedroom to cry.

The deep need to have friends and be one with peers is subtly cheated if neighbor mothers cool their relationships with the parents, and suddenly find that their own children's schedule demands a different playtime than before. Often it is difficult for the mother to know for certain whether the excuse for loss of neighborliness is real. The publicity given to virus as a cause of leukemia in mice has made many parents afraid. Sometimes the child's best friend moves; sometimes he switches to another "lane" in school; sometimes he has to practice or do his homework after school. One leukemic child was so excited when he made a new friend who was able to spend the night that he vomited.

Adolescents have a special problem with any manifestation that makes them different from their peers. A study of 182 adolescents with malignancies, 81 of whom had leukemia, at St. Jude's Hosital in Memphis, reports: "For both boys and girls, the loss of hair is a singularly distressing occurrence which immediately and obviously marks them as 'different,' Alopecia [baldness] ... to many adolescents is more bothersome than is his disease. To the girls it means loss of attractiveness and femininity; to the boys it signifies loss of sex appeal and virility."[59] These authors say that when an adolescent first learns his diagnosis, his immediate concern is not "Will I die?" but "How will this disease make me different?"

School

School is vital to children old enough to attend. Doing what everyone else does symbolizes normality. It further signifies that there will be a future, for which the child must prepare himself. Not only is school the major channel for social contacts and interests, but successful competition with peers determines self-esteem. Some parents react to a child's leukemia illness by thinking, "What difference does it make, if he is going to die? Why make him go to school, when he doesn't want to? Why not just let him stay home and enjoy himself?" The answer is obvious; he will not enjoy himself, brooding about the house alone when his peers are in school, his difference magnified.

There are obstacles to regular attendance and to successful competition. During the early part of remission, the child may still receive biweekly spinal injections and bone marrow punctures to monitor the leukemic process in the marrow. Children who attend distant clinics may be away for half a day or more each time. The child may for a long period receive weekly medication that nauseates him the next day. He needs to be guarded diligently against infection during the times his platelet count is low, which means keeping him away from other children during the many winter and spring periods when respiratory infections or childhood infectious diseases are frequent. Basketball games, auditorium events, and other large gatherings of children are hazardous sources of infection. Because of the danger of hemorrhage, he should not be kicked or jumped on. If he eventually becomes weak and miserable with bone pain, he may not be able to walk to school, go out at recess, or sit in class for a full session.

Psychological management at school also poses problems. If teachers do not fully understand the disease and its treatment, they may think the child is malingering, and resent the absences and interruptions. If they have been told the child's diagnosis, it may be difficult for them to treat the child normally. Some echoes of children's reactions to psychological problems at school have been heard in such statements as "All the kids knew, and they treated me as if I was already dead," or in expressions of strong feelings that they did not want the teacher or anyone else to know their disease. The St. Jude's study of adolescents reports that the young people went to great lengths to conceal their disease.[60]

Despite some hazards—such as the trauma and danger of infection—from school attendance, physicians recommend it because of the psychological gains. During well-established remissions when the platelet count remains stable, participation in strenuous sports is permitted. Individual schoolteachers are known to have provided thoughtful opportunities for children to attend school as long as possible, and for interrupted periods or partial sessions. Small children, shy over baldness or entering class late or sporadically, have been made to feel welcome. The tactful teacher can do much to prevent cruelty from other children, who have been known to grab the child's wig, or taunt, "You've got leukemia. You're going to die."

The school environment deserves almost as much social work attention as the home, when the child is school age. Some schools resist the child's attendance. In some cases, families of other children are afraid he will infect their children and, as one very good teacher said, "Any sick child is, frankly, a nuisance." Some mothers who are functioning adequately can communicate directly with the teacher or principal, with the help of a letter from the physician. Mothers who are distraught, disorganized, preoccupied, or unaccustomed to reaching out may need assistance if the school hesitates to permit the child's attendance.

The school social worker is the best person to acquaint an outsider with the personalities and relationships of the inner world of the school system. If there is no school social worker, the school nurse may be the best person to approach, since she will need to secure the physician's recommendations for first aid when nosebleeds, nausea, or other physical problems arise, and the nurse will be consulted by the principal and the teacher when they have doubts about the physical condition of the child. In schools that have trimmed off the "luxuries" of school counselors and nurses for lack of tax support, the principal is the person to approach. Conferences that include the teacher should be arranged, with sufficient opportunity for her to feel assured that she can manage and that she knows what to do if emergencies arise. Continuing contact with the teacher would appear to offer mutual assistance. Home teachers are not adequate substitutes for regular class attendance, but they are helpful adjuncts during interim periods when the child must stay home because of malaise or threat of infection; difference from peers becomes more disturbing and pronounced if the child is behind in his classwork.

The Family and the Early Terminal Stage

The "new" treatment, we are assured, will not permit a long downhill course, with its erosion of family life, since many of the children who have had multiple, simultaneous, heavy drug therapy and radiation at the beginning will die swiftly when the long remission ends. For many children who have not been treated with "total therapy" at onset, however, relapse signals the beginning of a downhill process. Shorter intervals of remission occur after each reinduction, with longer and more painful periods of illness and massive treatment.[61] The family can no longer thrust aside the anticipated loss of the child, and the crisis reactivates. Living with leukemia gradually merges into dying with it. One family described the period as an "emotional roller coaster." The Stanford pediatrics social work staff describes the entire experience with leukemia as "the siege." They caution families to conserve their energies, and to avoid making major decisions or changes while undergoing the battle, which becomes intense as the child starts downhill.

The worker in the community shares with hospital staff three goals for the family during the child's early terminal stage: first, prevention of the child's abandonment; second, help in coping with the many practical problems that compound stress; and third (and closely related to practical problems), the maintenance of maximum quality of family life during this period of extremity.

Abandonment. Psychologic or physical abandonment is the most serious possible threat to the child, particularly because the majority are young children to whom separation from parents is the deepest anxiety. The danger arises in part because mourning begins when loss of a loved one is anticipated. "Anticipatory grief" may result in premature feelings of actual bereavement; the parent's pain may be so great that he must separate himself emotionally from the child. Peretz says it well: "Acute grief may deprive both the dying patient and the bereaved-to-be of the possibilities still remaining in their relationship."[62] Aggravating the danger of premature bereavement, and thus psychological separation from the child, is the child's altered appearance and behavior. Swollen from steroid treatment, hair still scanty, lame from bone pain, lethargic, withdrawn, and eyes reproachful, the child does not resemble the vigorous person the parents remember. Still later, if he becomes bloated, bleeding, and tortured, he is only a caricature of himself.

Emotionally exhausted from rising hope during improvement and despair during relapses, the parent not infrequently wishes it was over, while the child still lives and increasingly needs parental love and protection. Depending upon the rapidity and nature of the child's dying, the parents may fervently want death to come. Psychological abandonment expresses itself in excuses to avoid visiting the child while he is in the hospital or, when there, by wandering around visiting other children or, with other parents, staying out of the child's room. In actuality, many reasons do exist why hospital visiting, if over a prolonged period, becomes very difficult. Earning a living, preparing meals, doing laundry, caring for other children must go on, and both physical strength and financial resources do dwindle or come to an end.

Practical problems. Help with the many practical problems of the family (which have been discussed chiefly under "Financial Problems," above) is a concrete way of bolstering the parents through the "siege." This help provides tangible evidence of caring, which is itself emotional support. Shared burdens are lighter, as sophisticated psychological explanations prove and folk wisdom has always known. Lessened pain means lessened danger of emotional exhaustion and premature separation from the child.

Helping the child remain at home as long as possible and minimizing the length of hospitalization do not ensure that the child will not be abandoned emotionally, but they eliminate some of the obstacles and make the greatest possible contribution to the quality of the child's life. Home care requires time-consuming, patient, and detailed liaison service to ensure adequate medical and nursing supervision in a makeshift setting.

Among the more urgent requirements are measures to minimize chances of infection. Restrictions on social activities of siblings, to reduce their exposure to crowds, colds, and chickenpox, may be hard to enforce. Some families have found their friends and relatives helpful in providing overnight stays, vacations, and outings for siblings. In families receiving assistance or on a marginal income, fuel, bedding, food, and decent shelter for the entire family may be the most difficult items to provide, a situation that tempts the social worker to urge hospitalization for the sick child as an easier solution. In some families, pride, or habituation to a very low standard of living, may make the mother unable to itemize what she needs. The public health nurse then becomes the key figure in assessing what the child needs to maintain optimum protection against infection in the home.

Private health agencies not infrequently have "patient care" funds from which equipment and special allowances can be authorized. And if repeated hospital stays and multiple blood transfusions exhaust the family's insurance provisions and savings, Crippled Children's Services or Medicaid applications may become necessary if they have not been earlier. All such agency referrals should be preceded by telephone inquiry regarding both probable acceptance and any documents needed for proof of eligibility. In any event, close cooperation between health and welfare agencies—an obvious necessity in these cases—may require substantial outreach by one agency to the other.

Transportation is one of the most difficult of the family's problems, especially where frequent trips must be made to medical centers located in urban areas poorly served by public transportation and inadequately equipped with parking space. A patient search for transportation facilities by telephoning community agencies, church and club groups may be necessary in behalf of parents with limited emotional or financial resources. In some communities, informal organizations provide the backbone of help to the very poor; in others, organized agencies such as the Cancer Society and the Red Cross help provide transportation for families of children with leukemia.

A television set is essential for both child and mother. This avenue for escape into an artificial but multifold social life is the most practical in American urban life. The worker should be alert to whether the family TV is in working order. Some clubs provide such items quickly, though the publicity sometimes attending club-funding drives may itself pose problems.

The increased survival times made possible by modern treatment place more leukemic children in school age before the end of their course. In such cases, provision for the child's partial school attendance affords the mother some respite, an opportunity to go to the store, the beauty parlor, etc. Other opportunities for the mother's escape from worry are sometimes provided by other parents, through cooperative sitting arrangements, or by parents of children who have died.

Quality of life. This third goal for the family is achieved in part by the alleviation of stresses, as we have seen; other contributions are the presence and emotional support of other persons, family closeness, and, for some persons, religion. The parents particularly need extended family and church as sources of support. Mexican American families and others whose culture includes closeness of extended family are fortunate. However, the urban mother who lives in an apartment where she knows few neighbors and who has no relatives in the community is especially lonely. In intact families where the father works and the mother stays home, her confinement to the dwelling provides little opportunity to share or channel her daily anxieties. Brooding without outlet during the day bottles up feelings and magnifies real or imagined changes in the child's appearance or behavior.

Some negative influences are integral to extended family relationships. Some parents have complained of the painful necessity of repeating to all the interested relatives the physician's latest reports, how the child is feeling, etc. Grandparents of the leukemic child may disagree with the medical treatment, what and how much to tell the child, or the manner in which the mother supervises the child. Grandparents may aggravate sibling rivalries by spoiling the ill child and plying him with gifts. The dormant or overt dislike between the mother and her own mother, or between in-laws and one parent, may blossom into feuds when such highly charged emotions are part of the constellation.

Three studies report relationships with grandparents as disappointing or difficult in a significant number of cases. Bozeman reports that only three of 14 maternal grandmothers gave emotional support to the mothers.[63] Friedman et al. find that the grandparents tended to question or disbelieve the diagnosis and to distort reality.[64] Binger et al. report that in ten of 20 families interviewed, one or both sets of grandparents were a burden or hindrance.[65] The problem that grandparents have in accepting the loss of a grandchild is illuminated by Peretz's discussion of loss. "Infancy and childhood are particularly vulnerable times for loss to occur. *Old age*, when defensive and adaptive skills are often diminished, is another time when loss which would otherwise appear surmountable may overwhelm the psychic apparatus."[66]

Nevertheless, extended family, including grandparents, often provide care of other children, help with errands, and frequently are essential sources of emotional support for siblings as well as parents. The social worker should be aware of the significant members of the extended family and become acquainted with them if feasible as she explores potential strengths in the family constellation. If a grandparent is actively involved with family life, she or he should attend the clinic with the mother and child and sit in on family conferences with the physician. This lessens the grandparents' frustrations over not knowing what is going on.[67]

Small church congregations or large churches with assistant pastors who specialize in counseling and pastoral visiting serve as extended family for many who do not have relatives in the geographical area. Church friends, however, tend to fall away if the parents do not attend church and church social activities over a period of time. Church attendance obviously is difficult or impossible when the child is in relapse or near death. The pastor can rekindle the interest of the congregation if it has flagged.

Religion itself may or may not be a source of strength, probably depending on two factors. First is the firmness of religious strength and second is the nature of the religious belief. Someone has said that most persons cultivate only a weak reed but at the end expect a strong oak. Crisis, when the personality is jarred and man reaches for a new means of coping, offers opportunity for spiritual growth if resources are available. Religion often means more to persons who are suffering than many healthy intellectuals appreciate. However, religious doctrines differ in the amount of comfort they offer at a time of anticipated loss. In some, redemption can be secured in a few minutes of repentance, and in others, earned only by a lifetime of effort. Some doctrines hold out life after death, and others do not. The most dangerous and seemingly frequent pitfall is reliance on prayer to achieve bodily protection. It is this concept that is shattered when the child's course is downhill and death ensues, often resulting in bitterness and loss of faith in God. Another dangerous form of religion is one with heavy emphasis upon punishment for sins.

The worker obviously should not provide religious counseling or impose her own beliefs. It is helpful, however, to invite discussion in order to learn what the parents believe or half-believe or may be worrying about. If feelings of guilt or punishment or expectations of a miracle are revealed, the worker should so inform the clergyman if there is one, or seek out clergy of the parents' background with the time and capacity to give guidance and the emotional support that accompanies it. All clergy are not comfortable about fatal illness, just as all physicians are not. Usually the Council of Churches staff know who are most helpful to grief-stricken families and will provide the worker with information about clergy if asked.

In cases where the worker herself is the main source of emotional support, she may worry, "What can I say?" Listening is more helpful than philosophizing; physical presence is more comforting than words. It is essential to reinforce hope, as contrasted with denial. Experts point out that the focus for hope narrows as the child's condition worsens. The parents may no longer hope the child will survive, but may hope he can come home from the hospital, or that he can become strong enough to have the visiting teacher again, or even that his headache will go away or his fever come down or his appetite improve. Parents have repeatedly said they live from day to day. If the parents are to convey some hope to the child, they must have something to hope for themselves, however small it may seem, and this needs to be echoed and reinforced by the worker.

Family closeness, another asset to be encouraged, is not achieved in the majority of cases, if the Stanford and University of California Medical Center experiences are any indication. However, notable family strength exists in some instances. How closely related this may be to verbal communication is not known; certainly shared tenderness toward each other and the child, compatible attitudes toward essentials, and respect for the needs of siblings are necessary. These depend on the accident of mutual emotional maturity in the parents, and may possibly vary in different geographical areas where subcultural differences support family life. One study, in which the parents were from intact families and at least moderate socioeconomic status, showed that the major source of emotional support to each parent came from the spouse.[68]

Great help comes from parents of other children suffering from leukemia, according to several observers. One source points out that parents fear they will go to pieces when the end comes, but that when they observe other parents who do not break down, their fears diminish. Even in outpatient clinic, friendships form between mothers whose sympathetic comprehension surpasses all others when a platelet count is reported or hospitalization is or is not recommended.

The Dying Child

A nursing doctoral student whose dissertation was based on psychological tests with fatally ill children found that some of their stories and interpretations of pictures showed not only preoccupation with death but feelings that nobody cared.[69] One girl told a story about the child in a picture who was dying but when she got to heaven God did not care. Because indirection is often used by children to express deep feeling, thoughtfulness is required in demonstrations of concern, not only for the child but for the objects of his projection. When he is hospitalized, the detachment and objectivity of the staff too frequently merge into psychologic abandonment as the child defeats their efforts at cure and lapses into the dying process. When he is at home, he sees less of his classmates and former friends. An assessment of his problem with respect to loneliness, as well as his mother's problem, is part of the reevaluation required by a change in the child's medical condition.

Securing visits from peers or adults is a difficult task. The awkwardness people feel about what to say contributes to a serious problem of loneliness and feeling of abandonment. Teachers may have their classes write letters to the house-bound child, and the home teacher's visits break the monotony. Assignment of schoolwork is a token that he is expected to return to normal. The social worker's visits and those she can stimulate from volunteers should not be addressed to the mother alone but to the child as well. A dog seems of great assistance. Pets of all kinds afford interests—something little that needs protection and care and that returns love and reassurance. Television personalities of daily shows provide substitute friends. "It's time for Jim (or Walter or Lucy) to come on" is the house-bound's visit from a friend.

The effect of religion upon the child's mental state is variable. School-age children not infrequently find religion boring. Little children may fear an all-knowing God as someone who knows what they did wrong and therefore is a punishing being. The kind of religious teaching, if any, the child has had will affect his concepts. Because children as well as adults can fear hellfire or devils, the area should be explored if feasible, to see what the child believes. In some instances, little children have expressed comfort—"I am going to Heaven, to be with Jesus"—and some adolescents have profound and deeply religious feelings about afterlife or continuity of spirit.

The last hospitalization may be long or short. The child may incur a raging infection that terminates his life within 24 hours; some children die quickly from a brain hemorrhage, or lapse into a toxic coma. One experienced nurse described the differing modes of dying as dependent in large part on whether death comes as the result of the disease or of chemotherapy during an attempted reinduction of remission. She described the relatively peaceful death of a child whose pain can be kept under control by sedation and who may die of slow internal bleeding, in contrast to one with two or three weeks of violent vomiting as a result of chemotherapy.

The terminal experience has been described as "hell" for many. Binger et al. report that 19 out of 20 parents interviewed after the death of their children felt they should have been more prepared for the end.[70] Possibly they could have given a greater degree of support to the child had they had time to incorporate some degree of dread before the terminal experience. However, the physician's difficulty in preparing a family for an experience so highly variable can be appreciated. Solnit and Green point out the difficulty of securing data about the communications and thus the needs of dying children. "It appears that adults fear the shattering impact if they allow themselves to see, hear, and regard the dying child's behavior."[71] However, all the evidence points toward the child's need to know that he has not been abandoned, and that someone will be there with him.

In a rare description of a dying child's last hours, Elizabeth Diaz, a hospital child-care worker, told of her activities with Anne, a four-year-old child with leukemia.[72]

I had once watched a dying leukemic child who had known what was coming the weeks and days before his death. The dilated pupils and strangely high-pitched voice had indelibly imprinted on my mind the terror that knowledge of death can bring to a seven-year-old child. Anne showed some of the same type of terror in her frantic cry for the play lady, "Me want somebody to stay with me," even a few weeks before her death.... Her hysterical screaming for her overburdened mother was another manifestation.

In this case Miss Diaz says the social worker "made a brief appearance" and brought the mother, who left after a short time. The play lady then remained, helping to wipe the blood from the child's mouth as she coughed, and continuing to tell her about Cinderella and hold her hand until she died.

"There is a strong need in most of us to flee from the reality of death," Peretz says,[73] which may account for the social worker's "brief appearance" even though she knew the mother could not (emotionally) remain with the child. Most staff reports agree that dying children tend to be placed at the far end of the hall in a private room and ignored as much as possible by all the staff; this corresponds with my own experience.

The warmth and comforting presence of his mother, or in some cases father, seems to be far the most important source of help to the dying child. One hospital social worker points out the need to anticipate the mother's exhaustion during the long process of death, and how helpful it is to arrange a substitute sitter for part of the time and to encourage the mother to go out for a break—or even just to lie down or walk around. Relatives who are caring for the other children at home may be able to relieve the mother for short periods, if this has been anticipated and worked out in advance.

Anticipation of the mother's ordeal and arrangements for her support can include arrangements with her doctor for the use of tranquilizers. One social worker says that she supports the mother in doing whatever the mother prefers; if she cannot bear to stay with the child, she supports her in leaving. It would appear that if this seems essential because no means of strengthening her is available, arrangements could be made for a substitute to stay with the child. At Stanford Hospital, a priest volunteered to stay with children whose parents abandoned them or whose parents could endure only short intervals of remaining at the child's bedside. Volunteers have been helpful in relieving the mother.

In mourning, part of the working out of grief consists in going back over every detail, again and again, and asking oneself whether one should have done more or acted differently. Surely the mother's mourning process is eased if she has been sustained and encouraged to stay with the child who screamed for her, instead of walking out because she could not endure the child's ordeal. Binger et al. report the anger some parents express against hospital staff for the treatment the child received at the end of his life.[74] They point out that this behavior reflects pain, not an insult to the staff. Conversion of terrible pain into irrational anger is indeed common, but it is also true that hospital care of a very ill person may include some painful procedures, occasionally performed from ineptitude but usually in an effort to prolong survival.

Arranging for the child's death at home is worked out in some cases, where the physician is willing to visit frequently and a nurse specialist can either teach a public health nurse or go herself to the home. Evaluation of psychological strengths and physical resources must precede such a plan, and the family must know that immediate hospital admission can be secured if they are not able to care for the child. They must also have complete confidence that the physician will come if an emergency arises. Home deaths have been described as infinitely more comfortable for the child, and as yielding growth experiences of great magnitude for the parents. The mourning process is said to include positive feelings that the child was a special child, who gave the family a unique gift of spiritual strength through courage shown and closeness developed. Families who can provide for a child's death at home obviously must be carefully selected and well located for convenient visiting of the physician and nurses.

The effect on siblings of a child's death at home is not known. The sibling's maturity and sense of being part of the family plan, and his ability to help, would be factors to consider. The availability of relatives or friends to care for siblings during unusually painful episodes would also need consideration.

The destructive effect of a child's death on family life is otherwise well documented, though the elements that make it thus have not been sorted out. Compassionate evaluation and carefully thought-out plans to minimize trauma and stresses for each family member would appear to lessen the wake of negative reactions. The social worker in the community can be a substantial source of help in the evaluations necessary, in finding resources to minimize concurrent stresses, in providing support to the mother by helping her to stay with the child, in giving attention to siblings' needs, and in cooperating with hospital staff and public health nurse to secure the best medical care available.

CHAPTER FIFTEEN

Muscular Dystrophy: Duchenne's Form

OF THE SEVERAL muscle diseases that affect children, the most common is *Duchenne's pseudohypertrophic muscular dystrophy*. Muscle diseases are similar in many respects but have important differences. This discussion will confine itself to the most common form, named for the man who first described it, a French neurologist, Guillaume Duchenne, in 1861.[1]

Duchenne's muscular dystrophy is primarily a disease of young boys, a mysterious muscle malady in which *striated* muscle (or striped muscle, that used in voluntary action) progressively degenerates, to be replaced by fat and fibrous tissue.[2] Progressive muscle weakness occurs as a consequence. Approximately 100 forms of therapy have been tried and found useless.[3] There is still no cure.

Fortunately, the disease is not common, its prevalence quoted variously at from 200,000 upward,[4] in the U.S. population. The topic is included in this book to represent the larger number of progressive neuromuscular conditions, and also to clarify the relationship between the fatal outcome of these diseases and the need for social services. A child welfare worker once responded to referral of such a child with the remark, "I couldn't accept the case. I looked up muscular dystrophy in the dictionary and saw it was fatal. My time is so limited, I must give priority to the living. I cannot afford to waste it on a child who is about to die." She did not know that the rate of progression, though relentless, is slow and does not bring death until 18 to 20 years of age in the majority of cases, or that a few live even beyond that age.[5]

Human care service workers will find on an occasional medical report reference to other neuromuscular diseases such as *facioscapulohumeral* or *Landouzy-Déjerine dystrophy*. This form usually has a later onset, creates less disability, and progresses more slowly than Duchenne's.

Another diagnosis is *Erb's Juvenile* form of *limb girdle* muscular dystrophy, which is intermediate between the severe Duchenne's and relatively mild facioscapulohumeral forms of muscular dystrophy.[6] There are other rare forms of muscle disease that one may sometimes identify from the words *myotonia* or *myotonic*, which refer to muscle spasm or rigidity, and *amyotonia*, lack of muscle tone, or flaccidity. Because each of the progressive neuromuscular diseases runs a distinctive course and affects a different set of muscles at different times, thus causing differing kinds of disabilities and outlooks, the worker should read about the specific disease affecting a given child in the *Merck Manual*[7] or a more detailed medical text. As indicated, the dictionary alone can be very misleading.

Duchenne's muscular dystrophy differs from the diseases presented in other chapters in several ways. Unlike children with impaired locomotion and wheelchair status from spina bifida or spinal cord injury, *children with muscular dystrophy have normal feeling even though they cannot move their limbs.* In addition, the child more nearly resembles a quadriplegic than a paraplegic, because of weakness in the shoulders and upper arms. The disease itself is painless. It has no remissions and allows no letup like arthritis. There are no good periods in which the family and child can regroup their psychic forces and renew their hopes. The rate of progression is generally predictable (though with a wide variation among some individuals). In most cases one can foresee what is going to happen and plan accordingly. Muscular dystrophy is an upside-down disorder, developmentally. Normal children grow stronger and more independent. Children with Duchenne's grow weaker and more dependent. The psychosocial implications can be surmised.

THE MEDICAL REALITIES

Cause and Hereditary Pattern

The cause of muscular dystrophy is still unknown. "It is thought the disease may be a deficiency disorder, caused by lack of one or more enzymes in the chain of biochemical events that occur in muscle cells."[8] In 1959 an enzyme, conveniently abbreviated CPK, was found to be in elevated blood levels early in the course of Duchenne's muscular dystrophy, and also in the majority of carriers tested.[9] Persons with muscular dystrophy have also been found to possess lower than normal concentrations of LDH-5, "an enzyme important in catalyzing the conversion of glucose to energy in muscle contraction."[10] Research on chickens and mice goes forward. One experienced neurologist says that recent breakthroughs permitting better classification of muscle diseases may unravel the mystery of the cause very soon.[11] Others express less optimism.

The muscular dystrophies are inherited. *Different forms have different hereditary patterns.* Duchenne's is carried on a sex-linked recessive gene, like hemophilia. The carrier mother is normal, but half her boys are dystrophic and half her girls are carriers. The other children are normal, with *no potential for developing or carrying the disease.*[12]

In a large number of cases, the mother gives no history of muscular dystrophy in her family. This is construed to mean a high mutation rate, or, in other words, a spontaneous development of the defective gene in the mother. It can be construed to mean a superficial history or ignorance or cover-up by the person giving the history. The mother's knowledge or lack of knowledge of her carrier status is significant to those concerned with the mother-child relationship. The CPK serum enzyme test is used to determine carrier status, with a reliability of approximately 70 percent.[13] This is a blood test, and some clinics repeat it at weekly intervals to secure an average, for the greatest possible accuracy. The CPK levels decrease with age, so that accuracy is greater in young women. Tentative findings can be confirmed with muscle biopsy or electromyography.[14] Both are major tests and involve minor to major discomfort depending upon the skill and equipment used by the physician or technician.

Symptoms, Diagnosis, and Course

Onset occurs usually before age three.[15] Early symptoms are a waddling gait, "toe-walking," frequent easy falling, and difficulty in climbing stairs. The toe-walking becomes more pronounced, and the child looks markedly swaybacked (*lordotic*) as his body compensates to keep its balance. He has difficulty in straightening up from a bent-over position and often has to use both hands to pull on the railing to drag himself upstairs. In getting up from a lying position, "he rolls over on his abdomen, gets on his hands and knees, and then rises by placing his hands alternately on his knees and thighs until he gradually brings his body into erect position."[16] This is sometimes described as "Gowering," after the physician who first described it.

The child with Duchenne's is so easily recognized by his symptoms by the time they become this pronounced that "the signs are unmistakable." Nevertheless, parents often complain of long delay in securing a diagnosis. Part of the problem of delayed diagnosis may be due to the healthy appearance of the muscles, which are large with fat, especially in the calves.[17] Neurologists insist that diagnosis should include a careful history, an enzyme test, urinary creatine-excretion test, electromyogram, and muscle biopsy. One neurologist states that many children brought to specialty clinics with a diagnosis of muscular dystrophy have other neurological or collagen diseases instead, and that extreme care is necessary in distinguishing the disease.[18]

Dr. Vignos, a specialist, divides the phases of the child's course into two, ambulatory and wheelchair, and further divides the ambulatory phase into early, terminating with loss of ability to climb stairs; late, terminating with loss of independent ambulation; and brace-walking. He states that the course is determined by the rate of muscle deterioration.[19] The late ambulatory phase occurs at about nine years of age, the brace-walking phase at 10 or 11 years, and the wheelchair phase begins between 10 and 12 years of age. Braces are not prescribed by all neurologists who specialize in care of children with muscular dystrophy, since the weight of the braces is thought to handicap the child as much as or more than the progression of muscle weakness.[20] One specialist states that usually wheelchair existence begins at age 10 but that the time can be extended to age 12 or 13 if the family will work with the child at home (providing exercises and insisting on proper posture and positions) to the degree necessary.[21]

Of great psychosocial importance are the rate and distribution of muscle weakness. The calves, buttocks, lower back, shoulders, and upper arm muscles are more severely affected first.[22] The retention of hand motion and use of the face and throat makes possible some important activities. However, a generalized weakness, including the muscles of the trunk, chest, upper back, and neck, sets in gradually and becomes disabling soon after the child becomes wheelchair-bound. If the child topples forward in his wheelchair, he cannot straighten up, or if his head flops back or to one side, he cannot pull it upright.

Slight weight gains or short periods of bed rest due to childhood diseases or ill-advised operations can cause loss of ambulation. Once a child goes into a wheelchair, he does not return to ambulation. (This term is not synonymous with walking, but instead means moving about at least in part by one's own effort.)

As the muscle weakness progresses to involve all the muscles, including those used in coughing, the child becomes completely helpless. He is vulnerable to respiratory infections. He dies from weakness of the heart muscle, or when the muscles necessary to respiration fail. He may be helpless, needing total care, for six to eight years, depending on how long he lives after weakness of all muscle groups begins and how carefully he is nursed when he has acute illnesses. Most children die in late teenage.[23]

Treatment

Treatment is designed to do two things—prolong the period of ambulation and prevent and/or treat complications. No drugs specific for muscular dystrophy are known, and surgery is used only selectively and sparingly.

Prolonging ambulation. Physical therapy and in some cases bracing, the use of other prostheses, and encouragement of appropriate activity and position are the means used to keep the child out of a wheelchair as long as possible. The importance of psychological support and attention to the family social situation is emphasized by everyone who comments on treatment, since these are essential to maintain the family's efforts.

Regular stretching exercises, conducted at home and/or school several times daily, proper positioning of the child in the wheelchair or bed, and standing are important. The stretching exercises counteract the tendency to contractures caused by imbalance in muscle pull, and standing decreases urinary complications and slows down "brittle bones," or *osteoporosis*. Vignos says the stretching should be applied to three different muscle groups, and that "maximum stretch must be maintained for at least 10 seconds and repeated 10 times, twice a day"; in addition, active resistive exercises are prescribed. He states that the techniques are complicated and require experienced therapists and "cooperative patients" (he later comments on the "negativism often shown" by the children). Too much exercise is actually harmful.[24]

In a symposium on the management of children with muscular dystrophy, a layman asked an expert whether the early stretching and use of night splints is of real value in retarding the development of contractures. His response was, "If the child is found early enough, and if the parents can be alerted to the fact that proper position and postural attitudes are important in the future development or control of contractures, you can definitely delay them.... When these patients get beyond a certain stage, it seems almost impossible to do anything at all. Treatment is sometimes too painful and sometimes productive of pressure sores."[25] At the same symposium, a carefully designed study was reported in which maximum physical rehabilitation measures were applied to a group of children at the New York State Rehabilitation Hospital. The findings were that "neither muscle reeducation, nor strengthening exercises, nor activity performance can apparently increase actual muscle strength ... [but that] most patients with progressive muscular dystrophy can improve their performance of activities of daily living by proper instruction and supervision *if they are not too severely disabled and are properly motivated.*"[26] (Italics added.)

The key to prolonging independent ambulation by physical therapy measures is not increase of muscle strength but prevention of contractures around the weight-bearing joints. "Do not wait for contractures to begin. It is a losing battle then, but if every muscle has been carefully evaluated, and one anticipates contractures through the warning signs, much can be done to prolong the child's functional capacity. However, it may be difficult to convince the family to perform the exercises."[27] Accordingly, the relationship of successful treatment to early diagnosis, access to skilled medical care, and parental cooperation is obvious.

Diet is an adjunct of physical therapy in prolonging ambulation. Because of limited physical activity, the child with muscular dystrophy can gain weight rapidly. The added weight creates a burden for weak muscles that may be the crucial factor in creating premature wheelchair existence. A calorie-restricted diet is therefore recommended. Therapeutic diets are not employed, having been found useless.

Management of complications. Contractures and pulmonary complications are the most prevalent. Surgery to release contractures of hips and knees should be postponed until the brace-walking stage or later, according to Vignos, in order to avoid the subsequent bed rest. He follows surgical treatment with prescription of steel, long leg, double-upright braces, weighing six or seven pounds, and by intensive physical therapy for four to six weeks.[28]

At a later stage, and in highly selected cases, some clinical teams may also prescribe surgery for correction of spinal deformity if a severe deformity cannot be ameliorated otherwise and if the child has a relatively good life prognosis.[29] Since such surgery requires approximately a month in the hospital and six months in a body cast, it obviously is a venture requiring the most thorough consideration of all factors involved, including the effect on the family. Collapse of the back muscles throws the child forward, thrusting the rib cage down on the pelvis and crowding all the organs. As the boy tries to settle into a comfortable position, he may twist around and become contracted and fixed in his position. A boy who suffers from this complication has greater difficulty coughing and breathing. Physicians differ in the extent to which they attempt correction by surgery or prescription of plastic body jackets. Some allow the child to be comfortable and happy as long as possible without interference, and others take maximum effort to make the child's body as straight as possible.[30]

Prevention and conscientious treatment of both acute and chronic problems are essential. Physical therapy to maintain chest muscles that are essential in coughing includes a variety of blowing and breathing exercises, such as blowing up balloons, blowing out candles, blowing toy horns. Teaching the child to stop and take a very deep breath and let it out slowly, every half-hour, is another means of helping him maintain chest muscle capacity. If the child contracts an infection in the lungs, mucus accumulates if he cannot cough it up. Antibiotics, postural drainage exercises, and instruction of the parents by a public health nurse in suctioning the child are prescribed. Vignos says, "We regard productive bronchitis as a relative pulmonary emergency in muscular dystrophy and feel that prompt medical treatment is essential to avoid possibly fatal outcome."[31]

Other complications are those common to all wheelchair and bed patients, such as pressure sores, urinary infections, and osteoporosis. Pressure sores are sometimes avoided by use of sheepskin pads or occasionally water beds, and require that the child learn to lift himself and shift position as long as he can, and later that he be shifted or turned at varying intervals from every half-hour to every two hours. Preventive measures for urinary complications include standing at a standing table or standing board; the same method is used to prevent osteoporosis. Medications (sulfa preparations and others) are used for treatment of urinary infections.

Equipment. Self-care aids, night splints, braces and crutches, standing boards, hydraulic lifts, motorized and collapsible wheelchairs, suction machines, washing machines if the child is bedfast, and, for families who can afford them, recreational vehicles or vans equipped with ramps and clamps for wheelchairs are among the major pieces of equipment needed by a child with muscular dystrophy at different stages of his career. Self-care aids and a motorized chair are indispensable in making life endurable for the child and in lightening the burden of his care. The wheelchair must have removable arms and swing-away leg rests. A portable chair needs to be lightweight so the mother can lift it. Bed and toilet seat must be of the same height as the chair seat, in order to facilitate transfer. A hospital bed or high bed facilitates the care of a heavy, bedfast child.

Among self-care aids are so-called "polio arms," or ball-bearing arms, that are fitted to the wheelchair, and support the upper arms in such a way that the child has almost full use of his lower arms and hands in feeding himself, brushing his teeth, etc. These custom-built, expensive prostheses must be built and fitted by experts, since they are no help if the fit is not exact. They are prescribed selectively, keeping in mind the child's motivation and family willingness to work with the device. Some physicians are better acquainted with their use than others and more prone to prescribe them. A common problem is the resistance of the child with muscular dystrophy to use of aids because they signify to him that his condition is worse. Children tend to fear any sign of lost ground. Motivation of both child and family is an integral part of the use of equipment.

Mental Status

Controversy exists on whether children with Duchenne's muscular dystrophy show higher incidence of mental retardation than other children. Certainly many function on a retarded level. A camp executive said he thought that half the children with muscular dystrophy were slow to respond, preoccupied, or mentally dull. The principal and vice-principal of a special school could not agree, since some of the students obviously were mentally bright and others functioned as retarded. Whether retarded functioning is due to pseudo-retardation from social isolation and anxiety, whether it is real and part of the disease, whether these children have perceptual difficulties that cause learning disability, or whether retardation progresses as the disease progresses have all been discussed and investigated.

Opinions have ranged from that expressed by an educator of exceptional children—"Severe retardation in the basic skills, such as reading and arithmetic, is due more generally to the mental inactivity caused by social, psychological and educational consequences of the disease than to the lack of intellectual capacity"[32]—to opinions that "about 25% of children with Duchenne's have mental retardation."[33]

A psychologist has developed the thesis that boys with muscular dystrophy suffer impaired development of body image at a critical period, between ages five and seven, because of muscle weakness that inhibits both normal mastery of the environment through motoric activity and father identification. Psychologists report that poor body image is related to abstraction difficulties and reading and number concepts; that these things, plus undesirable first-grade experiences, create the learning difficulties. The psychologist who has elaborated this idea does not believe that true mental deficiency is a "usual accompaniment of muscular dystrophy."[34] Two persons who work closely with children with this disease have voiced the same opinion in interviews with me. They acknowledge severe scholastic retardation, but do not believe it is due to mental retardation.

A study reported from Warsaw, Poland, seems to reflect the current accepted opinion.[35] The mean IQ of 100 boys in the study was 76, and of 30 others, 92. Mental retardation was not dependent on severity of muscle involvement or on environmental factors, but seemed to be genetic. In families with more than one affected child, the IQ was similar in the affected children. However, mental retardation among children with muscular dystrophy is a complex problem and much remains to be learned.

PSYCHOSOCIAL IMPLICATIONS

A disease that progressively disables a child creates changing problems for the parents. Their attitudes, relationships, and burdens shift during the different stages of onset, the child's weakness and partial crippling, then complete helplessness, and death. The family's life cycle changes and matures over this long period; other children may be born and incur problems, and various vicissitudes occur. Socioeconomic, ethnic, medical care, and community factors influence the situation. Dystrophic children themselves vary, in both physical stamina and emotional stability, creating different "inputs" and altering the constellation. Families demonstrate, therefore, many different ways of coping with muscular dystrophy, and they cope differently at different times. The point at which a helping person enters the family's life process will determine the special relevance of problems to be described here.

An attempt will be made to discuss some parental attitudes, physical burdens, need for respite, finances, housing, and transportation under the general heading of the family. A second section about the child will include effects on his personality, sibling and peer relationships, school, camp, out-of-home care, religion, and attitudes toward death. Because family's and children's reactions and behaviors are interrelated, the main topics are arbitrary and are divided in this way merely to simplify presentation.

The Family

When muscular dystrophy already exists in the family or among the mother's relatives, fear and dread during the pregnancy have been described, with a later guilt-ridden, sacrificial attitude of the mother toward the child. However, most parents do not come to the attention of those who have written about them until later in the child's course, so that only fleeting references are found in the literature to the anguish the mothers feel when the diagnosis is first made. One social worker reported that it was difficult to get information in this area.[36] In describing the behavior of the mothers in the study, she reported that they spend a great deal of energy on cooking and cleaning. They fear the child will not eat properly, they eat sparingly themselves, and keep children and home spotlessly clean. She described the parental state as one of "continual anxiety," so that this sacrificial reaction may have served a good purpose in maintaining the mother's balance. This study was performed 20 years ago.

Occasionally, overtly angry mothers are found, as in families of other chronically ill children. The angry, aggressive mother refuses to sympathize with her son; she forces him to fend for himself in every way possible, often refuses to cooperate with doctors and therapists, and may channel her energies into improved legislation and facilities; she is often in conflict with the school.

At present, many mothers are nervous, driven women, near the point of chronic physical and nervous exhaustion. Some cope by working outside the home and employing sitters as long as they can, which makes them even more tired but provides an escape that seems necessary.

It will be recalled that no family history of muscular dystrophy is given in many cases.[37] Wershow's in-depth study of 18 families indicated guarded replies in response to a question about dystrophy in the family background. "We would not know—an aunt or cousin might have had a child with dystrophy, but in the old days people kept children like that hidden. It wasn't the way it is now."[38] Families who reported living in dread of learning the child's diagnosis, aware that his clumsiness and slowness augured something serious, spoke of fears of cerebral palsy or retardation, not of muscular dystrophy. However, some members of half the families suspected the child had muscular dystrophy before the child was taken for diagnosis.[39]

There is no question that some families entertain no thought of muscular dystrophy, and during the child's preschool years they go from one doctor to another for a diagnosis. They may be told that the child will outgrow the condition, or receive misinformation about the cause, and they are stunned when they finally learn their child has the disease so well publicized in televised fund-raising events as crippling and fatal. Accepting the diagnosis is almost too much to endure. Two mothers have said they refused to believe the diagnosis, and put aside their concern until forced to come to grips with it later. Both were under great stress, one because she was pregnant again and the other because she had just lost a premature child; a blanket of denial protected them from collapse. One mother, who had lived through years of sadness and the death of her boy, said that at no time is the anguish so great as when one first learns and adjusts to the diagnosis.

One small study that reported a particular effort to learn the attitude of fathers said they expressed a feeling of need to "race against time" because of the child's expected early death. "They tended to emphasize striving for total cure." The investigator thought some fathers felt guilt or discomfort that they could not be of more help in caring for the child.[40]

Though no study is known of the difference in parental behavior toward children when hereditary factors are known and not known, it seems logical that a mother who knows she may pass on a dread disease to her child would have greater guilt than one who does not. A father who knows that his wife knew would seemingly feel greater anger toward her and less hesitation in burdening her with the child's care. A study in this area is badly needed. In practice, caution is indicated in probing because the subject is so charged with emotion.

A number of divorces do occur in families of children with muscular dystrophy. The father is usually the parent who cannot endure weakness and illness in a child, especially a boy, though cases are known in which the mother is unable to face her burden and leaves or abandons the child. However, muscular dystrophy's full impact on the family's life-style does not usually occur until the child is eight to 12 years old (when he falls a great deal and then goes into a wheelchair and must have substantial physical care). Thus the marriage escapes the impact of physical burdens until after it has had a chance to "set," and the partners have become accustomed to marriage as a child-rearing institution. Theoretically, muscular dystrophy should not break up as many marriages as the chronic diseases that distort family life-styles earlier. However, no facts are known; this is another area that needs study.

One destructive force that has been mentioned in studies is embarrassment because of the curiosity of neighbors and strangers, and shame, resulting in social isolation when the parents do learn the child has muscular dystrophy.[41] The studies were performed in the 1950's; it is possible that social attitudes have changed to make this less of a problem.

Because it does indeed take two or more persons to care for a child with muscular dystrophy, those families in which the father participates in rearing the boy produce obviously healthier situations. A father who adapts housing and equipment to facilitate the child's independence and relieve the mother of unnecessary burdens, who builds models or toy trains with the boy, who lifts and undresses and toilets him at night, is giving the boy reassurance that his weakness has not deprived him of his father's love, and is giving the mother physical and emotional help. In one case known, the father took the boy on separate vacations fishing and camping, which gave the mother complete respite for short periods at regular intervals; in another, the father used his mechanical skills to devise ingenious motorized equipment that gave the boy unusual mobility and independence.

The number of stepparent families is notable. Whether it is greater than in the normal population, again, is not known (see Chapter 2, p. 32). Stepfathers rarely seem to participate fully in the child's care, but they do provide an adult companion who gives the mother emotional support and who provides child care for the siblings while she takes the affected boy or boys to clinic or for therapy. Stepfathers both attenuate the intensity of mother-child relationship and divert the attention she could otherwise give to the child.

In some instances the father or stepfather has abdicated either by leaving or by busying himself elsewhere after work hours—"He plays handball a lot, so he's not here when it's time to put Johnny to bed," or "He gets extra pay by working overtime, and we need the money." In these cases the child is reared entirely by mother and siblings. His physical weakness defeats him in masculine identification, and realistic dependence on the mother grows greater as he matures. She finds him heavier to lift and increasingly unable to help himself, and tends to resent the burden. Equally, the child becomes aware of the hereditary nature of his disease and blames her. How overt the mutual resentment is, and how strong a thread in the total web of feelings, varies. Children usually blurt out their blame of the mother, or act it out, at some point, but give the impression that they keep their feelings to themselves most of the time.

The Physical Burden

A perceptive recreational therapist commented recently that children with muscular dystrophy can be difficult to work with because *they need so much*. The demands of a child who simply cannot get up when he falls—"Hey, somebody, I'm on the floor"—and who virtually must have another person's arms and legs to work for him after he reaches age ten to 12, is like a child-sized baby with a boy's desires and needs. When his elbows are propped on a table the right height for his wheelchair, he can feed himself, perform schoolwork, play table games, and perform craft activities. Although he can propel himself in a wheelchair, and later he can still move about if he has a motorized chair, providing there are no curbs or steps or narrow doors, in other ways he is helpless.

The extent of the physical burden depends on his conditioning, equipment, and housing facilities. Some boys are stronger constitutionally than others. They deteriorate less rapidly, have fewer colds and bouts of pneumonia. Physicians and therapists differ in how much they lay on the parents in terms of exercises and putting on braces and splints. Heavy expectations of home therapy often create guilt in the mother who is unable to put the child through all the exercises recommended, or result in negative attitudes toward medical care and/or the child. Stretching exercises are usually painful. The scenes and the resentments when the mother inflicts the pain often result in neglect of the exercises.

Housing affects the physical burden, and other factors crucial to well-being. A child marooned on the second floor cannot go to school or participate in recreational activities. He is always underfoot, intensifying resentments, pity, or other adverse feelings, and lack of stimulation diminishes his capacity to project feelings on a variety of persons and events.

In Bernstein and Malter's study of 34 New York City families, 15 had housing that was "inadequate for even minimal needs of the dystrophic patients,"[42] and Wershow's study of 18 Baltimore families showed that, as measured by his standards, "not one of the families had housing that was fully adequate."[43] His standards describe well the housing needs of a dystrophic child: (1) street level entrance, with ramp if necessary; (2) sleeping quarters and play area on the same floor with the bathroom, and not isolated from family activities; (3) doorways and halls wide enough for wheelchair maneuvers; and (4) bathroom large enough for wheelchair and mechanical lift.

In the San Francisco Bay Area, few families with dystrophic children are known who live in the hilly, compact city itself.[44] They seem to live instead in the suburban areas where space has been used extravagantly, thus permitting one-story homes. The problem of stairs, so defeating to all aspects of life for a paraplegic, has not been troublesome for the majority. However, lack of space for equipment and for use of the bathroom for toileting and bathing tends to create difficulties. If the child receives therapy at home, storage room for a standing table is necessary. A hydraulic lift and two wheelchairs also take space. The use of a commode in the child's bedroom can be substituted for the toilet if he does not share a room with others, but the lifting necessary for both bathing and toileting creates such a common problem that back injury is often reported among the mothers.

Moving to a more suitable location if housing is inadequate constitutes a complicated problem requiring thorough exploration. Substantial physical effort and time expenditure may be necessary to supplement the family's efforts, especially if the mother is the only parent and is exhausted from care of the child and employment or training for employment. Wershow believed that the families he studied were handicapped in learning about better housing by lack of extensive social contacts through which persons usually make their needs known and learn of someone who is moving or of a house available at moderate rental. A third of the families in his study would not consider moving because of the presence of helpful neighbors or relatives.[45]

In addition to possible feelings of fear, shame, inertia, or defeat, location in respect to jobs and schools is a paramount problem. Cost of adequate housing is perhaps the most difficult obstacle of all. Because of the many requirements of housing that serves the needs of all the family members, only partial improvement may be possible. The matter cannot be relegated to an aide or volunteer as a matter requiring time-consuming effort alone, though the assistance of such a person may be very helpful.

The *weight* of the child is another factor affecting degree of physical burden. Many children seem to become overweight during the first few years after they go into wheelchairs. Seeing the child deprived of so many pleasures, the parent finds it hard to deprive him of food to keep his weight down. However, during the end stages, wasting of the muscles often occurs and the child becomes like a skeleton, relatively easy to lift provided the mother has been instructed in proper methods. By then contractures and deformities frequently complicate the problems of physical care.

In addition to weight, the dystrophic child is hard to lift because of the flabbiness of his weakened muscles. The child "slips out of your hands, there is nothing to hang onto." Since his body lacks tension, "he is a dead weight." Furthermore, his shoulders may dislocate if an attempt is made to lift him in the ordinary manner of an embrace and tug under the arms, for his limb-girdle muscles do not function to protect the sockets. A special mode of lifting must be employed—as one carries a baby, not as one ordinarily lifts a child.

He can be plucked by the belt or tugged by his clothing. If his hands slide off the arm of the wheelchair, or his head falls forward, someone must be there to reposition him. During adolescence the boy's weakness has become so pronounced that he cannot put his penis in a urinal or pull up his zipper. Little or no embarrassment exists in respect to toileting between a totally loving mother and a boy whose security in her is complete. This is not always the case. Feeding the boy may not be beyond the mother, but toileting needs may not be within her capacity. Male siblings often are pressed into taking this responsibility, or the boy may have to wait to urinate until the father, an uncle, or a neighbor comes home from work. Penile appliances with leg bags, similar to those used for incontinent persons, may be practical substitutes. Depending on the boy's weight, he may be impossible for the mother and siblings to lift onto a bedpan or slide onto a toilet. Elevated toilet seats, chairs with removable arms, and other aids help.

The enormity of the physical burden on the mother is readily apparent.

Some parents seem to relax under the weight of impossible demands, compromise the ideal with what is practical for them, and let the problems of each day take care of themselves. Some avoid the responsibility through a variety of means. In most families with other children, the siblings usually share the responsibility with the mother. The effect on the siblings is discussed later.

However, the need for respite is great in all cases and is one reason why special schools and summer camps perform such important roles.

Public health nurses and physical therapists who come to the home are able to suggest home modifications and equipment that ease the burden. They often need the assistance of social agencies in securing needed devices or more appropriate housing or housing modifications. These concrete services that relieve stress have secondary gains of primary importance. They lessen tensions and resentments, and they build relationships that permit the parent and child to communicate with the worker. Out-of-home care becomes inevitable for many children as they grow into adolescence unless some relief to the mother is provided. Housekeeping service or attendant care or provision for sitters can prevent or delay the trauma and expense of nursing-home placement. Sometimes relatives are available who will come at regular times during the week and give the mother a chance to go shopping or to a church or club group.

Transportation

Transporting the limp-muscled child with muscular dystrophy from one locale to another requires special equipment and / or special manpower. In some communities the school buses are not so equipped, and the driver is not allowed to leave his seat when the child is picked up and brought home from school. This means that the mother must carry the child up and down the steps of the bus. In such instances, schooling ends when the mother falls down the steps with a too-heavy child in her arms, strains her back, or gives up. School buses increasingly are being equipped with ramps and clamps for wheelchairs, permitting placement of the child in the chair before he is loaded onto the bus. The U.S. Department of Transportation has issued permission for more buses to be specially equipped for the handicapped.[46]

Some agencies that provide transportation services, such as a local Red Cross, have minibuses equipped with motorized lifts or ramps and clamps. A community that has no such equipment may find one or more service clubs interested in providing a bus for the handicapped. "Indoor-outdoor" clubs provide manpower to take wheelchair-bound persons to special sports and cultural events.

Middle-class families with an interested father can adapt a recreational vehicle to carry a wheelchair, permitting the affected boy or boys to go with the others on family errands and outings. Most middle-class intact families seem to have such vehicles. Poor families must rely on the kindness of neighbors, relatives, or church members to provide manpower to wheel and lift; some out-reach service may be necessary to help them locate helpful youths or men. Limiting requests for aid to transportation for medical care alone deprives the boy of much needed socialization.

The importance of transportation facilities needs no elaboration. A child who has nothing to look forward to, who is continuously isolated with no stimulation, is an unnecessarily deprived person. Brooding, fears, fantasies, and mother attachment create resistance to anything new to the point of serious distortion.

Finances

Hospitalization for those children who have repeated respiratory infections or who have surgery to release contractures or correct deformities is usually a legitimate service of the Crippled Children's Services, Medicaid, Champus (military Medicaid), or private insurance. Wheelchair accidents requiring emergency room services are also covered. However, the family may be required to pay for part of the costs. Physical therapy is provided by the Crippled Children's Services, or by the Elks Club or other similar private organizations in many areas.

The largest expenses the family incurs are for equipment and its repair, doctor's visits and medication, and domestic service. The unusual generosity of the Muscular Dystrophy Association ordinarily relieves the family of expenses for purchase of basic equipment. The most expensive unmet need is that for domestic service, sitters, or housekeeping aid. Transportation and medication are additional sources of expense. Rent for suitable housing may also constitute a serious problem if the family cannot afford a downstairs apartment or house without steps, and one in which the hallways and bathroom permit a wheelchair.

Because a washing machine and sufficient bedding are essentials after the child becomes bedfast, these items must be kept in mind, in addition to the constant repairs that equipment requires. That the television needs to be kept in order is obvious. Wheelchairs with pneumatic tires get flat tires, and need repairs to various parts at times. They must also be replaced as the child grows. Because of foot drop, the child's toes drag on the ground if the chair is too small. A motorized chair is an incalculable aid after a boy progresses beyond the ability to wheel his own chair. He may be able to go to a regular school if his chair is motorized. He can go about the neighborhood, the yard, and house independently. His feelings of self-worth, and the reciprocal feelings of freedom from either obligation or guilt on the part of others, are enormous aids emotionally. However, such a chair is very expensive, and usually requires either a community enterprise, a substantial family debt and sacrifice, or a gift from a family whose invalid has died.

Coping with the Fatality of the Disease

Families of children with muscular dystrophy are variously described in the literature as "living in a prolonged state of anxiety and distress,"[47] or with a "constantly gnawing heartache"[48] or with "a great measure of acceptance,"[49] which, however, is defined as "taking care of the child without complaining or weeping, answering his questions realistically and understanding the inevitable course of the illness." An initial reaction of shock and distress is not disputed. Observation indicates that the early period varies considerably in length; that some parents remain chronically at the edge of upset; others separate themselves from the child physically or emotionally; others channel their anxiety into constant activity; some achieve great strength and solace from religion and perhaps thus more truly "accept" the tragedy. These basic elements undergird the reactions of all.

No one can remain at a high pitch of emotion of any kind over a prolonged period. Through repeated shocks from seeing other children in late stages of muscular dystrophy and the long gradual course of the disease, the parents learn to live with the situation with less acute grief. However, in a long-term progressive disease, certain benchmarks of progression occur that constitute crisis points. These stir up original anxieties. When the dystrophic child must quit regular school and go to a special school; when he can no longer attend special school but must stay home; when the mother can no longer lift the child; when the child contracts pneumonia; and when the beginning of the end announces itself through collapse of a lung or the child's failure to rally from repeated infections—these are common occasions when anxiety boils up again.

The very fact of an end in sight, even an end through death, aids the parents' endurance. The physical burdens, the anxieties, the financial sacrifices, all are going to come to an end. One mother revealed the component of anger in her mixed feelings by the tartly quizzical manner in which she said, "Death is only a transition, so what does it matter?"

Constant activity seems to be one of the most common ways of coping, perhaps because it is a natural response to the demands. Taking care of a dystrophic child, whether during the early stages of physical therapy and clinic appointments and school-related adjustments, or the intermediate stage of adapting the household and family to his wheelchair existence, or the still later stage of frequently positioning, turning, lifting, toileting, feeding, etc.—caring for the child and for the other members of the family requires a great deal of activity in itself. Because the child is home alone much of the time, the conscientious mother is forced into trying to devise means of keeping him occupied, and this means creating crafts and games, stimulating and enabling hobbies, enticing other children into the home through parties and special occasions, etc. Work in the parents' organization provides an opportunity to get acquainted with other mothers, which invites participation in their concerns and in common causes. Mothers who escape through work outside the home are carrying not only the two jobs of many of today's married women but the third job of caring for an invalid boy or youth.

The type of medical care makes a great difference in the mother's ability to tolerate the psychological and physical burden. An impersonal clinic may provide very little emotional support, in contrast to the strength available from a warm, long-continued relationship with a sustaining doctor. Continuity of care from a trusted physician aids both the child and the mother.

In stable marriages, the father is the mother's source of strength. The child himself may help sustain the mother. Mothers whose boys have died have shared their memories of precious moments when the affected child made unselfish gestures and thoughtful remarks, displayed courage, and gave them thrills of pride. The way a family felt upon the death of a loved teenager was expressed by a cousin, in part as follows: "Today is the day we say goodbye to Bob... today is the day we say hello to his living and loving memories. Thank you, dear Bob... thank you for all that you taught us about life. Thank you for all the happiness and strength you gave us. Thank you for sharing your life with ours.... Bob was crippled —but crippled only physically. His heart for love and his will for life were stronger and healthier than anything we will ever know. They haven't died, they will always be with us."

How the parents integrate the knowledge of eventual fatality determines how well they can answer the child's questions about death that come unexpectedly, with no opportunity to prepare a reply. The parents' attitude determines how perceptively they can respond to his fears of the dark, his need to sleep with someone, his fear of being alone or abandoned, his enuresis, his outbursts of anger. Most of all, parental integration provides a framework for communication. Children need to talk over "Why me and not my brother," "When am I going to die," "Will I be up there in heaven alone," but can only communicate the most frightening questions to someone they trust and in whom they have real security. Not all children voice their fears. They are taught by their parents that a hopeful attitude is the only one acceptable and they are not to open subjects that no one is able to handle.

The hyperactive, emotionally distant, or overtly disturbed mother cannot provide the security and trust the child needs. If the worker can succeed in establishing a relationship with her, and she is enabled to talk out her worries, guilt, and resentments, she is better able to meet her child's needs. However, her defenses, her ways of coping, are to be respected. Opportunity to unburden, not confrontation or destruction of what she hides behind, is to be sought.

Some mothers give up; this complaint against them is voiced by therapists and physicians who want the mother to continue exercises and to try new equipment, only to find themselves frustrated by excuses and delays. An attitude of giving in to ultimate fatality is destructive when it is conveyed to the child. If he senses that she believes all is hopeless and nothing is worthwhile, he is condemned to live inside himself with only fantasies for support. Other mothers, who refuse to give up and continue to strive for mastery over the inevitable, may turn to strange diets, astrology, or quack cures, vesting their hopes in whatever faddism comes their way. The mothers who are still working to overcome the child's destiny are still hopeful. Though their activities may be peculiar and result in deprivations for the child, they do convey to him that all is not lost; he can have hope; his mother is on his side. Finding that slim line between despair and "acceptance" must be very difficult indeed. What worker can say the parent's way is wrong?

Effects on the Child

The child with muscular dystrophy is even more influenced by family attitudes and circumstances than the majority of chronically ill children, because of his increasing helplessness and the amount of time he spends at home. However, he has had a better opportunity to build up a sense of trust and security than those children whose defect is obvious from birth or the early months, and fortunately his muscle weakness is not disabling until after the toddler period, when activity is an imperative of psychological development. If, therefore, the marriage is stable and the parents are mature, the child with muscular dystrophy has early psychological strengths on which to build. When he is intellectually well equipped, as many are, he has further assets. Some exceptionally fine, able young persons with this disease stand out in the memory of all who have worked with them.

The literature of the 1950's, when most of the published psychological explorations took place, is contradictory in regard to the serious nature and prevalence of emotional problems. That many children suffer emotionally is confirmed by experienced professional persons, and readily apparent upon observation of behavior, the language of childhood. One study of the nature and extent of psychological or social maladjustment reported that about half the children made a "satisfactory adjustment," and that these came from the "better adjusted" homes where parents displayed a realistic acceptance of needs and limitations.[50] In the other half, the children were termed emotionally immature, the immaturity expressed by withdrawal, lack of tolerance for frustration, and excessive dependence on the parents. One author, who claimed that children with muscular dystrophy display a relative absence of emotional problems, described the most frequent disorder as "spoiled child syndrome." "These are children who are always demanding new toys and games, yet are never happy with them. They usually whine incessantly and burst into tears at slightest provocation. They never know what to do with themselves. They give up before trying muscular activity that they are actually capable of performing."[51] This author blamed the situation entirely on the parents, and acknowledged no influence of the child's awareness of the implications of his disease and its frustrating limitations. Another study reported that the emotional reactions of the children were anxiety after falling and getting hurt, anxiety about being a "cripple," general anxiety or fear of everything, and resentment that well people did not appreciate their problem. "Sensitivity of body appearance was present in all patients. There was concern over progressive loss of freedom of activity and guilt over dependence on the mother but fear of losing her."[52]

Wershow, who has spoken of the "shy, fearful, withdrawn nature of this diagnostic group," but who prefaces his study with comments about his predilection toward seeing strengths not weaknesses, summarizes his findings: "many children did not seem to be frustrated and deprived because of their immobility." It will be recalled that all of his 18 study families but two were "relatively stable two-parent homes."[53] However, he pointed out that "the most striking thing about these children is their isolation ... they are marginal to any play groups and grateful for crumbs of relationship to other children." Factors not readily apparent must account for the lack of feelings of deprivation he described, in light of children's normal needs for relationships with other children.

Problems in managing aggression and anger are mentioned in the literature and are confirmed by a psychiatric social worker acquainted with children referred to her because of overt behavior problems.[54] She states that these children have difficulty getting along with peers because they do not want others to share toys, they strike out at others, and resist lessons and therapy. In light of what weak children suffer at the hands of physically normal, sometimes bullying peers, and of their constant fear of falling, problems in managing normal aggression would be expected. A psychiatrist says, "The situation is comparable to a person who has been attacked but is prevented from retaliating because he is bound hand and foot."[55] Whatever the proportion of overt behavior problems in the total population of children with muscular dystrophy, helping persons should be aware of potential areas of difficulty.

From approximately six to ten years of age, though earlier in many cases, the child's muscle weakness makes it impossible for him to run. One observer relates watching a child jump up and down in place while his playmates ran a relay race.[56] She tells of another child huddling behind a door or in a closet to avoid being knocked over when his classmates were physically active. Falls hurt. They are not the tumbles of babyhood. Children with muscular dystrophy break bones, incur sprains, cuts, and bruises when they fall. Inability to get up after a fall adds to the misery when muscle weakness advances. Nevertheless, ambulatory children fight to continue their tiptoe, swaybacked, precarious walking as long as possible. Although they do not articulate dread of the wheelchair, or knowledge of what it means, they act it out.

Sibling and peer relationships. No study is known, but an impression exists that ambulatory and early wheelchair-bound children with muscular dystrophy may be subject to more unkind treatment by peers than are children with other chronic illnesses. In the early stages they wear no outward badge of crippling—no crutches, no deformity—to spell out to their concretely thinking peers that they are physically unable to compete. They look weak rather than ill. This may be the reason for the taunts and physical abuse reported.* No parental account of the course of a child's development has failed to include anecdotes or comments about the unkindness of other children. "They push him over on his bike, and of course he can't get up," "Two boys dragged him out into the middle of the street and left him sitting there, but his little sister ran home and told me and I went and got him up," "They told him he waddled like a duck, and he came home crying," "They told him he only had three years to live," "Since he's been in his wheelchair they throw his toys on the ground, and he can't pick them up." One mother gave the boy's sibling karate lessons which he used effectively on the bullies who had been attacking the dystrophic child en route to school.

The reaction of the child to the frustration inherent in his situation, and to the rejection by schoolmates and neighbor children, depends on how sensitive he is, on his parents' support and reactions and the guidance they may or may not provide, on the point in his psychological development that traumatic events occur, and on many other factors. The most common reaction seems to be withdrawal. The philosophy of the physician or clinic influences the child's experience during this phase. Some physicians are so convinced of the importance of ambulation that they insist on delay of wheelchair use beyond the point where the child would benefit psychologically. Although the "captivity of the wheelchair" is an apt phrase, children can get around on level surfaces at home and in school with much greater ease in a chair than during the last phase of toe-walking. "An entirely changed personality" has been described when the child has given up the fight of staying on his feet, finds the joy of scooting around in a

* Dr. C. M. Binger, Coordinator, Children's Services, Langley Porter Neuropsychiatric Clinic, San Francisco, has pointed out that physically normal children suffer anxiety concerning body image and integrity when they see children with handicapping conditions; as a way of coping with their anxieties they may criticize or belittle the handicapped child.

chair, and is freed from constant fear of falling. The problem of the wheelchair is dependence on others to overcome the ever present obstacles of steps, shag rugs, curbs, hills, and rough places in the ground. A terrible patience seems to settle over most children as they learn from experience to wait until someone comes to push them.

Siblings are the most important peers in the child's life. Living under the same roof and bound by family ties, they care about him. They have grown up with his misfortune and take him for granted the way he is. Siblings are protectors from other children. Often an invalid child lives vicariously through their achievements. However, less is known probably about child-sibling relationships than any others. They are so taken for granted they are seldom verbalized. It is known that some dystrophic children would enslave their physically normal siblings—"Hand me this, pick up that"—if not restrained. Some are known to be abusive verbally toward physically normal siblings. Envy, and confusion why he is the one to bear the cross, not they, must be inevitable. An outstanding boy to be described later, however, made excuses for his siblings when they wanted to run out and play or failed to disguise their impatience about pushing him in his wheelchair.

The burdening of siblings in helping with physical care seems to be common. Some unfortunate effects have been seen. Siblings who have been overburdened not uncommonly leave home at 16 or 17. Signs of mounting resentment may be seen in the providing of hasty or unkind physical care. In other instances, a close-knit large family may regard the affected boy as their combined responsibility. School-age siblings, including younger children, help the boy to dress, push his wheelchair, and, if he goes to regular school, take him back and forth.

Though siblings' feelings have not been studied in depth, Solow comments that sibs may feel guilty about their good fortune and about the way they have treated the affected boy. He points out that when they face the reality that the boy is going to die, they must anticipate the loss of a very meaningful relationship.[57] Henley and Albam observed two main tendencies on the part of relatives and siblings of the group of boys they studied: spoiling or overindulgence of the dystrophic child, and an overt hostility on the part of younger siblings, related to the emotional deprivation of the younger, physically normal child.[58] Neglect of normal siblings has been reported in cases of extreme maternal preoccupation with the dystrophic boy: "Tommy, do you want some ice cream? Tommy, are you warm enough? Tommy, do you want to watch television?" In such cases the normal children may display hurt, or fleeting hurt and then anger, or may feign indifference.

How siblings feel when they watch the Telethon, or are part of the discussion of the boy's early death, is not known. They are hard to draw out in family interviews. The impression gained is that they are worried and saddened. Some siblings do take part in the Telethon; they actively interest their friends in the phenomenon of muscular dystrophy and channel their anxieties in a highly positive way. The desire to become a nurse, or member of the helping professions, has been known, as in brothers and sisters of children with kidney disease and other long-term, eventually fatal conditions.

One would assume that sisters bear a special weight of stress until they know whether they are carriers. This does not mean they do not intend to marry. One sister of three boys with muscular dystrophy, one of whom had died, said, "of course I intend to have children, whether they have muscular dystrophy or not. We all love my brothers very much." In other words, her brothers were worthwhile human beings. She discounted their suffering.

Concern about offspring is not confined to sisters. One brother who has married does not want to have children. Though he knows he cannot be a carrier, he has a general fear of having a defective child. He was close to his dystrophic brother, and was always fearful about his own health.

*School.** Depending on the facilities available in the particular locality, the child with muscular dystrophy may attend regular school, special school for the orthopedically handicapped, special classes in a regular or integrated (for handicapped) school, may have home teaching or no schooling at all. Twenty years ago, two surveys, one of children in metropolitan areas in New York, showed that a large proportion of school-age children received home teaching or none.[59] Wershow's study 15 years ago of children with muscular dystrophy in Baltimore and surrounding counties showed that the majority of city children went to special school, but the majority in the county area received home instruction or none.[60] The current situation is unknown, but it may be assumed that the large proportion of families now living in cities, the advances made in motorized equipment, and the greater public awareness of muscular dystrophy have resulted in a decrease in the number of children who cannot attend school.

Fortunately, most children can attend the psychologically crucial first grade at a regular school. Some will need special school facilities, usually between the ages of seven and ten, or by the time the contracted heel cords and lordosis make the child's balance precarious. Special classes in integrated schools seem to be ideal. Here the teachers of regular classes have elected to teach where some children have physical handicaps, and they receive training in meeting special needs. A special education counselor is

---

* For the opportunity to learn about the current programs of special and integrated schools, the author is especially indebted to Miss Marjorie Abbott, Principal of the Chandler Tripp School of Santa Clara County, Mrs. Gayle Rosenberry, the Vice Principal, and their staffs, and to the Principal, Mr. William Cencirulo, and staff of the Fremont Older School of Santa Clara County.

available to answer their questions about specific children—"Will he be able to go to the supplies cabinet and get his own materials?"—and to rescue them from situations beyond their capacity. Thus the teachers are relatively secure and knowledgeable. They are able to prepare the physically normal children. The child has the haven of special handicapped children's classes, special teachers, and all the facilities and auxiliary personnel for his home base. He can spend the lunch hour, the most hazardous time of day for rough play, with other handicapped children instead of out on the playground, if he prefers (as most do).

He is not continually in a situation where he meets defeat and isolation from peers. When one watches normal children on the playground with a handicapped child, his painful isolation is obvious. Some normal children will perhaps throw him a ball, but they need the time to discharge their own restless energies, and ordinarily leave him standing or sitting in one corner, by gate or fence, while they shriek and run together.

Moreover, the child who attends such an integrated school does not suffer from the inevitable negative forces in a school designed for handicapped children only. He is expected to do more academically, and if he is capable in certain areas, math or language, he can go ahead and receive recognition accordingly. He may be able to attend the same school with his siblings and neighbors and thus avoid the isolation at home that stems from not being part of the group that goes to school together.

Some type of schooling away from home is very important. The special schools for the handicapped play a constructive role for most children with muscular dystrophy who live in urban centers. Individualized attention, a high teacher-child ratio, special bus transportation, special physical facilities, and, in California, the availability of physical therapy at school are of great help to children and parents alike. Children who are unable to care for their own needs can have a socializing experience that must be witnessed to be appreciated. The stimulation, fun, learning, and normalcy of their daily routine minimize the severity of the psychological problems for both parents and children.

As children with muscular dystrophy get older and weaker, they either drop to home teaching or, in communities with good facilities, can enter a special high school program. In Santa Clara County, California, a federally funded three-year experiment called the "Life Experience Program" has been developed that is part recreation, part pre-vocational, and part teaching daily living skills. The program is now being developed in an additional 20 counties in California.[61] The curriculum includes the rules of different sports, how to select constructive TV programs, the building of collections, shopping, asking directions from strangers, using vending machines, calling a taxi, crossing busy intersections, etc. Some children are able to bowl and swim, with aid, and to play adapted forms of baseball.

Teachers have found that some children have never emptied cereal into a bowl for themselves, even though it is still possible physically, or opened a refrigerator or made a sandwich. They have never been inside a grocery store, because their mothers have left them in the car when they went to purchase food.

A ramp and clamps for wheelchairs or a motorized lift to get a child into a special school bus is a necessary part of the school's equipment. Not all have the necessary equipment, or community pressure to create special programs. Children then have either a few hours of home teaching a week or in some cases none at all.

Home teachers often provide the homebound child with the most important events of the week. Their coming is looked forward to because of the special attention, the break in the monotony, and the stimulation. They are greatly to be appreciated but are no substitute for special classes if any means can be devised to get the child to a school. The home teacher for the child with muscular dystrophy in some respects is easier to secure than for the child with remitting disease, because the scheduling can be done well in advance and the need is continuous except when the child has a respiratory infection. However, some teachers have said that muscular dystrophy is their greatest problem emotionally, because of the sadness of watching a child go downhill.

Camp and recreation. Camp is one of the events a child can look forward to and remember. Camp for 25 or 30 virtually helpless children in wheelchairs is a triumph of human resourcefulness. Owing to the unusual skill and generosity of the Muscular Dystrophy Association, camp experience is being made possible for an increasing number of dystrophic children. During 1973 an additional 59 camp sessions were financed by the MDAA.[62] Easter Seal camps for the handicapped also include some children with muscular dystrophy. Helping persons involved with families considering a camp experience for their children may want to inquire into the staff-child ratio and learn as much as possible about the facilities. The helplessness of dystrophic children could make camp a tragedy if it were inadequately administered. However, when well planned and conducted, summer camp can be an extraordinary source of delight and happy memories. The one or two weeks the child is away from home also afford badly needed respite for the family.

The child, and sometimes his mother, may resist the idea of his going to camp the first time, because it is so far removed from experience and is a fearful unknown. It breaks into the child's comfortable dependence on his mother for care of physical needs. In some instances, children who deny there is anything wrong with them do not want to associate with other crippled children, and their parents enable them to have enough stimulating and pleasant recreation with physically normal children so they do not have a need to go to a handicapped children's camp. Most children, however, should be encouraged to try a camp experience if it is available. Like other children, they will be homesick at first and have two or three days of psychic discomfort while adjusting to entirely new surroundings and dependence on strangers, but after a few days they will enjoy themselves and learn new activities and make new friends.

At the San Francisco Bay Area Muscular Dystrophy Association Camp, the child-counselor (college student volunteers) ratio is almost one to one, and the physical work necessary in preparation of craftwork has been performed before the child arrives. A hydraulic lift at the swimming pool, ramps, rafts, floats, ropes, and other needed equipment permit daily "swimming," modified "baseball," cookouts, many crafts, and special events. A session that the writer attended for children ages 10 to 12 included children ranging from 7 to 15, older and younger siblings of the major group. Four children were still walking and 28 were in wheelchairs.

Such a setting quickly demonstrates the *importance of fun*. Children who are obviously depressed, and come together as an aggregation of isolates, scream with laughter and shout to one another after swimming and baseball performed with the aid of the counselors' hands, feet, and strength. Wershow reported, "One has to know this diagnostic group of shy, fearful, seemingly withdrawn children to appreciate the enthusiasm and outgoing qualities they manifested in camp."[63] Approximately half the children at the Bay Area Camp session seemed to become a cohesive group after two or three days. The others spent their time with a special friend and their counselors, or remained largely preoccupied and alone, with the counselor nearby.

Influences other than depression in determining capacity for relationships included the amount of giving from the counselor, the child's temperament and intelligence, and whether the child was in discomfort from the variety of ailments, in addition to muscular dystrophy, that beset many children.

Camp, even more than attendance at a special school, provides an opportunity for group experience with others with the same disease, and thus an opportunity for observing those with more advanced conditions and for communicating their fears of concerns. Children who were still walking gave no indication that they were worried about the future. They used their energy running about, but watched their footing so they did not fall, playing active games with each other and performing the craft and group activities provided. They and the children in wheelchairs were concerned about the same things that make other children happy or unhappy, such as food, winning or not winning, whether their craftwork turned out well or displeased them, taking turns, etc. The older boys were interested in the pretty girl counselors, some of them boisterous about wanting a kiss, and joked enviously of the men counselors' prowess.

Since hand-motion activities are those in which dystrophic children can most readily amuse themselves, boys are fortunate whose mothers are interested in creative arts and who themselves gain pleasure from drawing, painting, stenciling, tie-dye, ceramics, etc. Particularly fortunate are boys whose fathers can devise some means to enable them to participate, and participate with them, in model building, photography, collections of stamps, coins, rocks, shells, bottles, matchbooks, or other things from which they can learn, and around which they can exchange ideas and trade with other children. Innate intelligence and creativity, motivation and some funds, but primarily *free energy from someone with hands, feet, and concern*—whether this be a parent, siblings, neighbor children, relatives, or a volunteer secured by a helping person—all these are the components of leisure-time activity.

Children who are not interested in crafts are sometimes interested in mathematics and electronics; others gain pleasure from radio talk shows they can make phone calls to and become identified with; others enjoy record players and learn to appreciate music. Youths interested in electronics have taken special pleasure in becoming ham operators. With civilian band equipment they can talk to each other, listen to police and emergency calls, and, by becoming members of civilian band clubs, make friends and maintain vital interests. The expensive equipment may be provided by a local ham operators' group or through a special fund-raising event of a service club, if the family or a helping person makes the need known.

Reading, the natural resource of the home-bound, is less often utilized than would appear natural, in part because of the scholastic retardation of many children with muscular dystrophy and in part because television has supplanted reading for a substantial part of the American public. However, reading remains a source of enjoyment for some children, and can be cultivated. Children can be encouraged to enter contests, to keep up on the records of sports stars, to memorize poems, etc. Children from families in which religion is important memorize the names of chapters of the Bible and verses from the Psalms and read the Bible. They look forward to Sunday school and church, social events, and visits from church members.

Keeping busy and as stimulated as possible not only enriches the child's life but makes him more interesting to other children, so that he is less apt to be socially isolated. Most important, in the long, downhill years, he escapes from brooding about his fate by occupation with the present and anticipation of pleasures in the future.

Reactions to knowledge of early crippling and death. Children with muscular dystrophy cannot be shielded from knowledge of their diagnosis and its implications because of the fund-raising literature and Telethon of the Muscular Dystrophy Association. Some performers and writers have emphasized early death to loosen purse strings. If children themselves do not see the Telethon, peers do, who tell them about it. Most dystrophic children seem to feel that this special event is theirs, and that the amount of money raised is related to their chance to live. "I hope the Telethon raises enough money to save me," a nine-year-old boy said. Several children have voiced their hope of life in a scientific breakthrough before death catches them. They think of the Telethon as the medium that will create the scientific advance. Accepting the pain of stretching, performing their blowing exercises, and accepting the discomfort of night splints are routines presented by parents as ways the child can stay healthy until the breakthrough comes.

Another source of hope for some children is heaven or an afterlife. Concrete thinking of the young or retarded more easily produces a picture of a place to go to than do abstract ideas of immortality. "It's going to be a better place than this, that's for sure," one boy said in response to a group session after the death of a classmate. Thoughtful attempts to turn funerals into "celebrations" of the transition to the better life meet with verbal acquiescence sadly given. "We had a celebration for Jim. But I miss him."

Although children with muscular dystrophy turn blank or change the subject when threatening thoughts are brought up by persons they have not tested, most seem to speak freely of death fears to those they trust. A recreation therapist at a convalescent home, who acts as a father figure for a number of boys with muscular dystrophy, states they are most prone to think of death and want to talk about it when they are tired, sick, or discouraged, or brooding for lack of anything to occupy their minds.[64] The death of another child with muscular dystrophy who attends the same school, with whom they have contact, depresses all. Acute reactions shown are refusal to go to sleep for fear of dying, refusal to get out of bed, refusal to go to swimming class for fear of catching cold.

The current emphasis on communication about death to counteract feelings of isolation has had some negative and some positive results. In one instance, a school psychologist urged the father to tell a nine-year-old boy he was going to die, which he did, though reluctantly. The child, already insecure, is now terrified of being left alone, is enuretic, afraid of the dark and of monsters, etc., and continues to ask such questions as "When am I going to die?" and "Will I be alone in Heaven?"

A *context of security* seems essential for communication about death, as does some *avenue for hope*. In a videotaped interview, a 19-year-old youth, Robert Mendenhall, talked with his teachers about his experience with muscular dystrophy and his views of death. He had had a secure, trusting, and open relationship with a wise mother of sincere religious views.

Though the retrospective account dimmed the problems Robert remembered from childhood, he told of how he felt like crying when the other boys teased him; how he had an invisible friend to play with when no one else would play with him, and to eat with, and how the mother always laid a plate for "Henry"; how he had accused his mother of being to blame for transmitting the disease when in early puberty she had denied him something he wanted. However, he never felt that "my mom was trying to get rid of me" when she had to place him in a nursing home, since she had discussed with him ahead of time that she had to work to support the family, but that she would stay home and take care of him and go on welfare in case he felt he simply could not go. Luckily, he lived in a community with nursing-home facilities for children and youth. Though he felt strange at first about being dressed and undressed by strangers, turned several times a night and toileted by them, he said that at the nursing home he now has friends—"There's someone to talk to"—and everyone is nice to him. When he goes home on weekends, he is bored and looks forward to returning to the home.

Early death "doesn't bother me. I see death all the time at the home, and you get used to it. It's been in my family [his mother's philosophy] that usually you die when your job is done and your purpose on earth has been accomplished. I asked my mom straight out when I would die, and she said, not that I *will* die at age 20, but she *thinks* at about age 20.

"I think people are scared because they wonder what it's like to lie under cold dirt or be burned [cremated]. Me, I just accept it. My mom says, Why worry now? When my time comes, it comes, but don't think about it until then. The only thing I'm worried about is my brother and sister. I don't want them to go to pieces; *I want them to carry life on, not to end it.* I don't think they will, but I want them to take care of my mom.

"I believe that when you die you rest—in this new world or whatever. I don't believe this is the end. It's a better life. I don't know... *I just believe it's a good place—that way I'm not scared.* I hope I remember this life; I think I'm helping other people, by explaining what handicapped people are like—just the same as everybody else, only weak."

In response to questions about when and how other children should be told of death, he said, "About nine- or ten-year-old kids would want to know, and parents should tell them, or get teachers to tell the parents what to say, because some parents might need a little assistance."

The compassionate, caring, and unselfish philosophy that Robert developed, and his courage, stemmed from the security he had in his mother and his good fortune in having exceptional teachers and an unusual nursing-home placement. Even he had a defense against fear of immediate death. He believed he would "get a sign," and until this came, he need not fear that death was imminent.

In a paper on cystic fibrosis outstanding for its compassion and involvement, Dr. Martin I. Lorin of the Babies Hospital at the Columbia-Presbyterian Medical Center, New York City, says "Even those [children] who are realistic about their disease and talk openly of death usually have hopes of at least one more remission, one more trip home."[65] He notes that a child's intellectual acceptance of death is qualified by *"not now—later."* (This could also be said of adults.)

Robert had wanted urgently to live long enough to go with his classmates on an elaborately arranged trip to Disneyland. He struggled through a near-fatal siege of pneumonia to do so. A sad source of satisfaction to his mother was that "Bobby got his last wish." Despite his acceptance of the nursing-home placement, he wanted to die at home, and did come home— uncharacteristically in the middle of the week—and died there that night.

In summary, children with muscular dystrophy have a long time to live with knowledge of early death. Their questions must be answered when they raise them, but discussions of death can be constructive only in a context of trust and security. Because their questions may come at unexpected moments, parents, foster parents, and trusted workers should prepare themselves in advance for the kind of philosophy they think they can honestly express, in a way that is not annihilating. Some hope must be left open. Setting definite ages of expected death is not sound. Some children do live well beyond age 20, and in fact a scientific breakthrough may possibly come before the death of children currently afflicted. Visualizing death, not as the end, but as the beginning of a new life, in a better world, is a definite help to many young persons who cannot tolerate the thought of extinguishment at what should be the threshold of their careers. Isolation and brooding allow time for destructive thoughts. All children need activities and something to look forward to. It may not be a trip to Disneyland, but if activities are part of the continuing social plan, it can be an outing to a sports event, a party, a trip to the planetarium, a church social, or whatever seems particularly pleasurable to that person.

CHAPTER SIXTEEN

Sickle Cell Anemia

SICKLE CELL ANEMIA is a painful, inherited blood disorder found predominantly in Black children. One of several genetic conditions characterized by racial discrimination,* the disease is among the most common chronic illnesses of this group.[1]

Sickle cell anemia is significant for social workers and other helping persons because of its scope, the frequently severe disability it causes, and the consequent havoc resulting to family and child. Moreover, one authority states that the child's survival is related to the severity of the disease and "in large part to environmental factors and in particular to the availability of medical care."[2] Severe limitations do exist on the extent to which medical management can alter the course of sickle cell anemia, and equally great limitations on the contribution of social services. "Limited goals" are not unusual, however, in the aims of helping personnel, and much can be done in preventing needless pain, hospitalization, crippling, early death, and family disorganization.

High in priority are educating the parents of children with sickle cell disease, enabling them to put into effect what they learn to do, and working to prevent the birth of additional children with this painful, life-limiting condition.†

Of major importance is a distinction that the worker should make between sickle cell *trait* and sickle cell *anemia*. The *trait* exists when the blood line of only one parent transmits the gene; the *disease* or *anemia* occurs when the person receives the gene from both parents. *The person with the trait is a carrier but is not ill*, whereas the person with the anemia has a variable but serious disease. Persons with the trait do not become worse

---

* Cystic fibrosis, Rh factor disease, and PKU (phenylketonuria) are some of the commonly known diseases of predominantly Caucasian distribution.

† Some Blacks do not agree with prevention as a goal, but I have consistently advocated prevention of transmissible disease, regardless of racial distribution.

and do not gradually develop the disease. This misconception exists among some groups and causes unnecessary worry and alarm. Nor is sickle cell anemia "catching," another misconception that can be laid to rest by the informed worker.

The incidence of sickle cell anemia among Blacks in the United States is estimated as one in 400 persons. The trait occurs in about 1 in 10 American Blacks. About 50,000 persons in the United States are thought to have sickle cell anemia, and about 2 million have the trait.[3] The frequency of the trait in a relatively small group of the population creates a risk that a sickle cell gene will be present in both parents unless carriers become aware of their inheritance and exercise caution against having children with another who has the trait.

Unfortunately, ignorance of the existence of the disease among the unsophisticated is compounded by attempts at secrecy by those who know of the condition but consider it a disgrace. Sickle cell anemia is sometimes called "bad blood" and thought of as a condition like syphilis.

THE MEDICAL REALITIES

Sickle Cell Disease

An abnormality of red cells gradually evolved in peoples living in certain regions of Africa that permitted them to survive malignant malaria. This once-protective mechanism has been transmitted to the genes of the descendants. The gene causes a disorder of the hemoglobin or oxygen carrying part of the red cell. At times, the normally round, flexible cells distort themselves into elongated crescents, or sickle shapes. The occasion for sickling is lack of enough oxygen in the cell, for causes to be elaborated later, or sluggishness of the blood, for reasons yet to be identified.

Normal red cells pass through the blood vessels smoothly, but sickle-shaped cells are rigid and will not pass through tiny vessels; instead they "logjam" the capillaries. Since oxygen is vital to all tissues, the area ordinarily fed by the blocked capillaries will suffer serious damage or die. These occasions are very painful, and are called *occlusive vascular* or *pain crises*. The body's natural defenses heal the dead areas with scar tissue, and scar tissue in lieu of normal functioning cells creates additional problems.[4]

According to L. W. Diggs, a specialist who has studied sickle cell disease for many years, the abnormal cells are fragile and die more quickly in the circulation than normal cells. "As a result of the imbalance between the rates of blood formation and destruction there are varying degrees of anemia, which for a given individual tend to remain fairly constant."[5]

In addition to chronic anemia occasioned by the short life span of abnormal red cells, children with sickle cell anemia can have sudden sharp drops in the number of cells their bone marrow manufactures. These drops come about if some infection or toxic substance, including drugs, injures the cells of the bone marrow.[6] These are called *aplastic crises*, and are fatal if not treated promptly.

In sickle cell anemia, nearly all the red cells are abnormal or subject to sickling, whereas in the trait, only about a third of the cells are affected, too small a proportion to create symptoms except in unusual circumstances. In addition to these two opposite extremes of sickle cell disease there are mid-forms, sometimes called *variants*. In these, sickle hemoglobin occurs in association with *thalassemia*, or with *hemoglobin C or D*. These conditions are usually of intermediate clinical severity; that is, the child has symptoms of sickle cell anemia but they may be of milder form.[7]

Significance of Sickle Cell Trait

The primary significance of the trait is genetic. Being a carrier has potential psychosocial hazards, discussed later, but has been believed of physical importance only if the person is subjected to extreme oxygen deprivation, as in riding in an unpressurized plane.[8] Bloody urine and severe damage to the spleen have been reported under such circumstances. However, in 1961, a pathologist associated with Diggs at the University of Tennessee, in reporting autopsy findings of over 1,200 Negroes over one year of age, stated that in 4 percent death was due to the trait, and in another 8 percent the trait was a contributory cause of death. "The real problem is that sickle cell trait, unlike classical sickle cell anemia, does not produce marked clinical signs and symptoms under usual living conditions. However, add the stress of anoxia [lack of oxygen] from congestive heart failure, shock from any cause, or even a mild respiratory tract infection, and fatal results may occur."[9] Alcoholism and surgical anesthesia, this pathologist states, are other conditions that may cause death when combined with the trait.

Since the Viet Nam war, four deaths have been reported among 4,000 Negroes at a basic training camp. The four had come from low altitudes to a camp at over 4,000 feet, and collapsed and died after moderate physical exercise during their first few days at the higher altitude. In three of the four cases no significant autopsy findings other than sickling were found. The reporting physician comments on the puzzling nature of why only four died (in light of the statistical probability that perhaps 400 had the trait).[10] At approximately the same time as this report (1970), the medical literature contained a letter from a physician regarding a woman with sickle cell trait who had a stroke while taking oral contraceptives. He commented that the contraceptive may have lowered the oxygen content of the hemoglobin in the brain sufficiently to activate the sickling potential.[11]

Thus it appears that as more is known about sickle cell anemia, the more complex the problem becomes. Possession of the trait does not shorten the life span under ordinary conditions. It is not yet clear how significant the trait may be under conditions of severe stress. However, the long-held view remains that persons with the trait are able to lead normal lives. It is important that neither the person, nor his family, nor the worker thinks of him as ill.

Pattern of Inheritance

The pattern of inheritance is Mendelian-recessive. This means that if both parents carry the trait, the general statistical odds are that one in four children will be born with the anemia, two in four will be carriers of the trait, and one will have neither the anemia nor the trait.[12] *Social workers and parents need to remember that inheritance patterns refer to statistical chances only and not to any particular family. A family cannot count on having normal children because they already have one child with the disease, or children established as carriers.* Many families have two, three, or more children with sickle cell anemia.

Symptoms, Course, and Outlook of Sickle Cell Anemia

The proportion of cells that sickle varies from person to person.[13] When two or more children in one family have sickle cell disease, some may have sickle cell anemia, and others the "variants" or mild forms. Of those with anemias, some children are well most of the time and able to lead relatively normal lives, whereas others are severely disabled. Many die in infancy or early childhood.

"In general, the disease appears to be more severe in childhood than later in life, and the earlier the onset of symptoms, the poorer the outlook."[14] Since affected babies have normal hemoglobin for the first few months of life, the symptoms do not appear until the latter part of the first year; diagnosis is usually made between the second and fourth year. The baby may be irritable, pale, and jaundiced, *fail to thrive*, have a poor appetite and distended stomach. The child is subject to weakness, abdominal pain, bone deformities, and heart enlargement, and may also have severe neurological disorders such as transient or permanent blindness, convulsions, or coma.[15] Experts emphasize that health and social workers should suspect the possibility of sickle cell anemia in Black children who are chronically sickly, and arrange an examination that includes sickle cell testing.

The *pain crises*, due to logjamming of cells, vary in severity and last from a few hours to two weeks, but usually several days. Their frequency varies unpredictably; sometimes they occur every few days or weeks, sometimes years apart.[16] The child's back, chest, arms, and legs may be painful; his joints may be swollen, and he is feverish, may be drowsy, unable to speak, have nosebleeds, bloody urine, or other symptoms, depending on the location and diversity of the occluded capillaries and destroyed tissue.

In severe crises the pain is so great the child must be hospitalized—he is unable to eat or sleep and needs narcotics for relief. However, many children have minor crises of short duration only and are often cared for satisfactorily at home. Dr. Powars of the Los Angeles Sickle Cell Center states that of the 300 children treated during a ten-year period some have been hospitalized only once.[17]

Hospitalization varies widely from case to case. The severity of the disease, the mother's alertness in detecting early symptoms of crises and ability to administer necessary care at home, and the physician's predilections are among determining factors. Some children are hospitalized innumerable times, for as long as ten days or two weeks, with many emergency-room visits in between. At the opposite end are occasional children who are hospitalized rarely. Frequency of clinic visits for supervision also varies from case to case and at different times. Some children attend the clinic every two weeks and others every two months, depending on how well they are getting along.

Toddlers and preschool children are most subject to crises, hence need close supervision, and are more prone to frequent hospitalization than older children. The young child has a characteristic "hand-foot syndrome," or painful swelling of hands and feet, and abdominal pain is frequent.[18]

Crises are precipitated by infection, chilling, dehydration, strenuous exercise, sweating, changes in barometric pressure, and other causes that increase the body's demand for oxygen. Diggs says that cold triggers painful crises in some patients. Even putting a hand in cold water may create pain and swelling; cold, damp weather results in an increased number of crises.[19] They may occur unpredictably, for no cause that can be identified. Stress and exhaustion seem to precipitate crises. Long bus or automobile rides, which cause sluggish circulation, and high-altitude trips including plane rides are felt to be hazardous because of the rarified air. Infections are the most common causes of crises. "The major offender is the common cold."[20] Infections are a frequent cause of death.[21]

Increased pallor or lethargy may signal increased severity of anemia, the possibility that a dangerous *aplastic crisis* has begun. Pallor in a Black is shown by a "grayish cast over the brown skin tone, most apparent in the same areas that white skin is lightest—the nose, cheekbones, wrists, hands, forehead, forearms, etc."[22]

Signs of increased anemia may signal another potentially fatal episode in young children, bleeding into the spleen. This *splenic sequestration* requires emergency medical care, for the child goes into shock from which he will die if it cannot be reversed quickly.[23]

Other serious episodes that workers caring for children should be aware of are liver (*hepatic*) crises, manifested by even greater than usual jaundice, dark urine, and lassitude; *retinal sickling* with visual impairment of mild to complete absence of vision; in older boys a distressingly painful erection of the penis called *priapism*; *sickling in the brain*, with various associated manifestations from headache to convulsions, coma, or stroke; *kidney disturbance*; and *sickling in the bones*, accompanied by severe pain.[24]

Children with sickle cell anemia develop chronic problems because of repeated capillary failures and tissue destruction, and their physical growth is retarded. Death, however, is not due to progressive deterioration, but is frequently sudden and unexpected, sometimes with no known causative factor but, as previously indicated, often precipitated by infection.[25]

"Survival to adulthood is not rare," according to the United States Public Health Service.[26] General agreement exists that the life span is considerably shorter than normal. It is lengthening because of improved capacity to treat symptoms.[27] Children usually die in their late teens, but general figures are misleading in individual cases and create grave apprehension among affected children and their families as the child nears the end of his teens. Of children with sickle cell anemia, 50 percent are said to survive to adulthood.[28] A Johns Hopkins study, reported in 1964, showed several patients over 40 years of age, and it projected an increased number of such persons in the future.[29]

Treatment

No cure exists for sickle cell anemia, and treatment is "symptomatic." British physicians say "the prevention of intravascular sickling is the most helpful way of treating the patient."[30] They point out the importance of keeping the child warm, of avoiding tight garments that impede circulation, and treating infections. Educating the mother to avoid circumstances that may precipitate a crisis, and to recognize symptoms of impending crisis, is believed to be the foundation of prevention.

The Los Angeles Sickle Cell Center staff attempts to teach parents the importance of maintaining good health habits and of teaching the child to drink an abundance of liquids regularly. The Los Angeles Center teaches the mothers to use "soaks," or to place the child in a bathtub of warm water if he complains of aching, or every morning during threatened crises. A Jacuzzi whirlpool is provided by the Center for use in the bathtub for children whose families cannot afford to buy one.

Experts emphasize the importance of prompt, vigorous treatment of infections.[31] The child cannot wait until infection is established, that is, for a fever to show that infection is under way. The physician should be called at the first sign of lethargy, sneezing, loss of appetite, or other sign that the child does not feel well. Dr. Powars points out that infections frequently mimic crises. Transfusions are necessary during aplastic crisis or bleeding into the spleen. In some cases transfusions are used to treat anemia or are administered on a prevention basis. Bed rest, warmth, pain medication, forcing fluids, and antibiotics are used for pain crises, in addition to specific treatment for complications that may arise, such as pyelonephritis, pneumonia, or meningitis.[32]

PSYCHOSOCIAL IMPLICATIONS

Too little is known of the psychosocial effects of sickle cell anemia to afford authoritative information. The condition has created widespread attention only recently; there is no collection of studies or reports of long clinical observation. Black social workers now working in sickle cell programs have given a substantial portion of their efforts to organization, administration, screening programs, and other broad-scale management problems; few Caucasian workers have been involved with a large number of families of children with this condition.

Added to the difficulty is the wide variation in meaning of the disease to individual children and families because of the variability of symptoms among affected children. The major limitations one child suffers differ from those of another. Furthermore, middle-class Blacks, the most articulate and able to describe their experiences, have a different constellation of circumstances surrounding the disease than the poor.

Certain aspects are, however, self-evident, and others recur often enough that some generalizations become possible. Parents of children with sickle cell anemia need accurate and detailed information. They may need help with housing and dietary problems because of the relationships of sickle cell crisis to infection and cold. Other areas of need arise from the importance of immediate medical attention when crisis threatens or occurs. Problems arise in many cases from repeated hospitalization of the young child, lassitude and retarded growth, delayed sexual maturation of the adolescent, and in some cases, the effects on child and family of repeated episodes of sudden, severe pain, and in others, the crippling that occurs as a result of destroyed tissue. Over all hang the lack of norms and the apprehension caused by expectation of the child's early death.

Stigma and Lack of Information

Though Linus Pauling discovered the basic defect in 1949 and the disease had been observed and described much earlier,[33] very little general information existed until recently. In a 1969 survey among the Black population in Richmond, Virginia, only 30 percent of the general population and 65 percent of the college graduates told the interviewers that they had heard of the disease.[34] A medical social worker at a sickle cell anemia clinic said that an undercurrent of half-truths does exist among the Black population; that sickle cell anemia is thought of as "bad blood" and families known to have it are avoided or ostracized.

However, many parents do not hear the term "sickle cell anemia" until a physician uses the term when diagnosing a child. Two serious problems may result. The parents may misconstrue the name and nature of the disease. One mother said that her sister, who was with her when the physician used the term "sickle cell anemia," asked much later, "How can a little child like that have syphilis cell anemia?"

Lacking an understanding of what to expect and of the importance of attempting to prevent or alleviate crises, the mother is not prepared to help the child. The mother quoted above said her sister's response to the second crisis was, "What, did he catch sickle cell anemia again? He already had it a year ago." This mother made the serious charge that the physician's failure to instruct her regarding symptoms of impending crises and the need to force fluids at this time led to the child's stroke. She had walked with him a long distance in the hot sun at the time the stroke occurred, having no knowledge of the importance of avoiding dehydration as a means of preventing obstruction of blood vessels by sickled cells.

As a result of recent publicity urging tests for sickle cell trait, and insufficient general public knowledge of genetics, some adverse side effects have occurred. Individuals may be taunted or groups may be discriminated against; emotional racial overtones can obscure realities. Sickle cell anemia has been termed the "first political disease." Attempts have been made to curry votes by promoting legislation or appropriations for testing and treatment.[35] It has been called a "prickly disease" because of the emotions that surround any condition that is predominantly confined to one racial group.

Financial Problems

Hospitalization creates the most costly feature of sickle cell anemia, especially if it occurs frequently. However, this expense may be met by private insurance, Medicaid, or Crippled Children's Services in the majority of cases. More difficult to secure are the funds necessary for long-term healthy living that prevents unnecessary sickle cell crises. Expenses for readily available transportation at times of crisis may also constitute problems, as may those for the mother's hospital visits or extended stays near the hospital.

A consideration of needs for suitable housing, clothing, and diet, which are outlined in the following sections, makes plain to experienced workers how difficult are the financial problems created by sickle cell anemia. A Supplemental Security Income allowance for a child of a family receiving assistance would appear to be essential in order to expand the capacity of the grant to provide suitable housing. If the child is denied SSI assistance on the basis of insufficient disability, the need for prevention of disability through funds for housing, clothing, and diet warrants an appeal. Families may need help in appeal procedures, and in taking advantage of food stamps and other means of making best use of income. They may need advocacy effort in order to secure public housing if a waiting list exists.

In one-parent families, a hidden cost is that the mother is unavailable for employment in most instances, especially during the child's preschool years, when he is most prone to physical problems and least able to detect and articulate symptoms that warn of impending crises. If the mother is upward-striving and accustomed to working, she may need opportunity to sort out her feelings about lowering her standard of living while the child is small, or she may need help in locating a fully reliable mother substitute for her child. If she lives in an area where welfare departments place great emphasis upon employment of all mothers, her child's needs may require more interpretation to the department than she can provide on her own.

Another expense requiring ingenuity and at times advocacy pertains to transportation. In Western cities dependent upon automobile transportation, an old car creates constant disruptions, financial problems, and delays among families in lower socioeconomic groups. More practical in some instances is an arrangement for agency help, including provision for cost of gasoline for a neighbor's car for night and weekend emergency visits to the physician or hospital.

Fortunately, the emergence of Sickle Cell Centers and inner-city agencies that emphasize service to ethnic groups has made possible more potential resources for help than in the past for families of children with sickle cell anemia. The worker's main needs may be an awareness of the relationship between social circumstances and the child's health, so that she can be an effective interpreter, and sophistication regarding the use of resources.

Housing and Diet

Keeping in mind that crises are precipitated by infection, and that infection furthermore is the most common cause of death, the relationship of housing and diet to the child's well-being readily appears. Middle-class families maintain life-styles and have funds to provide nourishing food and healthful housing, but the social circumstances of the poor—or half of all Black families—directly oppose the survival needs of the child with sickle cell anemia.

Sickle cell anemia is sometimes thought of as a "winter disease" because of the frequency of crises during flu season and cold weather, but summer heat brings its own special hazard, that of dehydration. Moving to another locality can be an issue in sickle cell anemia, as in asthma and other illnesses affected by environment; a child who has repeated crises in localities characterized by extremes of heat and cold may suddenly improve after moving to a milder climate. But if a child plays hard and is without supervision, or is under circumstances where insufficient fluid is supplied, he can incur serious hazard, including stroke. Important in preventing colds and other upper respiratory infections is clothing that protects against the elements—shoes with good soles, galoshes or rubbers, raincoats, sweaters, and in winter warm underwear, socks, caps, scarves, gloves or mittens, and coats or jackets. Clothing must be replaced when it is outgrown, worn out, lost, or stolen. It is essential that housing permit a relatively warm, stable environment, with hot running water, and room for the child to sleep in a bed by himself, away from the common colds of brothers and sisters. His bed needs to be comfortable enough that he can rest, and he needs sufficient bedding for warmth.

Against these needs are the familiar realities of the poor. Not only is crowding common, but the manager of the public housing complex or the apartment building may turn off the heat at certain hours to save money, or the heating system may break down and lack repair for an indefinite period. The plumbing may be shared and out of order. A hot tub bath every morning may be far removed from housing potential. The gas and electric company may turn off the family's heat because of nonpayment of bills. Makeshift neighborhood day-care facilities in basements, empty stores, or warehouses may be without adequate heat in winter; this can also occur in public schools.

Knowing that chill may precipitate a sickle cell crisis, the worker needs to take action quickly when a family's housing problem comes to attention. Extra clothing and an electric blanket are easier to provide than warm housing, and provide partial stop-gap remedies. However, the agency may need to interpret the medical problem to the gas company, the public housing administrator, apartment manager, or other persons responsible for heating the building. The worker may need to seek administrative exception to policies against payment of back bills or ceilings on rent payments. "Crisis intervention," with a case closing and return to income maintenance status, would not appear to be appropriate, for a recurrence of the social problem may be anticipated: if budget counseling or direct vendor payment of utilities is indicated, such circumstance will require long-term rather than crisis-oriented action.

Nutrition is a primary force in maintaining a high level of protection against infection. The needed high-protein, high-vitamin, adequate-iron diet requires careful planning. Milk, meat, and beans, usual sources of high-quality protein, are prohibitively costly for most families. Fortunately, fish, eggs, liver, and poultry have not been as badly affected by inflation. Middle-class educated families can take advantage of the flood of information on complicated vegetarian substitutes for meat proteins. Some can grow their own leafy vegetables in yard or community garden.

The aid of a dietician is often helpful. If the available dieticians are not oriented to low-budget problems, health aides on the staff of the health department may be of assistance in helping mothers plan menus that approximate the child's needs and are not too far removed from the family food habits.

Great variation exists in eating styles; the matter needs exploration, since marked physical improvement can occur when a child has the nutrition, warmth, protection, and rest his condition requires. In families where children snatch what food they can when they want it, and planned meals are not part of the life-style, intensive effort may be required to help the mother. If she is working, she may need to quit and devote herself to supervising and caring for the children. A capable family member, or friend, may be able to provide care, especially if paid to do so. A homemaker may be needed.

"Pushing fluids," a related dietary matter, requires teaching the child to drink water frequently, and keeping a bottle or pitcher of water and a glass out where he sees them and is therefore reminded to drink. Fruit juices are a welcome adjunct to the water, and should be available if at all possible. Soda pop and popsicles are used to tempt the child to drink, especially when he is in an incipient crisis and does not want to drink anything. Too much soda is probably unhealthy and is expensive but may induce the child to accept fluids at times of threatened sickle cell crises. The obvious problem pertaining to soda pop arises in respect to the other children.

Warm clothing, decent housing, good food, regular habits—these needs are so simple and self-evident that their importance may be overlooked. Services to enable families to achieve them can be so time-consuming and frustrating that they may be unconsciously passed over, or relegated to another agency or person. If the agency delegates environmental services to aides or requests the services of other agencies, follow-up is essential. The needs of some poor Black families are not only overwhelming but extremely complex; it seems unlikely that environmental services without counseling, education, and support will suffice.

Medical Care

When the first symptoms of infection or crisis begin, and the child is listless, uninterested in food, slightly feverish, aching, or too tired to play, the physician must be notified immediately. If he knows the mother and child well, he may prescribe medication by telephone, but he may wish to see the child without delay. This poses some practical problems. First, the parents must understand the disease and what is needed, and why. They must have prior arrangements for transportation at all times. The continuing child-care arrangements must permit early recognition of symptoms.

After diagnosis, some parents need help in returning to the physician for more information. They may have failed to absorb the highly charged information, or the physician may have used terms the parents did not understand. A parent who attends a busy clinic may have little opportunity to ask questions; she may see only an intern who does not know the full details about sickle cell anemia; she may be inarticulate or not know what to ask, or too shy to say she does not understand the words the doctor has used.

Some parents profit from the company of a person less emotionally involved, who has a list of questions that need exposition. Often a conference that includes both parents and the social worker helps all, ensuring the worker's capacity to reinforce what the physician has said on later occasions when fears come out and questions need more discussion. At times the worker may not be able to attend a joint conference with the physician. In such cases it may help to write down with the mother the questions that need amplification, or arrange for a hospital social worker to help the parents secure a conference with an appropriate physician. The worker can support the mother in her need to know and her right to ask questions.

Sickle cell anemia centers serve large areas, often far distant from the child's home. If distance is a problem, arrangements are necessary for some liaison medical care by a pediatrician who is quickly accessible. Finding a competent physician who is willing to take "welfare cases," if the family receives public assistance, and who has proved available on weekends and in the evenings is sometimes a time-consuming problem requiring substantial knowledge of medical resources. The medical consultant of the agency may prove helpful in arranging for a suitable pediatrician to accept responsibility, or the center social worker or physician may be able to make recommendations from experience with physicians in the locality where the child lives. A former resident of the medical center may have entered private practice in the locality and have special interest in sickle cell anemia and in keeping in contact with the medical center. Some Black physicians are especially interested in sickle cell anemia. The health department is another resource to investigate for locating a suitable local practitioner.

Private physicians are notably impatient with families who do not keep appointments, and may refuse further service after one or two experiences in which they have been inconvenienced. Parents who are dependent on neighbors for transportation may find the neighbor is not available at time of need, and may not have a telephone to notify the physician's office of inability to bring the child in. For this reason, in addition to the primary need to help the parents secure a physician's examination quickly, a worker involved in helping the family of a child with sickle cell anemia should give top priority to reliable arrangements for transportation to medical care.

A small child who is subject to crises needs close surveillance, if early symptoms are to be detected in time to prevent full-blown crises. Casual arrangements for child care while the mother works obviously are not suitable. Whereas older siblings may be acceptable to welfare departments as child-caring persons for usual families, and mothers frequently rely on neighbors to look after their children while they work, the busy neighbor or older child cannot be relied upon to detect early symptoms of crisis. Day-care arrangements subject the child to the hazard of exposure to other children's colds and childhood infections. The preschool-age child with sickle cell anemia needs his own mother or an approved substitute who is not caring for a number of other children.

Often the family is one in which the mother has many preoccupations in addition to the child with sickle cell anemia; she cannot devote her full attention to him. Not infrequently she has other children with varying degrees of disability from the same disease. The mother may be fearful of medical care, especially in a teaching center where she has heard "they experiment on you," or "they use your child as a guinea pig." A carefully individualized plan that is acceptable and practical is necessary during any period in which the child is having many crises.

Hospitalization

Fortunately, some children with sickle cell anemia require hospital care seldom or not at all. However, an infant or preschool child who is repeatedly removed from home for hospitalization at a time he is in pain, and whose trauma is compounded by immobilization and injections, may develop severe separation behavior similar to that of an autistic child. Workers in the community who are not familiar with hospital ward scenes may fail to appreciate why hospital staff who have observed these children rocking and banging their heads on the crib sides think wryly of the disease as spelled "sickle's hell." Prevention of the acute separation grief and its psychological consequences is sufficiently important to merit the needed thoughtfulness and expense. Some hospitals will permit the mother to remain with the child; many now permit the mother to feed the child and to take care of him during the day.

The child's need for mothering during hospitalization has become so well known, and the trauma of separation during a painful period noted by so many experts,[36] that further observation seems redundant. Yet in practice few poor mothers with large families do spend much time with their hospitalized children. Some might be able to take advantage of hospital policies if funds were available to pay a neighbor or friend for care of children at home. A sitter or homemaker can sometimes be arranged for by the agency if the worker has told the mother to let her know when the child is admitted to the hospital. Parents who live at a distance from a special sickle cell center may need extra funds to stay for a few days at a nearby guest house or motel. Many modifications are possible when the worker and the parent recognize the importance to the small child of having his mother with him. The worker often needs to take the initiative in discussing plans with the mother, especially if she seems to take for granted that nothing can be done, or has stopped trying to work her way out of various problems in daily life.

Children can be released from the hospital after a minimum amount of care if they are continued on antibiotics and receive recommended care at home during the convalescent period. However, lack of follow-through at home on treatment begun in the hospital may result in a serious prolonged relapse.[37] Thus coordination between the social agency in the community that is helping the family with care of the child at home and the hospital physician and/or social worker or liaison nurse becomes of paramount importance in preventing waste of care and unnecessary pain and injury to the child.

Family Adjustment

Added to the variability occasioned by the nature of the disease are family relationships, which vary according to the subcultural pattern of family living. There are extreme differences in Black family patterns just as in those of Caucasians and Orientals, but a fallacious tendency exists to lump all Blacks in the low socioeconomic group, with subsequent poverty patterns. The rapid growth and substantial number of middle-class and professional Black families in the North and West provide an entirely different web of circumstances to which a sick child relates from that of the urban ghetto family or the Southern rural family. The support offered by extended family relationships and deeply felt religious ties becomes weakened, while educated response to medical care and paternal sharing of family responsibility become strengthened. Anger and projection of blame may replace apathy and resignation. A younger generation, or the relatives in another section of the country, may hold new values, and an older generation cling to old, as the rapid upward mobility of the American Black adds to family complexities. Thus the "system" in which illness becomes a part, altering and being altered by other parts, is itself a shifting variable.

Whether a matriarchal culture pattern exists that affects paternal tendency to shift the burden of care of a sick child to the mother is not known. However, Black social workers have pointed out the tendency of the father to avoid facing his contribution to the child's disease or care. Added to the emotional burden common to parents of children with other hereditary disease is resentment over sickle cell anemia's being a problem primarily of Blacks. The fathers tend to feel they have enough rejection to cope with;

that the stigma of a unique genetic disease is too much to face. Accordingly, in many cases, one sees the familiar picture of the mother carrying the burden alone.

Welfare department and child-placement-agency case loads attest to the fact that the father is not always the parent who cannot bear the stress of caring for a child with sickle cell anemia. As happens in other burdensome disease conditions, mothers may face their inability to cope and ask for placement of the child in a foster home, or escape the problem through use of drugs or alcohol or by sending the child to relatives. Children who are neither wholly abandoned nor adequately cared for require frequent hospitalizations. Early interruption of this pattern of neglect, or of the mother's inability to cope with a sickly, crying child, is important. The child's life and emotional development depend on early, decisive action in either supplementing the mother's homemaking, child-caring resources or removing the child from her care.

Lack of communication between parents after learning of a child's serious and fatal disease is graphically described in an interview given by a mother to a magazine writer.[38] One of their three children with sickle cell disease died unexpectedly of a stroke.

After Gregory's death, my husband and I never really sat down and talked. Not because we didn't want to, but *we each were so caught up in our own sorrow that we couldn't realize what the other was going through,* and we both went in different directions when we should have stayed and pulled together. Maybe if we had had a drag-em-out talk or gone to see a family counselor or our minister, it would have helped. *Instead, we began hitting out at each other, and it's a terrible thing when two people try to torment each other.*

This mother went on to say that her husband lost his faith in God—"What kind of God would take my child away?"—and turned to drugs. When another child would go into sickle cell crisis, he would disappear, "strung out on drugs somewhere.... He would say, 'That's exactly why I'm where I am. I don't want to see it.'" Eventually he returned to work periodically, but "every time Shelton and Ramona would go through a very serious crisis he feared that they would never recover and he seemed to feel life wasn't worth living."

This same mother described the guilty feelings that lurk between parent and child, commenting on the child's questions about why he was born to suffer so much: "He said he would never say that to me because it is not my fault [he had of course said it].... I think it takes a lot of understanding, respect and courage to be able to keep from throwing it back at your parents and say, Why did you have me? Or, you knew we were like this, why did you have other children?"[39]

Continued reproduction of diseased children has been commented on in other chapters. In several instances of children with sickle cell disease, mothers have said that they and their husbands would not have married had they known the suffering their children would endure and what they would go through themselves; yet the number of families who have more than one child with sickle cell disease is substantial. One can speculate on the reasons: projection—"the doctors told us we couldn't possibly have another child with the disease"; ignorance—"we thought that after having one child with the disease and losing two in miscarriages, our chances for a normal child were good"; religious reasons; denial; or the strong urge to prove normality—all these may operate. Accidental conception adds to the number. The guilt cannot be erased, whatever the reason.

The "vulnerable child syndrome" is seen in sickle cell anemia. Guilt over transmission would appear to play a part. Added to this is the reality of hearing a child wake up screaming in pain and finding oneself helpless to do anything to relieve it, a painful experience reinforcing the feelings of the parents on hearing the physician say there is no cure and that the child will probably not survive until adulthood. The frequency of crises and how they are handled are other factors in the parental reaction. Strong emotional support, as well as practical help in preventing full-blown crises and in securing adequate medical care, is indicated in preventing the pathological overprotection arising from anxiety over the child's expected death.

One parent said the hardest thing for herself and her family about having a child with sickle cell anemia was learning to live from day to day. Neither parents nor children, both of whom had the disease, knew when a sickle cell crisis would occur, or what kind it would be, or how serious, or whether it would be fatal. They could not plan ahead for anything—vacations, company, special events, later schooling, careers—but rather had to live life only in the present. Otherwise they had too many disappointments. Though existentialism, "make today count," is a movement many young adults and older persons adopt, the denial of any future-oriented goals to children, who must be future-oriented to mature, is major pathology.

Anxiety is justifiable, and none can assure the parents or child that he will escape the crippling or early death they have seen occur in other children, or that he will not continue to have crises. But just as the negative cannot be ruled out, neither can the positive; the child may live to middle age, and may have little or no permanent crippling. Sensitive to the potential areas of self-blame, family friction, and mixed feelings, the worker will avoid bottling up destructive emotions with quick reassurance. She can find out from the physician whether the child in question has a severe form of the disease. She can provide opportunities for catharsis and avoid false reassurance, but at the same time reinforce hope. In addition to verbal emphasis on the positive, the worker can help bring about the child's chance of a good life by giving her attention to seemingly mundane but vital matters that prevent infections and full-blown crises, and ensure immediate medical care when they threaten.

School

Education is especially important for the child with sickle cell anemia because he will not be able to undertake unskilled labor or an outdoor job as an adult. Yet the fatigue that anemia creates is a major obstacle to his schooling and socialization. Fatigue varies in degrees and over time, but a general lassitude seems always present. Some children have periods when they cannot sit through a class period. Getting to school or walking between classes can be too tiring. Especially when loss of sleep from pain, and joint tenderness and swelling, add to the general fatigue, the child cannot attend. The child who is too tired to go to school and needs isolation from other children during winter months can perhaps attend summer school, day camp, or church school; good weather can be used as a compensation for seasonal slowdowns in the educational and socialization process.

A child with severe disease or one who is undergoing a series of infections and crises may need to stay out of school and have a home teacher, particularly during the winter months or the flu season, or during a period of childhood epidemics at school. Tele-teaching is used by some school districts to supplement the home teacher. Danger exists that the child will get behind in his studies, will feel alien, and want to remain at home; that his fatigue will gradually induce an indolent way of life. Unnecessary home-bound status reinforces the intensity of mother-child relationships and attenuates normal ego development.

The worker should keep in touch with the child's medical progress and encourage early return to school as soon as the physician advises it is feasible. If fatigue due to anemia interferes with school attendance, transfusions may restore the child to a temporarily improved level of functioning. Diet plays an important role in degree of anemia and thus of fatigue, so that the worker will need to determine the child's typical daily food intake and learn whether it includes sufficient iron.

When a child needs to remain at home over a prolonged period, deliberate attention to sources of stimulation is needed. The Los Angeles Sickle Cell Center has a tutorial program, sending Black tutors, some of them adults with sickle cell disease, into the homes to supplement the work of the home teachers and provide support, encouragement, and stimulation to the child. One mother showed the author her own resourcefulness in bringing the outside world into the child's room, by helping him paper his walls with posters and magazine cut-outs; a neighbor had given this child a high, swivel stool so that he could look out the windows, swiveling in the direction of activity.

When the child returns to school, coordination should be secured with the school nurse, if there is one, and recommendations from a physician with regard to competitive sports and physical education classes. Children frequently are allowed to engage in noncompetitive athletics but may be prohibited from body-contact sports. Bicycle riding and swimming are encouraged for some, although the chilling that may follow swimming may prevent this activity. In the classroom, teachers may need information about sickle cell disease.[40] The teacher ideally should be alert to signs that the child is feeling bad, and should become able to distinguish between real fatigue and manipulation. The worker needs to be aware of the possibility of misunderstanding about the nature of the disease on the part of the teacher or schoolmates. Pamphlets are readily available to the teacher (see notes).

Urban schools have restroom problems that may create special difficulty for the child whose regimen requires drinking an unusual amount of liquids and frequent urination. Older boys loiter in the bathrooms to smoke, frightening younger, smaller boys away from the toilets by attacking them. The small, poorly developed Black boy with sickle cell anemia is a likely target. Children frequently learn of certain times or restrooms that are safe, or they may reduce fluid intake and strive to avoid using the bathroom at school. The worker may need to help with special arrangements or suggestions from the school nurse, physical education teacher, or principal.

Long bus rides to school or clinic create problems. Sluggish circulation is a problem when a child sits with bent knees over a long period, and cannot get up and walk around. Sickling and occlusion may result. A conference with parents and the principal may be necessary to arrange school attendance close to the child's home. Since many ramifications can exist, including the child's feelings about where he wishes to attend, teachers' attitudes, availability of toilet facilities, etc., the subject warrants a visit or conference rather than a quick telephone call.

Effect on Personality

The burgeoning of interest in sickle cell disease is too recent to permit accumulation of solid data regarding the emotional growth of children with sickle cell disease. The severity of the disease, the number of hospitalizations and age of the child when they occurred, and how they were handled create substantial differences. Two preadolescent girls have been observed who are independent and self-assured, although small. One is quiet and the other an outgoing happy child; both have a number of interests such as music, photography, and sewing, in addition to their schoolwork. These are children who have had the advantage of loving, middle-class parents, intact homes, good schools and medical care, and who have not suffered crippling episodes during crises. They are still not entirely aware of the implications of their conditions, nor have they entered adolescence. A similarly normal boy has been seen, who has become quiet and seems bewildered by nightly painful priapism.

How soon the child should be burdened with the knowledge of implications of his disease is not known. One intelligent mother said it is like adoption, something the child should grow up knowing instead of learning suddenly from a fund-raising television program or cruelly from another child. She had provided her children with the comic book HEW has issued, "Where's Herbie—A Sickle Cell Story,"* and although her child had never alluded to its information that sickle cell disease cannot be cured, she thought the child had grasped its meaning.

Predictably, major problems become apparent at adolescence. Delayed sexual development, small size, and general fragility result in what Aaron Smith of the Peninsula Sickle Cell Foundation calls the "Peter Pan syndrome." At adolescence the boys tend to have feminine voices, small bones, and a childlike, immature manner. Both the physical manifestations of the disease and its consequences tend to keep him a child indefinitely. Jean Vavasseau, medical social worker and administrative assistant at the Los Angeles Sickle Cell Center, has expressed her impressions that passivity and excessive dependence on the mother are common.[41] She has observed the uncertainty and fear that accompany experience of unpredictable pain and helplessness to avoid it. At adolescence and early adulthood the dependence has a large hostile component, as would be expected, but need for the mother's help during painful episodes keeps the child close to her. Inability to break away reinforces the hostility.

Mrs. Vavasseau has also observed outward forms of social maladjustment, "acting out," in early adolescence. Retarded growth, delayed puberty, and social immaturity place the boy of junior high school age at special disadvantage with his sports-minded, active peers. Intervention to help him adjust at the time of entrance to junior high school may be needed.

Young adulthood has special problems connected with the misinterpretations that have grown up around expectation of death before the age of 20. Each crisis is vested with anxiety that death is at hand. Lack of norms and goals in young adults may exist because of ideas of both the child and his parents that he would not live to be an adult. "Now here I am; what do I do?" The child has not been prepared for adult responsibilities.

Among the increasing number of young adults who have survived are some, however, who are living relatively satisfying lives despite the handicap of frequent pain, fatigue, and crippling. Intense religious commitment

---

* U.S. Department of Health, Education, and Welfare, Office of Child Development, publication #1291-0177, National Institute of Health, Bethesda, Maryland.

may serve as a bulwark against fear of sudden death and provide opportunities for active social functioning. Sedentary, nontaxing employment has provided some with the chance to be productive and independent as well as mentally occupied. Black girls who can graduate from high school and who have the advantage of counseling and advocacy from an agency have various clerical employment opportunities; boys are less able to find sedentary employment not requiring physical strength.

Dating and employment both raise questions of secrecy about the disease. One girl said that she had never been able to get a job when she answered honestly the application questions about health problems, but after becoming employed she told her employer and found him sympathetic and understanding. In dating, the issue is probably less relevant. The chances are that a sickly or constantly tired young person is known among his group of friends to have sickle cell disease; that even though the couple may not talk about it, they know, and know the implications for marriage. The problem is different for the young person who has the trait. This matter is discussed later.

It is obvious that studies are needed of the emotional concomitants of sickle cell disease, but meanwhile community workers should be prepared to provide intensive and long-term psychological and vocational counseling for adolescents and young adults. Hostility, difficulty in achieving independence, passivity, and lack of norms are difficult but commonly encountered problems of various origins. Where drug dependence results, the use of pain medication for crises should be kept in mind as a possible cause and remaining need. The youth also needs to be able to depend on someone who cares enough to give physical aid when illness strikes. In vocational counseling, a further reality is the ever-present possibility of new or increased physical crippling, and the limitations in life span that still exist. The worker should be content to strive for limited goals in light of all the circumstances.

Implications for Marriage and Childbearing

Trait. Large-scale testing of young people for sickle cell trait has been advocated on the assumption that knowledge of carrier status would prevent a young person from mating with another known to have the sickle cell gene. Some states now require sickle cell trait tests on preschool children. Advocates believe that those who know they have the trait may be able to secure counseling and information, eliminating confusion and minimizing guilt and shame. The distinction between "trait" and "anemia" also can be made clear, alleviating needless anxiety over the person's physical state. This is important, because the term "sickle cell" has acquired such dread connotation that knowledge of carrying the trait may create hypochondria; all bodily discomforts are imagined to come from having the trait. Another advantage is that knowledge of having the trait can be conveyed to the person's physician, a fact the latter should know before using anesthetics.

A major advantage should include access to test-related resources for genetic counseling for persons contemplating marriage, pregnancy, sterilization, or abortion if pregnant. The mother of two children with sickle cell anemia said that she has now undergone sterilization; furthermore, that she and her husband have talked over their problem and decided they would not have married each other had they known that each carried the trait. Whether in truth they would not have married—at the time they were young and in love—is open to question.

Ann Landers, in her syndicated column, made a tersely relevant comment about genetic counseling and marriage. In response to an inquirer who wrote, "Why are people so stupid? Why do they marry without the slightest thought to family background?... Perhaps a course in genetics in our public schools might help," the columnist wrote:[42]

> *Dear Wanted:* The basis for most marriages is emotional, not rational. I know of no way to "smarten up" the emotions. Logan Clendenning said it best: Men are NOT going to embrace genetic findings. They are going to embrace the first attractive, trim-figured girl with limpid eyes and flashing teeth, despite the fact that her germ plasm might be reeking with cancer, hypertension, hemophilia, color blindness, hay fever, and epilepsy.

Those who question large-scale testing point to the lack of sufficient high-quality genetic counseling to accompany the tests, and to the boomerang effects that may occur, such as the possibility for discrimination in employment or insurance. One physician states that large-scale mandatory testing for other conditions that require laboratory facilities has been plagued by inefficient laboratory work. Neither the Los Angeles Center nor the National Association for Sickle Cell Anemia advocates compulsory testing; rather, they promote education that will help Blacks want to be tested. Problems encountered thus far include resistance, especially among some males who react with angry resistance to anything with a racial connotation, indifference, or feelings that they have enough problems without the possibility of adding another.

The time of testing raises questions. Waiting to test until applying for a marriage license is too late to prevent emotional havoc. Coupling sickle cell testing with that for venereal disease seems invidious. Testing preschool or school-age children has been called a waste of limited resources in that young children will not be concerned for years with issues pertaining to marriage and childbearing.[43] Adolescence is preferable from the standpoint of making the test a meaningful procedure; yet adolescence is not ideal in terms of the emotional storms this period brings.

Anemia. In recent years enough children have survived sickle cell anemia to the age of parenthood that this issue has become relevant. Genetic counseling appears vital for these young people. As has been pointed out in other chapters, chronically ill persons with poor self-images tend to want to prove themselves by having a baby. The irrationality of passing on to a child the suffering that the person has himself endured may not hold back an unconscious need to establish wholeness. The Public Health Service points out that there is a low fertility rate among women with sickle cell disease, but "many women who do become pregnant have serious complications. There is increased maternal mortality associated with such pregnancies, and the perinatal mortality rate is high."[44] Although the decision about childbearing is a precious and personal choice, it should be made with full knowledge of the realities. Help in finding resources for the couple's choice of contraceptive method should be provided if wanted.

Foster Care and Adoption

An unwed mother's relinquishment of her child for adoption frequently takes place soon after the child's birth, before symptoms of sickle cell anemia have had an opportunity to appear. Lack of information or sketchy information about the male parent is common in relinquishment and the child's genetic inheritance is unknown. Neither the worker nor the foster mother with whom the child is placed is prepared for the advent of serious illness in the child. Great havoc can occur if the foster parents expect to adopt the child. A foster mother who is unable to cope emotionally or physically with an infant who periodically requires day-and-night care and close medical supervision may ask to have the child removed. Separation from the foster mother adds to the child's trauma. Finding a suitable foster family quickly may be very difficult. The foster mother with nursing background may have several other children in the house who are potential carriers of infection.

Pre-relinquishment interviews should take into account the prevalence of sickle cell trait, variant, and anemia in the Black population. The mother who is a carrier may not be aware of carrying the trait, but her family may include siblings who have died early or there may be other possible indications of sickle cell problems in her family; when this is the case, the agency can be aware that the infant may have the trait, a variant, or anemia. Relinquishment proceedings and placement can proceed accordingly.

The first essential of the adoption plan is definitive diagnosis. Early detection of a sickle cell problem may not include differentiation between trait, variant, and anemia. The trait, obviously, is insufficient reason to prevent adoption, and a variant such as thalassemia may in some instances not discourage potential adoptive parents from accepting the child. The agency, however, may wish to hold the child in the care of an observant, reliable foster mother until the child is age two or older.

The agency will certainly then wish to have the pediatrician receive consultation from a pediatric hematologist with access to necessary laboratory facilities, before final decision about adoption is discussed with prospective adoptive parents.

A child handicapped by minority status and sickle cell anemia will have a difficult life, and his parents will also. The small, frail baby will lose his power to draw instinctive tender response as he grows into school age and adolescence; the burden of his illness will be inescapable. The notion "No child is unadoptable" finds challenge in the child with sickle cell anemia, and the agency may need to weigh carefully the merit of an adoptive home against finding long-term, stable, and medically subsidized foster care.

Sources of Information

The federal government has funded and promoted development of information and treatment centers throughout the country where a large number of Black persons live. Twenty-four Sickle Cell Screening and Education Clinics have been set up in urban areas throughout the Southern states, and in some Midwestern and Western cities, from New Orleans to Seattle.[45] In addition to screening clinics, there are 15 Comprehensive Sickle Cell Centers, which provide outpatient care, education of professional and paraprofessional persons, and outreach services, and conduct research.[46] The centers are located at the following universities and medical centers: University of Pittsburgh; University of Chicago; Children's Hospital Research Foundation, Cincinnati; School of Medicine, Miami; University of Southern California, Los Angeles; Downstate Medical Center, Brooklyn, New York; Medical College of Georgia, Augusta; University of Tennessee in Memphis; Indiana University, Indianapolis; University of Illinois, Chicago; Martin Luther King Hospital, Los Angeles; Howard University, Washington, D.C.; Harlem Hospital, New York City; Boston City Hospital, Boston; Children's Hospital, Detroit.

A national organization, the National Association for Sickle Cell Disease, Inc.,* has local branches in some areas and parent groups are being formed. Parent groups provide opportunity for speakers and promote parent interchange. Agency in-service training programs may secure speakers from these organizations. Often low-income parents need help in transportation or encouragement to attend meetings.

* Located at 945 South Western Avenue, Los Angeles, Calif.

CHAPTER SEVENTEEN

Spina Bifida: Myelomeningocele Form

SPINA BIFIDA is a term loosely used to describe its most significant manifestation, *myelomeningocele*. This massive birth defect has replaced poliomyelitis as the major cause of paraplegia in the young child. In addition to paralysis and deformities of the lower part of the body, children so affected frequently have hydrocephalus, are incontinent, and in some instances are mentally retarded. The defect is so grave that until mid-century children with myelomeningocele were allowed to die. Technical advances in neurosurgery on newborns coincided with release of energies and funds from the conquest of poliomyelitis. Now repeated surgery and intensive management prolong the lives of many children until adolescence and beyond. Social work faces an extraordinary challenge in helping families and children with this condition if the great cost in suffering of the children and their families, the financial outlay and the massive medical efforts, are not to be wasted.

This term, spina bifida, covers not only myelomeningocele (sometimes called *meningomyelocele* and sometimes *spina bifida cystica*) but lesser defects, *meningocele* and *spina bifida occulta*. It results from incomplete closure of the lower end of the bony spinal cord.[1] The contents of the cord, the nerve fibers, fluid and lining (*meninges*) bulge out in a sac covered by membrane. Hazard exists that infection to the brain, *meningitis*, will occur. Meningocele is not as serious as myelomeningocele because the nerve tissue itself usually is not damaged and the defect is subject to complete surgical repair. Spina bifida occulta is usually minor and often not even discovered except accidentally, by X ray.[2]

Hydrocephalus often occurs in conjunction with the defect, so that these children have the multiple handicaps resulting not only from spina bifida but also from hydrocephalus and the surgery to relieve it.

A remarkable variation exists in the frequency of spina bifida within various populations. Race and social class are vital factors, for reasons not understood. In the United States, rates in White families of low socioeconomic status are three times higher than in the upper socioeconomic groups. The Black population has low rates—less than half those of the White population.[3] Low rates among the Jews and high rates among the Irish, low among the Chinese and high among the Sikhs, add mystery to the nature of the environmental influences on this "multifactorial" genetic condition.[4]

Spina bifida and a related defect, anencephaly (in which the contents of the brain extrude through the back of the head), are even more common than cerebral palsy. They occur in between one and ten per 1,000 births, with a familial tendency and significantly higher risk to children in a family that has already had one child with the condition.[5] In such instances, the risk is one in 12 pregnancies,* but higher than this if the couple has had two children with spina bifida, hydrocephalus, or anencephaly.[6] Beginnings have been made in **intrauterine** detection by *amniocentesis* (see Chapter 5 on prevention). Selective births are possible among families that have access to special centers with the necessary facilities and want further children but are afraid to risk pregnancy unless it can be terminated if the fetus is found to be malformed.[7]

Each child with spina bifida is unique. A wide range of crippling exists, and the combination of handicaps differs within the group and from that of other multihandicapped children. A summary of some common medical realities, and then of some common psychosocial problems, provides a basis for considering the individual child.

THE MEDICAL REALITIES

Symptoms†

Because of the great variation in the implications of various forms of spina bifida and the range and combination of handicaps caused by myelomeningocele, the first task of the helping person is to secure clarification of the kind and degrees of handicaps of the individual child.[8]

The long-term picture in patients [with myelomeningocele] surviving to late childhood and adult life varies from bladder and bowel dysfunction alone, and moderate weakness and sensory loss below the knee, to flaccid paraplegia and anesthesia below the waist. Also seen are moderate to severe degrees of intellectual deficit as well as seizures and behavior disorders that may be proportional to the severity of the hydrocephalus.

In detail, this means that the child usually has medical problems as follows:

* This is a high figure; a lower rate is quoted at the Stanford Medical Center.
† The description of symptoms is adapted from Dr. John Lorber's booklet for parents, "Your Child with Spina Bifida" (London: A.S.B.A.H., 112 City Road), pp. 8–25 *passim*.

Bladder and bowel dysfunction. Children with myelomeningocele are usually incontinent of urine because of inability to contract the bladder. It overflows, and since they have no feeling they do not know when they are passing urine. In most cases, the distended bladder can be partially emptied several times a day by the Credé method (pushing in on the lower abdomen), but some urine still dribbles. This creates no problem in infancy but is a serious social problem later, and is physically dangerous because urine in the bladder harbors infection and may create back flow into the kidneys, which has serious consequences. Not all children have "overflow" incontinence, but they may have other forms of incontinence of urine.

Not only are nerves to the bladder damaged; nerves to the lower bowel and bowel sphincter are damaged as well. The child, having no sensation, does not know when he needs to evacuate, nor can he evacuate voluntarily. Thus he is incontinent of feces. Some children can develop automatic evacuation once a day by action of the upper bowel.

Paralysis and deformities of the lower extremities. Depending on the height of the spinal lesion and the damage to the nerve tissue in the spine, myelomeningocele creates absence of sensation in the lower extremities, muscle weakness, deformities, and tendency to fractures. However, many children are able to walk with crutches and braces if orthopedic surgery has corrected some deformities and suitable training has been instituted. Some have legs that are completely limp or *flaccid.* They may have dislocated hips and varying deformities of the legs and feet, depending on the areas of muscle weakness and counterpull of other muscle groups. Of special importance to social workers who may be involved in supervision of children with spina bifida is an understanding that fractures occur very readily because the bones are thin and brittle. They are particularly weak after having been in plaster casts for orthopedic treatment. The child has no feeling in his legs and therefore does not exert the protective actions a normal child would use.

Lorber states: *"Remember not to blame anyone if a fracture occurs; it can easily happen even with the best care."*[9] Repeated fractures *are not an indication for removing the child from his parents.*

Other physical deformities and symptoms. In addition to the major multiple handicaps of the child with spina bifida, there are others such as *scoliosis* and *kyphosis* of the spine, creating twisting or a hump, respectively. Children with severe myelomeningocele are short because of the spinal deformities and poorly developed legs. Because of inactivity and short stature, the child is prone to obesity. As in any person with lack of sensation and poor circulation, and especially in those who wear braces, sit in wheelchairs, etc., the skin breaks down easily from pressure, so that pressure sores are a constant hazard. Children with hydrocephalus have vision problems; those without hydrocephalus tend to squint.

Mental capacity. The Children's Hospital of Philadelphia reported that of 171 children admitted to their program, 115 had survived, were located and under active follow-up.[10] Two-thirds of their series of children had had shunts because of hydrocephalus. Almost 50 percent of the children with shunts who walk with braces or crutches had developmental or intellectual quotients of 80 or above. (Evidently about 70 percent of their follow-up group could get about.) Those unable to walk were also seriously retarded.

A very small series, 14 children, from Cornell University Medical Center, said not to be fully representative, were between seven and eleven years of age at the time of a study that was reported with great optimism.[11] Eleven children were ambulatory and six of the 14 were able to attend regular classes in school. Only six of the 14 were considered significantly retarded—the other eight having intelligence in the "low to high average range."

A study in England of 59 children about 15 years of age who had spina bifida and/or hydrocephalus quoted research that surviving children who do not have hydrocephalus compare favorably with the normal population.[12] This series verified this. Of the one-third who did not have hydrocephalus, the IQ ranged from 61 to 115, with a mean of 92 and a median of 94. Of the two-thirds with hydrocephalus, the IQ scores were about 10 points lower throughout, ranging from 55 to 108, with a mean of 84 and a median of 82. Both groups tended to be "slow but accurate in simple clerical tasks." The report concluded, "The majority of young persons handicapped by spina bifida or hydrocephalus will require special facilities if they are to feel part of the working community."[13]

In an extensive analysis in 1972 of 200 consecutive cases treated by Lorber and associates in Sheffield, England, 51 percent of the children had survived until ages seven to nine. Of these 103 children, one-fourth were able to attend regular classes. Lorber stated that only one-fifth of all admitted to this and another series, 263 children in all, had IQ's of 80 or over, and "very few have an IQ of 100 or more."[14]

Outlook

Untreated, the majority of these children are said to die from meningitis or hydrocephalus before they are one year of age.[15] Those who do not may linger for months or years.[16] Chronic kidney *(renal)* disease is the major cause of death in affected infants since the advent of neurosurgery.[17]

To avoid hazards of meningitis and increasing paralysis, English pediatric surgeons began in the late 1950's to close all myelomeningoceles on the first day of life or as soon as possible thereafter.[18] As described by Lorber, foremost of the early English enthusiasts, this operation was followed by surgery to insert a shunt in the ventricle of the brain whenever hydrocephalus existed or developed.

The practice of immediate surgery on all babies with myelomeningocele came to be widely adopted in the United States, and has been described recently as part of a "conservative" approach.[19] Meanwhile, Lorber and associates, who have accumulated experience on over 1,500 children, have had second thoughts, because long-term results were "disappointing," and "the policy of offering active treatment to all infants, irrespective of the type and degree of their physical condition and their social background resulted in great suffering for the patients and in grave family, social, educational, financial, and community problems."[20]

Analysis of results has convinced Dr. Lorber that four attributes or "adverse criteria" are ascertainable at birth and that the child should be permitted to die untreated if any of these exist. They include severe paralysis, gross enlargement of the head, kyphosis, and other abnormalities or birth defects. He believes the location of the myelomeningocele above the small of the back to be prognostic, and that this *thoracolumbar* location, or a severe degree of hydrocephalus, contraindicates treatment.[21]

However, some American pediatric neurologists are not willing to accept these criteria as definitive or as reasons for failing to operate on all babies with myelomeningocele.[22] Different approaches are used at different centers because of differences emerging in their own series of cases, philosophical differences among physicians, and the varying amounts of experience they have accumulated. Substantial controversy exists about the ethical problems involved.[23] Luzzatti at Stanford states that the outcome of medical intervention has been more positive in some respects in the United States than in England. Moreover, in England, more out-of-home-care facilities exist for untreated babies during what may be a long process of dying; this practical difference affects the amount of pressure that physicians receive from parents to take measures that make care easier and thus prolong life.

The ultimate life expectancy of children who survive the early years cannot be ascertained because of the recency of aggressive treatment. Lorber reported a recent series of 200 children in which 84 percent of the children with no "adverse criteria" and 41 percent of those with one or more adverse criteria had reached ages seven to nine years.[24] Half of the children with adverse criteria were dead by the age of two years, despite vigorous surgical and medical treatment. A different outcome has been reported by the Children's Hospital in Philadelphia. Although some of the children were lost to follow-up, of those who were known only 46 percent of the high-lesion group were dead and the overall mortality was only 19 percent. The median age of their series of children was not reported.[25] In a large southern California clinic serving 300 children with spina bifida, approximately 30 were adolescents. The literature reveals that the number of adolescents is increasing substantially. At the 4th International Conference on Birth Defects, held in Vienna in 1972, one study that was reported referred to 200 persons with myelomeningocele who were over 18 years of age.[26]

Treatment

Treatment requires the service of a large number of physicians and paramedical staff. Its aim is to prevent needless complications and enhance rehabilitation. Neurosurgery is performed first, to close the spinal-cord lesion and install a shunt in the ventricles of the brain if necessary. Orthopedic surgery to prevent deformities and increase the child's chance of walking with braces and crutches may be begun early in infancy or delayed, depending on the philosophy of the physicians. Genitourinary management is also necessary, because of bladder and kidney problems. The child may need the care of an ophthalmologist if eye problems also exist. A pediatrician is needed to manage the child's general health, instruct the family in the child's bowel training, and coordinate the work of the various surgeons, therapists, and technicians who work with them.

Neurosurgery. The neurosurgery to close the sac is usually begun within the first 48 hours after birth, and that to establish a shunt to drain the fluid from the enlarged ventricles within three months. The percentage of children who contract meningitis and the number of times a child contracts it during this early period seem to vary according to the medical treatment and the quality of care available at home and in the hospital. Not only is meningitis a painful, traumatic condition for the child, necessitating lumbar punctures and venipunctures and other painful treatment, but it adds to the hazard of mental retardation. Ventriculitis, or infection of the ventricle into which the shunt is inserted, is another problem affecting mental capacity. The prevalence of this complication varies at different treatment facilities.

Shunts must be revised as the child grows unless the hydrocephalus arrests spontaneously. No one can foresee which children will sustain spontaneous arrest and which will have trouble with the shunts. According to Dr. Lorber, very early shunts more frequently need revision; he emphasizes the advantage of avoiding a shunt if at all possible. Children who have shunt difficulties often have very severe trouble, including blindness, with repeated hospitalization for neurosurgery.[27]

Orthopedic treatment. The time at which orthopedic surgery is begun and the amount of surgery, like other aspects of management, vary from center to center. Children have as many as 20 or more operations. Dr.

Kopits, at the Johns Hopkins Birth Defects Treatment Center, begins splinting and casting before the child is six months of age, and performs major surgery to correct deformities of the hips and feet, if indicated, before the child is a year old, in order to ready the child for early standing (in braces) and gait training at approximately one year of age.[28] This parallels the English practice of "vigorous" neurosurgical and orthopedic treatment from the beginning, but contrasts with the practice described by the Philadelphia Children's Hospital team, where the baby's impaired and deformed lower extremities are swaddled, then braced, and not operated on until after he is walking.[29]

Kopits says that paralytic dislocation of the hip, due to imbalance of muscle power about the hip, is "one of the most disabling conditions in the patient with meningomyelocele."[30] A tendon-transfer operation is used to stabilize the hip. Unfortunately, the child cannot flex his hip sufficiently to walk upstairs after this is done; he has an out-toeing gait, and is subject to pathological fractures of the lower legs during recovery from the operation.[31] However, repair of the hips is deemed essential.

The knees if deformed are splinted, and the mother or surrogate is taught exercises to be performed on the child's joints several times a day. "The manipulation has to be gentle because the bones are brittle."[32]

Feet are deformed in over 90 percent of the children, Kopits states, with a variety of deformities requiring different appropriate treatment measures, including tendon transfer, fusions, and other operations.

Some deformities do not lend themselves to completely satisfactory surgical results and frequently are accompanied by difficulties in convalescence. Nevertheless, extensive orthopedic surgery seems relatively common in treatment of children with myelomeningocele, as precursor to the emphasis on ambulation during the preschool years.

Ambulation is not a synonym for walking, but is defined as "the process by which a person displaces himself from one point to another in his environment by his own will, and *to an extent*, under his own power."[33] Children with myelomeningocele "ambulate" to different degrees, depending on their lesions, deformities, and other factors. Their capacity ranges from ability to walk for many activities, though most need crutches and braces, to the ability to get about only in a wheelchair. Standing is emphasized even for those who cannot walk or stand unassisted, because of the physiological and psychological benefit of the standing position. It aids the urinary system, reduces the proclivity to fractures, helps the circulation, and gives the person a different perspective and response from other persons than from chair or bed position. However, opinions differ regarding the amount of surgery, casting, bracing, pain, expense, therapy, etc., that is justified to create ability to stand by a child who will never be able to walk. If a child will inevitably use a wheelchair because his condition does not permit him to move his legs independently, it would appear that the minimum necessary should be done, in light of the many other forms of treatment the child must undergo.

Bracing and surgery of the spine are orthopedic measures necessary if the child develops paralytic scoliosis caused by absence of muscle strength. Sidewise curves may become very severe and disabling if not halted by bracing and ultimately spinal fusion. The latter is postponed until growth has stopped if possible. The operation, followed by a body cast for three to six months, is not successful in many cases, according to Kopits, and pressure sores from the cast are apt to develop.[34] One form of spinal deformity that may develop in wheelchair-bound children is *lumbosacral lordosis*. It is untreatable once the deformity has become fixed, and must be prevented by muscle surgery and bracing before the child's body is pulled forward over the thighs.[35]

Children who have had orthopedic surgery frequently are sent home with lower extremities in plaster casts. They will need to remain in bed unless a coaster can be purchased or devised (plyboard on wheels or wagon with attached plyboard) that enables the child to go where his siblings are or be with his mother while she is working in the house. Care of an incontinent child in a leg or hip cast demands knowledgeable, close care and supervision. Urine and fecal matter on the cast weaken it and soon create a stench. Furthermore, inactivity of the child creates constipation, which in turn eventually causes impaction and a form of diarrhea. Lifting and turning the child in a heavy cast can harm the mother's back. Appropriate care of the child's skin to avoid pressure sores is essential. Therefore, the mother needs to be taught cast care before the child leaves the hospital and needs the continuing help of a public health or visiting nurse.

Management of Bladder and Bowel Incontinence*

During infancy the bladder problem is not complicated. Some centers teach the mother to "Credé" the baby before the child leaves the hospital so that she can express the urine in a safe and efficient manner several times a day. Other management teams do not believe this is necessary. One medical group has reported that dribbling and wet diapers are no special problem until the child enters school, when the authorities may object to the odor. The hindrance to acceptance and social development during the preschool period was not mentioned.

Urologists differ with regard to "conservative" management, which means leaving girls in diapers indefinitely and utilizing penile appliances and collecting bags for boys. Some urologists advocate indwelling catheters

---

* The reader will want to compare the discussion of bladder and bowel control (pp. 485–90) in the chapter on spinal cord injury, since medical staffs differ on what they consider optimum programs in these areas.

for girls, which can be attached to collecting bags anchored to the thigh. The former group fear the increased dangers of infection that indwelling catheters introduce. In some areas, surgery is performed on both boys and girls, or on girls only, to divert the passage of urine through a conduit to a "spout," or *stoma*, on the lower abdomen, to which a collecting bag can be attached. The surgery is referred to as "diversionary." The diversion is performed to bypass the bladder. Various operative procedures are used, the two most common being the *ureterostomy* and the *ileal-loop bypass*. In the former, the ureters are brought out directly to the surface of the skin. In the latter, a loop of small intestine is separated from the rest and brought out to the abdominal wall; the ureters are implanted in this loop. The operation, whether ureterostomy or ileal-loop bypass, may be done during the preschool years or later. Careful attention to hygiene is necessary whether penile appliances or collecting bags at the stoma site are used, since skin irritation and infection occur unless the skin is kept dry and clean, a difficult task when constant dribbling occurs. Odor develops in the collecting bag unless it is cleansed thoroughly and frequently on a regular schedule.

Surgery on the urinary tract may be performed not only for social reasons but to prevent or alleviate damage to the kidneys and ureters. Lorber describes the necessity of frequent urine cultures and prolonged treatment of any infection, "intensive investigative monitoring," because "damage to the upper renal tract is usually silent until the trouble is far advanced."[36] In some clinics, medication is given on a preventive basis, and surgery is performed only when there is evidence of serious infection.[37] *Hydronephrosis*, a common problem, can lead to kidney (*renal*) failure and death.

The practice at the Stanford Medical Center Birth Defects Clinic was described by the clinical nurse specialist, Sherrie Wilkins, who trains parents in home management of bladder and bowel incontinence. She stresses two aspects. These are the goal of independence in the child, and early beginning in training.

Ileal-loop surgery is delayed until the child is old enough to participate in the decision, unless kidney pathology forces surgery earlier. The rationale is that an ileal loop is mutilating, and second, care of the site of the stoma or "spout" and of the collecting bag requires a high degree of motivation. Adolescents are careless or frequently have conflicting feelings about cleansing the bags, and carry the odor of stale urine, which makes them socially unacceptable. Selected girls about seven years or older are taught a new method of "intermittent catheterization," which is gaining favor as a result of reports of cases studied in which urinary infection had not become a significant problem.[38] This method requires insertion of a clean catheter three to four times a day, and wearing a pad for dribbling. At the Stanford Medical Center families are carefully screened to select girls for whom intermittent catheterization is suitable; about 25 percent are believed to be suitable.[39]

Early training has been found to be of critical importance for success in teaching bowel evacuation on schedule.[40] Bowel training is begun before bladder training because the male child cannot wear a urinary appliance while in diapers. At around 18 months of age, when a physically normal child would be starting bowel training, the parents are instructed to insert a suppository into his rectum before dinner, and after dinner put him on a potty in squat position with a balloon to blow up to make him strain. This must be done at the same time every night. Consistency and timing are keys to success. If the child's diet contains sufficient bulk and fluids, and if nothing interferes with the regimen over a sufficiently long period, the child will have a nightly bowel movement. Some clinics advocate enemas or digital evacuation of feces, especially the latter, but these methods are not taught at the Stanford clinic because of negative side effects.

Children who are not referred to the clinic until they are older are placed on a regimen similar to that described for young children.

The management of bladder incontinence varies for boys and girls according to whether the bladder is flaccid or spastic. Until the infant is about 18 months of age, his care is essentially the same as that of a physically normal infant. At 18 months the Credé method (pressure or sharp blows on the lower abdomen) is begun several times a day, and girls are placed in "adaptive" pants or "Everett Guard" plastic pants, with liners. At school age the girl can wear normal pants over the Everett Guard.

If the bladder is flaccid, the girl and family are evaluated to determine whether intermittent catheterization can be taught. If the bladder is spastic, the girl is not a candidate for intermittent catheterization and will have to wear an Everett Guard until she is old enough to help decide whether she wants an ileal-loop diversion.

In case of kidney pathology, the child may require an indwelling catheter for a temporary period. This will need to be changed by a public health nurse once a month.[41]

Boys are fitted with a penile appliance. First the mother and later the child are taught to insert the penis into a sheath to which a urinal is attached that drains through a tube to a collecting bag strapped to the leg. Cleanliness, skin care, adequate fitting of the sheath and emptying of the bag are all essential; excoriations and ulcerations of the penis occur if it is bathed in urine or the sheath is too tight.

Emphasis throughout is placed on the child's learning to take care of himself. Mrs. Wilkins regards as a "therapeutic failure" a ten-year-old child calling for his mother to change him. She believes that boys and girls of normal intelligence can learn without difficulty to take down their adaptive pants, remove soiled and insert clean liners, and that boys can fit their own appliances and empty and cleanse their own collecting bags. As will be described later, there is some disagreement over this degree of optimism.

Some urologists do not advocate use of the penile appliance for boys on the basis that skin breakdown occurs even with the best of care.[42] For this reason they recommend diversionary surgery when the child is between two and four years of age. The care of the stoma and surrounding skin and cleansing of the pouch require instruction and conscientious care. A "faceplate" of a substance similar to moleskin is applied around the stoma, and the pouch is then applied to the faceplate. Unless the faceplate is fitted carefully, urine dribbles under it and causes skin breakdown. However, if the skin is properly cleansed and powdered and the plate is fitted correctly, it may be left on for a week. The pouch needs to be emptied every three to four hours. Care is necessary in removing the faceplate to avoid injury to the skin. Fresh pouches are needed every two weeks. They must be soaked and cleansed thoroughly every week with soap and vinegar solution and a scrub brush. It is conscientious attention to this process that makes the difference in social acceptability.[43]

Coordination of Treatment

The foregoing paragraphs provide a glimpse of the urgent need for coordination of medical procedures. Those described did not include the laboratory procedures coincident to the treatment of various systems, ranging from intravenous pyelograms to shunt X rays, blood counts, urinalyses, and electroencephalograms, nor did they indicate the supervision of the dermatologist, the ear, nose, and throat specialist, the dentist, audiologist, and ophthalmologist, the brace fittings, the occupational therapy visits, and the long-continued physical therapy. Some birth defects clinics employ a coordinator, and some hold multipurpose clinics with the various specialists in attendance, so that the mother and child can be seen by each of the many concerned persons on one day. Extra expense, time, and transportation are unavoidable if no one coordinates the multiple visits and examinations. One specialist's program may interfere with another's. Freeman says that havoc results from lack of coordination, and describes "the imperatives of multidisciplinary care."[44]

PSYCHOSOCIAL IMPLICATIONS

Even a cursory review of the burdens that spina bifida or myelomeningocele imposes on the child and his family makes plain the mountainous psychosocial hazards. The physician's conflict over saving the lives of severely affected children is readily understood. Acquaintance with some of the appealing, cheerful toddlers and mentally alert schoolchildren, however, explains the determination of some medical groups and the National Foundation–March of Dimes to give children with spina bifida a chance to live. Awareness of the problems of adolescents, of some of the less fortunate small children, and of the families goes far toward understanding the feelings of other physicians that surgical intervention is not warranted where the defect is most severe.

Nurses and social workers who work with families of children with spina bifida remark on the wide range of behaviors and problems encountered. Not only is the medical condition in itself highly variable, owing to the variable nature of the spinal lesion, but the child's feelings about himself, and his consequent behavior, reflect the family's attitude toward him almost as much as the degree of his disability. The children who develop problems are those requiring social work attention, and thus some of the common problems merit examination.

Family Adjustment

Parental attitudes change over time. Different problems exist as the child grows. The immediate period after the child's birth is one of shock and revulsion and may be accompanied by overt rejection. One mother told of seeing something peculiar on her child's back like a piece of liver when the infant was held up upon delivery. She asked if the child was all right and the doctor said, "It's breathing." A nurse ran from the delivery room crying. In another instance, a father told how he walked the streets for a week in a daze, after the doctor had told him that his son would never walk, would be blind, incontinent, and retarded. He did not know what to tell his wife; this the doctor had left to him. The mother remembered hearing the nurses argue about what floor—surgery, medicine, or where—to take her to after delivery: "She can't go back here, she's had a bad baby." One father told what it was like when relatives of other babies pointed to his and said in shocked tones, "See that little one over there? What's wrong with it? Has it got two heads?" He said he was ashamed at feeling ashamed.

One experienced social worker states that she believes all parents of severely handicapped children reject them in part. Certainly many parents wish the child would die when they realize what an overwhelming defect he has. A few parents refuse to take the child home from the hospital. In other instances a father or mother may desert the family if the other insists on bringing the child home.

Social class may have a bearing on parental acceptance. Dr. John James, Chief of the Myelodysplasia Service at the Los Angeles County Hospital and the Rancho Los Amigos Hospital, has expressed his impression that mothers from lower socioeconomic classes, often unwed, accept what fate or God has brought them. Expecting little, they can accept little. Difference in role expectations from role performance has long been known to create problems in general, so that this observation appears logical. That it does not always hold true is obvious, for many poor persons have driving ambition while only dimly understanding limitations in children.

The decision whether to operate and thus attempt to save a baby with indications of severe deformity is made by the physicians alone, on the basis that the parents could not possibly participate intelligently in decision making: they are too stunned to think; they cannot take in what lies ahead even if the probabilities are described in detail, and they later feel guilty about having made a decision to let a child die. These reasons have validity, and one could add another problem, that of lifelong disharmony between parents if one had acquiesced to the other's feelings against his own feelings or desires. "You were the one who wanted to let her live" might be silently or actively thrown at the other during many painful episodes in the future. However, if decisions regarding surgery were postponed a week or ten days, and discussions were held that offered opportunity for explanations and assessment of parents' true feelings, it seems conceivable that decisions regarding active measures to save the child might be made by the physicians on the basis of parental desires. Parents have rights and obligations that obviously should be taken into account in some way.

Helping persons who are involved with unwed mothers or other parents at the time of the birth of a child with myelomeningocele will need to support the parents as fully as possible so they can make their own decisions, if given the opportunity. The worker may unwittingly influence the decision in a substantial manner by helping or not helping the parent locate out-of-home-care resources. If the parent does not want the child, every effort should be made to secure placement in a nursery. Both the Supplemental Security Income (SSI) disability provisions and those of the developmental disabilities programs technically are available for financing such care. Whether they are, in fact, depends on local administration and sometimes on the persistence and ingenuity of the worker.

The majority of parents who receive early support through the first weeks and months tend to bury their feelings and postpone coming to grips with the overwhelming nature of the handicap. Once the child's meningocele sac has been repaired and his hydrocephalus reduced through a shunt, his care may not require a great deal more effort than that of any other baby; when he is dressed, he looks like any child with a slightly large head.

To what extent and just how the parents should be confronted with the child's future at infancy may be debated. Use of denial as a defense until shock can be incorporated would seem to be indicated. However, some experienced persons believe that early involvement with the nature of the hazards ahead promotes active preparation to meet problems involved. Educational group discussions (as contrasted with confrontation or gestalt-type groups) offer one acceptable device. They give different persons different ways of coping with their anxiety. Some parents may hide in silence behind dark glasses while listening to the lecture and discussion by others, or they can channel their grief and worry into verbalization and into parent-group organization matters. A realistic problem the social worker faces with regard to organizing a group is that, except in areas of very high population density, there are few parents of children with spina bifida in any one age-group.

An Australian physician, describing a careful social management program at a myelomeningocele service in the Sydney suburbs, has reported that parents are not invited to group discussions until the child is six months old, because the first six months are accepted as a period of grief and mourning, in which the parents' reactions are confused.[45] The mothers' groups were brought together on the basis of the social worker's and physician's knowledge of their personalities and needs, and discussion was directed to a prearranged number of subjects that included the mothers' experiences on first seeing the child, their reactions and those of their relatives, their thoughts and fears for the future, and how the child has affected their lives. The venting of hostile feelings is encouraged. Some groups evidently interacted better than others; in the more effective groups, a decrease of anxiety was apparent in many mothers, along with better adjustment to reality.[46]

As in working with any parents suffering from grief and shock, the social worker will be guided by her own sensitivity about when they can express their feelings. They need to do so, but at a time when they can without being overwhelmed. The burden on the marriage is very great; it is necessary for the social worker to back off when signs indicate that one of the partners could tolerate the defective nature of his offspring. As in other impairments or disease conditions, the father often has difficulty accepting that his boy child is not normal. The father's sense of maleness may be threatened. Understanding and supportive cooperation in helping the parents meet the practical problems posed by frequent hospitalizations and extra burdens on home care build the foundation for the parents' capacity to express doubts and resentment and thereby come to a better resolution of feelings.

Denial, often a second phase after the first period of shock and horror, cannot be maintained if the child's head grows to great proportions, if he cries and is fretful, or if the family meets with constant turmoil caused by hospitalizations for shunting procedures and orthopedic surgery. They may live for months or years in recurrent anxiety over the child's survival and with constant transportation, financial, and child-care problems.

This third phase, that of turmoil and anxiety, has potential negative results. Anger and frustration may be projected onto the spouse, causing marital friction; they can lead to despair and separating the self from the child. One father said, "Spina bifida is a study in futility." He referred to the repeated operations on the child that never led to functional results: after all the child's suffering, the expense, and family disruption, he could never answer colleagues' or relatives' questions about anything tangible being accomplished. Deformities or worse complications were being prevented, but prevention cannot be seen; only if the surgery had enabled the child to walk or to become continent would the father and relatives and colleagues feel that the surgery had accomplished something substantial.

The turmoil of the active treatment period, often during the preschool and early years, is lightened or heightened by the concurrence of other stresses, such as illness of other family members, by the accessibility and helpfulness of relatives, financial strain or capacity to hire help, and the maturity of the marriage. Some marriages are strengthened by the ordeal.

Extraordinary involvement of the father in the care of some severely handicapped children contrasts with the behavior of many who abdicate responsibility. The father's importance is evident in providing a manly model to a little boy, in physically caring for a heavy, awkwardly casted child, and in emotionally sustaining the mother. These very helpful attributes, though springing from the father's emotional maturity and sound marriage relationships, are enhanced by the model a caring physician provides. A deliberate policy of involving both parents in responsibility for decisions about the infant from the beginning, and of treating them as jointly caring and responsible, enhances their ability to express the many positive aspects of their own feelings toward the child. When the parents observe that persons they respect express pleasure in the progress the child is making and regard him not as an object of revulsion but a child to be enjoyed, they receive renewed strength. Perhaps any faltering in their own self-esteem as parents of a deformed baby is checked when they themselves are treated with respect.

Helping the mother secure some form of attendant care or domestic service may be important during the early period in preventing intolerable stress, especially when the other children are ill or if she is pregnant or trying to cope with a number of other problems at once. This too can help the parents' attitude toward the child and each other.

If the child survives early shunting and orthopedic surgery, and if bowel training and bracing and exercise procedures have been successfully incorporated into family routines, the parents may then go on to the next step and see the child thriving, growing, and going to school, and they may start to worry about the future. Now that they feel the child is going to live, they wonder what will happen to such a severely handicapped child during the teenage years. The realization that the child probably will not marry begins to dawn; often they, like the parents of retarded children, worry whether they can look forward to a day when the child is self-supporting and they can be relieved of responsibility. Indeed, what will happen when they die? Will one of the siblings have to take care of the child? In other words, a new phase begins, once the parents can relax their tensions over the child's survival; now many begin to worry about the future. Resentment against the trap they are in sometimes contaminates their management of the child.

Financial Problems

Another practical problem with which the worker may help is in regard to financial resources. Financing the many hospitalizations and surgical procedures and therapy treatments is outside the potential of all but a few families. Group insurance materially helps if parents are employed. Public provision of many thousands of dollars is needed to supplement insurance, and to provide the bulk of care for the uninsured. Crippled Children's Services often meet most of the financial need for surgery and physical therapy and some of the cost of equipment. Those health and welfare departments that compute a "liability" or portion that the family should pay for hospital and medical care according to its income level should take into account the long-term magnitude of the financial burden. Excessive pay-back requirements limit the family's ability to visit the child and to take care of him at home between periods of hospitalization; they may add to reasons for rejection. A family that deprives its normal children of usual clothing, food, or recreation and pours all of its substance into the crippled child may make him into a scapegoat later: "We could have lived in a nice house if it had not been for all the money we had to spend on you."

Expenses not met by insurance that may be met only in part or not at all by Crippled Children's Services include wheelchairs (ranging from $500 to over $1,000), braces, home equipment, and transportation for clinic and hospital visits.

Transportation costs may be substantial if the child is cared for at a medical center hospital or special clinic in a city far from the family's home. The funds spent are important in permitting maintenance of family ties and providing the limited satisfactions of being parents on which continued responsibility is built. Care of other children at home, provision to stay overnight if the hospital is at a distance, automobile expenses, and time away from work are some of the commonly encountered obstacles to frequent visiting. They become good excuses not to visit the child if they are realistic and help has not been provided. Finding financial resources to help the family meet needs in actual medical care requires patience and attention to minutiae, in part because of the large number of shifting hospital staff. Wasted effort results from misunderstandings unless the social workers make deliberate efforts to coordinate hospital and social agency arrangements.

Incontinence

One of the group of expenses myelomeningocele occasions is a range of equipment related to management of incontinence. Constant dribbling creates need for diapers or disposable liners for plastic pants. A washing machine and, in rainy areas, a dryer have to be available in most cases to avoid the piling up of wet diapers with objectionable odor. Where appliances are used, they must be alternated, cleansed, and replaced, and require tubing, adhesive, and other accessories. Bowel incontinence is inexpensively managed only if digital evacuation or enemas are used, both considered undesirable. Inexpensive suppositories available through public medical care provisions are usually ineffective, and Ducolax suppositories, used over a period of months and years, create substantial expense.[47]

The budget for diapers and appliances can be computed only after learning from the physician or clinical nurse what methods are used and taught at the clinic. The genitourinary specialists who resist prescription of catheters and advocate use of diapers instead, because of concern over kidney infection, say wet diapers need not have an odor if the child drinks a great amount of fluid; dilute urine does not have an odor. However, taking in a large amount of fluid results in many diapers and a large daily washing.

Another realistic problem is the urine smell that plaster casts develop when fractures require casts that extend to the groin, or when casts are applied after hip surgery. From comments of hospital staff and parents, the stench evidently is difficult to prevent, and can be overwhelming. When dribbling and odor constitute major problems in the child's acceptance, helping persons should inquire of the family and physician to learn the possibility of a different form of medical management of the urinary problem. Diversionary surgery may run counter to the physician's usual practice, or he may not ordinarily recommend the use of an indwelling catheter; however, he may reconsider if the child's psychosocial needs are drawn to his attention.

A serious common problem of older children with spina bifida is the smell of urine that envelops them. The rationale for delay in diversionary surgery until the child can participate in the decision is that meticulous cleansing of the appliance is essential to avoid the odor of stale urine. The careless child or adolescent who fails to care for his stoma, tubing, and appliance conscientiously and on schedule is in trouble. The skin around the stoma ulcerates, and in addition he walks in a pervasive cloud of urine odor; he is a social outcast. This is less of a problem when others take responsibility for his care. Thus the care of the stoma and appliance becomes involved in the independence struggle of adolescence, and can be a constant source of friction with parents or caretakers. For the younger child, care of either a stoma or a penile appliance is a worrisome burden for parents.

Bowel incontinence is said to be largely controllable in all but a few cases, and one experienced medical specialist states that in his experience most children achieve "social control" by the time they are adolescents.[48] The right combination of medical management, social conditions, motivation, and intelligence is required; if this combination does not exist, the consequences can be socially disastrous. The matter is not too delicate for exploration with child and family; it is in fact vital.

One clinical nurse specialist has pointed out that usually no success occurs in children of "lower-lower" income families because parental lifestyles preclude consistency, the essential ingredient of early bowel training.[49] Not until the child himself wants to achieve bowel control does she consider any effort to help him worthwhile. A child of normal mentality who wants to attend regular school, and cannot until he no longer has bowel accidents, is motivated to learn how to evacuate on schedule.

The Stanford method described has several requisites. A child who attends his own toilet must have arms long enough to do the necessary reaching, and he must be able to bend, which assumes he is not in a cast. He must be able to transfer himself from chair to toilet, and have access to a bathroom he can have to himself for an hour or so, without other persons pounding on the door and needing to get in. If the family shares a bathroom with other families, this is not possible. A commode chair can be secured and used in a bedroom at a time when others do not need to use the room. If the child cannot transfer himself, he can be lifted onto the commode, if his mother is able and willing to lift him, and left alone if he is sufficiently motivated to take care of himself.

Because it is much quicker and easier for a mother to perform a manual evacuation than for the child to wait for a suppository to work or try to use manual evacuation on himself, often the mother does not teach the child to become independent in caring for his evacuations. When mental retardation or perceptual motor difficulty compounds the problem of the child's understanding and dexterity (as is often the case), only an exceptional mother will expend the necessary effort over a long period of time.

One mother told me that bowel training had been the worst problem she had encountered in the care of her child. She had received no instructions during the first few years, and then she blamed herself, saying that she had been working from the wrong concept. She had assumed she could assist him to achieve an evacuation schedule in only a few months, whereas in actuality years of consistent training were required. No illness, no vacation, no attendance at other children's special occasions—nothing could be allowed to interfere.

Children who persistently have bowel accidents may do so for physical or psychological reasons. Some have enough feeling to know when they are going to have a movement, but others with no feeling do not know their bowels have moved. They therefore lack discomfort, and the phenomenon of olfactory satiety prevents their nostrils from being assailed as those of others around them are. Therefore the child is not motivated to change his diaper. In addition, psychological reluctance to take care of his diapering may stem from increasingly painful awareness of his difference from others and thus add to a child's natural disinclination for distasteful chores. Some believe that occasionally children use bowel accidents to gain attention, or to flaunt their cruel difference, or to manipulate others. The behavior may be symptomatic of spoiled, immature development or of a family life-style that pays little attention to hygiene.

Where control is not achieved, it causes friction and may mount into a serious social problem. A child who is perceived as repulsive, and especially one who becomes the object of contention between parents or mother and stepfather and siblings, may receive his final rejection because bowel or urinary incontinence has not received adequate management. The next time the child is hospitalized for a fracture or surgery, the family find they cannot take him home again. The child then joins the group of severely handicapped children placed in a nursing home or awaiting foster care, miserable with longing to go home to parents who have decided they can no longer put up with him.

This chain of events can be prevented through close attention to the management of incontinence. The social worker cannot close herself off from this greatest social disability by assuming that matters of hygiene are not her function. She should insist on finding the medical and nursing resources necessary to teach child and family proper management, and should herself examine the social problem of bladder and bowel care.

Diet

Because of inactivity, and disproportionate amount of time spent in a sitting or lying position, children with myelomeningocele tend to constipation. They also incline to obesity. Diet needs careful regulation to avoid these problems and also to avoid bowel looseness or diarrhea. Because the child is deprived of so many satisfactions, some parents are unwilling to deprive him of candy and cookies, even though his obesity will create a serious problem in lifting him.

Foods that cause flatulence, such as beans and gas-forming vegetables of the cabbage family, are to be avoided for social reasons. Intelligently planned diet becomes more difficult as inflation mounts. A dietician's advice should be sought, but mediated by a person of practical wisdom if the diet list given seems highly technical or not feasible economically. The public health nurse or homemaker service may be useful to the mother or foster mother, especially if obesity, psychological deprivation, or bowel problems seem to add to management difficulties.

School

Not infrequently young adults crippled early in life substitute fantasy for effort in respect to goals. The child who wears a brace almost as heavy as himself learns to avoid physical activity. Motivation dulls to suit his capacity. Lazy habits develop in part from emotional deprivation and physical limitations, and also from having been excused from effort because of disability. If the child is deprived by overprotective parents, teachers, siblings, or other children of deserved rewards and punishments, he feels that he was not deemed capable of achievement, or he feels that the parent or teacher did not care enough about him to take the trouble to discipline him.

Children who go to special classes attended by a majority of mentally retarded children may not be required by their teachers to do normal classwork. Many classes for the multihandicapped have a curriculum made up predominantly of arts and crafts. A frequent parental complaint is of inadequate scholastic content and lack of structured, disciplined effort. When this is true, the child may develop characterological inferiority and laziness as additional serious handicaps.

For those children who will live to adulthood, schooling is of utmost importance. Vocational potential will be entirely dependent on mental equipment; the ability to earn a living and to get along independently will rest on early education and training. In England, special schools for children with spina bifida and similar handicaps have been established with staff available to provide for medical and nursing needs. This is done to prevent unnecessary loss of schooling for children who at best will lose much school time because of repeated operations and illnesses.

An individualized plan is necessary for optimum schooling for each child. Regular schools are indicated for children with minimal to moderate physical handicap whose incontinence has been brought under control by diversionary surgery, the use of appliances, and appropriate diet and regimen. If the child is not rejected by his peers and can obtain at least minimal social satisfactions, such schooling probably prepares him best for adult life. However, if he is teased because of bowel accidents or urine-smelling casts or appliances, is ignored or left out of social events, and if he must miss a good deal of schooling because of illness, a special school for the handicapped appears to be more appropriate. In California, the staffs of special schools include physical therapists in addition to matrons who change diapers, etc. Many obvious advantages accrue in such schools, not least the conservation of parental energies that might otherwise be spent taking the child back and forth for physical-therapy sessions.

Adolescence

Adolescence brings its strain of usual adolescent disturbances. One cheerful nurse emphasizes the normality of these problems, in light of the age-group involved—the mood swings, interest in the opposite sex, resentment of adult authority, desire for independence and for good times. An experienced social worker has commented on the variety of wholesome interests among the adolescents she knows with spina bifida. Some adolescents have achieved remarkable self-sufficiency and reflect family attitudes that, though handicapped, they are not disabled. These children have been loved, and have been expected to give and take in the same manner as their brothers and sisters.

However, adolescence is a time when the child arrives at a cognitive grasp of his handicap and its implications. The full impact of his plight collides with the peak of emotional instability. It is no wonder, then, that persons experienced in working with them remark almost universally on the difficult problems adolescents have. They include physical deterioration—as in children with kidney failure, an eventually fatal condition—or problems that center around psychological difficulties. Severe physical handicap thwarts the normal psychological achievements of adolescence—that beginning of independence, sexual maturity, and vocational choice. Dr. Lorber has commented on the anguish of the youth who realizes there will be "no love, no marriage, no job, no independence" for him. Overt despair—"Why did this happen to me?"—seems to be less common than masked or flippant revelations of feelings. "I guess I'll have to marry another crip—no one else would have me." The anxieties, confusion, and anger the youth feels may come out in resentment, bravado, ill-conceived ideas, moodiness.

The child who has been getting about on crutches may decide to use a wheelchair. Although the upright position is physiologically desirable, the adolescent may find that he can get around more quickly and easily in a chair. Some of them believe that the image they project is more normal when sitting than when dragging around a paralyzed body on crutches. The chance of embarrassment from dribbling or bowel accidents is less and the catheters and appliances are more easily managed. A standing program at home can be substituted for crutch-walking.

Bedsores, mentioned earlier as a constant hazard, can be avoided if the child has been taught to move his position frequently and if he does what he has been taught. Motivation is necessary. An opposite motivation may operate, unconsciously or subconsciously. Large bedsores require surgery and often long hospitalization. When life becomes too difficult, a large bedsore may provide opportunity to escape into the protected environment of a hospital where dependency needs are met and the other adolescents are also different from the norm.

One adolescent, in telling how he helped educate his schoolmates that he is no different from them just because he is in a wheelchair—"It might happen to you tomorrow; I'm no different than you are"—repeatedly used the pronouns "we" and "they" to distinguish between handicapped and nonhandicapped persons.

Two forms of unreality seem to be not uncommon among counselors or helping persons. One is to encourage the adolescent to consider himself perfectly normal, and no different from others. He is different, and he knows it. Delusions do not help him, nor does their encouragement promote an honest relationship. That he can be worthwhile though unique, or a member of a minority group, and accepted and loved for what he is seems to be a more rewarding approach. However, the awareness of difference is a torture to the adolescent, especially if he has been rejected in early life. His sensitivity to social stigma is a weak spot in the fabric of personality, as brought out in Chapter 3.

Another related form of unreality is to encourage the severely handicapped youth to strive for independent living. His urge for independence is great, but in reality he needs physical help on a secure, continuing basis. That provided temporarily by a roommate, or by a series of attendants or aides, is not enough. The young person who cannot live at home needs out-of-home care, not a lonely apartment where the washing machines are not the right height for his wheelchair use and companionship is not available. The young person with myelomeningocele has physical dependencies. Reliable provision should be made for them.

In commenting on the emotional maturity of an adolescent, a psychiatrist said, "He's 17, going on 8." The boy had been reared by intellectual parents, who had overemphasized the early independence preached by medical teams and textbooks while denying fulfillment of the child's dependency needs because of their rejection. Their anxiety to relieve themselves of the perpetual burden of a chronically dependent child had forced him into premature assumption of self-care. He responded with desperate bids for attention and suicidal depression.

Emotional immaturity commonly springs from inadequate socialization. The child who has been often hospitalized, who remains indoors and is unable to move about without effort, does not learn how to play or to develop the give-and-take of the active child. Mothers who reject and overprotect children, as seems common, foster dependency. The adolescent with myelomeningocele is often unready for teenage stress. An observation that has not been confirmed but comes from different sources is that children with spina bifida mature early sexually. Learning to cope with menses and ejaculations may rouse more conflict in the mothers than in the children. However, the children should receive medical or nursing instruction especially because of the interrelationship with the management of urinary incontinence (unless diversionary surgery has been performed).

At adolescence the need for recreation becomes especially intense. If the child has gone to a special school and did not develop neighborhood friendships, he is particularly subject to isolation. Wheelchair status does not invite the active involvement of other youth. Reality demands that the young person with spina bifida learn to enjoy solitary pursuits and that he find means of communicating with other handicapped young persons.

A telephone is essential. A great deal of social interchange can be maintained with those he knew in the hospital or sees at clinic, and with the few he has met with whom he has developed a relationship at school or church. Urban communities have "indoor sports" clubs, and some hospitals and communities have developed peer groups. Hobby clubs are other channels for friendships that can be maintained largely by telephone. Transportation frequently is an obstacle to attendance at sports events, club meetings, and other potential sources of interest and stimulation. Volunteers should be secured to provide transportation if parents or relatives are not able to do so.

Girls who learn to sew and cook and do handwork find outlets that are not inhibited by wheelchair existence. Hobbies and collections can be a source of enrichment and satisfaction to boys and girls, and a means of developing friendships with the nonhandicapped. Television is the great pacifier for the handicapped. It is as essential as a telephone and a washing machine. However, the child who does nothing but watch television is cultivating loneliness and unreality.

Out-of-Home Care

Out-of-home care includes day care, state hospital or institutional placement, small-nursery care, and foster home care. One clinic reports that day care is utilized frequently. In the author's locality, day care for the "atypical infant" has begun, but group-care facilities usually will not admit handicapped or chronically ill children. The emphasis that Head Start has begun to place on inclusion of handicapped children in their programs may open more doors. Certainly day care of the preschool child with myelomeningocele offers respite to mothers from the physical and emotional burdens that heighten feelings of rejection and provides opportunities for badly needed socialization.

The only study known that describes the frequency of out-of-home placement is a study of custody, and therefore pertains to institutional and foster home care.[50] Thirty of the 173 children followed in the Seattle myelodysplasia clinic had been so placed, a statistical incidence "forty-two times greater than for children in the U.S. at large." One child had been adopted, five had been placed in institutions for the retarded, and the remainder were placed in foster homes. Over half had been placed by single mothers, which is a telling documentation of the thesis that "it takes two" to care for a severely affected child. Ten infants, or one-third of the placed group, had gone to institutions or foster homes directly from the hospital at the time of birth, either because they had been selected as children for whom surgical intervention was not warranted or because their mothers relinquished them. Almost all the others were placed between ages two and four, which the authors of the study point out corresponds to the age when the child "fails to meet developmental landmarks."[51] This probably means that the parents gave the child up when they found for themselves that the child could not talk, could not be toilet-trained, and in some cases possibly that he was mentally retarded.

In direct contradiction to observations of Dr. James[52] and others that rejection occurs less frequently among lower socioeconomic groups, the Seattle study showed that over half of the placing parents were from the lowest socioeconomic class, and only one-fifth from the top three classes combined. Rejection and relinquishment are not necessarily synonymous. In five of the 30 placed children, someone brought court action to force relinquishment, which must have been a judgment of severe neglect. (Whether neglect means rejection is moot.) This may or may not concur with Dr. James's observation that the mortality rate is higher among children of lower socioeconomic classes (which he, however, did not ascribe to home conditions but to "failures in the medical care system").

The point receiving greatest emphasis in the report of this study was that the placed group consisted by and large of those with the most severe defects or worst prognosis. There was a significant correlation between placement and a combination of severe paralysis and mental retardation.[53]

That many older children must be placed in foster homes or nursing homes has been observed by hospital and child welfare workers. Three reasons have been conveyed in interviews. First is the build-up of stress upon the mother owing to other critical events in the family, such as desertion by the husband or illness or death of another child. Another is the mother's inability to cope with uncontrolled bowel incontinence, revulsion over washing diapers of large children and the odor, lack of knowledge of how to train the child or his lack of amenability to training due to retardation or psychological problems. A most unfortunate third is removal of the child at the instigation of the hospital because of the child's repeated leg fractures (see p. 457, Dr. Lorber's caution against blame when repeated fractures occur).

The need for a special child welfare unit, appropriately funded, as in Los Angeles County, was discussed in Chapter 4. Practical wisdom confirms the Seattle study[54] in regard to the proportionately large number of children with myelomeningocele who are placed in out-of-home care. The reader is referred to Chapter 4 for a review of the problems and needs in placement.

The difficulty in finding foster homes for children with myelomeningocele is so great that even in Los Angeles some young children are placed in nurseries who should be in foster care. The need for a high board rate because of the great expense is obvious. Without it, the quest is virtually hopeless.

Help from a special school in daytime training of the child relieves the foster mother of the total burden. She is relieved of his care for several hours a day and can get other work done and achieve respite from his emotional turmoil. Earlier we discussed the projection onto the foster family of the child's hurt over rejection by his own parents—his inability to understand or accept the mother's inability to care for him. "Why did you throw me away?" one boy asked his mother over and over. Among older children placed in foster homes, refusal to cooperate in bowel training or in care of appliances, getting drunk, smoking, and using any form of acting out available to the wheelchair-bound have been reported. These problems emphasize the finding of the Los Angeles unit for placement of physically handicapped children that timing of placement for quick school entry and choice of foster home near a good school are essential to successful foster placement of the severely handicapped child. The foster mother needs the school's help.

When infants with extreme defects are placed in nurseries or institutions, the exposure to infections and lack of mothering tend to hasten their death. Selecting a child for death by institutional placement is not consonant with surgical treatment of orthopedic deformities or hydrocephalus. It is therefore part of a total plan that should not be made by the social worker alone. Absence of surgical intervention is not the same as lack of medical care. The child who is to be allowed to die needs pediatric supervision for prescription of pain-relieving drugs and medical decision regarding what constitutes the minimum of humane care.

It has been said that the ugliness of the deformity of the child with myelomeningocele is a factor that professionals need to guard against in decision making about an appropriate course of care. Social workers in community agencies who have not had opportunity to come to terms emotionally with physical abnormality overreact at times. Teams who are able to evaluate multiple-handicapped children are usually available through developmental disabilities programs or atypical infant divisions of the federally funded child development offices, in special spina bifida clinics at medical centers, or, in some rural areas, crippled children's clinics of the health department. If, after such an evaluation, the decision is made that the child should be treated and afforded a chance to live, foster home care, not small- or large-nursery care, would seem to be a vital part of the plan.

Foster care workers often do not utilize the help of public health nurses. They may have found that a nurse tried to take over the relationship with the foster mother or was too authoritative and alienated the foster mother, or the worker may not be aware of what the nurse can do. Unless the child is placed in a community geographically close to a special spina bifida clinic and the foster mother has access to a clinical nurse specialist there for frequent advice, a public health nurse would seem to be a valuable ally in helping foster mothers with bowel and bladder care training, diet, cast care and bracing, skin care and avoidance of pressure sores. Frank discussion between nurse and social worker of mutual areas of responsibility would seem essential in preventing the kind of friction or avoidance that has characterized some child welfare and public health nursing organizations. Each has its own area of special expertise.

CHAPTER EIGHTEEN

Spinal Cord Injury

SPINAL CORD injury occurs most frequently among those given to risk-taking, adolescent boys and young men. Since the virtual control of poliomyelitis, it has become the primary cause of paraplegia and quadriplegia among older children and youths. Paraplegia, or paralysis below the waist, and quadriplegia, or paralysis below the neck, may occur as the result of other conditions, such as poliomyelitis, spina bifida, and muscular dystrophy. Children of all ages, and some girls and women, are also found among those with spinal injury. The medical problems differ according to diagnosis, and the total meaning differs according to social factors. This chapter emphasizes the problems of youths, especially adolescent boys, who are victims of spinal cord injury.

Since the damage to the neural fibers is not always complete, spinal cord injury does not always result in complete paralysis below the site of the injury. However, the usual person with a "transected cord" is permanently paralyzed and without sensation below the level of the injury. He may be paraplegic, or in the case of a high spinal injury, he may be quadriplegic. Loss of capacity to feel pressure, touch, or pain has more ramifications than are readily apparent. Not only is the person unable to move his legs but he cannot tell whether his feet are touching the ground. "Proprioception," or the ability to tell where one is in space, is lost, as well as the protective warnings that pressure and pain provide. The disability is in fact so great that suicide is a major cause of death among this group.

THE MEDICAL REALITIES

Automobile accidents, surfing and diving accidents, and gunshot wounds are common causes of fractures of the bony spine, with resultant impingement upon, and bruising and bleeding or stretching and twisting of, the

NOTE: For the Medical Realities section, the descriptions of the cord and its function, medical problems arising from transection of the cord, and medical treatment of the cord-

cord. The cord itself is rarely severed, but the nerve pathways die as a result of the pinching, hemorrhage, or other injury. Since spinal-cord nerve pathways do not regenerate, injury to the cord is permanent. Thus the interruption in function of the neural pathway to the brain has been compared to a permanent break in the main line carrying electricity to a house.[1]

Prognosis for ultimate return of some feeling or motion cannot always be ascertained until approximately two months after the injury. The cord is in shock for the first few weeks. When in shock, it does not function. After the shock wears off, the paralysis may improve.

The Spinal Cord

Those involved in helping a cord-injured person need some understanding of the spinal cord's function and the effect of the mishap upon it. The complexity of neurology—even more difficult to understand because different sets of terminology exist for the same items—defeats an attempt to master detail. Selected facts that have practical meaning for the injured person, his family, and the helping persons follow.[2]

The normal cord is a chalk-sized cable of millions of tiny nerve fibers and cells, encircled by a bony tube made up of a series of rings. These rings or vertebrae are numbered in three series—*cervical, thoracic,* and *lumbar*—beginning at the top of the neck and going down. There are seven cervical, twelve thoracic, and five lumbar vertebrae. At the bottom is the *sacrum* and *coccyx,* or tailbone. In a grown man the true cord does not come all the way down the spine but ends at approximately the top of the lumbar region. It ends in a mass of nerve roots that supply the lower part of the trunk and the legs.

Emerging from each side of the bony rings, in holes called *foramina,* are nerves that are numbered according to the vertebrae from which they protrude. Hence "C_4" refers to the site of spinal nerves that supply impulses to the lower part of the neck, "C_5" to the shoulders, "T_4" to the nipple line, "T_{12}" to the trunk muscles, etc.

An understanding of the relationship of feeling and movement to the function of the spinal cord readily makes apparent that the higher the injury the more extensive the paralysis. A person with a "broken neck" at the level of C_4, for example, is not able to breathe without outside power, since the muscles involved in breathing are paralyzed. He is unable to cough and bring up mucus if he has a cold. Each inch of spine or

---

injured person are from Drs. E. Shannon Stauffer, Alice Garrett, and Elaine Wilcox. They have described the rehabilitation of spinal cord–injured persons in lectures, tapes, personal communications, and report of work, under SRS Grant RD 2114M-68-C2 to the Attending Staff Association of the Rancho Los Amigos Hospital, Downey, Calif., entitled "Interdisciplinary Clinical, Educational, and Research Aspects of a Regional Center for the Rehabilitation of Spinal Cord–Injured Persons," issued in September 1969.

approximately each vertebra is of great importance in the functioning of the person (especially if he is sent to a rehabilitation center where he is taught to make use of his unaffected muscles). Thus a person who has a fracture severing the spine at C_4 is completely dependent, whereas one whose injury is at C_5 can bend his elbows and has some movement in the shoulders; if the injury is at C_6 he can also extend his wrist; if the injury is at C_7 not only can he bend his elbows but he can straighten them out, he can bend as well as extend his wrists and has some weak function in his hands.[3]

The person whose injury is in the middle back, and who therefore has normal function in his arms and chest, is obviously much less disabled than the person with a high neck injury, except in two important areas, sexual performance and bladder control. Owing to the fact that the cord itself does not come far enough down to supply the nerves that go to these areas, no reflexes exist that can be capitalized on. Thus the paraplegic who can walk with braces and a cane may in some instances have as great a social disability as the person who has sustained an injury that weakens his entire trunk and arms.

The inner make-up of the cord is of interest in that two separate bundles of nerve fibers transmit sensory information via the peripheral nerves to the brain, and motor information from the brain back down the cord to the muscles and skin in the same area. When information such as pain, touch, cold, and pressure comes into the cord on peripheral nerves, it is conveyed across the cord up to the brain via many connections called *synapses*. Not only are all voluntary movements wired or programmed into the spinal cord prior to birth, but the autonomic nervous system that controls the sweat glands, bladder, bowel, and blood vessels is also "fired" in the spinal cord.

At least half the connections in the cord are said to be those that prevent movement. The importance of prevention or control of motion is easily understood in respect to the bladder. Persons with spinal cord injury are also subject to spasms because of the loss of inhibitory motor mechanisms.

Reflexes differ from other movements in that the sensory information does not go up to the brain for command and down again to the nerves and muscles, but rather the sensation "arcs" across the cord from one connection to another and then to the muscles supplied by the nerves in that area. Reflexes are important in spinal cord injury because those that exist can be utilized in training.

Treatment

Early referral to a rehabilitation center is a key to good care. The complexity of medical management requires a team of physicians from different specialties and allied health professionals such as physical therapists, occupational therapists, rehabilitation nurses, psychologists, social workers, and vocational counselors. Few private physicians or general hospitals have the facilities, the professional staff, the expertise, or the equipment required.

Rehabilitation center care is extremely expensive. Social agencies justifiably weigh the potential advantages against high expenditures. The relative expense of care in a rehabilitation center, balanced against many years of expensive maintenance of a completely dependent individual in a custodial facility, is highly economical in the long run, provided, of course, that follow-up ensures maintenance at home of the program begun there.

A strengthening program for arms and shoulders is one of the main features of a treatment program. In order to reduce the burden on other people and build up the capacity for independence, spinal cord–injured persons who retain upper-extremity function can be taught to swing themselves out of bed to a wheelchair or commode, and even to transfer themselves from a portable wheelchair into a car with hand controls. These activities, however, are athletic feats, achieved after months of grueling effort.

Watching the tremendous effort required of a paraplegic learning to lift his own dead weight must inevitably be a deeply emotional experience for a parent or spouse. Allowing him to do it himself in order to build his physical strength and independence requires their strength of will. However, adolescents who can mobilize their psychic energy toward independence and have the opportunity for skilled teaching from a physical therapist can develop very strong arms and considerable ingenuity in taking care of themselves. By learning "curb hopping," a method of flipping themselves in a wheelchair up over a curb, they may also acquire mobility in the community, to the extent that steps and narrow or revolving doors do not prevent use of buildings.

Corollary to the strengthening program is treatment designed to stretch the hamstring muscles, which connect the buttocks to the knees, so that the person can sit with his legs straight out in front of him. This position permits the person to dress himself and also to take care of bowel and bladder mechanics.

Equipment carefully tailored to the weaknesses and strengths of the person's muscles and motivation is important in the goal of independent self-care. Specialists at a rehabilitation center devise equipment of the right size and capacity. Electric wheelchairs permit mobility for all, including those who are able to use only a tongue-switch control. The heaviness of the electric wheelchair, however, makes necessary an additional, lightweight portable chair, unless the person is completely house-bound, since an electric chair is not suitable for transporting.

A "hi-low bed" with appropriate mattress and slings and bars is another piece of major equipment essential in promoting maximal self-care activities of the person with a high-level injury. Adapted feeding and grooming equipment, raised toilet seats and toilet arm supports, grab bars, ramps, crutches, hand splints, arm supports, urinal clamps, corsets, braces, and splints are other frequently used pieces of equipment to help the person help himself.

The expense, sometimes amounting to more than $5,000 for a person who needs and can utilize many expensive appliances,[4] is either wasted or economical according to the availability of attendants to help the person utilize them after he returns home from the treatment center, and according to accessibility to professional personnel for repairs and modifications of the equipment as required.

Complications

One of the most important contributions a rehabilitation center makes to a person and his family is to educate them in preventing hazardous, expensive, and uncomfortable complications.[5] The person learns to inspect his skin twice daily for impending signs of pressure sores, and to shift weight frequently to avoid pressure. He is taught exercises he can do himself. The family should be taught those they can do to prevent permanent contractures and deformities. If instructions at the center are adequate, he and his family will also be taught a bowel program and catheter care to prevent serious social and genitourinary problems.*

Bladder problems are the leading cause of death in spinal cord–injured persons. A catheter is necessary until the person can be trained to void without one. However, catheters heighten the danger of infection. *Pyelonephritis* or *hydronephrosis* (see Chapter 7) may develop, requiring vigorous treatment—if possible by a urologist. *Bladder and kidney stones* are also common.

A major urological problem is *dysreflexia*. The condition constitutes a medical emergency, since it can lead to cerebral hemorrhage and death unless relieved immediately. It occurs most frequently during the first year after the accident, but remains a danger for persons whose cord is injured at or above the nipple line. The dysreflexic state is one in which sudden high blood pressure occurs as a result of the distention of any organ or a variety of stimuli such as pain or change in temperature. The condition is accompanied by sweating, shakiness, and headache. Blockage of the catheter may be the cause. Immediate examination of the catheter is essential. If the blockage is not of the catheter but is inside the body,

---

* The reader will want to compare the discussion of bladder and bowel control (pp. 462–65) in the chapter on spina bifida, since medical staffs differ on what they consider optimum programs in these areas.

medication is necessary with close attention to blood pressure. Intravenous administration of medication by a physician to lower the blood pressure is necessary to save life if the attendant does not overcome the rise in blood pressure through care of the catheter.

Pressure sores constitute another serious complication. They are not innocuous, as the terms "pressure sores" and "bed sores" commonly denote. On the contrary, they can cause death from infection, and in any instance they are large, ugly, oozing wounds that take many weeks or months to heal and must sometimes be closed surgically. (It has been estimated that a pressure sore costs at least $10,000, because of the hospitalization, surgery, and delay in treatment that arise.) Social workers, like everyone else involved in working with the youth, are responsible for helping him to prevent pressure sores. They are caused by impaired circulation and death of the skin from loss of oxygen that occurs at the site of bony prominences if he remains in one position for more than two hours. They occur not only when he lies in bed without being turned often enough, but when there is pressure from braces or even wrinkles in clothing. By inspecting his body with a hand mirror, the youth himself can watch for signs of redness, the precursors of pressure sores, and with proper equipment can be taught to shift his weight unless he is completely helpless.*

Continuing follow-up of urological function, skin condition, orthopedic problems, respiratory status (if the breathing muscles have been involved), and care of equipment is necessary throughout the lifetime of the person. Transportation to physicians' offices or clinic usually requires a bus-type automobile or van and sometimes ramping equipment to the vehicle.

Bladder Control

Control of bowels and bladder is necessary for social acceptance. It divides the children who can go to school from those who have to stay home; the youths who can be cared for by their families from those who must go to nursing homes; those who can be tolerated from those who suffer crushing humiliation. The satisfactory management of incontinence therefore becomes the pin on which social planning turns for those whose disability includes loss of bladder or bowel control or both.

A bladder separated from the brain's control by an interruption in the neural pathway of the spinal cord is referred to as a *neurogenic bladder*.[6] The injured youth cannot void without assistance until trained to do so, and even then he is incontinent. Nor can a return of voluntary continence be the goal, for, as has been stated, nerve regeneration or repair is impos-

---

* A "Primer for Paraplegics and Quadriplegics" has been prepared by the Institute of Physical Medicine and Rehabilitation of the New York Medical Center, 400 E. 34th St., New York, New York. Every paraplegic and his family should have one of these inexpensive (50 cents), instructive booklets if possible.

sible. The only exceptions occur when early incontinence has been caused by shock, which wears off, bringing with it partial bladder control.*

Urological examination, including X rays, is required before evaluation of the most suitable method of management of a neurogenic bladder. Private physicians frequently do not have experience in teaching bladder training and management. Admission to a rehabilitation center for this vital aspect of care should be arranged if at all possible. After a short period of in-patient care, the training can be continued on an out-patient basis if transportation and other difficulties can be overcome.

Urologists differ on means of bladder control best employed by paraplegics. An in-dwelling or "Foley" catheter provides a means of mechanical control that dulls the edge of the social and psychological burden but is unfortunately unhealthy. An in-dwelling catheter permits a person with paraplegia to be mobile, accident-free, odor-free, and, if he can use his arms, entirely independent of others in caring for his urinary function. A good nursing teacher can teach most persons to irrigate and reinsert their own catheters, providing the disabled person has use of arms and hands and has normal intelligence. Males have fewer problems in catheter care than females. Family members may be taught catheter care if their reliability has been established. Catheters must be changed every two weeks and should be irrigated twice a day. Hence the task of care is substantial. Furthermore, signs of abnormalities, such as blood or mucus or gravel in the urine, indicate the person needs to be seen by a physician.

Catheters stimulate kidney stones and infections; their prolonged use deteriorates the kidneys and reduces life expectancy. Although an older person can perhaps afford to ignore urological ill health, on the assumption that death will arrive before his kidneys fail, the adolescent boy should be encouraged to choose the healthier alternative, namely training his bladder to empty itself. Girls sometimes retain the use of catheters, as discussed later, in spite of the detriment to health.

The kind of bladder training or management that is feasible depends on the site of the cord interruption, for the site determines the physiological response. It will be recalled that the spinal cord ends in a mass of nerve roots in the lower middle of the back (at the first lumbar vertebra). An injury or cord affection above this site creates an "upper motor neuron" bladder. An injury below it creates a "lower motor neuron" bladder. The upper motor-neuron bladder is sometimes referred to as a "spastic" or "automatic" or "reflex" bladder; the lower motor-neuron bladder is called "flaccid" or "mechanical" or "atonic" or "a-reflexic." Most persons who have incurred a spinal cord injury (and some with brain tumors, multiple

* A person with paraplegia because of multiple sclerosis may for inexplicable reasons get better at times, and his temporarily improved general functioning may include improved bladder control. Otherwise it may be said that the incontinent person cannot hope for cure but rather must learn to cope with this socially overwhelming disability.

sclerosis, strokes, or muscular dystrophy) have upper motor-neuron injuries.

In this instance, conditioning is employed to teach the primitive control center in the lower part of the brain to empty the bladder automatically without conscious control, in the manner of an infant. The method includes having the patient drink a specified amount of water during a specified interval during which the catheter is kept clamped. The catheter is released for a few moments at regular intervals. The routine must be performed around the clock until the bladder learns to empty itself automatically. A month may be long enough for a bladder to "train" itself, although in some persons it will not learn to empty without the aid of a catheter under a year of training.

In the case of a lower injury and a lower motor-neuron bladder, a more difficult management problem occurs. Mechanical means are used for emptying. The person is taught to push on his lower abdomen and strain in such a way as to force the bladder to discharge its contents. This is called the Credé method.

"Training" the bladder teaches it the life-saving task of emptying itself without the irritation of a catheter; it does not teach the bladder to empty at socially convenient times. Partial security for two or three hours can be achieved if the person empties his bladder before an important event. However, even the "trained" bladder expels urine unexpectedly—a sneeze or cough or chill or a push on the abdomen or some other stimulus may cause voiding. Thus appliances are necessary.

The male appliance is a long, narrow, flat rubber bag worn on the upper leg and attached externally to the penis. This can be emptied once a day. In an emergency the bag may be worn as long as three days without emptying. Since the bag does not show under the pants leg and since almost any normally intelligent person can be taught to apply and take care of it, the male who has use of his arms can become entirely independent in respect to care of the bladder. However, proper application of the device is imperative, for skin breakdown and gangrene of the penis can result from too tight or improper application.

The girl has a more difficult problem psychologically and physically, for no external appliances are satisfactory and she must wear a padded diaper covered by rubber panties. If she has sufficient strength in her arms and has been taught the mechanics of moving her body on and off a diaper, she is able to change herself. The diaper needs to be changed at least four to six times a day because of inevitable problems of dribbling or leakage. Odor is said not to be an inherent problem if there is no infection and if the person drinks enough water to keep the urine dilute and therefore odor-free. However, because feelings often revolt against the ignominy of living in wet diapers, girls not infrequently refuse them, utilizing catheters indefinitely despite the injury to health.

Under *optimal* circumstances the purchase, use, care, and maintenance of catheters and appliances are not difficult; that is, if the youth is intelligent, is mobile, has access to funds, and access to a specialist or rehabilitation center whose staff includes a helpful teaching nurse, and if the home provides (1) room for an undisturbed sterile tray with necessary bowls, medications, sprays, pads, forceps, syringe, etc., and (2) privacy for the disabled person's daily attention to his catheter and to care of appliances or to changing of diapers.

Youths who have suffered brain damage, or who cannot use their arms, or who live in crowded conditions, or whose family budgets do not include extra funds for needed equipment may labor under social handicaps that destroy self-respect and gravely affect personality and relationships with others.

Bowel Control

The bowel problems[7] of the spinal cord–injured person have obvious ramifications for his social relationships and his feelings about himself. Whether a young person can aspire to live alone, how much care a family member can provide, and the suitability of attendants are affected by the realities of the bowel problem and the kind of management it requires. The necessary diet affects the budget. A visiting nurse will need to supervise the program, and the injured youth may be more comfortable discussing the specifics of management with a nurse.

The so-called "neurogenic bowel" of the paraplegic should be maintained on a regime similar to that maintained before the injury. If the person is accustomed to having bowel movements more than once a day, he can be placed on a once-a-day routine; if he usually evacuates only once a day, he can usually be put on an every-other-day or twice-a-week routine, a nursing expert advises.[8]

Diet is an obvious corollary to the bowel routine. A high-protein diet is necessary for paraplegics, and they must drink a large amount of fluids for satisfactory management of both bowel and bladder. Some physicians and nutritionists believe the intake of calcium through milk products should be kept low to reduce the problem of kidney stones. Furthermore, the right combination of bulk and of foods that may be laxative or binding must be worked out for the individual and then maintained.[9]

Persons with upper motor-neuron problems should be started on a suppository program. Such a program may require as long as two hours a day. Laxatives are not as satisfactory as suppositories because they create unpredictable bowel movements and may be followed by leaking or a small movement. The mildest and least expensive suppositories are glycerin suppositories; they are not difficult to use provided the person is taught to get them high enough up into the rectum, into the second sphincter and up against the wall of the bowel. The suppository should be used at the same time as the person usually has a bowel movement; he will have a movement within an hour, and he does not have to sit on the toilet all this time.

After two or three weeks of daily suppositories, the person should be able to maintain a regular bowel schedule by adhering to a regime of proper diet and sufficient fluids, and using the same time to go to the toilet. While the patient is establishing a schedule, he may have to use more expensive strong suppositories and take a stool softener three to four times a day, in addition to adhering to recommended food and fluid intake. The suppositories and stool softeners required may not be in the formularies of official medical-care agencies and can be enough of an expense to warrant special consideration in the budget.

The embarrassment of diarrheal accidents or unexpected bowel movements, or the very unpleasant experience with an impacted bowel, is so great that teenagers will ordinarily be motivated to adhere to a bowel program despite its trying nature.

More of a problem is the bowel management of persons with lower motor-neuron injuries (which includes most persons with spina bifida, as well as those with low-level spinal cord injuries). Some centers teach a method referred to as digital stimulation and manual evacuation of feces. Although this method is particularly upsetting to some persons, Rancho Los Amigos Hospital has found that the method can be taught even to persons with a dull-normal mentality or to preschool-age children. Digital stimulation requires a well-lubricated gloved finger for pressure on the rectal sphincter. The time required for the evacuation is 20 to 45 minutes, after the person has learned the routine. After a year or so on the routine, the program is said to require little time and to be a relatively easy matter. However, because bowel and bladder and sexual functions are tied together in people's minds, manual evacuation of feces is especially upsetting to some persons and to those from some cultural groups.

The person who has use of his upper extremities and can perform the evacuation himself is in less danger of being hurt than if he is unable to take care of his bowel program and must rely on someone who may be careless. If the paraplegic must rely on a careless attendant or on a family member who is not reliable or who finds the digital evacuation too objectionable, he can be maintained on a suppository program with less handling of the stool.

Enemas are said to be inadvisable because they tend to stretch out the bowel and impair peristalsis. Use of enemas will upset the bowel program for two or three weeks. A very upsetting interruption to the bowel program occurs if the person takes one of the new broad-spectrum antibiotics that change the bacterial flora and cause diarrhea. If the antibiotic is given in milk or if buttermilk is used later, the difficulty can be alleviated.

Sexual Problems of the Paraplegic Youth

The phrase "a paraplegic is a paraplegic" regardless of diagnosis is not correct. Of obviously enormous import, especially to the adolescent boy or young man, is a difference in sexual capacity according to the extent of damage to the spinal cord. For example, the poliomyelitis virus destroys only the anterior horn cells of the cord and therefore permits retention of sensation. The spinal cord injury that destroys the total cord destroys sensory as well as motor functions. A person who can feel is in an entirely different situation from one who cannot. Though the paraplegic from poliomyelitis may have paralyzed hips and lower trunk muscles, he can feel sexual impulses and have an erection. Although his sexual partner must be the aggressor in sexual relationships, adapting her position to his needs, he nevertheless can retain the vital function of manhood. The person with a complete spinal cord injury, however, cannot have erection or orgasm except in a small percentage of instances where it can be stimulated by reflex action. Persons with incomplete destruction of the cord may retain some aspects of sexual capacity.

The problem of urinary incontinence affects sexual relationships. A catheter in the female need not interfere physiologically with her sexual ability, since the catheter tubing does not lie in the vagina but in the urinary outlet. However, catheters are psychologically inhibitory to sexual relationships. It is said that this fact encourages some young persons to accept the handicaps of automatic bladder functioning in contrast to dependence on a catheter.

Girls who have sustained spinal cord injury can become pregnant, and deliver normal infants in a natural manner.

The symbolic destruction of manhood that occurs at the same time the person has lost bowel and bladder control and use of part of his body seems a possible cause of the high rate of suicide among young men who have sustained spinal cord injury.

PSYCHOSOCIAL IMPLICATIONS

The Person and His Grief

Those who have observed the anguish of the paraplegic and those who have themselves experienced this catastrophe tell us that immediately after the injury and onset of paralysis the person is psychologically paralyzed and may in fact be speechless.[10] He undergoes a period of depersonalization in which he is like an observer of himself or like a robot, feeling as if he is in a fog.

After the period of chaos, the injured person starts to work over what has happened to him, dreaming about it and needing a listener, since he wants to talk about it over and over. Because the customary feeling of omnipotence—"It can't happen to me; those things happen to other people"—is shattered, there is a tendency for the psyche to project omnipotence onto professional persons, expecting that the physician will be able magically to help him become well. This may create anger and difficulty when the inevitable disappointments occur. The person may become actually psychotic at night or when hospital morale is poor, or he may hold up until time of discharge and then collapse. A great variety of reactions are possible, interlaced with guilt feelings and anxiety.

Dealing with these feelings takes the person's psychic energies. He denies reality for the first several weeks or months, the denial serving a valuable function in postponing some of the psychic work that has to be done. He expects a miracle, and is not interested in realistic plans. The helping persons involved need to encourage the injured person, giving him something to hang onto and yet not reinforcing unreality. Listening without interrupting as he works over his feelings can be very helpful. Experience with severely affected poliomyelitis patients led one authority to suggest that adults too pained even to talk about themselves can be greatly aided by indirect means—providing gradual opportunities for them to test themselves and others in ordinary social situations, such as going to the hospital canteen or purchasing a birthday gift.[11] This method doubtless applies to adolescents as well.

A phase of actual grieving for the lost body image follows the denial. It must precede restoration to a relatively healthy psychological functioning, in the same manner that "grief work" is essential to a bereaved person before he can return to a new mode of functioning. How long the grief and depression last varies, depending in part upon the previous personality structure.* The person becomes depressed only when he has begun to give up hope of walking again and has begun to look at other patients to compare himself with them and to consider reality. Grief work and adaptation may require as long as two years.

It has been suggested that the injured person needs to be involved in activity during this period but that he should not be pushed. Those who wish to help, or whose responsibility it is to help, gain nothing by giving way to the impatience and frustration they are bound to feel. Consistent support, the sharing of reality problems, the encouragement of ingenuity,

* Myron Feld, "Psychiatric-Psychological Survey of 1,000 Cases of Spinal Cord Injury," *Proceedings* of meetings of the Institute on Spinal Cord Injury held at the Veterans Administration Hospital, Long Beach, Calif., October 19, 1960. Dr. Feld states that the acute stage or delirium lasts approximately one month, the denial stage about three to four months. The second stage of depression, with hostility and antisocial behavior, lasts until approximately a year after the injury, with resentment against dependency and urge to exert the self following this period during the next six months. These reactions are described among the "normal" patients: "It takes 18 to 24 months, perhaps; some people less, some people 12 months" (p. 65). Persons with abnormal personality patterns, Dr. Feld states, react according to their preexisting patterns.

and planning and sustaining the youth through these months are all difficult for the social worker and other professionals involved. It is important that the professional person's own unconscious feelings of guilt and anxiety do not unwittingly feed into the injured youth's problems.

Family Adjustment

The strain on the family at the time the boy is injured can be readily understood. Hope for some improvement may be realistic during the first two months, unless, as indicated, early surgery has revealed permanent damage to the spinal cord. Suspense, sorrow, and frequently guilt are compounded by physical stress in making financial arrangements for hospital care, visiting the injured youth, attending to legal affairs related to the accident, etc. Whereas the boy is too dazed to face reality as the early weeks elapse, the parents and/or young wife more quickly see and accept the irreversibility and totality of the catastrophe.

Tenuous family relationships including adolescent marriages may be expected to break. The young spouse who "didn't intend to marry a crip," or the father who is unable to bear the sight of a paralyzed son and who leaves the scene, is not an uncommon situation. They of course help to shatter even further the world of the injured person. Intensive and continuous emotional support is needed by both family members and the patient. Meeting the family members' regressive dependency needs during their crisis, and providing acceptance and understanding along with help with financial and physical needs, may hold a family together.

If the father withdraws into work or deserts the family, another male figure may provide some support. A "big brother," minister, scout leader, student volunteer, or relative may be enlisted. The idealism of youth can be capitalized upon in securing peer support if the person has a few friends who are willing to visit and able to sustain him over the early months.

Sibling relationships and the interaction between siblings and parents should be watched as the family settles into the long-term adjustment. The tendency for the mother to give special attention to the injured boy or for the father to withdraw or to develop a special relationship with his physically normal children creates particular problems during adolescence. The injured youth's resentment over normal siblings' activities and capacities is heightened if his father pays less attention to him; the favoritism he receives from the mother is resented by his brothers and sisters. Many families do succeed in maintaining a balance but the hazards are real; minor preventive intervention may make major adjustments unnecessary later.

Drugs are part of the picture for many paraplegic adolescents. Not infrequently the youths have been introduced to pills and marijuana in school and may have been under the influence of drugs at the time of the accident. If the person remains long in a hospital or rehabilitation center with other young persons, he will be introduced to drugs by his new friends and those who come to visit them, if he has not been introduced to them earlier. Drugs not only dull pain and offer escape from a horrible and bleak world, but may symbolize the rebellion that is part of adolescence. The use of drugs is to be discouraged if for no other reason than that the paraplegic or quadriplegic has to rely on a clear head and dares not risk toxic brain damage. The marijuana that may have seemed so harmless on some occasions may act unpredictably, creating delirium leading to falls and fractures.

Financial Problems

Families often do not live in houses suited to wheelchair locomotion. Enormous unnecessary outlays may be made for extended hospitalizations, or nursing home care, while the family looks for a suitable place it can remodel or adapt to. The search is slowed down by reluctance to even consider bringing the boy home during the initial period after his injury, since his care seems too overwhelming to contemplate. Helping family members understand the resources that will be available and encouraging them to look for a home without steps and with wide halls and doors, or one that can be remodeled, are urgent matters.

They will need room for an attendant and for massive equipment, as well as requiring suitable architectural features and a pleasant environment for 24 hours a day. Coordination with the rehabilitation center is essential to learn the size of the equipment, how wide doorways need to be, etc. Since the burden on the family, and the independence the boy can achieve, will depend on the suitability of the home, the financing necessary to secure adequate housing should become one of the social worker's main concerns.

Social workers not infrequently encourage families to get along without a paid attendant, assuming that the mother, father, brother, or sister can give the paraplegic or quadriplegic youth the care he needs, and not wishing to draw upon public funds any more than absolutely essential. Such an economy proves shortsighted, for the physical strength required, feelings of revulsion and pity or resentment over the burden, the daily, continuing sacrifice have limits. The two-way process of interaction between the injured boy's feelings about his dependency, at the time that his psychological growth is bursting with need for independence, and his anger against the world will inevitably invade the matter of physical care with an intensity of feelings that defies constructive handling.

To prevent either a family break-up or a crisis resulting in nursing home placement, an attendant is needed to aid the youth with toileting and dressing until he is able to transfer from bed to wheelchair and toilet and take care of his own bowel and bladder program. If this is literally impossible, arrangements need to be made for a visiting nurse to come to the house to help with the bowel and bladder program, and to aid with other aspects of hygiene as well as to supervise skin care and repair and care of equipment.

Equipment that facilitates care reduces the amount of attendant care, but it cannot be assumed that the equipment purchased is working. All too often the family needs more instruction in its use or the appliance or rental company needs pressure to return and re-fit some part.

Transportation is another major social problem and one upon which social adjustment depends. Morale and motivation toward independence depend on the person's ability to think of himself as part of the mobile world about him. A car is very important, as soon as the boy is able to transfer himself from bed to wheelchair to car seat. It can be a goal and reward for the effort needed to learn to "transfer." Financing a car with hand controls or a bus-type automobile may be undertaken by a church group or a service club; flexibility in budgeting of public assistance grants to include transportation costs is possible in some counties if the transportation is part of a rehabilitation or work plan.

Recreation

The conversation of wheelchair youth testifies to the imperative of recreation during adolescence. Physically normal children are constantly on the go. The guitar lessons, basketball games, surfing, debate club, rock dance, or riding about in a car and stopping for a snack at the drive-in—these serve to channel restless energy and the drive to get away from home and develop identity with peers.

The wheelchair-bound adolescent is tormented by his need to be out with the others. It is a token of acceptance, of really living, to go places with them. The severely handicapped youth "forgets" he might be a burden; he can ignore the stares of strangers; he hates those who would restrict or remind him that he is different. The boy who lives close to others his age or is part of a lively church group is not left behind, providing he has something to offer the crowd because of his interest in things and people, and providing he is neat and financially able to pay for gas, admission fees, and snacks.

Unfortunately, many paraplegic youths do not have the necessary assets. They may be emotionally depressed, do poorly in school, or have little at home to enliven their interests or provide things to talk about. Some smell bad because of lack of bowel and bladder management, or do not have clothes or the allowance necessary for transportation, snacks, and fees. Some live in remote areas, or in second-floor housing with no way to get downstairs.

Necessary enabling services, which are fundamental but time-consuming, require first attention. Volunteers may sometimes be enlisted to assist in helping the boy develop interests in photography, guitar, ceramics, or school politics, which will enrich his life and attract other youths to him. Volunteers may also transport him to games and special events until he can make his own opportunities to go out. They may help the family look for more suitable housing. These tasks may sometimes be asked of paraprofessionals, church groups, service clubs, or other groups.

The Junior League of Los Angeles, and undoubtedly similar organizations in other communities, developed directories of recreational opportunities for the handicapped. "Around the Town with Ease," the Los Angeles Directory, describes curbs, steps, seats, width of restroom doors, parking facilities, etc., of funlands, stadiums, museums, art galleries, and parks, as well as seasonal programs and other points of interest including universities. Such a guide is of great value in planning trips and activities for wheelchair youth.

When trips are organized, two handicapped youths are support for each other, whereas more than two draw attention and make them feel conspicuous, alienated, and hateful of their condition.

Vocational Preparation

Vocational preparation is the focus for great conflict in the older teenager. The youth who has not thought seriously about a job and with no work experience does not know what he can do or what he wants to do. He cannot be expected to think of himself as a permanent cripple for many months, during the period of denial while the organism is coping with survival and adjustment. Refusing to consider himself in need of any special training because of the tenacious hope for a miracle, the spine-injured youth is not interested in learning to type with a stick between his teeth or thinking seriously about what he can do from bed or wheelchair to earn a living. Premature attempts to involve him in vocational preparation are futile and lead only to anger and disappointment on the part of all involved.

In light of automation's increasing pressure upon those with marginal vocational capacities, the goal for the paraplegic teenager should be a life that offers opportunities for self-respect and healthy rewards, not necessarily one that will bring money and a career. A careful evaluation of the person's aptitudes, drive, and family motivation, his interests and scholarly bent, should precede action.

Work with head and hands does offer an opportunity for achievement of wholesome goals in the case of many paraplegics. Persons whose intelligence and family's interests are compatible with professional career goals can ultimately find satisfying identities as vocational counselors, social workers, psychologists, lawyers, physicians, etc. However, these are the exceptions. Quadriplegics can have little realistic hope for employment unless they are persons of exceptional drive and exceptional resources.

One of the problems encountered is the practice in vocational rehabilitation agencies of giving credit to counselors according to the number of persons they place in employment. They need a great deal of encouragement and exceptional supervisory assistance if they are to spend the time required in aiding a paraplegic or quadriplegic youth.

If the youth does not have the capacity for rehabilitation to a profession or competitive employment, he may be a person who can be helped to attend a special school and later a sheltered workshop. There he may find the "social corset" that work offers the normal person. By providing relief from monotony, creative outlets, daily goals, social relationships, stimulation, opportunities for learning, and respite for the family, these activities fill many needs.

Notes

1. Introduction

1. Russell Baker, "How the Photograph Lies," syndicated column from the *New York Times*, in the *San Jose Mercury*, July 16, 1974.
2. Selma Fraiberg, author of *The Magic Years* (New York: Scribner, 1959), is Professor of Psychiatry and Director, Child Development Project, University of Michigan.
3. Benjamin S. Bloom, *Stability and Change in Human Characteristics* (New York: Wiley, 1964), Preface, p. vii.
4. Florence Hollis, "The Psychosocial Approach to the Practice of Casework," in Robert W. Roberts and Robert H. Nee, eds., *Theories of Social Casework* (Chicago: University of Chicago Press, 1970), p. 37.
5. Erik H. Erikson, *Childhood and Society* (2d ed.; New York: Norton, 1963), p. 37.
6. *The Health of Children, 1970*. Selected Data from the National Center for Health Statistics, DHEW Publ. no. (HSM) 73–1211, p. 25.
7. Hyman Goldstein, "Demographic Information in Maternal and Child Health," in Helen M. Wallace et al., *Maternal and Child Health Practices* (Springfield, Ill.: Thomas, 1973), p. 123.
8. *Examination and Health History Findings among Children and Youths 6–17 Years of Age, 1973*. Vital and Health Statistics series 11, no. 129–08. DHEW Publ. no. 74–1611, p. 26.
9. Quoted in Aubrey L. Ruess and Edward F. Lis, "Prevalence of Handicaps in Children: Considerations and Issues," in Wallace (note 7), p. 943.
10. "Social and Rehabilitation Service," Medical Services, DHEW, mimeo., August 1, 1974.
11. Ake Mattsson, "Long-Term Illness in Childhood," *Pediatrics* 50 (1972): 801.
12. Helen Wallace, "How to Evaluate the Services and Care Offered Handicapped Children," *Public Health Reports* 85 (1970): 647.
13. Russell J. Blattner, "Congenital Defects: Impact on the Patient, Family and Society." Paper presented at the Second International Conference on Congenital Malformations, International Medical Congress, New York, N.Y., 1963, p. 365.
14. *Health of Children of School Age*. Children's Bureau Publ. no. 427, HEW, 1964, pp. 5, 6.
15. Mattsson (note 11).

16. Harry A. Sultz et al., "Erie County Survey of Long-Term Illnesses: Incidence and Prevalence," *Amer. J. Public Health* 58 (1968): 491–98 *passim*.

17. Goldstein (note 7).

18. I. Barry Pless, "Epidemiology of Chronic Disease," in Morris Green and Robert J. Haggerty, *Ambulatory Pediatrics* (Philadelphia: Saunders, 1968), p. 764.

19. *Prevalence of Chronic Circulatory Conditions, U.S., 1972* (DHEW Publ. no. HRA 75–1521), Table 15, p. 34.

20. John Kosa et al., eds., *Poverty and Health* (Cambridge: Harvard University Press, 1969); information reported from U.S. National Center for Health Statistics, "Disability Days, United States, July 1963–June 1964," Vital Statistics: data from the National Health Survey, series 10, no. 24, 1964, pp. 29–33.

21. "Disability Days, 1971." Vital and Health Statistics, U.S. HEW, PHS, June 1974, p. 6.

22. *Los Angeles Times*, February 2, 1969. Report of a speech by Dr. Malcolm Todd, President, California Medical Association, at the American Academy of Pediatrics. *Health of Children of School Age* (note 14). Arthur J. Lesser, "Concepts and Content of Maternal and Infant Care Projects from a National Viewpoint," *Amer. J. Public Health* 56 (1966): 726. Ellen Winston, "Medical Assistance under Title XIX of the Social Security Act," *Welfare in Review*, August and September, 1965, U.S. HEW, p. 14.

23. *Examination and Health History Findings* (note 8), p. 27.

24. Howard R. Newman, Commissioner, Medical Services Administration, Social and Rehabilitation Service, Washington, D.C.; speech before the National Health Forum, Boston, March 12–13, 1974.

25. Kosa et al. (note 20); information reported from "Medical Care, Health Status, and Family Income, United States," Vital Statistics: data from the National Health Survey, series 10, no. 9, 1964, pp. 53–64.

2. A Conceptual Foundation

1. Benjamin S. Bloom, *Stability and Change in Human Characteristics* (New York: Wiley, 1964), pp. 214–15.

2. From Alexander Pope's "Just as the twig is bent the tree's inclined."

3. Florence Hollis, *Social Casework in Practice* (New York: Random House, 1964), pp. 5–6.

4. Charles Wahl, *New Dimensions of Psychosomatic Medicine* (Boston: Little, Brown, 1964), pp. 8–10.

5. Roy R. Grinker, *Psychosomatic Research* (New York: Norton, 1953), p. 188.

6. Hans Selye, *The Stress of Life* (New York: McGraw-Hill, 1956).

7. Ronald McKeith and Joseph Sandler, *Psychosomatic Aspects of Pediatrics* (New York: Pergamon, 1961), pp. 40–41.

8. For a summary of the literature and statement of principles, see Irma L. Stein, "The Systems Model and Social System Theory; Their Application to Casework," in Herbert S. Strean, *Social Casework* (Metuchen, N.J.: Scarecrow Press, 1971).

9. B. F. Skinner, *Beyond Freedom and Dignity* (New York: Knopf, 1971); Eric Berne, *Games People Play* (New York: Grove, 1964); Erving Goffman, *Stigma* (New York: Aronson, 1974); and Thomas A. Harris, *I'm OK, You're OK* (New York: Harper & Row, 1969), p. xv.

10. See Charles Loomis, *Social Systems* (Princeton, N.J.: Van Nostrand, 1960), pp. 30–36.

11. See E. T. Hall, *The Silent Language* (Greenwich, Conn.: Fawcett World Library, 1963).

12. George E. Ruff and Sheldon J. Korchin, "Adaptive Stress Behavior," in Mortimer H. Appley and Richard Trumbull, *Psychological Stress, Issues in Research* (New York: Appleton-Century-Crofts, 1967), p. 297.
13. Appley and Trumbull (note 12), p. 7.
14. Irene M. Josselyn, *Psychosocial Development of Children* (New York: Family Service Association, 1948), p. 27.
15. Roy Grinker and John P. Spiegel, *Men under Stress* (New York: McGraw-Hill, 1945), p. 82.
16. Thomas French, *Integration of Behavior* (vol. 1; Chicago: University of Chicago Press, 1952), p. 57.
17. Leon J. Saul, *Emotional Maturity* (2d ed.; Philadelphia: Lippincott, 1960), p. 189.
18. For comprehensive analysis of the literature, see *Deprivation of Maternal Care* (Geneva: World Health Organization, 1962), especially Mary D. Ainsworth, "The Effects of Maternal Deprivation: A Review of Findings and Controversy in the Context of Research Strategy," pp. 97–159. For later comments, see Harry Munsinger, *Fundamentals of Child Development* (New York: Holt, Rinehart & Winston, 1974), p. 261.
19. R. A. Spitz, "The Role of Ecological Factors in Emotional Development in Infancy," *Child Development* 20 (1949): 145. See also R. A. Spitz and K. M. Wolf, "Anaclitic Depression," in *Psychoanalytic Study of the Child* (vol. 2; New York: International Universities Press, 1946), p. 113.
20. Saul (note 17), pp. 197–211; and Levi Lennert, *Stress and Distress in Response to Psychosocial Stimuli* (New York: Pergamon; International Series of Monographs on Experimental Psychology, vol. 17, 1974), p. 14.
21. D. H. Funkenstein, *Mastery of Stress* (Cambridge: Harvard University Press, 1957), pp. 277–79.
22. French (note 16), p. 57; and Michael Harrington, *The Other America* (Baltimore: Penguin, 1963), pp. 134–36.
23. French (note 16), p. 57.
24. Grinker and Spiegel (note 15), pp. 144–45.
25. Lydia Rapoport, "Crisis-Oriented Short-Term Casework," *Social Service Review* 41, no. 1 (1967): 35.
26. Rosemary Creed Lukton, "Crisis Theory: Review and Critique," *Social Service Review* 48 (1974): 394.
27. *Ibid.*, pp. 394–96 *passim*.
28. Rapoport (note 25), p. 38.
29. Saul (note 17), p. 42.
30. See Susan H. Dawson, "A Developmental Approach to Helping: The Epigenetic Model Applied to the Period of Early Childhood," *J. International Association of Pupil Personnel Workers* 17, no. 4 (1973): 176–80.
31. Paul Mussen, John Conger, and Jerome Kagan, *Child Development and Personality* (3d ed.; New York: Harper & Row, 1969), pp. 43–60 *passim*.
32. *Ibid.*
33. See William R. Thompson and Joan E. Grusec, "Studies of Early Experience," in Paul H. Mussen, ed., *Carmichael's Manual of Child Psychology* (3d ed., vol. 1; New York: Wiley, 1970). See also Munsinger (note 18), p. 227.
34. Josselyn (note 14), p. 22.
35. Ruth Munroe, *Schools of Psychoanalytic Thought* (New York: Holt, Rinehart & Winston, 1955), p. 175.
36. For two of the many discussions on the development of trust, see Erik Erik-

son, *Childhood and Society* (2d ed.; New York: Norton, 1963), pp. 247–51 *passim*; and Bruno Bettelheim, *The Empty Fortress* (New York: Free Press, 1967), pp. 27–33.

37. Benjamin Spock, *Baby and Child Care* (rev. ed.; New York: Pocket Books, 1968), pp. 214–17.
38. Munroe (note 35), p. 175; and Josselyn (note 14), p. 47.
39. Erikson (note 36), pp. 247–74 *passim*.
40. Bloom (note 1), pp. 88–89.
41. C. W. Breckinridge, "Intellectual Growth and Development," in *Tulane Studies in Social Welfare* (New Orleans, La.), vol. 3, 1961, p. 54.
42. Selma Fraiberg, *The Magic Years* (New York: Scribner, 1959), p. 118.
43. Jean Piaget, *The Origins of Intelligence in Children* (New York: Norton, 1952), p. 331.
44. Unpublished lecture by Mrs. Muriel Mizisin, Psychologist, San Diego, January 15, 1965.
45. Fraiberg (note 42), p. 125.
46. *Ibid.*, p. 121.
47. Bloom (note 1), pp. 88–89.
48. Mary Acker, Ph.D., Psychologist, Child Development Center, Valley Medical Center, San Jose, Calif., personal communication, February 7, 1975.
49. Margaret Mead, "Four Families," National Film Board of Canada; 2 parts, 30 minutes each, 1960. Distributed through McGraw-Hill.
50. *Ibid.*
51. Kurt Lewin, *Resolving Social Conflicts* (New York: Harper, 1948).
52. T. Adeoye Lambo, M.D., Deputy Director-General, World Health Organization, Geneva, paper presented at the 17th International Congress of Schools of Social Work, Nairobi, Kenya, July 6–9, 1974.
53. *Statistical Abstracts of the United States*, 1973 (Washington, D.C.: Bureau of the Census, Department of Commerce), Table 355, p. 223.
54. *Ibid.*, Table 354.
55. *Handbook on Women Workers*, 1965 (Washington, D.C.: U.S. Department of Labor), Bulletin 290, pp. 24–50.
56. *Ibid.*
57. *Ibid.*
58. *Economic Report of the President*, 1965.
59. *Handbook on Women Workers* (note 55).
60. "More and More Broken Marriages," *U.S. News & World Report*, August 14, 1973, p. 30.
61. Paul C. Glick and Arthur J. Norton, "Frequency, Duration and Probability of Marriage and Divorce," in *Marriage and the Family* (Population Division, Bureau of the Census, May 1971), pp. 307–17.
62. *Ibid.*
63. *Statistical Abstracts of the United States*, 1973 (note 53), Table 91, "Percent Distribution of Single and Never Married."
64. "More and More Broken Marriages" (note 60).
65. *Ibid.*
66. 1975 Delegate Assembly Issues Papers, Children's Rights Statement, *NASW News* 20, no. 3 (1975): 13.
67. *Day Care and Child Development Reports* 3, no. 11 (May 27, 1974).
68. *Child Care Arrangements of the Nation's Working Mothers*, 1965 (Washington, D.C.: U.S. Department of Health, Education, and Welfare), pp. 3–6.

69. Ibid.
70. Frances Lomas Feldman and Frances H. Scherz, *Family Social Welfare* (New York: Atherton, 1967).
71. Sarane S. Boocock, Ph.D., "Is the U.S. Becoming Less Child-Oriented?," address at the annual meeting of the American Society for the Advancement of Science, 1974, excerpted in the *National Observer*, February 22, 1975.
72. Helen M. Wallace, *Health Services for Mothers and Children* (Philadelphia: Saunders, 1962), pp. 102, 105.
73. Bloom (note 1), p. 218.
74. Publilius Syrus was a Latin writer who flourished in the first century B.C.
75. Gerald Caplan, "Emotional Implications of Pregnancy," in *Concepts of Mental Health and Consultation* (Washington, D.C.: Children's Bureau, U.S. Department of HEW, 1959).
76. Lydia Rapoport, "The State of Crisis, Some Theoretical Considerations," in Howard J. Parad, *Crisis Intervention* (New York: Family Service Association, 1965).
77. Bloom (note 1), p. 196.
78. Lewin (note 51), p. 67.
79. Dawson (note 30), p. 177.
80. Ainsworth (note 18), p. 149.
81. *The Sydney* (Australia) *Sun*, November 29, 1953.
82. Josselyn (note 14).
83. Bloom (note 1), p. 196.
84. Ibid.
85. John Bowlby, "Separation Anxiety," *International J. Psychoanalysis* 41 (1960): 89–113.
86. Ibid.
87. Rapoport, "The State of Crisis" (note 76) and "Working with Families in Crisis," *Social Work* 7 (1962): 48–53, and Erich Lindemann, "Symptomatology and Management of Acute Grief," in Parad (note 76), pp. 22–31, 129–39, 9–21.

3. The Experience of Chronic Illness

1. Albert Solnit and Morris Green, "Pediatric Management of the Dying Child," *Pediatrics* 40 (1967), Special Supplement, Part II, pp. 222–24.
2. Matthew Debuskey, *The Chronically Ill Child and His Family* (Springfield, Ill.: Thomas, 1970), p. 13.
3. Audrey T. McCollum and A. Herbert Schwartz, "Social Work and the Mourning Parent," *Social Work* 17, no. 1 (1972).
4. Elliott Podoll and Kenneth Smith, "Problem of Parent-Child Dependencies in One-Parent Families, Including Psychosymbiotic Relationships," paper presented at meeting of the American Orthopsychiatric Association, San Francisco, April 11, 1974.
5. Carolyn Baum, Cedars Sinai Medical Center, Infants' Consultation Service, "The One-Parent Family," paper presented at meeting of the American Orthopsychiatric Association (note 4).
6. Lola M. Irelan, ed., *Low-Income Life Styles* (Washington, D.C.: U.S. Dept. of HEW, Welfare Administration), p. 21.
7. Jerome Cohen, School of Social Work, University of California at Los Angeles, "Alternative Life Styles," paper presented at meeting of the American Orthopsychiatric Association (note 4).
8. Rose Grobstein, Genetic Counseling, Child Care Conference for Nurses, Stanford University Hospital, Stanford, Calif., March 13, 1973. Also Barbara Field,

"The Child with Spina Bifida," *Medical J. Australia*, December 2, 1972, p. 1287.

9. S. Olshansky, "Chronic Sorrow," *Social Casework* 43 (1962): 191-93.

10. Charles Hurt, Clinical Social Worker, Orthopedic Hospital, Los Angeles; personal communication, March 20, 1970.

11. Sylvia Schild, "The Challenging Opportunity for Social Workers in Genetics," *Social Work* 11 (1966): 22-28.

12. Podoll and Smith (note 4).

13. Clifford Burnett et al., "Neonatal Separation: The Maternal Side of Interactional Deprivation," *Pediatrics* 45, no. 2 (1970): 197.

14. C. M. Binger, "Childhood Leukemia—Emotional Impact on Siblings," in E. James Anthony and Cyrille Koupernik, eds., *The Child in His Family*. Vol. 2, *The Impact of Disease and Death* (New York: Wiley, 1973), pp. 195-207.

15. Erik H. Erikson, "Eight Ages of Man," in *Childhood and Society* (2d ed.; New York: Norton, 1963), pp. 247-74 *passim*.

16. John Bowlby, *Child Care and the Growth of Love* (London: Penguin, 1953). Anna Freud, "The Role of Bodily Illness in the Mental Life of Children," *Psychoanalytic Study of the Child* 7 (1952): 69-81. James Robertson, *Hospitals and Children, A Parent's Eye View* (New York: International Universities Press, 1963). Mary D. Ainsworth et al., *Deprivation of Maternal Care, A Reassessment of Its Effects* (Geneva: World Health Organization, 1962).

17. Sula Wolff, *Children under Stress* (London: Penguin, 1969), p. 58.

18. Thesi Bergmann and Anna Freud, *Children in Hospital* (New York: International Universities Press, 1966).

19. Erikson (note 15).

20. Roberta Simmons et al., "Disturbance in Self Image at Adolescence," paper presented at meetings of the Midwest Sociological Society, April 1972, pp. 22-24.

21. Erving Goffman, *Stigma, The Management of Spoiled Identity* (Englewood Cliffs, N.J.: Prentice-Hall, 1963), p. 17.

22. Beatrice A. Wright, *Physical Disability—A Psychological Approach* (New York: Harper & Row, 1960), p. 191.

23. Donald Brieland and students, "States of Severely Handicapped Young Adults," master's essay, University of Chicago, 1966.

24. Wolff (note 17), Introduction, p. 11.

25. Florence Blake and F. Wright, *Essentials of Pediatric Nursing* (Philadelphia: Lippincott, 1963), p. 32.

26. Bergmann and Freud (note 18), p. 142.

27. Anthony and Koupernik (note 14), p. 17.

28. Ake Mattsson, "Long-Term Physical Illness in Childhood: A Challenge to Psychosocial Adaptation," *Pediatrics* 50 (1972): 803-5.

29. *Ibid.*, p. 805.

30. Solnit and Green (note 1).

31. Max Sugar, "Disguised Depression in Adolescents," in Gene L. Usdin, ed., *Adolescence, Care and Counseling* (Philadelphia: Lippincott, 1967), p. 78.

32. Harold M. Visotsky et al., "Coping Behavior under Extreme Stress," *Archives of General Psychiatry* 5 (1962): 423-48 *passim*.

33. Michael el Jabala et al., "Surgical Management of the Burned Child," in Debuskey (note 2), p. 93.

34. Ruth F. Odgers and Burness G. Wenberg, *Introduction to Health Professions* (St. Louis: Mosby, 1972), p. 4.

35. *Ibid.*, p. 2.

36. Vivian Mazur, "The Child's Adaptation to the Hospital," in Evelyn K.

Oremland and Jerome D. Oremland, eds., *The Effects of Hospitalization on Children* (Springfield, Ill.: Thomas, 1973), pp. 28–30.

37. *Low-Income Life Styles* (note 6), p. 2.

38. Blake and Wright (note 25), pp. 33–34.

4. Community Resources

1. Arthur J. Lesser, "Trends in Maternal and Child Health," in Helen M. Wallace, *Health Services for Mothers and Children* (Philadelphia: Saunders, 1962), p. 48.

2. *Ibid.*, p. 47.

3. *San Jose Mercury* (Washington Post Service, November 24, 1972).

4. *Ibid.*

5. Tom Fulton, "Congress Studies Spate of National Health Insurance Bills," *NASW News* 19, no. 6 (1974).

6. Ellen Winston, "Medical Assistance under Title XIX of the Social Security Act," *Welfare in Review*, September 1965, p. 15.

7. Barbara S. Cooper et al., "National Health Expenditures," *Social Security Bulletin*, March 1974, p. 8.

8. Barbara S. Cooper and Paula A. Piro, "Age Difference in Medical Care Spending, Fiscal Year 1973," *Social Security Bulletin*, May 1974, p. 3.

9. *Ibid.*

10. Klaus J. Roghman et al., "Anticipated and Actual Effects of Medicaid on the Medical-Care Pattern of Children," *New England Journal of Medicine* 285 (1971): 1053–57 *passim*.

11. See table, National Center for Social Statistics, Office of Program Innovation, Medical Services Administration, Department of Health, Education, and Welfare, Washington, D.C., mimeo., 1974.

12. Government Research Corporation, *National Journal Reports* (Washington, D.C.) 6 (1974), no. 26: 969–73.

13. California State Department of Health Regulations, Title 17, part 1, chap. 4, subcategory 13, 1975, Child Health and Disability Prevention Program.

14. Cooper et al. (note 7), p. 10.

15. Lesser (note 1).

16. Marjorie Smith Mueller, "Private Health Insurance in 1972, Health Care Services, Enrollment and Finances," *Social Security Bulletin*, March 1974, p. 21.

17. *Ibid.*, p. 22.

18. Alfred M. Skolnik and Sophie R. Dales, "Social Welfare Expenditures, 1972–73," *Social Security Bulletin*, January 1974, p. 12.

19. *APWA Washington Report* (American Public Welfare Association) 10, no. 2 (1975): 2.

20. Skolnik and Dales (note 18), chart 3, p. 18.

21. Ray Ribal, Eligibility Work Supervisor, II, Income Maintenance, Santa Clara County, Calif., Department of Public Welfare; personal communication, September 3, 1974.

22. *APWA Washington Report* 9, no. 1 (1974).

23. DHEW, SSI Letter no. 111, 11, Supplement 1, "Evaluation of Child Claims."

24. The simplified version of the food stamp represented here is taken from information supplied by Mrs. Lillian Russell, Coordinator of Food Stamps, Santa Clara County, Calif., on July 14, 1974. Many details have been omitted. As in inquiry about other public assistance programs, specific inquiries should be made of the local public assistance office.

25. *NASW News* 20, no. 2 (1975): 11.
26. *Ibid.*
27. Skolnik and Dales (note 18), p. 4.
28. Jack Stumpf, "Getting a Slice of the General Revenue-Sharing Bread for Human Care Services," *J. Alternative Human Services* 1 (1974): 14.
29. *Ibid.*, p. 8.
30. "A National Program for Comprehensive Child Welfare Services," Child Welfare League of America, 67 Irving Place, New York, N.Y.
31. *Ibid.*, pp. 2–3.
32. Bernice Boehm, "Protective Services for Neglected Children," in Alfred Kadushin, *Child Welfare Services* (New York: Macmillan, 1970), p. 1.
33. *U.S. Federal Register* 34, no. 18 (1969): 1351.
34. Mary R. Lewis, "Day Care under the Social Security Act," *Social Service Review* 48, no. 3 (1974): 443–45 *passim*.
35. "In-Home Services, Toward a National Policy," Working Conference, Urban Life Center, Columbia, Maryland, May 31–June 2, 1972, p. 48.
36. Arthur Fleming, Working Conference (see note 35), p. 44.
37. "Costs of Homemaker, Home Health Aide Service and Alternative Forms of Service," National Council for Homemaker, Home Health Aid Service, 1974, p. 33.
38. Lewis (note 34).
39. *Ibid.*, p. 433.
40. Friends Committee on Legislation, *Newsletter* 23, no. 8 (1974).
41. Mrs. Leonora Wilson, Health Planner, Consultant to Day Care Centers, Santa Clara County, Calif.; personal communication, October 10, 1974.
42. Milton Willner, "Unsupervised Family Day Care in New York City," in "The Changing Dimensions of Day Care" (Child Welfare League of America, 1970), p. 58.
43. Jerome Bruner, "Overview of Development and Day Care," in *Day Care: Resources for Decision* (Day Care and Child Development Council of America, Washington, D.C., 1971).
44. DHEW Publication no. (OHD) 75-1070, "Handicapped Children in Head Start Programs."
45. *Head Start Newsletter* 7, no. 6 (1974).
46. "Standards for Foster Family Care Service" (Child Welfare League of America, 1959), p. 41.
47. Mary James, Supervisor, Special Foster Care Unit for Physically Handicapped Persons; paper presented at the Regional Conference, Child Welfare League of America, Los Angeles, April 16, 1970.
48. *Ibid.*
49. Studies of successful placements of physically normal children disagree on the factor of age of the foster parent's own children. See Jonathan Kraus, "Predicting Success of Foster Placements of School-Age Children," *Social Work*, January 1971, p. 71.
50. John Bowlby, "Separation Anxiety, A Critical Review of the Literature" (Child Welfare League of America, 1964); Therese Benedek, *Insight and Personality Adjustment* (New York: Ronald, 1946).
51. Regional Conference (see note 47).
52. "Standards" (note 46), p. 9.
53. *Children Waiting, State Social Welfare Board Report on Foster Care* (California Health and Welfare Agency, Summary of Recommendations, 1972), Preface.

54. *San Jose Mercury*, November 23, 1974.
55. Donald Brieland, "Children and Families," *Social Work* 19, no. 5 (1974): 573.
56. Janet L. Hoopes et al., *A Follow-up Study of Adoptions* (Child Welfare League of America), vols. 1 and 2.
57. Alice Hornecker, "Adoption Opportunities for the Handicapped," *Children*, July–August, 1962.
58. News release, January 15, 1969, Child Welfare League of America.
59. Lillian Ripple, "A Follow-up Study of Adopted Children," in Kadushin (note 32), p. 399.
60. Alfred Kadushin, *Adopting Older Children* (New York: Columbia University Press, 1970), p. 67.
61. Fred Massarik and David S. Franklin, "Adoption of Children with Medical Conditions" (Children's Home Society of California, 1967).
62. *Ibid.*, p. 3.
63. Kadushin (note 60), p. 210.
64. Massarik and Franklin (note 61).
65. Kadushin (note 60), pp. 46–47.
66. *Ibid.*
67. Hoopes et al. (note 56), vol. 2, pp. 63–81 *passim*.
68. *White House Conference on Children* (Washington, D.C.: Government Printing Office, 1970).
69. Alice M. Varela, "Toward the Integration of Health, Education, and Welfare Resources for Mothers and Children at the Level of Delivery of Service," in Alice M. Varela, ed., *Emerging Patterns of Health Care for Mothers and Children* (Institute sponsored by the Graduate School of Social Work, Rutgers University, New Brunswick, N.J., 1967), p. 3.
70. Milton Markowitz and Leon Gordis, "A Family Pediatric Clinic," *Children*, January–February, 1967, p. 25.
71. *Ibid.*, p. 30.
72. Yvonne L. Fraley, "Implications for Social Workers in New Jersey," in *Emerging Patterns* (note 69), p. 52.
73. John J. Horwitz, *Education for Social Workers in the Rehabilitation of the Handicapped*, Council on Social Work Education, vol. 8 of *A Project Report of the Curriculum Study*, 1959.
74. Werner Boehm, "The Relationships of Social Work to Other Professions," *Encyclopedia of Social Work*, 1967.
75. George C. McGhee, "A Bright Side of Welfare," *Saturday Review–World*; reprinted by the *National Observer*, September 21, 1974.
76. Frances Lomas Feldman and Frances H. Scherz, *Family Social Welfare* (New York: Atherton, 1967), p. 264.
77. Naomi Brill, *Working with People, the Helping Process* (Philadelphia: Lippincott, 1973), pp. 34, 38–41 *passim*.
78. Frances R. Morrow, M.S.W., Deputy Director, San Mateo County, California, Department of Health and Welfare; personal communication, October 2, 1974.
79. Fern W. Jaffee, "A Non-Traditional Pattern of Collaboration in Maternity Care," in *Emerging Patterns* (note 69), p. 13.
80. Ruth Wade Cox and Mary Hamilton James, "Rescue from Limbo," *Child Welfare* 49, no. 1 (1970).
81. Madelon George, Kazuyoshi Ide, and Clara E. Vambey, "The Comprehensive Health Team: A Conceptual Model," *J. Nursing Administration*, 1971.

82. "Visiting Nurse Service of New York: A Descriptive Study," *Chronic Illness Newsletter* 18, no. 3 (1967).

83. *Ibid.*

84. Dorothy E. Johnson, "The Role of a Pediatric Nurse," *Nursing J. India* 47 (1956): 118–19, quoted by Beatrice R. Moore in "When Johnny Must Go to the Hospital," *American J. Nursing* 57 (1957).

85. Leonard M. Linde, M.D., Pediatric Cardiologist, St. Vincent Medical Center, Los Angeles; paper presented at a Conference on the Effective Role of the Medical Social Worker on the Pediatric Cardiac Team, Los Angeles, September 20, 1974.

5. *The Unborn Child and the Mother*

1. Virginia Apgar, "Birth Defects—A Word from a Doctor," in *With Best Wishes for a Happy Birthday from the National Foundation* (National Foundation–March of Dimes, 622 Third Avenue, New York, N.Y.).

2. Stewart Clifford, "Prevention of Prematurity the Sine Qua Non for Reduction in Mental Retardation and Other Neurologic Disorders," *New England J. Medicine* 71 (1964): 243–49 (reproduced by the Children's Bureau, Department of Health, Education, and Welfare, Washington, D.C.).

3. Arthur J. Lesser, "High-Risk Mothers and Infants: Problems and Prospects for Prevention," in Florence Haselkorn, ed., *Mothers at Risk* (Perspectives in Social Work, vol. 1, no. 1; Adelphi University School of Social Work Publications, Garden City, N.Y., 1966), p. 15.

4. Joseph P. Rossi, "High-Risk Babies: Determining the Problem," paper presented at the 30th New England Health Institute, June 19, 1964; reprinted by the National Foundation.

5. *Scientific American*, February 1973, p. 228.

6. Provisional Vital Statistics, Monthly Vital Statistics Report, National Center for Health Statistics, Department of HEW, p. 1.

7. *National Observer*, June 1974, p. 22.

8. "Why the Poor Are Fewer," *Newsweek* 79: 62 (March 13, 1972).

9. *Ibid.*

10. Ernest B. Attah, *Science* 180 (1973): 1150.

11. June Sklar and Beth Berkov, "The Effects of Legal Abortion on Legitimate and Illegitimate Birth Rates: The California Experience" (International Population and Urban Research Institute of International Studies, University of California, Berkeley, Report no. 436, 1973), p. 286.

12. *Ibid.*

13. Helen M. Wallace, *Health Services for Mothers and Children* (Philadelphia: Saunders, 1962), pp. 80–82. See also Donald C. Smith, "Principles of Prevention, Identification and Management," in Helen M. Wallace et al., *Maternal and Child Health Practices* (Springfield, Ill.: Thomas, 1973), pp. 933–34.

14. Arthur J. Lesser, "Trends in Maternal and Child Health," in Wallace et al. (note 13), p. 51.

15. *Ibid.*

16. Hyman Goldstein, "Demographic Information in Maternal and Child Health," chap. 4 in Wallace et al. (note 13), p. 87.

17. *Ibid.*

18. "World Health and Population," Planned Parenthood release, May 1974.

19. A. Frederick North, "The Influence of Poverty on Maternal and Child Health," in Wallace et al. (note 13), p. 156.

20. *Ibid.*, p. 162.
21. Wallace (note 13), pp. 80–82.
22. Lesser (note 3), p. 17.
23. Wallace (note 13), p. 85.
24. *Ibid.*
25. Lucille Hurley, "The Consequences of Fetal Impoverishment," *Nutrition Today*, December 1968, pp. 3–10; "Nutrition During Pregnancy and Lactation," California State Department of Public Health, 1960. See also "Evidence Shows that Poor Diet Causes Mental Ills, Early Death," *San Diego Union*, October 30, 1969. Also Delbert H. Dayton, "Early Malnutrition and Human Development," *Children* 16 (1969).
26. Food and Nutrition Board, National Academy of Sciences, National Research Council, Washington, D.C. Standards issued in 1963.
27. Elaine Heil, Nutritionist, San Diego County Department of Public Health; lecture given at San Diego State University, School of Social Work, October 20, 1969.
28. Neville R. Butler and Eva D. Alberman, eds., *Perinatal Problems: Report* (London: Livingstone, 1969), pp. 40–41.
29. W. T. Tompkins, D. G. Wiehl, and R. M. Mitchell, "The Underweight Patient as an Increased Obstetric Hazard," *Amer. J. Obstetrics & Gynecology* 69, no. 1 (1955): 114.
30. Thomas H. Brewer, *Metabolic Toxemia of Late Pregnancy* (Springfield, Ill.: Thomas, 1973), pp. 933–34.
31. Jerry Plummer, "Hunger," study of clients of Aid to Families with Dependent Children (AFDC), presented to William S. Hay, Director of Sacramento County, Department of Public Welfare (mimeo.), September 1969.
32. *Smoking and Health—Report of the Advisory Committee to the Surgeon General of the Public Health Service* (U.S. Department of HEW, PHS Publ. no. 1103, January 11, 1964, pp. 343–44.
33. John D. Thompson et al., "Obstetric Antecedents of Perinatal Mortality and Morbidity," in Wallace et al. (note 13), p. 269.
34. Jane S. Lin-Fu, *Neonatal Narcotic Addiction* (Washington, D.C.: Children's Bureau, HEW, 1967).
35. Thompson (note 33), p. 270.
36. California State Department of Public Health, Statistical Bulletin, 1969.
37. Sklar and Berkov (note 11), p. 285.
38. *Ibid.*
39. "Report of a Conference on Parenthood in Adolescence," sponsored by Yale University, the University of Pittsburgh, and the Children's Bureau, Washington, D.C., January 22–24, 1970, p. 42.
40. *Ibid.*, p. 44.
41. Mohammed Hassan and Frederick H. Falls, "The Young Primipara," *Amer. J. Obstetrics & Gynecology* 88 (1964): 256–69.
42. James P. Semmens and William M. Lamers, Jr., *Teen-Age Pregnancy* (Springfield, Ill.: Thomas, 1968), p. 107.
43. F. C. Battaglia et al., "Obstetric and Pediatric Complications of Juvenile Pregnancy," *Pediatrics* 32 (1963): 902–10 *passim*.
44. Howard J. Osofsky and Rojan Reuga, "The Adolescent Pregnancy," in Wallace et al. (note 13), p. 886.
45. Semmens and Lamers (note 42).
46. Osofsky and Reuga (note 44). See also H. E. Chase, *The Relationship of*

Certain Biologic and Socio-Economic Factors to Fetal, Infant and Early Childhood Mortality (U.S. Department of HEW, Children's Bureau, 1964).

47. Elizabeth Herzog, "The Young Family: Some Perspectives," in "Report of a Conference on Parenthood in Adolescence" (note 39), p. 23.
48. "New Families, New Life Styles," in "Report of a Conference on Parenthood in Adolescence" (note 39), p. 53.
49. Wallace (note 13), p. 85.
50. Semmens and Lamers (note 42), quoting from National Vital Statistics Division.
51. *Statistical Abstract of the United States,* 1973 (U.S. Government Printing Office, Washington, D. C.), Table 70.
52. *Population and the American Future,* Report of Commission on Population Growth, Washington, D.C., John D. Rockefeller, Chairman, transmitted 1972 (Department of Documents, U.S. Government Printing Office), p. 88.
53. Sklar and Berkov (note 11), Table 5, p. 285.
54. Goldstein (note 16), pp. 110, 128.
55. Haselkorn (note 3), p. 17.
56. Beth Berkov and Paul W. Shipley, "Illegitimate Births in California, 1966–67," State of California Department of Public Health, Bureau of Maternal and Child Health, Bureau of Vital Statistics Regulation, March 1971, pp. 20–23 *passim.*
57. Blanche Bernstein and Mignon Sauber, "Deterrents to Early Prenatal Care Among Women Pregnant out of Wedlock," New York State Department of Social Welfare, Albany, 1960.
58. *Ibid.,* p. 109.
59. Osofsky and Reuga (note 44), p. 889.
60. *Ibid.,* pp. 890–91.
61. Bernstein and Sauber (note 57).
62. "Welfare Mothers for Fewer Births," *New York Times,* April 14, 1968; report of a study on "Fertility, Illegitimacy, and Birth Control," by Lawrence Podell, New York City University Center for Social Research.
63. Lee Rainwater, *And the Poor Get Children* (Chicago: Quadrangle Books, 1960), pp. 28–59 *passim,* 170–71 *passim.*
64. Sklar and Berkov (note 11), p. 286.
65. *Family Planning Digest* 1, no. 4 (1972): 3.
66. Michael Harrington, *The Other America, Poverty in the United States* (Baltimore: Penguin, 1963), p. 135.
67. Butler and Alberman (note 28), pp. 36–38 *passim.*
68. William Dieckmann, *Toxemias of Pregnancy* (St. Louis: Mosby, 1952), p. 53.
69. *Ibid.*
70. Brewer (note 30), Preface.
71. *Ibid.,* p. 3.
72. See Semmens and Lamers (note 42) vs. Brewer (note 30). Brewer says, "I am convinced there is nothing about teenage pregnancy per se that causes difficulty." Dr. Brewer thinks the unwed mother's tendency to starve herself to hide pregnancy as long as possible is the reason the rate is high in teenagers.
73. Dieckmann (note 68), p. 20.
74. Brewer (note 30), p. 71.
75. *Ibid.*
76. "Pregnant Weight Watchers Risk Harm to Babies," *Public Health Reports* 85 (1970): 964.
77. Dieckmann (note 68), p. 580.

78. *Ibid.*, p. 455.
79. Jorgen Pederson, *The Pregnant Diabetic and Her Newborn* (Baltimore: Williams & Wilkins, 1967), p. 48.
80. Henry Dolger and Bernard Seeman, *How to Live with Diabetes* (New York: Norton, 1965), p. 161.
81. *Ibid.*; and Pederson (note 79), pp. 42–43.
82. Elaine P. Rolli, *Management of the Diabetic Patient* (New York: Putnam, 1965), pp. 153–57.
83. *Ibid.*
84. Priscilla White, "Childhood Diabetes, Its Causes and Influence on the Second and Third Generations," *Diabetes* 9 (1960): 345–53.
85. *Ibid.*
86. *Ibid.*
87. Pederson (note 79), p. 157.
88. White (note 84).
89. Pederson (note 79).
90. Wallace et al. (note 13), p. 46.
91. Curtis Lester Mendelson, *Cardiac Disease in Pregnancy* (Philadelphia: Davis, 1960), p. 47.
92. *Ibid.*
93. Mendelson (note 91), p. 107.
94. American Heart Association, "Heart Disease and Pregnancy," 1963, p. 5.
95. Leon M. Gordis and Milton Markowitz, "Rheumatic Heart Disease and Pregnancy in Adolescent Rheumatic Fever Patients," *Pediatrics* 40 (1967): 104–5.
96. American Heart Association (note 94), pp. 13–14.
97. Mendelson (note 91), p. 107.
98. *Ibid.*, p. 108.
99. *Ibid.*, p. 5.
100. "Viruses and Pregnancy," *Therapeutic Notes* (Parke Davis Co., Detroit, Mich.) 74 (1967): 59–60 *passim*.
101. *Ibid.*, p. 61.
102. Janet B. Hardy, "Rubella and Its Aftermath," *Children* 16 (1969): 90–96.
103. Alice Chenowith, "Planning a Mass Attack on Rubella," *Children* 16 (1969): 95.
104. Jane S. Lin-Fu, M.D., U.S. Department of HEW, Children's Bureau, October 1966.
105. *Ibid.*
106. Arthur Lesser, "Trends in Maternal and Child Health," in Wallace et al. (note 13), p. 69.
107. Mary Clark, M.D., Deputy Director, Santa Clara County, California Department of Public Health; personal communication, June 6, 1974.
108. Chenowith (note 103), p. 96.
109. West's Annotated California Codes, 1974, Section 4301, Premarital Examinations.
110. Leaders Alert, Bulletin No. 26, National Foundation, New York, N.Y.
111. Clark (note 107).
112. Lesser (note 106), p. 67.
113. Wallace (note 13), p. 22.
114. Clark (note 107).
115. Lesser (note 106).
116. Billy Andrews, M.D., quoted in "Key Issues in Infant Mortality, Report of

a Conference in Washington, D.C.," National Institute of Child Health and Human Development, Bethesda, Md., April 1969, p. 50.

117. Bernice Giansiracusa, M.D., Director of Maternal and Child Health Services, Santa Clara County, California Department of Public Health; personal communication, June 1974.

118. R. L. Tips and H. T. Lynch, "The Impact of Genetic Counseling upon the Family Milieu," *J. Amer. Medical Association* 184 (1963): 183.

119. Sylvia Schild, "The Challenging Opportunity for Social Workers in Genetics," *Social Work* 11 (1966): 22–28.

120. *Ibid.*

121. Richard M. Nixon, "Presidential Message on Population," July 18, 1969, Population Crisis Committee, Washington, D.C., p. 18.

122. "What You Should Know about the Pill," a new American Medical Association bulletin, 0438–382–1; 75M, Op. 291.

123. *Ibid.*

124. HEW publ. no. HSM 73–16002.

125. John Letts, M.D., Chief of Obstetrics and Gynecology, San Mateo County Department of Health and Welfare; personal communication, May 1974.

126. Giansiracusa (note 117), personal communication, September 17, 1974.

127. Letts (note 125).

128. HEW publ. (note 124).

129. Letts (note 125).

130. Warren Miller, "Psychological Vulnerability to Unwanted Pregnancy," *Family Planning Perspectives* 5, no. 4 (1973): 199–201.

131. Aubrey Milunsky, *Prenatal Diagnosis of Hereditary Disorders* (Springfield, Ill.: Thomas, 1973), p. 158.

132. Karen Zuzich, Coordinator of Information, Referral and Service Center for Pregnant Girls, San Mateo County, California Health and Welfare Department; personal communication, February 22, 1974.

133. Alan Guttmacher, *Reader's Digest*, November 1973.

134. Lawrence Lader, *Abortion* (Indianapolis: Bobbs-Merrill, 1966), p. 39.

135. R. Bruce Sloane, "The Unwanted Pregnancy," *New England J. Medicine* 280 (1969): 1206–13.

136. Zuzich (note 132).

137. Sloane (note 135), quoting M. Ekblad, "Induced Abortion on Psychiatric Grounds: Follow-up Study of 479 Women," *Acta Psychiatric Scandinavia*, Supp. 99, 1955, pp. 1–238.

138. *San Jose Mercury News*, October 8, 1972.

139. Zuzich (note 132).

140. Sklar and Berkov (note 11), p. 283.

141. Letts (note 125), personal communication, February 22, 1974.

142. "The Physician and Contraception Sterilization," Association for Voluntary Sterilization, 14 W. 40th Street, New York, N.Y.

143. *Family Planning Population Reporter* 3 (1974): 25.

144. Statement of Prepare and Program, Association for Voluntary Sterilization, New York, N.Y.

145. "Voluntary Male Sterilization," *J. Amer. Medical Association* 204 (1968), editorial.

146. Giansiracusa (note 117), personal communication, November 26, 1974.

147. For example, see Robert W. Laidlaw and Medora Bass, "Voluntary Sterilization as It Relates to Mental Health," *Amer. J. Psychiatry* 120 (1964): 1176–79.

148. "Sterilization, Population Report, January 1973," Series C, no. 1, Department of Medicine and Public Affairs, George Washington University Medical Center, Washington, D.C.

149. C. R. Scriver, J. L. Neal, R. Saginur, and A. Clow, "The Frequency of Genetic Disease and Congenital Malformation among Patients in a Pediatric Hospital," *Canadian Medical Association J.* 108 (1973): 1111.

150. C. O. Carter, "Changing Patterns in the Causes of Death at the Hospital for Sick Children," *Great Ormond Street J.* 11 (1956): 65.

151. D. F. Roberts, J. Chevez, and S. D. M. Court, "The Genetic Component in Child Mortality," *Archives of Diseases of Childhood* 45 (1970): 38.

152. R. Saginur, A. Clow, C. R. Scriver, and F. C. Fraser, "Admission for Genetic Disease to a Pediatric Hospital," *MRC Prenatal Diagnosis Newsletter* (Montreal) 1 (1972): 13–15; as quoted in Carol L. Clow, F. Clark Fraser, Claude Laberge, and C. R. Scriver, "On the Application of Knowledge to the Patient with Genetic Disease," in A. G. Steinberg and A. G. Bearn, eds., *Progress in Medical Genetics* (New York: Grune & Stratton, 1973), vol. 9, p. 162.

153. Howard M. Cann, Associate Professor of Pediatrics and Genetics, Stanford University School of Medicine; personal communication, 1974.

154. Isaac Asimov, *The Genetic Code* (New York: Orion, 1962). See also George and Murial Beadle, *The Language of Life* (Garden City, N.Y.: Doubleday, 1966).

155. Asimov (note 154).

156. L. C. Dunn, "Sex Linkage and Sex Determination," *Encyclopaedia Britannica* (Chicago: Benton, 1960), p. 111C.

157. Joseph B. Warshaw and Lewis B. Holmes, "Congenital Malformations—Some Genetic, Embryological and Environmental Considerations," *Genetics and the Perinatal Patient* (Mead Johnson Symposium on Perinatal Developmental Medicine, held at Vail, Colo., June 12–14, 1972), no. 1, p. 18.

158. Lechaim Naggan and Brian MacMahon, "Ethnic Differences in the Prevalence of Anencephaly and Spina Bifida in Boston, Massachusetts," *New England J. Medicine* 277 (1967): 1123.

159. Cann (note 153).

160. M. Neil Macintyre, "Counseling in Cases Involving Antenatal Diagnosis," in Albert Dorfman, ed., *Antenatal Diagnosis* (Chicago: University of Chicago Press, 1972), p. 64.

161. Warshaw and Holmes (note 157), p. 17.

162. Scriver et al. (note 149), p. 1111.

163. Michael M. Kaback, "Perspectives in the Control of Human Genetic Disease," *Genetics and the Perinatal Patient* (Mead Johnson Symposium on Perinatal Developmental Medicine, no. 1, 1972), p. 55.

164. Cann (note 153).

165. Charles J. Epstein, Edward L. Schneider, Felix A. Conte, and Stanley Friedman, "Prenatal Detection of Genetic Disorders," *Amer. J. Human Genetics* 24 (1972): 216.

166. John W. Littlefield, "Recent Experience with Prenatal Genetic Diagnosis," *Genetics and the Perinatal Patient* (Mead Johnson Symposium on Perinatal Developmental Medicine, no. 1, 1972), p. 26.

167. Cann (note 153).

168. Littlefield (note 166), p. 26.

169. *International Directory, Birth Defects, Genetic Services* (4th ed.; New York: National Foundation, March 1974).

170. Kaback (note 163), p. 56.

171. Wallace (note 13), p. 39.
172. *Ibid.*
173. *Ibid.*
174. Jean Travers, "A Study of Prenatal Attendance at Santa Clara Valley Medical Center," ms, Santa Clara County Department of Public Health, San Jose, California, 1973.
175. Aline B. Auerbach, "Having a Baby—The Emotional Aspects of Pregnancy," Child Study Association of America, New York, N.Y., undated.
176. Tompkins et al. (note 29).
177. *Ibid.*
178. Helene Deutsch, "Pregnancy," chap. 6 of *Motherhood*, vol. 2 of Helene Deutsch, *Psychology of Women* (New York: Grune & Stratton, 1945), pp. 126–201 *passim*. See also Gerald Caplan, *Concepts of Mental Health and Consultation* (Children's Bureau Publ. no. 273, U.S. Department of HEW, U.S. Govt. Printing Office, 1963), chap. 4, "Emotional Implications of Pregnancy," pp. 44–56, and "Origin and Development of Mother-Child Relationships," pp. 57–78 *passim*. Also Auerbach (note 175); and Marcel Heiman, "Pregnancy, Interwoven with People and Problems," *Medical Insight*, August 1970, pp. 17–21 *passim*.
179. Caplan and Heiman (note 178).
180. Caplan (note 178).
181. *Ibid.*, p. 59.
182. M. Hultin and J. O. Ottosson, "Pregnancy and Delivery of Unwanted Children," and "Perinatal Conditions of Unwanted Children," *Acta Psychiatric Scandinavia*, Supp. 221, 1971.
183. *Ibid.*
184. William R. Thompson and Joan E. Grusec, "Studies of Early Experience," in Paul H. Mussen, ed., *Carmichael's Manual of Child Psychology* (3d ed.; New York: Wiley, 1970), vol. 1. See also Harry Munsinger, *Fundamentals of Child Development* (New York: Holt, Rinehart & Winston, 1974); and Roman Rechnitz Limner, *Sex and the Unborn Child* (New York: Pyramid Books, 1969).

6. Asthma

1. Clara G. Schiffer and Eleanor P. Hunt, *Illness Among Children* (data from the National Health Survey, Children's Bureau, U.S. HEW, 1963), p. 14.
2. Frederick Speer, *The Management of Childhood Asthma* (Springfield, Ill.: Thomas, 1958); and Louis Tuft and Harry Louis Mueller, *Allergy in Children* (Philadelphia: Saunders, 1970), p. 30.
3. Speer (note 2), pp. 36–37.
4. John M. Sheldon et al., *A Manual of Clinical Allergy* (Philadelphia: Saunders, 1967), pp. 21–30.
5. Tuft and Mueller (note 2), pp. 13–35.
6. Speer (note 2).
7. Sheldon et al. (note 4), pp. 437–38.
8. Samuel M. Feinberg, "Allergies from the Air and What to Do about Them," *Today's Health*, August 1961, p. 4. Reprint issued by the American Medical Association, 535 N. Dearborn Street, Chicago.
9. Susan Dees, "Asthma," in Edwin Kendig, *Disorders of the Respiratory Tract in Children* (Philadelphia: Saunders, 1967), pp. 449–87.
10. Susan Dees, "Development and Cause of Asthma in Children," *Amer. J. Diseases of Children* 93 (1957): 228–33.

11. Albert D. G. Blanc, *So You Have Asthma* (Springfield, Ill.: Thomas, 1966), p. 47; and Tuft and Mueller (note 2), p. 30.
12. Dees (note 6).
13. *Ibid.*, and M. Harry Jennison, "A Practical Approach to the Problems of Asthma," paper presented at the Children's Hospital at Stanford, Palo Alto, February 4, 1972.
14. Jennison (note 13).
15. Birt Harvey, "Asthma," in E. E. Bleck, *Physically Handicapped Children: Medical Atlas for Teachers of Chronically Ill Children* (New York: Grune & Stratton, 1975), p. 31.
16. Leon Gordis, *Epidemiology of Chronic Lung Disease in Children* (Baltimore: Johns Hopkins Press, 1973), p. 27.
17. Irvin Caplin, *The Allergic Asthmatic* (Springfield, Ill.: Thomas, 1968), p. 10; and Harvey (note 15), p. 8 of draft.
18. Blanc (note 11), pp. 56–59 *passim*.
19. Dees (note 6).
20. Harvey (note 15), and Blanc (note 11).
21. Discussion with pediatric allergy staffs at Children's Hospital at Stanford and Oakland Children's Hospital, August 1968.
22. Caplin (note 17), pp. 13–14.
23. Warren T. Vaughan and J. Harvey Black, *Practice of Allergy* (3d ed.; St. Louis: Mosby, 1954), pp. 1008–9.
24. Harvey (note 15).
25. Ernest Harms, ed., *Somatic and Psychiatric Aspects of Childhood Allergies* (New York: Macmillan, 1963).
26. *Ibid.*
27. Leon J. Saul and James G. Delano, "Psychopathology and Psychotherapy in the Allergies of Children—A Review of Recent Literature," in Harms (note 25), p. 1.
28. Kenneth Purcell: (a) "A Preliminary Comparison of Rapidly and Persistently Steroid-Dependent Asthmatic Children," *Psychosomatic Medicine* 23 (1961). (b) "Distinctions: Some Parent Attitude Variables Related to Age of Onset of Asthma," *J. Psychosomatic Research* 6 (1962): 251–58. (c) "Distinctions: Psychological Test and Behavior Rating Comparisons," *J. Psychosomatic Research* 6 (1962): 283–91. (d) "Distinctions Between Subgroups of Asthmatic Children's Perception of Events Associated with Asthma," *Pediatrics* 31 (1963). (e) "Some Observations on Psychosomatic Studies of Asthma," paper presented at meetings of the Society for Research in Child Development, Berkeley, Calif., 1963.
29. Sara Dubo et al., "A Study of Relationships Between Family Situation, Bronchial Asthma and Personal Adjustment in Children," *J. Pediatrics* 59 (1961): 402.
30. Jeanne Block et al., "Interaction Between Allergic Potential and Psychopathology in Childhood Asthma," *Psychosomatic Medicine* 26 (1964): 307.
31. Constance Nathanson and Marie Britt Rhyne, "Social and Cultural Factors Associated with Asthmatic Symptoms in Children," *Social Science and Medicine* (Oxford: Pergamon) 4 (1970): 293–306.
32. William Kaufman, "Food-induced Allergic Illness in Children," in Harms (note 25), p. 109.
33. Minoru Yamate, "Treatment of Bronchial Asthma," paper presented at meeting of the American Academy of Pediatrics at Stanford Hospital for Children, July 1971.

34. Tuft and Mueller (note 2), pp. 347–73 *passim*.
35. Caplin (note 17).
36. Speer (note 2).
37. Vincent J. Fontana et al., "Effectiveness of Hyposensitization Therapy in Ragweed Hay Fever in Children," *J. Amer. Medical Assn.* 195 (1966).
38. Yamate (note 33).
39. Speer (note 2).
40. *Ibid.*
41. Dees (note 9); and Gordis (note 16), p. 41.
42. Gordis (note 16), p. 11.
43. Caplin (note 17), p. 62.
44. *Ibid.*, p. 64.
45. Minoru Yamate, M.D., Chief, Pediatric Allergy, Children's Hospital at Stanford; personal communication, February 22, 1974.
46. *Ibid.*
47. See the article issued by the Committee on Children with Handicaps, American Academy of Pediatrics, "The Asthmatic Child and His Participation in Sports," *Pediatrics* 45 (1970): 150.
48. Michael L. Hirt, *Psychological and Allergic Aspects of Asthma* (Springfield, Ill.: Thomas, 1965), p. 211.
49. Gordis (note 16), pp. 28–30 *passim*.
50. *Ibid.*, pp. 32–33.
51. Marie Britt Rhyne, "The Atopic Child," in Matthew Debuskey, ed., *The Chronically Ill Child and His Family* (Springfield, Ill.: Thomas, 1970), p. 126.
52. Nathanson and Rhyne (note 31), p. 303.
53. U. Bronfenbrenner, "The Changing American Child—A Speculative Analysis," *Merrill-Palmer Quarterly* 7 (1961): 75; as quoted in Nathanson and Rhyne (note 31), p. 303.

7. Chronic Kidney Diseases

1. Harris D. Riley, Jr., "Pyelonephritis in Infancy and Childhood," *Pediatric Clinics of North America* 11 (1964): 731.
2. "How Your Kidney Foundation Can Affect You and Your Family," and "How Kidney Disease Can Affect You and Your Family," pamphlets of the National Kidney Foundation, 116 East 27th Street, New York, N.Y., p-30-71 and p-42-71, unpaged.
3. "Your Kidneys," National Kidney Foundation, 116 East 27th Street, New York, N.Y.
4. "Kidney Diseases, A Guide for Public Health Personnel," U.S. Department of HEW, Public Health Service Publication No. 1384, 1965, p. 5.
5. "Your Kidneys" (note 3).
6. "Kidney Diseases" (note 4).
7. "Kidney Diseases" (note 4), pp. 9–12 *passim*.
8. John Maloney, M.D., Chief, Pediatric Service, Valley Medical Center, San Jose, Calif.; personal communication, February 22, 1973.
9. Mitchell I. Rubin, "Pyelonephritis, Certain Aspects," *Pediatric Clinics of North America* 11 (1964): 650.
10. Bernice Widrow, M.D., Director, Renal Care Unit, El Camino Hospital, Mountain View, Calif.; personal communication, February 1973.
11. "Kidney Diseases" (note 4), p. 14.
12. Rubin (note 9), pp. 649–50.

13. Mary Clark, M.D., Deputy Director, Santa Clara County, California, Department of Public Health; personal communication, April 12, 1973. See also Rubin (note 9), p. 663.
14. "Kidney Diseases" (note 4), p. 14.
15. Rubin (note 9).
16. Clark (note 13); and Milton Gross, M.D., internist, San Jose, Calif., personal communications, February 1973.
17. Clark (note 13).
18. Edward H. Kass, ed., "Proceedings of a Conference on Chronic Diseases, Boston, Mass., June 4-6, 1969," *Milbank Fund Quarterly* 47 (July 1969), part 2. A wide-ranging discussion among experts revealed that the relationship between urinary tract infection and chronic renal diseases is established, but that large-scale community preventive methods through screening and follow-up are costly and not subject to general agreement among the medical profession because of insufficient definitive knowledge of cause-and-effect relationships.
19. Lawrence R. Freedman, "Whither Pyelonephritis," paper presented at the Annual Meeting, American Society of Pediatric Nephrology, San Francisco, May 16, 1973.
20. "Kidney Diseases" (note 4), p. 14.
21. Rubin (note 9), p. 664.
22. Thomas A. Stamey, "Urinary Infections in Infancy and Childhood," in *Urinary Infections* (Baltimore: Williams & Wilkins, 1972), chap. 5.
23. Maurice B. Strauss and Louis Welt, *Diseases of the Kidney* (2d ed.; Boston: Little, Brown, 1971), vol. 2.
24. Victor Vaughan and R. James McKay, eds., *Nelson Textbook of Pediatrics* (10th ed.; Philadelphia: Saunders, 1975), p. 1244.
25. *Ibid.*, pp. 1244-51 *passim.*
26. Donald E. Potter, Assistant Professor of Pediatrics, University of California, San Francisco; personal communication, July 12, 1973.
27. Florence G. Blake and F. Howell Wright, *Essentials of Pediatric Nursing* (7th ed.; Philadelphia: Lippincott, 1963), p. 260.
28. Waldo E. Nelson et al., *Textbook of Pediatrics* (9th ed.; Philadelphia: Saunders, 1969), p. 1035.
29. *Ibid.*, pp. 1035-42.
30. Wallace W. McCrory and Madeka Shibuya, "Post-Streptococcal Glomerulonephritis," *Pediatric Clinics of North America* 2 (1964): 645.
31. Strauss and Welt (note 23), p. 1367.
32. Chester M. Edelman, Jr., "Glomerulonephritis," in Henry L. Barnett and Arnold H. Einhorn, eds., *Pediatrics* (14th ed.; New York: Appleton-Century-Crofts, 1968), p. 1345.
33. Robert L. Vernier, "Chronic Glomerulonephritis and the Nephritic Syndrome," *Milbank Fund Quarterly* 47 (July 1969), p. 67.
34. "Kidney Diseases" (note 4), pp. 13-14. See also Malcolm A. Holliday, Donald E. Potter, and Robert S. Dobrin, "Treatment of Renal Failure in Children," *Pediatric Clinics of North America* 18 (1971).
35. "Childhood Nephrosis," National Kidney Foundation, undated. Also Bruce M. Tune, M.D., Assistant Professor of Pediatrics, Stanford University School of Medicine; at pediatric grand rounds, June 29, 1973.
36. "Childhood Nephrosis," National Kidney Foundation, undated. See also Sidney Levin, "Nephrotic Syndrome in Childhood," in Matthew Debuskey, ed., *The Chronically Ill Child and His Family* (Springfield, Ill.: Thomas, 1970).

37. Levin (note 36), p. 68.
38. Chester M. Edelman, Jr., "Treatment of the Nephrotic Syndrome," paper presented at meeting (note 19).
39. Malcolm A. Holliday, M.D., Professor of Pediatrics, University of California, San Francisco; personal communication, May 2, 1973.
40. "Acute Glomerulonephritis," National Kidney Foundation, 1971.
41. Holliday et al. (note 34).
42. H. Richard Tyler, "Neurological Complications in Renal Failure," in Louis G. Welt et al., eds., *Symposium on Uremic Toxins* (Chicago: American Medical Association, 1970), p. 781.
43. *Ibid.*, p. 783.
44. *Ibid.*, p. 785.
45. *Ibid.*
46. "High Blood Pressure and Your Kidneys," National Kidney Foundation, p-38-71.
47. Ellin Lieberman, "Hypertension in Childhood," paper presented at meeting (note 19).
48. Allan J. Erslev, "Anemia in Renal Failure," in Louis G. Welt et al., eds., *Symposium on Uremic Toxins* (Chicago: American Medical Association, 1970), p. 774.
49. S. W. Stanbury, "The Treatment of Renal Osteodystrophy," *Annals of Internal Medicine* 65, no. 5 (1966): 1133.
50. *Dorland's Pocket Medical Dictionary* (20th ed.; Philadelphia: Saunders, 1959).
51. Stanbury (note 49), p. 1136.
52. Holliday et al. (note 34), p. 616.
53. *Ibid.*, p. 618.
54. Malcolm A. Holliday, "Calorie Deficiency in Children with Uremia; Effect upon Growth," *Pediatrics* 50 (1972): 71.
55. Darla R. Erhard, "Nutritional Aspects of Growth," paper presented at meeting (note 19).
56. Carl F. Anderson et al., "Nutritional Therapy for Adults with Renal Disease," *J. Amer. Medical Association* 223 (1973): 68.
57. *Ibid.*, p. 69.
58. *Ibid.*, p. 70.
59. Joanne Hattner, Dietician, Stanford University Medical Center, Stanford, Calif.; personal communication, February 13, 1973.
60. Benjamin T. Burton, "Diet Therapy in Uremia," *J. Amer. Dietetic Association* 54 (1969): 477.
61. Donald E. Potter, M.D., Assistant Professor of Pediatrics, University of California Medical Center, San Francisco; personal communication, July 11, 1973.
62. Tracy La Rose, Renal Dietician, University of California School of Medicine, San Francisco; personal communication, July 11, 1973.
63. Barbara M. Korsch et al., "Experiences with Children and Their Families during Extended Hemodialysis and Kidney Transplantation," *Pediatric Clinics of North America* 18 (1971): 625–37.
64. Holliday et al. (note 34).
65. "The Tenth Report of the Human Renal Transplant Registry," prepared by the Advisory Committee to the Renal Transplant Registry, published in the *J. Amer. Medical Association* 221 (1972): 1496, 1499.
66. Richard N. Fine et al., "Renal Homotransplantation in Children," *J. Pediatrics* 76 (1970): 356.

67. Holliday et al. (note 34), pp. 613–21 *passim.*
68. "The Tenth Report of the Human Renal Transplant Registry" (note 65).
69. Malcolm A. Holliday and Donald E. Potter, "Long-Term Projections for Treating Renal Failure in Children," paper presented at meeting (note 19).
70. Fine et al. (note 66), pp. 347–57 *passim.*
71. Folkert O. Belzer, "Surgical Complications of Transplantation," paper presented at meeting (note 19).
72. C. M. Grushkin, "Medical Complications of Transplantations," paper presented at meeting (note 19).
73. Holliday and Potter (note 69); and Fine et al. (note 66), p. 356.
74. G. Raimbault, "Psychological Problems in the Chronic Nephropathies of Childhood," in E. James Anthony and Cyrille Koupernik, eds., *The Child in His Family: The Impact of Disease and Death* (Vol. 2; New York: Wiley, 1973), p. 66.
75. William S. Langford, "Physical Illness and Convalescence: Their Meaning to the Child," *J. Pediatrics* 33 (1948): 244.
76. Barbara Korsch and Henry L. Barnett, "The Physician, the Family and the Child with Nephrosis," *J. Pediatrics* 58 (1961): 710.
77. Raimbault (note 74).
78. Barbara Korsch et al., "Pediatric Discussions with Parent Groups," *J. Pediatrics* 44 (1954): 703, 707.
79. Raimbault (note 74).
80. Carol A. Levin, Clinical Social Worker, Renal Dialysis and Transplant Unit of the University of California Medical Center, San Francisco.
81. Roberta Simmons, Florence Rosenberg, and Morris Rosenberg, "Disturbance in the Self-Image at Adolescence," paper presented at the Midwest Sociological Society meetings, April 1972, p. 19.
82. *Ibid.,* p. 24.
83. Sherrill Hammer, "Management of Adolescents with Chronic Handicapping Conditions," Workshop, 13th Annual Meeting, Ambulatory Pediatrics Association, San Francisco, May 17, 1973.
84. Max Sugar, "Disguised Depressions in Adolescents," in Gene L. Usdin, ed., *Adolescence: Care and Counseling* (Philadelphia: Lippincott, 1967), p. 78.
85. Larry H. Dizmang, "Loss, Bereavement and Depression in Childhood," in Edwin S. Shneidman and Magno J. Ortega, eds., *Psychological Aspects of Depression* (Boston: Little, Brown, 1969).
86. Aman U. Khan et al., "Social and Emotional Adaptations of Children with Transplanted Kidneys and Chronic Hemodialysis," *Amer. J. Psychiatry* 127 (1971): 1197.
87. John E. Schowalter et al., "The Adolescent Patient's Decision to Die," *Pediatrics* 51 (1973): 87–103.
88. Roberta G. Simmons and Richard L. Simmons, "Sociological and Psychological Aspects of Transplantation," prepublication ms, p. 365. (Later published in David M. Hume and Felix T. Rapaport, eds., *Clinical Transplantation* [New York: Grune & Stratton, 1973].)
89. Penny Adler, Social Worker, El Camino Hospital, Mountain View, Calif.; personal communication, February 22, 1973.
90. Lois Christopherson, Clinical Social Worker, Stanford Medical Center, Palo Alto, Calif.; Workshop, "Taking Life in Your Own Hands," January 1973.
91. Facts regarding Medicare provisions were provided in personal communication from Leonard Ott, Staff Officer in State Operations Branch, and Ora Scott, Staff Officer in the District Office and Program Groups Branch, Bureau of Health

Insurance, Social Security Administration, San Francisco Regional Office, October 9–10, 1973.

92. Lillian Pike Cain, "Casework with Kidney Transplant Patients," *Social Work* 18 (1973), No. 4: 80.

93. Levin (note 80).

94. Guest Conference on Dialysis and Transplant in Children, University of California Medical Center, San Francisco, May 18, 1973; staff reports of dialysis and transplant from the Toronto Hospital for Sick Children.

95. Barbara Korsch, "Psychological Aspects of Kidney Transplantation in Children," paper presented at the 13th Annual Meeting, Ambulatory Pediatrics Association, San Francisco, May 17, 1973. See also Mary Crittenden, Ph.D., in Guest Conference (note 94).

96. Mary R. Crittenden and Carol A. Levin, "Psychosocial Growth of Children during Dialysis and after Renal Transplantation," unpublished report of preliminary findings.

97. Korsch (note 95).

98. Carol A. Levin, personal communication, February 1973.

99. Mary R. Crittenden, paper presented at meeting (note 19).

100. Korsch et al. (note 63), p. 11.

101. Roberta G. Simmons and Susan D. Klein, "Family Noncommunication: The Search for Kidney Donors," *Amer. J. Psychiatry* 129 (1972): 687.

102. Dorothy M. Bernstein, "After Transplantation—The Child's Emotional Reactions," *Amer. J. Psychiatry* 127 (1971): 1189.

103. Donald E. Potter, M.D., Assistant Professor of Pediatrics and Director, Pediatric Dialysis Unit, University of California Medical Center, San Francisco; personal communication, August 1973.

104. Simmons and Simmons (note 88), p. 381.

105. Carol Levin, personal communication (see note 80).

106. Bernstein (note 102), p. 113.

107. Simmons and Simmons (note 88), p. 381.

108. Khan (note 86), Bernstein (note 102), Simmons and Klein (note 101), and Korsch (notes 63 and 95).

109. Robert M. Eisendrath, "The Role of Grief and Fear in the Death of Kidney Transplant Patients," *Amer. J. Psychiatry* 126 (1969): 3.

110. Korsch et al. (note 63).

111. Simmons and Simmons (note 88), p. 361.

8. Congenital Heart Disease

1. Waldo E. Nelson et al., *Textbook of Pediatrics* (9th ed.; Philadelphia: Saunders, 1969), p. 964. See also Alexander S. Nadas, *Pediatric Cardiology* (2d ed.; Philadelphia: Saunders, 1969), p. 340.

2. John D. Keith, Richard D. Rowe, and Peter Vlad, *Heart Disease in Infancy and Childhood* (2d ed.; New York: Macmillan, 1967), p. 3.

3. Edward C. Lambert and Arno R. Hohn, "The Pediatrician and Congenital Heart Disease," *J. Pediatrics* 70: 833.

4. Helen M. Wallace, *Health Services for Mothers and Children* (Philadelphia: Saunders, 1962), p. 340.

5. Lambert and Hohn (note 3), p. 834.

6. Keith et al. (note 2), p. 170.

7. Wallace (note 4), p. 356.

8. Nadas (note 1), p. 966.

9. *Ibid.*
10. Lambert and Hohn (note 3), p. 834; and Keith et al. (note 2), p. 3.
11. Nadas (note 1), p. 349.
12. *Ibid.*, p. 353.
13. *Ibid.*, pp. 356–65 *passim.*
14. Lambert and Hohn (note 3), p. 837.
15. *Ibid.*
16. Dan G. MacNamara, "Management of Congenital Heart Disease," *Pediatrics Clinics of North America*, November 1971, p. 1197.
17. Nadas (note 1), p. 371.
18. Lambert and Kohn (note 3), p. 837.
19. Keith et al. (note 2), p. 76.
20. Nadas (note 1), p. 135.
21. Nedra B. Belloc, "Deaths from Congenital Heart Disease in California, 1945–64," *Public Health Reports* 82 (1967): 621–26.
22. Gary Gathman, M.D., Associate Chief of Pediatric Cardiology, Santa Clara Valley Medical Center; personal communication, February 17, 1972.
23. Arthur Selzer, *The Heart, Its Function in Health and Disease* (Berkeley: University of California Press, 1966).
24. John H. Mazur, M.D., Chief, Pediatric Cardiology, Mercy Hospital, San Diego; personal communication, July 1968.
25. Gary Gathman (note 22); personal communication, February 17, 1972.
26. *Annual Report of Cardiac Centers* (Bureau of Crippled Children's Services, California State Department of Public Health), 1970.
27. *Ibid.*
28. R. Newell Finchum, "Rehabilitation Following Cardiac Surgery," *Circulation* 43 (1971): 1–151 *passim.*
29. Belloc (note 21), p. 623.
30. *Ibid.*, pp. 623, 625.
31. *Vital Statistics Records of the California State Department of Public Health*, Department of Finance, Census Population, 1960 and 1970, as provided by Mrs. Patricia Miller, Statistician for the Crippled Children's Division, on September 15, 1972.
32. *Ibid.*, p. 62.
33. *Ibid.*, p. 16.
34. *Ibid.*, p. 24.
35. *Ibid.*, p. 26.
36. Lambert and Kohn (note 3), p. 846. Also Thelma Quinn, M.D., District Public Health Officer, Santa Clara County, California, Department of Public Health; personal communication, June 1972.
37. Lambert and Kohn (note 3), p. 845.
38. MacNamara (note 16), p. 1197.
39. Lambert and Kohn (note 3), p. 845.
40. Gary Gathman, M.D. (note 22), lecture to the Intensive Care Unit staff, Valley Medical Center, San Jose, Calif., March 8, 1972.
41. *Ibid.*
42. Keith et al. (note 2), p. 644.
43. Gary Gathman (note 22), personal communication, March 1972.
44. Keith et al. (note 2), p. 723.
45. *Ibid.*, p. 213.
46. *Ibid.*, p. 225.

47. Carlos I. Ibarra et al., "Recoarctation of the Aorta," *Amer. J. Cardiology* 23 (1969): 778–84.
48. Keith et al. (note 2), p. 293.
49. *Ibid.*, p. 367. See also Selzer (note 23), pp. 231–36 *passim*.
50. Keith et al. (note 2), p. 356.
51. Aldo Castenada, M.D., Professor of Surgery, University of Minnesota, lecture to the Department of Pediatrics staff, Valley Medical Center, San Jose, Calif., June 21, 1972.
52. Annual Report of Cardiac Centers (note 26), p. 24.
53. Keith et al. (note 2), pp. 403–21 *passim*.
54. Nadas (note 1), pp. 384–91 *passim*.
55. *Ibid.*, pp. 392, 394.
56. Keith et al. (note 2), p. 200.
57. *Ibid.*
58. *Ibid.*, p. 634.
59. Stanley John et al., "Total Surgical Correction of Tetralogy of Fallot," *Thorax* 27 (1972): 66.
60. Keith et al. (note 2), p. 631.
61. *Ibid.*
62. G. M. Maxwell and Sally Gane, "The Impact of Congenital Heart Disease upon the Family," *Amer. Heart J.* 64: 451.
63. *Ibid.*, pp. 453–54. See also Elliot C. Brown, Jr., "Casework with Patients Undergoing Cardiac Surgery," *Social Casework* 52 (1971): 611–16 *passim*.
64. Brown (note 63), p. 614.
65. Roberta Peay, "What Social Services Offer to Patients Who Undergo Heart Surgery," *Public Health Reports* 78, no. 12 (1963): 1050.
66. David Baum, M.D., Chief, Division of Pediatric Cardiology, Stanford Medical Center, Stanford, Calif.; personal communication, August 1972.
67. Maxwell and Gane (note 62), p. 452.
68. Michael Heffernan and Pat Azarnoff, "Factors in Reducing Children's Anxiety about Clinic Visits," *Health Services, Mental Health Administration Reports* 86 (1971): 1135.
69. Helen H. Glaser, Grace S. Harrison, and David B. Lynn, "Emotional Implications of Congenital Heart Disease in Children," *Pediatrics* 33 (1964): 373.
70. Morris Green and Albert Solnit, "Reaction to the Threatened Loss of a Child: A Vulnerable Child Syndrome," *Pediatrics* 34 (1964): 50.
71. Florence Bright Roberts, "The Child with Heart Disease," *Amer. J. Nursing*, June 1972, p. 1081.
72. Glaser et al. (note 69), p. 371.
73. *Ibid.*
74. Gary Gathman (note 22).
75. Glaser et al. (note 69), pp. 375–76.
76. Peay (note 65), p. 1046.
77. Roberts (note 71).
78. Sula Wolff, *Children under Stress* (London: Penguin, 1969), pp. 51–74 *passim*. See also Selma Fraiberg, *The Magic Years* (New York: Scribner, 1959), pp. 202–9.
79. Harold A. Richman, "Casework with a Child Following Heart Surgery," *Children* 11, No. 5 (1964): 184–85.
80. Paul R. Lurie, M.D., Professor of Pediatrics, University of Southern California, and Head, Division of Cardiology, Children's Hospital, Los Angeles, Calif.; personal communication, July 1972.

Notes to Pages 262–76

81. Leona M. Bayer and Saul J. Robinson, "Growth History of Children with Congenital Heart Defects," *Amer. J. Diseases of Children* 117 (1969): 564–72 *passim*.

82. Robert H. Feldt et al., "Growth of Children with Congenital Heart Disease," *Amer. J. Diseases of Children* 117 (1969): 578.

83. Maurice Chazan et al., "The Intellectual and Emotional Development of Children with Congenital Heart Disease," *Guy's Hospital Reports* 100 (1951): 332.

84. *Ibid.*, p. 333.

85. Nina Rausch de Traubenberg, "Psychological Aspects of Congenital Heart Disease," in E. James Anthony and Cyrille Koupernik, eds., *The Child in His Family* (vol. 1; New York: Wiley, 1970), p. 76.

86. Helen B. Taussig et al., "Long Term Observations in the Blalock-Taussig Operation," *Johns Hopkins Medical J.* 129 (1971).

87. De Traubenberg (note 85), pp. 77–79 *passim*.

9. Cystic Fibrosis

1. "Cystic Fibrosis," National Cystic Fibrosis Research Foundation, Medical Information, 521 Fifth Ave., New York, N.Y., 1970.

2. Carl F. Doershuk and LeRoy Mathews, "Cystic Fibrosis—Comprehensive Therapy," *Postgraduate Medicine*, 40 (November 1966): 561.

3. "Cystic Fibrosis" (note 1).

4. "Your Child and Cystic Fibrosis," National Cystic Fibrosis Research Foundation, New York, N.Y., 1967.

5. Paul A. Di Sant'Agnese, "Cystic Fibrosis of the Pancreas," *Amer. J. Medicine*, 21, no. 3 (1956): 406. Birt Harvey, former Chief, Pulmonary Disease Service, Children's Hospital at Stanford, Palo Alto, Calif.; personal communications.

6. Di Sant'Agnese (note 5), p. 411.

7. *Ibid.*, p. 412.

8. Paul A. Di Sant'Agnese, "Pathogenesis and Physiology of Cystic Fibrosis of the Pancreas," *New England J. Medicine* 277: 1287–95, 1343–52, 1399–1408.

9. Birt Harvey, "Cystic Fibrosis," in E. E. Bleck, *Physically Handicapped Children: Medical Atlas for Teachers* (New York: Grune & Stratton, 1975), p. 111.

10. Jack Wolfsdorf, David L. Swift, and Mary Ellen Avery, "Mist Therapy Reconsidered: An Evaluation of the Respiratory Deposition of Labelled Water Aerosol Produced by Jet and Ultrasonic Nebulizers," *Pediatrics* 32 (1969): 799. Samuel K. Bau, Norman Aspin, Donald E. Wood, and Henry Levison, "The Measurement of Fluid Deposition in Humans Following Mist Tent Therapy," *Pediatrics* 48 (1971): 605. E. K. Motoyama, L. E. Gibson, and C. J. Zigas, "Evaluation of Mist Tent Therapy in Cystic Fibrosis," *Pediatrics* 50 (1972): 299.

11. Harvey (note 5).

12. L. W. Mathews et al., "A Therapeutic Regimen for Patients with Cystic Fibrosis," the report of an investigation supported by the Cystic Fibrosis Foundation. See *J. Pediatrics* 65, no. 5 (1964): 679–93.

13. Harvey (note 5).

14. Harry Schwachman et al., "Studies in Cystic Fibrosis," *Pediatrics* 46 (1970): 335.

15. Leon Cytryn, "Factors in Psychosocial Adjustment of Children with Chronic Illness and Handicaps," paper presented at the Seventh Annual Congress of the International Association for Child Psychiatry and Allied Professions, 1970, Jerusalem, Israel, pp. 200–201.

16. Juanita Turk, "Impact of Cystic Fibrosis on Family Functioning," *Pediatrics* 34 (1964): 69.

17. Audrey T. McCollum and Lewis Gibson, "Family Adaptation to the Child with Cystic Fibrosis," *J. Pediatrics* 77 (1970): 572–76 *passim*.

18. Chancellor B. Driscoll and Harold A. Lubin, "Conferences with Parents of Children with Cystic Fibrosis," *Social Casework* 53 (1972): 140.

19. Alan Mitchell, "Plans for Tomorrow," paper presented at the Region XIV Conference, National Cystic Fibrosis Research Foundation, 1972, Oakland, Calif.

20. McCollum and Gibson (note 17).

21. Harvey (note 5).

22. Harry A. Schwachman et al., "Studies in Cystic Fibrosis: A Report of 65 Patients over 17 Years of Age," *Pediatrics* 36 (1965): 5.

23. *Ibid.*, pp. 4–5.

24. Erik H. Erikson, *Childhood and Society* (rev. ed.: New York: Norton, 1964), p. 361; and *Identity: Youth and Crisis* (New York: Norton, 1968), pp. 188–91 *passim*.

25. Mitchell (note 19).

26. Cytryn (note 15), p. 209.

27. McCollum and Gibson (note 17), p. 577.

28. R. H. Lawler et al., "Psychological Implications of Cystic Fibrosis," *Canadian Medical Assn. J.* 94 (1966): 1044.

29. Driscoll and Lubin (note 18).

30. Alan Tropauer et al., "Psychological Aspects of Care of Children with Cystic Fibrosis," *Amer. J. Diseases of Children* 119 (1970): 431.

31. McCollum and Gibson (note 17), p. 566.

32. Paul R. Patterson et al., eds., *Psychological Aspects of Cystic Fibrosis* (New York: Columbia University Press, 1973).

33. Martin I. Lorin, "The Twilight Hours," in Patterson et al. (note 32), p. 28.

34. Harvey (note 5), personal communication.

35. Mimi M. Belmonte and Yolande St. Germain, "Psychological Aspects of the Cystic Fibrosis Family," in Patterson et al. (note 32), p. 86.

10. Head Injury

1. John Mealey, Jr., *Pediatric Head Injuries* (Springfield, Ill.: Thomas, 1968), p. 3.

2. *Ibid.*

3. Joyce Brink et al., "Recovery of Motor and Intellectual Function in Children Sustaining Severe Head Injuries," *Developmental Medicine and Child Neurology* 12 (1970): 565–71. See also E. B. Hendrick and D. C. Harwood-Harsh, "Head Injuries in Children; Survey of 4,465 Consecutive Cases at the Hospital for Sick Children, Toronto, Canada," *Clinic Neurosurgery* 11 (1963): 45–65.

4. Roger J. Meyer and David Klein, eds., "Childhood Injuries: Approaches and Perspectives," Report of the Second National Childhood Injuries Symposium, American Academy of Pediatrics, Charlottesville, Va., 1968. Published in *Pediatrics* 44, part 2 (1969).

5. Joyce Brink, M.D., Associate Clinical Professor of Pediatrics, University of Southern California School of Medicine; and Chief, Pediatric Service, Rancho Los Amigos Hospital, Downey; personal communication, June 19, 1974.

6. Byron W. White, "The Control of Child Environment Interaction," in Meyer and Klein (note 4), pp. 799–801.

7. Nancy E. Wood, *Delayed Speech and Language Development* (Englewood Cliffs, N.J.: Prentice-Hall, 1964).

8. See the readily understood description of how the brain works, in Sol Adler,

The Non-Verbal Child (Springfield, Ill.: Thomas, 1964), or in a popular work such as "Inside the Brain, the Last Great Frontier," SR Special Section, *Saturday Review*, August 9, 1975, pp. 13–33 *passim*.

9. Mealey (note 1), p. 13.
10. Hendrick and Harwood-Harsh (note 3).
11. Brink et al. (note 3).
12. *Ibid.*
13. *Ibid.*; also Harold Dillon and Robert J. Leopold, "Children and the Post-Concussion Syndrome," *J. Amer. Medical Assn.* 175 (1961): 86–91; and comments by the Pediatrics Professional Staff, Rancho Los Amigos, January 1970.
14. See Perry Black et al., "The Post-Traumatic Syndrome in Children," in A. E. Walker et al., eds., *The Late Effects of Head Injury* (Springfield, Ill.: Thomas, 1969), pp. 142–47 *passim*.
15. White (note 6).
16. John H. Read, "Traffic Accidents Involving Child Pedestrians," in Meyer and Klein (note 4), pp. 847–48.
17. See Richard S. Lewis, "The Brain-Injured Child" (National Society for Crippled Children and Adults, Chicago), p. 13, for a description of behavioral manifestation of brain injury.
18. Sheldon R. Rappaport, ed., "Childhood Aphasia and Brain Damage" (Pathway School publication, Livingston Publishing Co., Narberth, Pa.), p. 120.

11. Hemophilia

1. "A Total Program for the Patient with Hemophilia," collection of papers from a symposium, *J. Amer. Physical Therapy Assn.* 46, no. 11 (1965). See Andon A. Andonian et al., "Medical Aspects of a Total Program for the Patient with Hemophilia," *J. Amer. Physical Therapy Assn.* 46, no. 12 (1966).
2. Andonian et al. (note 1). Estimate taken from experience at the Orthopedic Hospital in Los Angeles.
3. Andonian et al. (note 1), p. 1269.
4. Jessica H. Lewis, "The Inheritance of Hemophilia," *Hemophilia* 1 (1966), no. 2.
5. "Hemophilia" (National Hemophilia Foundation, 25 W. 39th Street, New York, N.Y.).
6. Florence B. Goldy and Alfred H. Katz, "Social Adaptation in Hemophilia" (National Hemophilia Foundation).
7. Carol Kasper, Director, USC Coagulation Research Laboratory for Hemophilia Rehabilitation; lecture on "An Overview of Hemophilia," March 20, 1970, at the Institute for Rehabilitation Counselors, University of Southern California, Los Angeles.
8. "Hemophilia" (U.S. Govt. Printing Office, 1966; Public Health Service Publication no. 1420); and Ake Mattsson and Samuel Gross, "Adaptational and Defensive Behavior in Young Hemophiliacs and Their Parents," *Amer. J. Psychiatry* 122 (1966): 1349–56.
9. Max Negri and Donna Boone, Institute for Rehabilitation Counselors, USC; paper presented at the Orthopedic Hospital, Los Angeles, March 20, 1970.
10. Kasper (note 7); see also "Hope for Bleeders," *Wall Street Journal*, March 1968; and Martin C. Rosenthal, "Management of Hemophilia," National Hemophilia Foundation, reprint from *Drug Therapy* 1, no. 3 (1971).
11. Jack Lazerson, "The Prophylactic Approach to Hemophilia A," *Hospital Practice*, February 1971.

12. Charles Hurt, Clinical Social Worker, Regional Hemophilia Center, Orthopedic Hospital, Los Angeles; personal communication, March 20, 1970.
13. Donald Avoy, Medical Director, Central California American Red Cross Blood Center, San Jose, Calif.; personal communication, August 30, 1974.
14. *San Jose Mercury*, May 4, 1973.
15. *Ibid.*, October 6, 1973.
16. Tess Forest, "The Paternal Roots of Male Character Development," *Psychoanalytic Review* 54 (1967): 61–67 *passim*.
17. *Ibid.*, p. 63.
18. Mattsson and Gross (note 8), pp. 1345–56 *passim*.
19. *Ibid.*
20. Alfred Katz, *Hemophilia: A Study in Hope and Reality* (Springfield, Ill.: Thomas, 1970).
21. Charles Hurt, personal communication.
22. Katz (note 20).
23. *Ibid.*, p. 42.
24. *Ibid.*, p. 48.
25. Goldy and Katz (note 6); and Charlotte Taylor, Rehabilitation Counselor, Regional Hemophilia Center, Orthopedic Hospital, Los Angeles.
26. Katz (note 20), p. 84.
27. Mattsson and Gross (note 8).

12. *Juvenile Rheumatoid Arthritis*

1. Ross Jeremy et al. "Juvenile Arthritis Rheumatoid Persisting into Adulthood," *Amer. J. Medicine* 45 (1968): 419–34.
2. Earl J. Brewer, Jr., *Juvenile Rheumatoid Arthritis* (Philadelphia: Saunders, 1970), pp. 2, 43.
3. John Calabro and Joseph Marchesano, "The Early History of Juvenile Rheumatoid Arthritis," *Medical Clinics of North America*, 1969, p. 567.
4. Brewer (note 2), pp. 4, 5.
5. William Parker et al., "Comparative Study of Patients with Rheumatoid Arthritis and with Rheumatic Fever" (Group Project, Applied Research, University of Chicago, 1966).
6. Sidney E. Cleveland et al., "Psychological Factors in Juvenile Rheumatoid Arthritis," *Arthritis and Rheumatism* 8 (1965): 1152.
7. John J. Calabro and Joseph Marchesano, "Current Concepts in Juvenile Rheumatoid Arthritis," *Medical Intelligence*, 277, no. 13 (1967): 696. Brewer (note 2), p. 2.
8. Brewer (note 2), pp. 11, 45. Calabro and Marchesano (note 7), p. 698.
9. Elizabeth Barkley, "Home Treatment Program," in Brewer (note 2), p. 137.
10. Brewer (note 2), pp. 25–44.
11. Calabro and Marchesano (note 3), p. 587.
12. Jeremy et al. (note 1), p. 421.
13. Brewer (note 2), p. 44.
14. John J. Miller III, Chief, Rheumatic Disease Service, Children's Hospital at Stanford; personal statement, August 15, 1971.
15. Calabro and Marchesano (note 3). Miller (note 14), September 14. Brewer (note 2), p. 45.
16. Miller (note 14), September 1.
17. C. G. McNamara, "Carditis with Rheumatoid Arthritis," in Brewer (note 2).
18. Brewer (note 2), pp. 27–28.

19. "Aspirin for Arthritis," Arthritis Foundation, 10 Columbus Circle, New York, N.Y., 1970.
20. Miller (note 14), September 14.
21. Calabro and Marchesano (note 3).
22. *Ibid.*
23. Miller (note 14); personal statement, September 14, 1971.
24. Calabro and Marchesano (note 3), p. 585.
25. Elizabeth Barkley, "Home Treatment Program," in Brewer (note 2), pp. 137–55.
26. Miller (note 14), August 18.
27. Malcolm Granberry, "Orthopedic Management of Juvenile Rheumatoid Arthritis," in Brewer (note 2), pp. 156–79.
28. Miller (note 14), September 14.
29. *Ibid.*
30. Granberry (note 27).
31. Joan Morse, "Involving Fathers in the Treatment of Patients with Juvenile Rheumatoid Arthritis," *Social Casework*, May 1968, pp. 281–87.
32. Miller (note 14), September 14.
33. "Aspirin for Arthritis" (note 19).
34. Harold Wolff, *Pain* (2d ed.; Springfield, Ill.: Thomas, 1958), p. 8.
35. Arnold H. Buss and Norman W. Portnoy, "Pain Tolerance and Group Identification," *J. Personality & Social Psychology* 6 (1967): 106.
36. *Ibid.*, p. 76.
37. Anna Freud, "The Role of Bodily Illness in the Mental Life of the Child," *Psychoanalytic Study of the Child* 7 (1952): 69–81.
38. Leon J. Saul, *Emotional Maturity* (2d ed.; Philadelphia: Lippincott, 1960), p. 123.
39. Freud (note 37), pp. 71–72.
40. Thesi Bergmann, "Observation of Children's Reactions to Motor Restraint," *Nervous Child* 4 (1945).
41. Freud (note 37), pp. 74–76.
42. Gaston E. Blom and Grace Nichols, "Emotional Factors in Children with Rheumatoid Arthritis," *Amer. J. Orthopsychiatry* 24 (1954): 588–601.
43. Cleveland et al. (note 6), p. 1154.

13. Juvenile Diabetes

1. Stephen E. Dippe, "Incidence and National Consequence of Diabetes Mellitus," Third Allied Health Postgraduate Course in Diabetes (American Diabetes Association and University of California), San Francisco, April 1971.
2. "Facts about Diabetes," County Diabetes Association, Santa Clara County, Calif.; fact sheet, undated.
3. Peter H. Forsham, "Diabetes, 1971," Third Allied Health Postgraduate Course (note 1).
4. Henry Dolger, *How to Live with Diabetes* (New York: Pyramid Books, 1965), pp. 13–17 *passim*.
5. Luther B. Travis, *An Instructional Aid on Juvenile Diabetes Mellitus* (Squibb, 1969), pp. 3–14 *passim*.
6. William B. Weil, Jr., "Current Concepts of Juvenile Diabetes," *New England J. Medicine* 278, no. 15 (1968): 829. *The Merck Manual of Diagnosis and Therapy* (12th ed.; Rahway, N.J.: Merck, 1972), pp. 213, 215. Paul B. Beeson and Walsh McDermott, eds., *Cecil Loeb Textbook of Medicine* (11th ed.; Philadelphia:

Saunders, 1963), pp. 1304–5. Julian Myer, ed., *An Orientation to Chronic Disease and Disability* (New York: Macmillan, 1965), p. 214.

7. Charles Epstein, "Genetic Counseling," Third Allied Health Postgraduate Course (note 1).

8. Albert E. Renold et al., "Diabetes Mellitus," chap. 4 in John B. Stanbury et al., *The Metabolic Basis of Inherited Disease* (3d ed.; New York: McGraw-Hill, 1972), p. 86.

9. William B. Weil, Jr. (note 6), p. 829. William B. Weil, Jr., "Diabetes Mellitus," in Morris Green and Robert J. Haggerty, eds., *Ambulatory Pediatrics* (Philadelphia: Saunders, 1968), pp. 690–95 *passim*. Robert L. Jackson and James K. Pickens, "The Child with Diabetes," in Garfield G. Duncan, ed., *Diseases of Metabolism* (5th ed.; Philadelphia: Saunders, 1964), pp. 1084–1105 *passim*.

10. Robert O. Christiansen, M.D., Assistant Professor of Pediatrics and Human Development, and Director, Pediatric Metabolic Service, Stanford Medical Center, Stanford, Calif.; personal communication, June 1971.

11. *Ibid*.

12. Priscilla White, "Childhood Diabetes—Its Cause and Influence on the Second and Third Generations," *Diabetes* 9 (1960): 345–53 *passim*.

13. E. Larson et al., "Long-Term Prognosis in Juvenile Diabetes Mellitus," *Acta Pediatrica*, Supplement 130, 1962.

14. Robert O. Christiansen (note 10). See also Priscilla White, "Natural Course and Prognosis of Juvenile Diabetes," *Diabetes* 5 (1956): 445–46.

15. Dolger (note 4).

16. Weil (note 6).

17. Larson et al. (note 13). Robert O. Christiansen, "Criteria for Control of Juvenile Diabetes Mellitus," American Academy of Pediatrics Postgraduate Course No. 1 (Stanford University School of Medicine and Children's Hospital at Stanford, Palo Alto, Calif.), July 13, 1971. Monroe Gross, M.D., President, Santa Clara County Diabetes Society; personal communication, May 1971. Robert Sharkey, M.D., former Chief of Pediatric Clinic, Santa Clara Valley Medical Center; personal communication, June 1971.

18. Christiansen (note 17).

19. Christiansen (note 10), July 1971.

20. Travis (note 5), pp. 60–65 *passim*.

21. Christiansen (note 10), July 1971.

22. *Ibid*.

23. Travis (note 5).

24. "Diet and the Diabetic," Upjohn Drug Co., 1970.

25. Margaret Bennett, *The Peripatetic Diabetic* (New York: Hawthorne, 1969), pp. 38, 104.

26. Evette Hackman, Dietician, Stanford University Medical Center, Department of Pediatrics, Palo Alto, Calif.; personal communication, June 1971. See also Travis (note 5), p. 66.

27. Travis (note 5), p. 69; Bennett (note 25); and Christiansen (note 10), at group meeting of parents of diabetic children, July 1971.

28. "What the Teacher Should Know about the Child with Diabetes," New York Diabetes Association, undated.

29. Christiansen (note 10).

30. Hackman (note 26); Jackson and Pickens (note 9); and mothers of members of Frisky Frescas, a group of diabetic teenagers, Santa Clara County, Calif., July–August, 1971.

31. Dolger (note 4), p. 112.

32. Euell Gibbons and Joe Gibbons, "If Your Child Has Diabetes," adapted from Euell Gibbons and Joe Gibbons, *Feast on a Diabetic Diet* (New York: McKay, 1969; reprint from the American Diabetes Association). See also Jackson and Pickens (note 9).

33. Douglas Frazier, M.D., Chief, Pediatric Metabolic Service, University of Southern California School of Medicine; personal communication, February 1970.

34. L. Baker et al., "Beta-adrenergic Blockade and Juvenile Diabetes," *J. Pediatrics* 75 (1969): 19.

35. Christiansen (note 17).

36. A. Marble and S. B. Rees, "The Pathological Physiology of Microangiopathy in Diabetes," reprinted by the National Foundation from *Triangle, The Sandoz J. of Medical Science* 7, no. 1 (1965): 10.

37. Priscilla White (note 14).

38. Vincent C. Diraimondo, "Chronic Complications," Third Allied Health Postgraduate Course (note 1).

39. Jerry Plummer, "Hunger Survey," Sacramento County Department of Public Welfare, Sacramento, Calif. (mimeo.), September 1969.

40. Richard V. Kaufman and Betsy Hersher, "Body Image Changes in Teenage Diabetics," *Pediatrics* 48 (1971): 123–27.

41. White (note 14).

42. Alan J. Crain et al., "The Effects of a Diabetic Child on Marital Integration and Related Measures of Family Functioning," *J. Health and Human Behavior* 7 (1966): 122–27 *passim*.

43. Jeanne Carolyn Quint, "Becoming Diabetic: A Study of Emerging Identity" (University of California D.N.S. dissertation, 1969; University Microfilms, Ann Arbor, Mich.).

44. Marian W. Metz, "Special Problems of the Emotionally Deprived Diabetic," Third Allied Health Postgraduate Course (note 1).

45. J. A. Birnbeck et al., "Emotional Disturbances in Juvenile Diabetics," *Diabetes*, Supplement 1, June 1968, p. 317.

46. Leon Gordis and Milton Markowitz, "Rheumatic Heart Disease and Pregnancy in Adolescent Rheumatic Fever Patients," *Pediatrics* 40 (1967): 104–5.

47. Jorgen Pederson, *The Pregnant Diabetic and Her Newborn* (Baltimore: Williams & Wilkins, 1967), p. 48. See also White (note 12).

48. Alan J. Margolis, "The Female Diabetic," Third Allied Health Postgraduate Course (note 1).

14. Leukemia

1. R. Lee Clark, in *Neoplasia in Childhood*, Proceedings of the Twelfth Annual Clinical Conferences on Cancer, 1967, at the University of Texas, M. D. Anderson Hospital and Tumor Institute at Houston (Chicago: Year Book Medical Publishers, 1969). See also *Essentials of Cancer Nursing* (American Cancer Society, 521 W. 27th St., New York, N.Y., 1963), p. 23.

2. Edward S. Henderson, M.D., "The Therapy of Acute Leukemia," paper presented at the Eighth Annual Clinical Cancer Conference on Continuing Education, "Perspectives in Cancer Chemotherapy and Bone Marrow Transplantation," San Francisco, March 16, 1973.

3. Alvin M. Mauer, *Pediatric Hematology* (New York: McGraw-Hill, 1969), p. 335. See also S. B. Friedman et al., "Childhood Leukemia" (National Cancer Institute, U.S. Public Health Service, National Institute of Health, HEW), 1972.

4. Friedman et al. (note 3), p. 4.
5. Mauer (note 3), p. 340.
6. Sigismund Peller, *Cancer in Childhood and Youth* (Bristol: Wright, 1960).
7. *Leukemia* (American Cancer Society, 1963).
8. Mauer (note 3), p. 340.
9. *Ibid.*, pp. 4–5, 333–34.
10. *Ibid.*, pp. 333–34.
11. *Cancer Source Book for Nurses* (American Cancer Society, 1963), p. 84.
12. Henderson (note 2).
13. Arthur Ablin, M.D., Associate Clinical Professor of Pediatrics, and Head, Pediatrics Hematology, University of California Medical Center; personal communication, March 15, 1973.
14. Mauer (note 3).
15. Donald Pinkel et al., "Nine Years' Experience with 'Total Therapy' of Childhood Acute Lymphocytic Leukemia," *Pediatrics* 50, no. 2 (1972): 249; and Rhomes Aur and Donald Pinkel, "Total Therapy of Acute Lymphocytic Leukemia," in Irving Ariel, ed., *Progress in Clinical Cancer* (New York: Grune & Stratton, 1973), vol. 5, p. 161.
16. Donald P. Pinkel, "Acute Leukemia," in Sydney S. Gellis and Benjamin M. Kagan, *Current Pediatric Therapy* (6th ed.; Philadelphia: Saunders, 1973).
17. *Progress Against Cancer*, Report by the National Advisory Council, 1969 (National Cancer Institute, HEW), p. 30.
18. Round Table Discussion, Eighth Annual Clinical Cancer Conference, University of California Continuing Education in Health Sciences, San Francisco, March 15–16, 1973.
19. Jordan R. Wilbur, M.D., "Combination Chemotherapy and Radiation Therapy of Childhood Neoplasms," paper presented at the Eighth Annual Clinical Cancer Conference (note 18).
20. C. Gordon Zubrod, M.D., "Strategy for Conquest of Malignant Disease," paper presented at the Eighth Annual Clinical Cancer Conference (note 18).
21. Henderson (note 2).
22. T. John Gribble, M.D., Associate Professor of Pediatrics, Division of Hematology, Stanford University School of Medicine; personal communication, July 17, 1973. Also Mauer (note 3).
23. Gerald P. Bodey and Eva M. Hersh, "The Problem of Infection in Children with Malignant Disease," in *Neoplasia in Childhood* (note 1), pp. 135, 139, 142–43.
24. Margaret P. Sullivan, "Complications in the Treatment for Acute Leukemia," in *Neoplasia in Childhood* (note 1), p. 259.
25. Bodey and Hersh (note 23), pp. 135–37 *passim*. See also Mauer (note 3), p. 326.
26. Emil J. Freirich et al., "Platelet Replacement," in *Neoplasia in Childhood* (note 1), p. 129.
27. *Ibid.*, p. 131.
28. Pinkel (note 16).
29. J. V. Simone, "Acute Lymphocytic Leukemia in Childhood," *Seminars in Hematology* 11 (1974): 25.
30. John C. Probert, M.D., M.A., B.M.B.C.H., Fellow, Faculty of Radiology, Stanford University Hospital; personal communication, October 5, 1972.
31. Ablin (note 13), personal communication, November 15, 1972.
32. *Ibid.*
33. *Ibid.* See also Henderson (note 2).

34. Audrey T. McCollum and A. Herbert Schwartz, "Social Work and the Mourning Parent," *Social Work* 17 (1972): 35.

35. Alfred G. Knudson and Joseph M. Natterson, "Practice of Pediatrics: Participation of Parents in the Hospital Care of Fatally Ill Children," *Pediatrics* 26 (1960): 482–90.

36. *Ibid.*

37. C. M. Binger, M.D., Coordinator, Children's Services, Langley Porter Neuropsychiatric Clinic, San Francisco; personal communication, November 14, 1972.

38. David M. Kaplan, "The Family in Illness and Death," symposium of the Department of Community and Preventive Medicine, Stanford University Medical Center, April 17, 1972.

39. Binger (note 37).

40. Mary F. Bozeman et al., "The Adaptation of Mothers to the Threatened Loss of Their Children Through Leukemia," Part I, *Cancer*, January–February, 1955.

41. Rose Grobstein, M.S.W., Chief Pediatric Social Worker, Pediatrics Department, Stanford Medical Center; at meeting of the American Academy of Pediatrics.

42. David M. Kaplan et al., "Family Mediation of Stress," *Social Work* 18 (1973): 62.

43. Cynthia Mikkleson, Clinical Social Worker, Department of Social Work, University of California Medical Center, San Francisco; personal communication, November 15, 1972.

44. James R. Morrissey, "Children's Adaptation to Fatal Illness," *Social Work*, October 1963, pp. 85–87 *passim*, 88.

45. Arnold T. Sigler, "The Leukemic Child and His Family: An Emotional Challenge," in Matthew Debuskey and Robert H. Dombro, eds., *The Chronically Ill Child and His Family* (Springfield, Ill.: Thomas, 1970), p. 55.

46. Albert J. Solnit and Morris Green, "The Pediatric Management of the Dying Child. Part II, The Child's Reaction to the Fear of Dying," *Pediatrics Special Supplement*, "Care of the Child with Cancer," Vol. 40, No. 3, September 1967, p. 224.

47. John E. Schowalter, "The Child's Reaction to His Own Terminal Illness," in Bernard Schoenberg et al., eds. *Loss and Grief: Psychological Management* (New York: Columbia University Press, 1970), pp. 53–59 *passim*. See also H. Donald Dunton, "The Child's Concept of Death," in Schoenberg et al., pp. 355–57 *passim*.

48. Binger (note 37).

49. Schowalter (note 47), p. 59.

50. *Ibid.*, p. 51.

51. Ablin (see note 13).

52. Pinkel (note 16).

53. C. M. Binger, "Emotional Impact on Siblings," paper presented at the 21st Annual Postgraduate Seminar on Management of the Chronically Ill Child, Children's Hospital Medical Center, Oakland, Calif., January 26, 1973.

54. John E. Schowalter, "The Child's Reaction to His Own Terminal Illness," in Schoenberg et al. (note 47), p. 53.

55. Elizabeth Kubler-Ross, Medical Director of Mental Health and Family Services of South Cook County, Chicago Heights, Ill., remarks at a Symposium on Death and Dying, February 17, 1972.

56. James Robertson, *Hospitals and Children: A Parent's Eye View* (New York:

International Universities Press, 1963). See also Anna Freud, "The Role of Bodily Illness in the Mental Life of Children," in Ruth S. Eissler et al., *The Psychoanalytic Study of the Child*, Vol. 7 (New York: International Universities Press, 1952), pp. 69–81 *passim*.

57. E. Omer Burgert, Jr., "Emotional Impact of Childhood Acute Leukemia," *Mayo Clinic Proceedings* 47 (1972): 273–77 *passim*.

58. *San Jose Mercury*, November 13, 1974.

59. Dan C. Moore et al., "Psychologic Problems in the Management of Adolescents with Malignancy," *Clinical Pediatrics* 8 (1969): 468.

60. *Ibid.*, p. 466.

61. Ablin (see note 13).

62. David Peretz, "Reaction to Loss," in Schoenberg et al. (note 47), p. 26.

63. Bozeman et al. (note 40), p. 12.

64. Stanford B. Friedman et al., "Behavioral Observations on Parents Anticipating the Death of a Child," *Pediatrics* 33 (1963): 610.

65. C. M. Binger et al., "Childhood Leukemia: Emotional Impact on Patient and Family," *New England J. Medicine* 280 (1969): 414.

66. David Peretz, "Development, Object Relationships and Loss," in Schoenberg et al. (note 47), p. 6.

67. Mikkleson (see note 43).

68. Binger et al. (note 65), p. 416.

69. Eugenia Waechter, R.N., Ph.D., Assistant Professor of Nursing, University of California Medical Center, "The Patient's Reaction to Disease and Death," paper presented at the 21st Annual Postgraduate Seminar (note 53).

70. Binger et al. (note 65).

71. Solnit and Green (note 46), p. 225.

72. Elizabeth Diaz, "A Death on the Ward," *Hospital Topics*, May 1969, p. 86.

73. David Peretz, "Development, Object Relationship and Loss," in Schoenberg et al. (note 47), p. 18.

74. Binger et al. (note 65).

15. Muscular Dystrophy

1. Elizabeth Ogg, *Milestones in Research* (Muscular Dystrophy Association of America, 1971, unpaged).

2. "The Muscular Dystrophies," *Pfizer Spectrum*, April 1972, p. 2 (reprinted by the Muscular Dystrophy Association of America [MDAA], 1790 Broadway, New York, N.Y.).

3. Wayne S. Zundel and Frank H. Tyler, "The Muscular Dystrophies," *New England J. Medicine* 273, nos. 10 and 11 (1965), p. 11 (March of Dimes reprint).

4. "The Muscular Dystrophies" (note 2), p. 2. Leona Miu, Patient Services Coordinator, MDAA, San Francisco Regional Office; personal communication, March 26, 1975.

5. Zundel and Tyler (note 3), p. 4. Also Hans J. Zwang, M.D., Director, Muscular Dystrophy Clinic, Herrick Memorial Hospital, Berkeley, Calif.; personal communication, April 5, 1975.

6. Zundel and Tyler (note 3), pp. 7, 8.

7. *Merck Manual of Diagnosis and Therapy*, David N. Holvey, ed. (12th ed.; Rahway, N.J.: Merck, 1972).

8. Sharon Golub, "An R.N. Refresher, Muscular Dystrophy," *RN*, April 1968, unpaged (MDAA reprint).

9. Ogg (note 1).

10. Golub (note 8).
11. Stanley A. Skillicorn, former Chief of Neurology, Valley Medical Center, San Jose, Calif.; personal communication, May 23, 1974.
12. Zundel and Tyler (note 3), p. 2.
13. "Research Dividend No. 1, Prevention," Santa Clara County Chapter, MDAA.
14. *Ibid.*
15. Paul J. Vignos, "Management of Duchenne's Progressive Muscular Dystrophy," in Morris Green and Robert Haggerty, *Ambulatory Pediatrics* (Philadelphia: Saunders, 1968), p. 741.
16. "The Muscular Dystrophies" (note 2), p. 2.
17. *Ibid.*
18. Skillicorn (note 11).
19. Vignos (note 15), p. 742.
20. Zwang (note 5), personal communication, February 28, 1975.
21. Dr. John Shu, M.D., Assistant Chief, Spinal Injury Service, Rancho Los Amigos Hospital, Downey, Calif.; personal communication, January 15, 1975.
22. "The Muscular Dystrophies" (note 2).
23. Skillicorn (note 11); and Zundel and Tyler (note 3). See also Golub (note 8), Vignos (note 15), and "The Muscular Dystrophies" (note 2).
24. Zwang (note 5), personal communication, April 5, 1975.
25. *Proceedings* of the Third Medical Conference of MDAA (New York, 1954), p. 141.
26. Morton Hoberman, M.D. (in note 25), p. 115.
27. Skillicorn (note 11).
28. Vignos (note 15), p. 744.
29. Shu (note 21).
30. Zwang (note 5). Also Clara Fleming, Physical Therapist, Chandler Tripp School, San Jose, Calif.; personal communication, February 25, 1975.
31. Vignos (note 15).
32. Elena Gall, Ph.D., "Special Educational Needs of Children with Muscular Dystrophy," paper delivered at the 35th Annual Convention of the International Council on Exceptional Children, May 1957.
33. Charlotte Thomson, M.D., lecture to staff meeting, Children's Hospital, San Diego, April 18, 1968.
34. Judith S. Mearig, "Some Dynamics of Personality Development in Boys Suffering from Muscular Dystrophy," *Rehabilitation Literature* 34, no. 8 (1973): 226–28 *passim.*
35. Anna Kozkka et al., Neurology Department, School of Medicine, Warsaw, Poland, "Mental Retardation in Muscular Dystrophy," in *J. Neurological Science* 14 (1974): 209–13 *passim.*
36. See Thomas F. Henley and Bertha Albam, "A Psychiatric Study of Muscular Dystrophy, the Role of the Social Worker," *Physical Medicine* 34, no. 1 (1955), unpaged (MDAA reprint).
37. Herbert Bernstein and Sidney Malter, *A Social Survey of Muscular Dystrophy* (MDAA, 1957), p. 2.
38. Harold J. Wershow, "Familial Problems in Living with Childhood Muscular Dystrophy: A Study of Eighteen Families," doctoral dissertation, University of Pennsylvania, 1960 (Ann Arbor, Mich.: University Microfilms), p. 76.
39. *Ibid.*, p. 59.
40. Henley and Albam (note 36).

41. Bernstein and Malter (note 37), p. 3. See also Robert S. Morrow and Jacob Cohen, "The Psychosocial Factors in Muscular Dystrophy," *J. Child Psychiatry* 3, no. 1 (1954), unpaged.
42. Bernstein and Malter (note 37), p. 6.
43. Wershow (note 38), p. 55.
44. Leona Miu, personal communication (note 4).
45. *Ibid.*
46. Kenneth Hashimoto, Chief Therapist, Santa Clara County, Calif., Crippled Children's Services; personal communication, February 26, 1975, pertaining to notification from the Board of Supervisors on January 30, 1975, that permission had been obtained from the U.S. Department of Transportation to purchase specially equipped buses for the handicapped.
47. Henley and Albam (note 36).
48. Morrow and Cohen (note 41).
49. Wershow (note 38), pp. 122–23.
50. Morrow and Cohen (note 41).
51. Justin L. Greene, *Emotional Factors in Muscular Dystrophy* (MDAA, 1957, unpaged).
52. Henley and Albam (note 36).
53. Wershow (note 38), pp. 141, 147.
54. Beatrice Tanzer, Psychiatric Social Worker, Santa Clara County Department of Mental Health, Children's Division; personal communication, February 26, 1975.
55. S. Mouchly Small, "Emotional Reactions to Muscular Dystrophy," *Proceedings* of the First and Second Medical Conferences of MDAA, 1951–52, 1957.
56. Mearig (note 34), p. 227.
57. Robert Solow, "The Emotional and Social Aspects of Muscular Dystrophy," paper presented at the Symposium on Muscular Dystrophy for Special Education Personnel, September 25, 1971, p. 5.
58. Henley and Albam (note 36).
59. Bernstein and Malter (note 37); and Morrow and Cohen (note 41).
60. Wershow (note 38).
61. Marjorie Abbott, Principal, Chandler Tripp School, Santa Clara County, California; personal communication, February 26, 1975.
62. *Annual Report*, 1973, MDAA.
63. Wershow (note 38), p. 45.
64. Gary Capen, Recreation Therapist at Westgate Convalescent Hospital; personal communication, February 15, 1975.
65. Martin I. Lorin, "The Twilight Hours," in Paul R. Patterson et al., eds., *Psychosocial Aspects of Cystic Fibrosis* (New York: Columbia University Press, 1973), p. 28.

16. Sickle Cell Anemia

1. "Sickle Cell Anemia, What It Is, What Can Be Done," U.S. Department of Health, Education, and Welfare, publication no. 72-5108, 1972, p. 9.
2. Alvin M. Mauer, *Pediatric Hematology* (New York: McGraw-Hill, 1969), p. 100.
3. Roland B. Scott and Althea D. Kessler, "Sickle Cell Anemia and Your Child," pamphlet issued by the Department of Pediatrics, Howard University School of Medicine, Washington, D.C., 1967.
4. T. John Gribble, M.D., Associate Professor of Pediatrics, Division of Hema-

tology, Stanford School of Medicine, Stanford, Calif., at Sickle Cell Anemia Workshop, Palo Alto, Calif., May 9, 1973.

5. L. W. Diggs, "Sickle Cell Crises," *Amer. J. Clinical Pathology* 44: 1.

6. *Ibid.*, p. 14.

7. Jane F. Desforges et al., "Improving the Odds for Your Patient," *Patient Care* 6, February 15, 1972.

8. Editorial note: M. Robert Cooper and James F. Toole, "Sickle Cell Trait: Benign or Malignant," *Annals of Internal Medicine* 77 (1972): 997.

9. William F. McCormick, "Abnormal Hemoglobin. II, The Pathology of Sickle Cell Trait," *Amer. J. Medical Sciences*, March 1961, p. 329.

10. Stephen R. Jones et al., "Sudden Death in Sickle Cell Trait," *New England J. Medicine* 282 (1970): 323–25 *passim*.

11. J. G. Greenwall, "Stroke, Sickle Cell Trait and Oral Contraceptives," *Annals of Internal Medicine* 72 (1970).

12. "Two Common Diseases of Blacks," Midpeninsula Sickle Cell Anemia Foundation, Stanford, Calif., 1971, p. 6.

13. Gribble (note 4).

14. "Sickle Cell Anemia, What It Is" (note 1), p. 5.

15. Andrew D. White, M.D., General Practice, Menlo Park, Calif., at Sickle Cell Anemia Workshop (note 4).

16. Diggs (note 5), p. 3.

17. Darleen R. Powars, "Sickle Cell Disease: Ending Some Misconceptions and Complications," *Consultant*, November–December, 1969, p. 1.

18. Desforges et al. (note 7), p. 105.

19. Diggs (note 5), p. 7.

20. Scott and Kessler (note 3), p. 11.

21. "Sickle Cell Anemia, What It Is" (note 1), p. 5.

22. Desforges et al. (note 7), p. 106.

23. *Ibid.*

24. Diggs (note 5), *passim*.

25. M. E. Jenkins et al., "Studies in Sickle Cell Anemia," *J. Pediatrics* 56 (1960): 30–38.

26. "Sickle Cell Anemia, What It Is" (note 1), p. 5.

27. Gribble (note 4).

28. Desforges et al. (note 7), pp. 111–12.

29. Mauer (note 2), p. 100.

30. H. Lehmann and R. G. Huntsman, "Sickle Cell Anemia," *Nursing Times*, April 17, 1969, p. 493.

31. Powars (note 17); Gribble (note 4); and White (note 15).

32. *Ibid.*

33. Jane S. Lin-Fu, "Sickle Cell Anemia, A Medical Review," U.S. Dept. of HEW, publication no. 72-5111, p. 1; reviewed 1972.

34. "Sickle Cell Anemia, What It Is" (note 1), p. 9.

35. Tabitha M. Powledge, "The New Ghetto Hustle," *Saturday Review of the Sciences*, February 1973, pp. 38–46 *passim*.

36. James Robertson, *Young Children in Hospital* (London: Tavistock, 1958). See also D. G. Prugh et al., "A Study of the Emotional Reactions of Children and Families to Hospitalization and Illness," *Amer. J. Orthospsychiatry* 23 (1953): 70.

37. Powars (note 17).

38. Genevieve Duncan, as told to Ponchitta Pierce, "You Can't Kiss the Pain Away," *McCalls Magazine*, January 1973, p. 56.

39. *Ibid.*, p. 134.

40. Scott and Kessler (note 3).

41. Jean Vavasseau, Medical Social Worker, University of Southern California, Los Angeles County Hospital, Sickle Cell Center, June 7, 1973, personal communication.

42. Ann Landers syndicated column, *San Jose Mercury News*, October 22, 1973.

43. Charles F. Whitten, "Sickle Cell Programming—An Imperiled Promise," *New England J. Medicine* 288 (1973): 318.

44. "Sickle Cell Anemia, What It Is" (note 1), p. 16.

45. "Sickle Cell Screening and Education Clinics," Bureau of Community Health Service, U.S. Dept. of Health, Education, and Welfare, 1975.

46. Personal communication from Aaron Smith, Mid-Peninsula Sickle Cell Foundation, quoting telephone communication from the Office of the Director, Sickle Cell Disease Program, National Institutes of Health, Bethesda, Md., August 26, 1975.

17. Spina Bifida

1. Patrick F. Bray, *Neurology in Pediatrics* (Chicago: Year Book Medical Publishers, 1969), p. 127.

2. *Ibid.* See also Miklos Sugar and Mary B. Ames, "The Child with Spina Bifida Cystica: His Medical Problems and Habilitation," *Rehabilitation Literature* 26 (1967), no. 12: 362–66. Reprinted in Dwayne Douglas Peterson, ed., *The Physically Handicapped: A Book of Readings*, The MSS Educational Publishing Co., 19 E. 48th Street, New York, N.Y., 1969.

3. Brian MacMahon, "Environmental Influences on Congenital Defects," *Medical Opinion and Review*, February 1970, p. 58.

4. *Ibid.* See also Lechaim Naggan and Brian MacMahon, "Ethnic Differences in the Prevalence of Anencephaly and Spina Bifida in Boston, Massachusetts," *New England J. Medicine* 277 (1967): 1121–23. Also Luigi Luzzatti, M.D., "Myelomeningocele," paper presented at the American Academy of Pediatrics Postgraduate Course, Palo Alto, Calif., July 14, 1971.

5. Naggan and MacMahon (note 4).

6. John Lorber, M.D., "Your Child with Spina Bifida," Association for Spina Bifida and Hydrocephalus, 112 City Road, London.

7. Norman Fast, M.D., John Lorber, M.D., John Freeman, M.D., and Panel, "Decision Making in Infants with Birth Defects," discussion at the American Academy of Pediatrics meeting, San Francisco, October 22, 1974.

8. Bray (note 1), p. 132.

9. Lorber (note 6), p. 23.

10. Mary D. Ames and Luis Schut, "Results of Treatment of 171 Consecutive Myelomeningoceles—1963 to 1968," *Pediatrics* 50 (1972).

11. Alfred L. Scherzer and Gail Garner, "Studies of the School-Age Child with Myelomeningocele," *Pediatrics* 47 (1971): 424–30.

12. J. G. Parsons, "Assessments of Aptitudes in Young People of School-Leaving Age and Handicapped by Hydrocephalus or Spina Bifida Cystica," *Developmental Medicine and Child Neurology*, Suppl. 27, 1972, p. 101.

13. *Ibid.*, p. 107.

14. John Lorber, "Spina Bifida Cystica," *Archives of Disease in Childhood* 47 (1972): 854–72.

15. Sugar and Ames (note 2), pp. 192–93.

16. John M. Freeman, "Is There a Right to Die—Quickly?" Editor's Column, *J. Pediatrics* 80 (1972): 904–5.

17. Rainer M. E. Engel, "The Genitourinary Tract," in John Freeman, *Practical Management of Meningomyelocele* (Baltimore: University Park Press, 1974), p. 166.

18. R. B. Zachary, M.D., Leeds Consultant, Pediatric Surgeon, Children's Hospital, Sheffield, England, "Ethical and Social Aspects of Treatment of Spina Bifida," *Lancet* 11 (1968): 274-76. See also Bray (note 1), p. 131.

19. Ames and Schut (note 10).

20. Lorber (note 14), p. 854.

21. *Ibid.*, pp. 854-55.

22. Fast et al. (note 7). Also John A. James, M.D., Professor of Pediatrics, University of Southern California School of Medicine; personal communication, January 14, 1975. Also Luigi Luzzatti, M.D., Director, Birth Defects Center, Stanford University Medical Center.

23. Robert E. Cooke, "Whose Suffering?" *J. Pediatrics* 80, no. 5 (1972): 906-8.

24. Lorber (note 14), p. 857.

25. Ames and Schut (note 10).

26. K. A. Evans and C. O. Carter, "The Offspring of Survivors of Spina Bifida Cystica," *Excerpta Medica*, no. 297, 4th International Conference on Birth Defects, Vienna, September 2-8, 1972.

27. Lorber (note 14).

28. Steven E. Kopits, "Orthopedic Aspects of Care of the Child with Meningomyelocele," p. 106 in Freeman (note 17).

29. Ames and Schut (note 10), p. 468.

30. Kopits, p. 127 (note 28).

31. *Ibid.*, p. 132.

32. *Ibid.*, p. 134.

33. *Ibid.*, p. 145.

34. *Ibid.*, p. 125.

35. *Ibid.*

36. Lorber (note 14), p. 865.

37. Ames and Schut (note 10), p. 468.

38. Engel, in Freeman (note 17), p. 186.

39. Sherrie Wilkins, R.N., Clinical Nurse Specialist, Birth Defects Center, Stanford University Medical Center; personal communication, October 1974.

40. John J. White and Issam Shaker, "The Management of Fecal Incontinence" in Freeman (note 17), p. 215.

41. Wilkins (note 39).

42. Engel, in Freeman (note 17), p. 176.

43. *Ibid.*, p. 194.

44. Freeman (note 17), p. xii.

45. Barbara Field, M.D., B.S., Coordinator, Meningomyelocele Clinic, Royal Alexandra Hospital for Children, Camperdown, Sydney, Australia, "The Child with Spina Bifida: Medical and Social Aspects of the Problem of a Child with Multiple Handicaps and His Family," *Medical J. Australia* 2, no. 2 (1972): 1286.

46. *Ibid.*, p. 1287.

47. Susanne Houghton, R.N., Liaison Nurse, Pediatric Service, Rancho Los Amigos Hospital, Downey, Calif.; personal communication, January 14, 1975.

48. John A. James, M.D., Professor of Pediatrics, University of Southern California School of Medicine; personal communication, January 14, 1975.

49. Houghton (note 47).

50. Patricia W. Hayden et al., "Custody of the Myelodysplastic Child: Implications for Selection for Early Treatment," *Pediatrics* 75 (1974).

51. *Ibid.*, p. 255.
52. James (note 48).
53. Hayden (note 50), p. 254.
54. *Ibid.*

18. *Spinal Cord Injury*

1. "Spinal Cord Injury Handbook," Rancho Los Amigos Hospital, 1601 E. Imperial Highway, Downey, Calif., 1968, p. 3. This handbook contains an excellent bibliography for paraplegic and quadriplegic persons and their families.
2. Synthesis from lectures at the Institute on Spinal Cord Injury, Rancho Los Amigos Hospital, March 5, 1970, by Eric Holmes, Associate Professor of Psychology and Neurology, University of Southern California School of Medicine; and Paul Muchnic, Regional Spinal Cord Injury (SCI) Service.
3. Edwin Edberg, Physical Therapy Supervisor, Regional SCI Service, Rancho Los Amigos Hospital; personal communication, March 6, 1970.
4. Edwin Edberg, "Equipment and Estimate Cost," Rancho Los Amigos Hospital, Form RD 172, issued February 1969.
5. Complications discussed by Richard Boggs, Chief of Neurological Sciences, Regional SCI Service, March 5, 1970.
6. The description of the neurogenic bladder and its training was provided through personal communication with Bernice B. Gunderson, Liaison Nurse, Urology Department, Rancho Los Amigos Hospital, on March 15-21, 1970. See "Interdisciplinary Clinical, Educational, and Research Aspects of a Regional Center for the Rehabilitation of Spinal Cord–Injured Persons," Attending Staff Association of the Rancho Los Amigos Hospital; excerpts from final report (SRS Grant RD 2114M-68-C2), September 1969, pp. 18-21 *passim*.
7. Annie Grdgen, Liaison Nurse, SCI Service, Rancho Los Amigos Hospital, on January 21, 1970, provided the bowel program described.
8. *Ibid.*
9. Judith Krenzel and Lois Rohrer, "Paraplegic and Quadriplegic Individuals," *Handbook of Care for Nurses* (Chicago: Wallace Press; The National Paraplegic Foundation), p. 25.
10. George Dillinger, M.D., Douglas Young Clinic, La Jolla, Calif., and Herbert Rigoni, Ph.D., Chief, Psychological Services at Rancho Los Amigos Hospital, have described the psychological reactions of the paraplegic. Jean Mitsuhate, M.S.W., Regional Spinal Cord Injury Rehabilitation Center, Rancho Los Amigos Hospital, has shared her experiences regarding the family.
11. Esther White, "The Body Image Concept in Rehabilitating Severely Handicapped Patients," *Social Work* 6 (1961): 51-58.

Index

Index

Abandonment: during dialysis and transplant, 231; in fatal disease, 318, 377, 394–95, 399, 400–401

Abdication of father, 53, 55; in asthma, 175, 191; in cystic fibrosis, 275, 279; in hemophilia, 301, 309–10, 318; in arthritis, 328; in diabetes, 363; in muscular dystrophy, 413; in sickle cell anemia, 445–46; in spina bifida, 469; in cord injury, 493

Abnormalities, congenital: prevalence of, 5f, 119; and drug use, 127; and maternal diabetes, 138; and maternal oxygenation, 141; and maternal viral infection, 142; and inheritance, 153, 154–55, 301; and rejection of pregnancy, 162–63; of urinary tract, 199–200; multiple, 234, 265–68; in hemophilia, 300. *See also* Chaps. 8 and 17

Abortion, 134, 148–51, 162–63; illegal, and maternal death, 139; methods of, 150; selective, 156–57, 316, 456; therapeutic, 139, 148f

Accidents: in dialysis, 208; vs. disease as cause of death, 287; bowel, as weapon in spina bifida, 473. *See also* Chaps. 10 and 18

Acting out, 68, 297f, 450

Activity: as need of toddler, 58–59; as treatment, 69, 272f, 308, 428, 431; in groups, 284, 344, 366; after head injury, 291; and hemophilia, 301, 303, 315; in arthritis, 326; and need for insulin, 346, 353; effect of treatment on, in muscular dystrophy, 407; as coping mechanism, 418–19

—limitation of: prevalence of, 5; and socioeconomic status, 6; and teenage pregnancy, 140; in kidney disease, 201; by dialysis shunt, 224f; in heart disease, 241, 258; in arthritis, 334–40, 341; in sickle cell anemia, 438

Adolescence: and importance of experience, 37; and death, 47; and chronic illness, 61–64; and hospitalization, 73, 476; and drug abuse, 127; and pregnancy, 127–30; and illegitimate pregnancy, 131–32, 133, 140; and unwanted pregnancy, 147; and asthma, 164, 187; and kidney disease, 203, 215–18; and dialysis, 207–8, 220, 225f; and transplant, 210–11, 229–30; and independence, 215, 226, 471–72; and heart disease, 245, 257; and cystic fibrosis, 282–86; and head injury, 284, 296–99; and hemophilia, 315–16; and arthritis, 332, 336–37, 339; and diabetes, 348, 359–60, 365; and hair loss, 391f; and muscular dystrophy, 415; and sickle cell anemia, 450; and spina bifida, 460, 463, 471–72, 475–77; and cord injury, 481–97 *passim*

Adoption: adoptability, 98–104; and heart murmur, 236; in hemophilia, 318–19; in sickle cell trait or anemia, 453–54

Advocacy, 318, 376, 442

Age distribution: of chronic conditions, 4; of asthma, 164, 166; of glomerulonephritis, 200; of head injury, 287; of diabetes, 343; of leukemia, 368; of cord injury, 481

Age of child: and severity of trauma, 2; and prevention, 4–5; and impact of experience, 11–12, 37, 39–40; and capacity for stress, 18–19, 40; and stages, 24–27; and specificity of need, 38–39; and complexity of experience, 39; and number

of allergens, 165–66; and meaning of asthma, 175, 180; and reaction to treatment for asthma, 193; and importance of help to family, 194; as variable in kidney disease, 197, 201, 211–18; and place of dialysis, 207; and dependency in dialysis, 226; and nervous system maturation, 289; and need for mother at home, 306–7; and pain, 336–37; and activity limitation, 338–39; and adjustment to diabetes, 358–59; and fear of mutilation, 389; and impact of hair loss, 391–92; and phases of muscular dystrophy, 405–6; and severity of sickle cell anemia, 435; and placement in spina bifida, 478
—and death anxiety: in chronic illness, 47; in leukemia, 381, 383, 389
—and outlook: in adoption, 100; in asthma, 166, 168, 174–75; in nephrosis, 202; in kidney transplant, 209; in heart surgery, 236–43 *passim*; in head injury, 289
—and self-care: in asthma, 183–84; in hemophilia, 303–4; in diabetes, 348
—and surgery: in kidney disease, 200, 209, 220; in heart disease, 236–43 *passim*; in spina bifida, 460–61, 463
—and understanding of implications: in asthma, 192; in kidney transplant, 220, 230; in hemophilia, 302, 317; in leukemia, 381; in sickle cell anemia, 450; in spina bifida, 475

Age of death: in cystic fibrosis, 274, 286; in diabetes, 346; in muscular dystrophy, 403, 406; in sickle cell anemia, 437; in untreated spina bifida, 458

Age of mother: and drug abuse, 127; and risk to mother and child in pregnancy, 127–30, 133–34; and illegitimacy, 128, 130f; and use of abortion, 134; and Down's Syndrome, 149; and tetralogy of Fallot, 234

Age of onset: nephrosis, 202; kidney failure, 203; hemophilia, 301; arthritis, 321; diabetes, 345; muscular dystrophy, 405; sickle cell anemia, 435
—and inheritance, in allergies, 166
—and management problems, in heart disease, 239–40
—and outlook: in cystic fibrosis, 283; in arthritis, 323; in diabetes, 346
—and schooling, 61
—and severity: in allergies, 165; in cystic fibrosis, 271; in sickle cell anemia, 435
—and stage of development: in kidney disease, 211–18; in arthritis, 327–28, 339; in muscular dystrophy, 420

—and stress on marriage, in arthritis, 328; in muscular dystrophy, 412

Age of siblings: and effect of chronic illness, 56; and implications of leukemia, 388

Age-related tasks, and chronic illness, 57–64

Aggression: perception of treatment as, 193; after head injury, 291, 297; expression of, and overprotection, 308–9; in muscular dystrophy, 421

Alienation from peers, 212–13, 265, 297, 421f

Allergy, 165–66; interacting allergens in, 172; in infancy, 178; and convenience foods, 178f

Alopecia, 202, 370ff, 391–92

Altitude: and congenital heart disease, 234; and sickle cell trait, 434; and sickle cell anemia, 436

Amniocentesis, 156–57; in elderly mothers, 149; in spina bifida, 456

Analytic theory, 169f

Anemia: maternal, and infant mortality, 125; in kidney disease, 201, 204; in cystic fibrosis, 270; in leukemia, 368; in sickle cell anemia, 433

Anencephaly, 154–55, 456

Anesthesia: and sickle cell trait, 434, 452; in spina bifida, 456f

Anger: of parents, 52, 54, 192, 276, 280, 362, 401, 411; of child, 281, 317, 336–37, 360, 421, 451f. *See also* Resentment

Angiogram, 236–37, 290

Anomalies, *see* Abnormalities

Anti-hemolytic factors, *see* Clotting factors

Anxiety, *see also* Fear
—of child: in asthma, 171; in kidney disease, 217; and age, 260, 336, 381, 389; and perception of pain, 260, 336; and surgery, 260; and test scores, 264; in cystic fibrosis, 281–86; in hemophilia, 302, 317; in leukemia, 381, 388–92; in muscular dystrophy, 421; in sickle cell trait, 451–52
—of family: in kidney disease, 213f; in dialysis and transplant, 231; in heart surgery, 254–57; in cystic fibrosis, 276, 280–81; in hemophilia, 308; in sisters of hemophiliacs, 311; in muscular dystrophy, 411, 418; in sickle cell anemia, 447; in spina bifida, 469–70

Aorta, 196, 234; stenosis of, 235; coarctation of, 237f, 242f; in transposition of great vessels, 243

Apathy, 59; in kidney disease, 203, 207,

INDEX

217f; on dialysis, 227; in leukemia, 369; in sickle cell anemia, 437f
Appetite: in kidney disease, 202–3, 205; after transplant, 229–30. *See also* Hunger
Appliances: braces, 303f, 326, 329f, 334, 406, 409, 461–62; splints, 326, 334, 407; eyeglasses, 356; polio arms, 409; penile, 415, 462–65 *passim*, 471, 488
Atresia, tricuspid, 238, 242
Atrial septal defect, 235, 238, 240, 244–45
Attendant care, *see* Household assistance
Attitude, *see also* Emotions
—of child: toward immobilization, 69, 421; toward dialysis, 226; toward mist tent, 282; toward hemophilia, 316–17; toward injections, 348; toward diabetes, 358–61; toward overprotection, 474
—of family members: toward abortion, 149; toward pregnancy, 161–63; in asthma, 184, 188–89; toward autonomy in kidney disease, 212; toward cost of asthma, 222; in heart disease, 253–54; after dramatic heart surgery, 257–58; in hemophilia, 307–12; toward cost of spina bifida, 470
—of hospital staff, in leukemia, 376
—of teachers: in asthma, 185–86; in hemophilia, 313
Autonomy, 59, 211, 220, 276, 317

Baldness: in nephrosis, 202; in leukemia, 370ff; emotional impact of, 391–92
Battering, factors associated with, 288
Behavior, 28, 40; patterned, 16; of child, related to love in parents, 55; problems in adoption, 101; asthma attacks as, 189–90; as language, 190; experience vs. sensitivity in, 259; effect of chronic illness on, 259–60; after head injury, 291–98 *passim*; in muscular dystrophy, 421; conditioned, in cord injury, 487–88
Behaviorist theory, 169–70
Bioethics, 8–9, 267–68
Birth: trends in rate of, 120f, 128, 134; defects, *see* Abnormalities; Chaps. 8 and 17
Bladder, 196f; infection, 198; extension of, 200; in head injury, 290; in spina bifida, 457, 462–65, 471–73; in cord injury, 485, 486–89. *See also* Urinary tract
Blame: of self by child, 212; after heart surgery, 255; of physician, 255, 374, 439; of mother by self and in-laws, 307, 309; of mother by son, 413; of parents by child, 446; for fractures in spina bifida, 457
Bleeding: and maternal death, 139; in cystic fibrosis, 270; in head injury, 290; into joints, 300, 302f, 312; sites of, in hemophilia, 301f, 304; in leukemia, 369, 371, 387, 393
Blood: oxygenation of, 141, 234f, 244, 433f; filtration of, 196; banks, policies of, 303, 305, 385; replacement of, 305–6, 385; cost of, 385
—cells: and kidneys, 196, 204; functions of, 368; in sickle cell disease, 433–34
—pressure: in toxemia, 136f; and oral contraception, 146; role of kidneys in, 196; and kidney disease, 199, 201, 204; during dialysis, 207; after transplant, 210; in cord injury, 485
—transfusions: and Rh sensitization, 143; in kidney disease, 204, 208; in heart disease, 242; in sickle cell anemia, 437f, 448
Body image: in kidney disease, 211, 215f; in heart disease, 265; in head injury, 295; in hemophilia, 317; in muscular dystrophy, 410, 421; in spina bifida, 475; grief for, in cord injury, 492. *See also* Self-image
Bowel management: in chronic illness, 59; during dialysis, 208; in head injury, 290; in spina bifida, 457, 462–65, 471–73, 478; in cord injury, 489–90
Brain, 288–89; complications in kidney diseases, 203; and diagnostic procedures (heart), 237; bleeding into, 302, 316; sickling in, 437; in anencephaly, 456. *See also* Chap. 10
Bruising, 369; and end of remission, 390
Budgeting, *see* Special needs
Burden: prospect for surcease, 19, 213, 275, 418, 470; of chronic illness, 43; of asthma, 175–80 *passim*; of kidney disease, 195–96; of dialysis and transplant, 230–31; of heart disease, 247, 252–57; of cystic fibrosis, 269, 275–77, 292–99; of hemophilia, 305–12; of arthritis, 327–29; of diabetes, 361–63; of leukemia, 373–81, 385–88, 394–99; of muscular dystrophy, 411–20; of sickle cell anemia, 445–48; of spina bifida, 466–70; of cord injury, 493–94. *See also* Financial problems; Time burden

Camps, 364–65, 366, 426–27
Carriers: vaccinated children as, 143; in X-linked disease, 154, 307f, 404; detection of, 157, 301, 405, 439, 451; in hemophilia, 301; girl siblings as, 311, 424; in muscular dystrophy, 404–5; in sickle cell anemia, 432; awareness of, and mate selection, 451f

Catheterization: urinary, 212, 241, 462–63, 463–64, 485, 487, 491; cardiac, 236–37
Cause: toxemia, 136; asthma, 164, 169–70, 187; urinary infections, 198; nephrosis, 202; renal failure, 203; heart trouble in children, 233; heart defects, 234; head injury, 287; hemophilia, 300; arthritis, 321; diabetes, 344; leukemia, 368; muscular dystrophy, 404; sickle cell anemia, 433; sickle cell crisis, 436; cord injury, 481. See also Death, cause of
Chemotherapy, 370–73
Child Welfare Services, 86–88
Christmas disease, 300–306 passim
Clergy, 47, 117–18, 254, 397f
Clotting factors, 302–3, 305f; concentrate, 302–3; cryoprecipitate, 302–18 passim
Clubbing, 235f
Collaboration, 104–18; in care, 293–94, 341, 460, 465; home-hospital, 445; multidisciplinary, 465; agency-hospital, 470–71
Coma: in kidney disease, 203f; in cystic fibrosis, 285; in head injury, 290–92; in diabetes, 345, 349, 352–53; in sickle cell anemia, 435, 437
Communicability: of leukemia, 368, 392; of sickle cell anemia, 433, 439
Communication: experience as, 15, 16–17; with child about death, 47–48, 284–85, 429f; between parents, 55–56, 176, 275–76, 446; within health team, 108–9; wheezing as, 190, 192; nonverbal, 190, 299, 381; language and culture barriers to, 213; between family and center, 219–20; with potential kidney donors, 228; of medical information by worker, 293; conspiracy to avoid, 311; about reproduction in hemophilia, 316; forced, about death, 383f; informing siblings of outlook, 387–88; child's need for, 419
Competition: with like-sexed parent, 62–63; limitation of, 183, 241, 338; in physical activity, 186, 326; and socialization, 312; scholastic, obstacles to, 392–93
Conceptualization: and development, 27f; and cooperation, 174; in diabetes, 358; of death, 383
Concussion, 289–90
Congenital conditions, see Abnormalities; Chaps. 5, 8, and 17
Constitution: and personality, 22–23; and behavior, 259
Contraception, 146–47; attitudes toward, 121; and age, 121, 134; and class, 134; in heart disease, 139; in diabetes, 365; in sickle cell trait, 434
Convulsions: in kidney disease, 203f; during dialysis, 208, 224; in heart disease, 235; after head injury, 291; in diabetes, 351; in sickle cell anemia, 435, 437
Coping mechanisms, 65–69; asthma as, 190, 192; playing-out of hospital experience, 214; of family in leukemia, 378; in muscular dystrophy, 418–19
Credé method, see Urination
Crippled Children's Services, 80; in heart disease, 248; in cystic fibrosis, 277, 282; in hemophilia, 305; in arthritis, 330; in leukemia, 384, 396; in muscular dystrophy, 417; in sickle cell anemia, 439; in spina bifida, 470
Crippling: suddenness of, in head injury, 295; in hemophilia, 300, 302f, 312, 316; in arthritis, 320ff; in sickle cell anemia, 447, 451. See also Deformity; Disability
Crisis: theory of, 20–21; and experience during, 37; unpredictability of, 45; of unwanted pregnancy, 147; pregnancy as, 161; heart surgery as, 233; and defenses in cystic fibrosis, 280; early head injury as, 293; in hemophilia, 308; in diabetes, 361; diagnosis as, 367, 377–80; and accessibility, 376; sequentiality of, 378; and spiritual growth, 398; in progression of muscular dystrophy, 419; in sickle cell anemia, 433f, 435–37, 441f, 444; and family's dependency needs, 493
Cryoprecipitate, 302–18 passim
Culture: poverty as, 30; transmission of, 30–31; and food allergens, 179; and attitude toward treatment, 253. See also Ethnicity
Cyanosis, 235f, 241, 246
Cystoscopy, 197

Day care, 33, 89–91; in cystic fibrosis, 279f; in arthritis, 338; in diabetes, 364; in sickle cell anemia, 444; in spina bifida, 477
Deafness: and socioeconomic status, 7; in hemolytic disease of the newborn, 143; in rubella syndrome, 234, 266; after head injury, 291
Death: philosophies of, 8–9; parents' and child's experience of, 46–49; siblings' reactions to, 56–57; fear of, 164, 226, 381, 429, 446; vs. dialysis and transplant, 206–7; diagnostic procedures in heart disease and, 237; institutionalization and, 268, 479; wish for, 275, 395, 418; preoccupation with, 283, 284–85, 399; in

cystic fibrosis, 284–86; from arthritis or treatment, 323; from leukemia, 373, 383, 399–402; age-related concepts of, 383; preparation of parents for, 400; at home, 401–2; child's questions about, 419; from sickle cell trait, 434; expectation of early, 450
—cause of: in infancy, 124, 233–34; after transplant, 210; heart surgery as, 238; in hemophilia, 302; diabetes as, 343; in diabetes, 345, 354; leukemia as, 367; in muscular dystrophy, 406; in sickle cell anemia, 436f; in spina bifida, 458; in cord injury, 485, 491
—infant: and race, 6; and prematurity, 124; and maternal age, 129; and illegitimacy, 131; and toxemia, 136; in maternal sickle cell anemia, 453
—maternal: and age, 128; and marital status, 131; causes of, 139; and diabetes, 139; in sickle cell anemia, 453
—rate: and race, 6; in asthma, 175; in kidney disease, 195; in heart surgery, 238–46 *passim*, 267; effect of heart surgery on, 240; in cystic fibrosis, 269; in head injury, 287; in leukemia, 368; in spina bifida, 478. *See also* Age of death; Life, prolongation of

Decision making: in adoption of handicapped, 101–2; about reproduction at risk, 144–46, 155; about prolongation of life in kidney disease, 218–20; and socioeconomic status, 219; by child in kidney disease, 220; specificity in, 220; about setting for dialysis, 226; about surgery in heart defect, 239, 256–57; for multihandicapped, 267–68; about prolongation of life in cystic fibrosis, 285; in daily life in hemophilia, 306–7, 317; by mother vs. hospital in arthritis, 329; about spina bifida surgery, 459, 463–67 *passim*, 471, 480. *See also* Responsibility; Self-determination

Deformity: in kidney disease, 204; after head injury, 290; in hemophilia, 302; in arthritis, 322, 325–26, 339; in muscular dystrophy, 407f; in sickle cell anemia, 435; in spina bifida, 455, 457, 461f. *See also* Crippling; Disability

Denial: in siblings with same disease, 56–57; as a coping mechanism, 66; in kidney disease, 212, 226; vocational preparation as, 283; by mother in hemophilia, 308; by sisters in hemophilia, 311, 316; and "forgetting" medication, 332; in diabetes, 360; of leukemia diagnosis, 380–81; during remission of leukemia, 386;
of diagnosis in muscular dystrophy, 412; and reproduction in sickle cell anemia, 447; in spina bifida, 467f; duration of, in cord injury, 492n

Dental care: in heart disease, 241, 248; in hemophilia, 303f

Dependence, 21, 55, 63, 66–67, 211, 214f; of single-parent mother, 51; in pregnancy, 161; in asthma, 171, 189, 191–92; in kidney disease, 211, 226; in crisis, 294; in hemophilia, 308, 310, 317; in muscular dystrophy, 404, 413, 422; in sickle cell anemia, 450f. *See also* Independence

Depression: as natural response, 67–68, 337; treatment of, 69–70; after diet lapse, 171; wheezing as symptom of, 190; in all adolescents, 216, 217–18; in kidney disease, 216–18; on rejection of kidney, 228; in cystic fibrosis, 283; after head injury, 291; in arthritis, 341–42; in muscular dystrophy, 427; length of, in cord injury, 492n

Deprivation: maternal, 38, 55, 58; of family, 181f, 191, 263, 276, 279, 294, 310, 363, 423; diet viewed as, 358

Desensitization, *see* Hyposensitization

Development: crises of, 20–21, 23–24; basic tenets of, 21–36, 37; irreversibility of, 24; sequentiality of, 24, 28, 38–39, 57–64; effect of illness on, 211–12
—physical: in heart disease, 235–36; in cystic fibrosis, 271; in sickle cell anemia, 450
—sexual: in sickle cell anemia, 450; in spina bifida, 476–77
—stages of: and age, 24–27; and need for protection, 193; and discipline in heart disease, 258; and cystic fibrosis, 276; and bleeding in hemophilia, 317; and onset of arthritis, 321

Diabetes: as risk factor in pregnancy, 138–39; and oral contraceptives, 146; urinary complications of, 199, 202; after transplant, 210; maturity onset, 344. *See also* Chap. 13

Diagnosis: and adoption, 101, 103; prenatal genetic, 156–57; major procedures, 195–96, 236–37; tests in kidney disease, 197–98; need for early, 199, 201, 269, 275, 368, 407; complexity in heart disease, 236–37; difficulty of, in arthritis, 322; imparting of, 376, 379, 381–84, 387–88; as an experience, 377–80; reaction to, in fatal illness, 377–81, 411, 418; child's questions about, 381–84; denial of, 412; age of, in sickle cell anemia, 435; need for information on, 443

Dialysis, *see* Kidney
Diet: as burden, 43; in pregnancy, 124–27, 129, 137f, 140, 160; macrobiotic and Zen, 126–27; allergens in, 165–66; in asthma, 173–74, 177–79; in kidney disease, 202, 205–6, 214; Giovanetti, 206; before vs. during dialysis, 208, 223–24; in cystic fibrosis, 272, 278, 282; in diabetes, 350–51, 355–56, 359–60, 366; in muscular dystrophy, 407–8; in sickle cell anemia, 440, 441–42; in spina bifida, 473–74; in cord injury, 489. *See also* Nutrition
Difference, feelings of, 61, 193, 265, 281, 317, 359f, 365, 391–92, 473, 476
Disability: long-term, in heart disease, 259–60; in hemophilia, 302; in adult after juvenile diabetes, 345, 353–54; in sickle cell anemia, 439. *See also* Crippling; Deformity
Discipline: in heart disease, 257–59; in hemophilia, 308–9; in arthritis, 329; in leukemia, 379, 386–87; in spina bifida, 474
Discrimination, in sickle cell trait, 452
Disruption: of development, 57–64; by dialysis, 224, 226; by hemophilia, 301–2, 317, 319; by spina bifida, 469
Divorce: rate, 32, 129; effect of, on child, vs. death, 50. *See also* Family, one-parent
Down's syndrome, 153, 156, 234, 245, 267, 368
Drugs: exposure to, in pregnancy, 122, 127, 149, 154, 234; in leukemia, 370–72; dependence on, in sickle cell anemia, 451; as escape in cord injury, 493–94
Dysreflexia, 485

Eclampsia, 137
Eisenmenger's complex, 244
Emotional support: in avoiding allergens, 179; and heart surgery, 255; to cystic fibrosis parents, 280; at death, 285, 400f; in crises, 293, 308; in accepting brain-damaged behavior, 297; in diabetes, 358; from affected child, 419
Emotions, 12–14, 19f, 24–27, 28, 30, 171, 289; and asthma, 164, 169–71, 189; and pets, 181, 391, 399
—problems of: and abortion, 149f; after sterilization, 151; in pregnancy, 163; in allergy, 166; in asthma, 169–70, 172, 182, 187, 191, 194; and malformations of genitalia, 200; in dialysis and transplant, 219; after head injury, 291; in hemophilia, 308, 315ff; in diabetes, 343, 353; in muscular dystrophy, 420–21. *See also* Attitude; *and separately indexed feelings such as* Guilt
Employment: of mother, 31–36 *passim*, 178f, 250–51, 275, 293, 306–7, 339f, 362, 411, 419, 440, 444; of father, 277, 305. *See also* Vocational future
Endocardial cushion defect, 245, 267
Endocarditis, bacterial, 241
Enuresis, 167, 276, 345
Environment, 2, 29, 37–38, 39–40; and malformations, 154; and asthma, 164f, 170, 174, 180, 182, 190; and brain damage, 295, 298; in development of diabetes, 344; and retardation, 410; in causation of spina bifida, 456
Enzymes: in pregnancy diet, 126–27; in prenatal diagnosis, 156; in cystic fibrosis, 270, 272, 277, 282; in muscular dystrophy, 404f
Epigenetic model, 22, 24
Equipment: for cystic fibrosis, 273–74, 278; for hemophilia, 304; for diabetes, 356; for muscular dystrophy, 409, 414, 417, 426; for spina bifida, 470; for cord injury, 484–85. *See also* Appliances
Erythroblastosis, 143
Ethnicity: and pregnancy diet, 125; and neural tube defects, 154–55. *See also* Culture; Race
Exercise as treatment: in cystic fibrosis, 273; in hemophilia, 303; in arthritis, 325f, 333–34; in muscular dystrophy, 407f, 414; in spina bifida, 461. *See also* Physical therapy
Exertion: in asthma, 169, 186ff; in glomerulonephritis, 201; in arthritis, 326
Eye and vision problems: after maternal virus infection, 142, 234, 265–66; as side effect of steroids, 202, 210; after head injury, 291; in arthritis, 321, 323–24; in diabetes, 345, 347, 353–54, 356, 365–66; in sickle cell anemia, 435, 436–37; in hydrocephalus, 458; in spina bifida, 460

Family: and transmission of culture, 30–31; life cycle of, 30f, 176, 252–53, 321, 328, 412; structure of, 31–35, 49–52, 413; pairing in, 34; scapegoating in, 34–35, 258, 363, 470; pathology, and severity of illness, 170, 194; isolation of, 181, 276, 308, 412; history, and attitudes, 307–8, 411f; and medical team, 374–76; and prolonged stress, 377
—extended: as support, 179, 230–31, 396–97, 445; attitudes in X-linked disease, 307–8

—one-parent: and race, 32; and experience of illness, 36, 182, 251; and child's experience of illness, 50–52; and dependency, 55; and placement, 478. *See also* Pregnancy, illegitimate

—relationships, 52–57; in asthma, 171, 175–76, 181, 191–92; in kidney disease, 218; in head injury, 292, 294–95; in hemophilia, 307–12; in diabetes, 361–63; in leukemia, 377, 378–79, 387–88, 389, 390, 397, 398–99; in muscular dystrophy, 411–14; in sickle cell anemia, 445–48; in cord injury, 493. *See also* Burden; Marriage; Parents; Siblings

—size of: and child's experience of illness, 52; attitudes toward, 120; and poverty, 123; and abortion, 149; and avoidance of food allergens, 178

Father: attitude of, toward child, 53, 55, 216, 300–301, 308, 412, 468; in relinquishment, 103; in pregnancy, 161; participation of, in care, 175f, 225, 309, 412–13, 445–46; substitutes for, 318, 493. *See also* Abdication of father; Employment; Parents

Fatigue: in pregnancy, 122; in kidney disease, 203, 207; and test scores, 264; in leukemia, 369; in sickle cell anemia, 448

Fear, *see also* Anxiety
—in child: with asthma, 164, 171, 192; of physicians, 213; of heart surgery, 260–61; with cystic fibrosis, 281; of predicted death, 382; with muscular dystrophy, 409, 421–22; expression of, and trust, 429
—in family: during pregnancy, 160–61, 411; of asthma attack, 175; perceived as anger by child, 192; in heart disease, 263; and leukemia remission, 385–86
—in others, of sick child, 193, 313, 392f

Feeding difficulties, 214, 236, 290

Fertility, 121; and anti-leukemia drugs, 202; in cystic fibrosis, 282; in diabetes, 344, 365; in sickle cell anemia, 453

Financial problems, 44, 81–84; in asthma, 180, 182–83; in kidney disease, 214–15, 220–23; in heart disease, 248–49; in cystic fibrosis, 277–78; in hemophilia, 303, 305–6, 319; in arthritis, 329–30; in diabetes, 355–57; in leukemia, 377, 384–85; in muscular dystrophy, 415, 417; in sickle cell anemia, 439–42; in pay-back requirements, 470; in spina bifida, 470–71; in cord injury, 484, 494–95

Food: stamps, 83–84; ethnicity in, 125; as allergens, 165–66, 171, 173–74, 177–78; families of, 178; convenience, 178–79; refusal of, as self-control, 214; absorption of, in cystic fibrosis, 270; related to activity and insulin, 346. *See also* Diet; Nutrition

Foster care, *see* Out-of-home care

Fractures: while on steroids, 202; in head injury, 289f; in spina bifida, 457, 461, 478

Gait: ataxia after head injury, 290; in arthritis, 322; in muscular dystrophy, 405

Genetic disease, 152–55; and parental guilt, 54, 279, 308, 368, 411f, 446f; and mental retardation, 145; counseling in, 145, 155, 452f; prevention of, 152–57; and extended family attitudes, 307–8. *See also* Heredity

German measles, *see* Rubella

Gestation: and prematurity, 123f; and rubella damage, 142

Giovanetti diet, 206

Globulin, anti-Rh, 143–44

Glomerulonephritis, 137, 197, 200–201, 202f

Glucagon, 351–52

Goals: and early death, 283, 450; and maturation, 447

Grandparents, *see* Family, extended

Grief, 40, 468, 491–93; anticipatory, 377, 394–95

Growth retardation: in rubella syndrome, 142; in asthma, 187; in kidney disease, 196, 202–3, 204f, 208, 210f, 216; in heart disease, 235, 242, 245f, 262–63; in cystic fibrosis, 271, 282; in arthritis, 324; in diabetes, 347; in sickle cell anemia, 435, 437, 450; in spina bifida, 457

Guilt: and chronic illness, 52; and genetic disease, 54, 279, 308, 411f, 446f; and initiative, 60; after diet lapse, 171; appeal to, by parents, 188; appeal to, by child, 190; fantasies of, 197; due to lack of information, 213; in adolescent dependence, 217; and discipline, 257; after relapse, 275; and working mother, 293; in sib responsible for head injury, 294; for resentment, 310; baseless, in leukemia, 368, 378; for nonparticipation in care, 412; for exercise lapse, 414; for being unaffected, 423; after decision to allow death, 467

Glycosuria, 347

Head Start, 477

Health Maintenance Organizations, 81

Heart, 234; in pregnancy, 139–41, 365–66; in status asthmaticus, 168; in kidney disease, 201, 207; failure of, 235, 242, 245–

46, 324f; diagnostic procedures, 236–37; in arthritis, 324f. *See also* Surgery; Chap. 8; *and under specific heart defects*

Hemarthrosis, 300, 302f, 312

Hemoglobin, 125, 433f

Hemolytic disease of the newborn, 143–44

Heredity: in diabetes, 138, 153, 344; in arthritis, 153; in Down's syndrome, 153; in kidney disease, 153; in spina bifida, 153, 154–55, 456; in asthma, 153, 164; in heart disease, 153, 234; in leukemia, 153, 368; in allergy, 165f; in urinary tract abnormalities, 199; in cystic fibrosis, 270; in hemophilia, 301, 316; in diabetes, 344; in muscular dystrophy, 404–5; in mental retardation in muscular dystrophy, 410; in sickle cell anemia, 435; in spina bifida, 456. *See also* Genetic disease

Home care: in hemophilia, 303–4, 306, 311–12, 315, 317; after arthritis surgery, 339–40; in early diabetes, 354–55, 362, 366; vs. hospital, in leukemia, 395; until death, 401–2

Home health aide, *see* Household assistance

Homemaker service, *see* Household assistance

Hope, maintenance of: in fatal illness, 281, 283, 381f, 384, 431, 447–48; narrowing of, 384, 398, 430; in mother, 420; and afterlife, 429ff

Hospitalization, 70–74; positive feelings toward, 73, 476; for abortion, 150; for discontinuance of steroids, 173; in asthma, 182; in urinary infections, 195; in kidney disease, 198, 202, 207, 213; in heart disease, 237f, 248; in cystic fibrosis, 277; in head injury, 287, 290; parents' experience of, 293; in hemophilia, 300, 303f; in arthritis, 327, 329, 334; in diabetes, 345, 353, 355, 365; parent participation in, 375–76; behavior after, 389–90; final, 400; in sickle cell anemia, 436, 439, 444–45, 469; in spina bifida, 476

Household assistance, 88–89, 140, 179, 251, 279f, 417, 469, 494–95

Housing: adaptation of, 44; in cardiac pregnancy, 140; in asthma, 179–80; in heart disease, 249; in cystic fibrosis, 278–79; in arthritis, 330; in diabetes, 362; in muscular dystrophy, 414–15, 417; and Supplemental Security Income, 439; public, 440; in sickle cell anemia, 440–41; after cord injury, 494. *See also* Location of family

Hunger, 125–26; in cystic fibrosis, 270, 276; in diabetes, 345, 352. *See also* Appetite

Hydrocephalus, 455f, 458ff

Hypoglycemia, *see* Insulin reaction

Hyposensitization, 172–73, 174, 274

Identification: achievement of, in adolescence, 61–64, 283; destruction of mother's, 176; with the aggressor, 212–13; as a lovable person, 284; of worker with client, 316; with medical personnel, 318; spoiled, 318; need for, in diabetes, 356–57; sexual, in muscular dystrophy, 413

Illegitimacy, *see* Pregnancy, illegitimate

Immobilization: of toddler, 58–59; and depression, 69; postoperative, 260; in arthritis, 337–38, 339–40; feelings toward, 421; in cord injury, 495

Immunosuppression, 210. *See also* Steroids

Incidence, 4; birth defects, 5; prematurity in poverty, 124; maternal death from heart disease, 139; neural tube defects, 154–55, 455–56; congenital heart defects, 233, 244; cystic fibrosis, 269; central nervous system leukemia, 371; sickle cell anemia, 433; sickle cell trait, 433. *See also* Prevalence

Incontinence, 159, 290, 457, 462–65, 471–73, 478, 486–90

Independence, 21, 188; in adolescence, 215, 226, 282; in young adult, 283, 298; in spina bifida, 463, 464–65, 471–72, 475–76; after cord injury, 484–85, 488, 494f. *See also* Dependence

Induction, 369, 370, 372, 375, 394

Infancy: socialization in, 25; as stage of development, 26, 57–58; and the vulnerable child, 55; tasks of, 57–58; high risk, 120, 124, 127, 131, 136, 138, 141; diet in, 127, 165–66; defect or disease in, 175, 198, 212f, 233–46 *passim*, 270f, 460–61, 467; and mother, 213; surgery in, 270; response to pain, 336

Infantilization, 66–67, 183–84

Infection: in pregnancy, 140, 141–43, 149; as allergen, 165f, 173, 187; in nephrosis, 200, 202f; after transplant, 210; in heart disease, 236, 241–42, 248–49; and placement of multihandicapped, 268; in cystic fibrosis, 270–71; in arthritis, 321; in diabetes, 344, 353; in leukemia, 369, 372, 393, 395; in muscular dystrophy, 408; in sickle cell anemia, 436f; in spina bifida, 455, 460; in cord injury, 485–86. *See also under* Urinary tract; Viruses

Institutionalization: for pregnant, unwed, cardiac teenager, 140; for multihandicapped, 268; for brain-damaged youth, 298; in spina bifida, 473, 477–79

Insulin, 344, 348; and age, 345, 347; related to food and activity, 346; types of, 347–48; insulin reaction (shock), 347, 349, 351–52, 360; storage of, 348

Insurance: private health, 80–81; dental coverage, 248; entrapment by, 277, 305; and blood costs, 305; and mother's employment, 306; discrimination in sickle cell trait, 452

Intelligence: development of, 27–30; testing, 30; effect of, on impact of asthma, 184–85, 188; post-transplant surge of, 229; scores in heart disease, 264; after head injury, 291–92; in muscular dystrophy, 409f; in spina bifida with hydrocephalus, 458. *See also* Mental retardation

Intensive care experience, 261–62

Intrauterine devices, 146–47

Intrusive procedures, 196f, 211, 317, 348; child's view of, 212; determinants of pain in, 332

Isolation, 44–45, 181, 203, 276, 308, 382, 386, 412, 421, 477

Ketosis (ketoacidosis), 345, 347, 352–53

Kidney, 196–97; artificial (dialysis), 196f, 201, 204, 206–8, 218–27, 229, 230–32; and pregnancy, 136f, 365; tests, 197–98; failure, 198–203 *passim*, 215, 463; in diabetes, 343, 353–54, 365–66; in leukemia, 370, 372; in sickle cell anemia, 437f; in spina bifida, 458, 463; in cord injury, 485, 487, 489. *See also* Transplant, kidney; *and* Chap. 7

Life, and death, 8–9
—expectancy: and socioeconomic status, 7; and pregnancy in diabetes, 139; with kidney transplant, 209; in unoperated heart defects, 245f; in cystic fibrosis, 269, 274, 283; in hemophilia, 300, 302; in diabetes, 343, 345–46, 366; in leukemia, 369, 373; in sickle cell trait, 434; in sickle cell anemia, 437, 451; in spina bifida, 458, 459–60; in cord injury, and use of catheters, 487
—prolongation of: by dialysis and transplant, 201, 206–7, 208, 218–20, 231; in multiple handicaps, 266–68; in cystic fibrosis, 285f; in leukemia, 369; in spina bifida, 458–59, 465–66, 467; resources for decision, 480

Location of family: and allergens, 180–81, 182; and access to care or schools, 223, 230, 249, 278, 296, 307, 319, 415; and climate, 440

Loneliness, 175–76, 180, 190, 396–97, 399

Loss, significance of, 40, 147–48, 217, 228, 255–56

Lung involvement: after transplant, 210; in heart disease, 235, 241–42, 244; in cystic fibrosis, 270–74; in muscular dystrophy, 408

Marriage: and divorce, 32, 129; during pregnancy, 129, 131; abortion within, 149; and genetic counseling, 452
—of affected child: and severity of handicap, 62; in cystic fibrosis, 283; in diabetes, 365; in sickle cell trait, 451–52; in sickle cell anemia, 453; in spina bifida, 470, 475; in cord injury, 493
—of parents, 35, 191; remarriage and the ill child, 50, 413; in asthma, 176; in heart disease, 252–53; in cystic fibrosis, 276, 279; in hemophilia, 306f, 316; and oversold adoption, 319; in arthritis, 328; in diabetes, 361, 362–63; in leukemia, 378, 387; and discipline, 387; in muscular dystrophy, 412; in sickle cell anemia, 446; in spina bifida, 467ff
—of siblings: in hemophilia, 311; in muscular dystrophy, 424

Maternal care projects, 80

Meconium ileus, 270

Medicaid, 77–79, 248, 277, 305, 330, 384, 396, 417, 439

Medical care: access to, 6–7, 249–50, 300ff, 318, 366, 432; resources for, 76–81; use of, 123, 135; perceptions of, 193; and chronicity, 195; fear of, 444; during institutionalization, 479
—in centers: and socioeconomic status, 6, 218–19, 222, 301; size of, and surgical mortality, 240–41; difficulties of attending, 249–50, 251; as determinants of family location, 278; social workers in, 285; proximity to, and adoption, 319; philosophies of, 375; staff stability of, 375; services of, 448, 454
—and treatment: of asthma, 171–74, 176–77, 192; of urinary tract disease, 198–99, 201f, 211; in heart disease, 237–39, 241–47; in cystic fibrosis, 269, 271, 272–74, 277; in hemophilia, 302–4; in arthritis, 324–27, 330, 332; in diabetes, 346–48; in leukemia, 370–73; in sickle cell anemia, 437–38; criteria for, in spina bifida, 459, 460–62; in cord injury, 483–85. *See also*

Orthopedic complications and care; Prenatal care; Surgery
Medicare, 220, 221–22, 225, 277–78
Memory loss, 288, 290, 296
Meningitis, 289; in leukemia, 371; in sickle cell anemia, 438; in spina bifida, 455, 460
Mental retardation: after maternal infection, 142; in hemolytic disease of newborn, 143; and subsequent reproductive behavior, 145; and Down's syndrome, 267; after head injury, 289, 291–92; after insulin reaction, 351; in muscular dystrophy, 409–10; in spina bifida, 455f, 458, 460; and placement, 478. *See also* Intelligence
Mist tent, 273–74, 277, 282
Mongolism, *see* Down's syndrome
Mother: marital status of, 32, 149, 150; deprivation of, 38, 55, 58; separation from, 38f, 169, 189, 213, 251; in chronic illness, 53–55; ambivalence in, 54; and hospitalization, 72, 224, 281, 444; and risks of pregnancy, 120–44, 154; in causation of asthma, 169; dependency on, 171, 189, 282, 308, 310, 413; loneliness of, 175–76, 396–97; identity of, 176; and infantilization, 183–84; and self-responsibility in child, 184; abandonment of, by father, 191–92; dependency of, on child, 192; as punisher and depriver, 212, 358; and diet, 214; in dialysis team, 225; as kidney donor, 228; abandonment by, 231; and anxiety of dialysis, 231; and adolescent, 282, 360; and safety control, 292; reaction to stress in, 293; feelings of responsibility in, 306, 308; need for support of, 358, 396–97, 401; and physician, 360; and awareness of carrier state, 405; reaction to diagnosis in, 411–12; resentment of and by child, 413; in prevention of crises, 436f; and placement, 446, 478; in bowel training, 472; and cord-injured child, 493. *See also* Employment; Family, one-parent; Parents; Pregnancy; Chap. 4
Motivation, 59; in treatment, 407, 472f
Mucoviscidosis, 269
Multihandicapped child, 265–68
Mutation, 153, 301, 405
Myelomeningocele, 455

Needling, 196f, 212, 317, 332, 348
Nephrectomy, 210, 227–28
Nephritis, 197
Nephropathy, diabetic, 354
Nephrotic syndrome (nephrosis), 195, 201–3, 212

Nervous system: central, 203, 288–89, 371, 482–83; autonomic, 289, 483
Neural tube defects, 154–55, 456. *See also* Chap. 17
Neurological involvement: in kidney disease, 203–4, 207, 224; in head injury, 290; in hemophilia, 302f, 316; in diabetes, 354; in leukemia, 371; in sickle cell anemia, 435; in spina bifida, 457, 459, 478; in cord injury, 481, 482–83, 491
Normalcy: regression in illness as, 26; conception as proof of, 54, 145, 316, 365, 447, 453; of family life, in chronic illness, 176, 179, 269, 275; need for, in child, by parent, 258; effect on, of home care in hemophilia, 303, 306, 313; school as symbol of, 392; of life with sickle cell trait, 435
Normlessness, 59, 438, 450f
Nutrition: prenatal, 122f, 124–27; and toxemia, 136f; and asthma, 173–74; in diabetes, 350–51; in leukemia, 387. *See also* Diet

Obstruction: urinary, 199f; bowel, 270
Odor: in cystic fibrosis, 281; in spina bifida, 462f, 471
Oedipal complex, 59–60
Onset: and separation from mother, 189; in hemophilia, 308; in arthritis, 320, 321–22; of diabetes, 344–45, 358; in leukemia, 373; in muscular dystrophy, 405. *See also* Age of onset
Oral gratification and chronic illness, 58
Orthopedic complications and care: in kidney disease, 204–5, 208; after head injury, 291; in hemophilia, 300, 302, 312; in arthritis, 322, 324, 326–27, 334–35; in leukemia, 393; in muscular dystrophy, 407ff; in sickle cell anemia, 435; in spina bifida, 457, 459, 461f. *See also* Fractures
Osteitis fibrosa, 204
Osteodystrophy, renal, 204
Osteoporosis, 322, 407ff
Outlook: pregnancy with diabetes, 138–39; asthma, 174–75; kidney disease, 195, 199, 202, 213; of kidney transplant, 210; in heart defect, 242–47 *passim*; in cystic fibrosis, 283; child's questions about, 285, 381–84; in head injury, 289, 290f; in hemophilia, 300, 318; in arthritis, 320, 322–23; in diabetes, 346; in leukemia, 369; informing siblings of, 387–88; in sickle cell anemia, 435–37, 447–48; in spina bifida, 458–60, 478; in cord injury, 482

Out-of-home care, 91–98, 103–4; in asthma, 183; for multihandicapped, 268; in cystic fibrosis, 279; for brain-damaged, 298; for adolescent with arthritis, 337; after sudden removal, 364; in muscular dystrophy, 416, 430; in sickle cell anemia, 453–54; in untreated spina bifida, 459, 467; in spina bifida, 473, 476, 477–80. *See also* Adoption; Day care

Overprotection: normality of, 193, 302; and social development, 265; and death wish, 275; and expression of aggression, 308–9; and death anxiety, 447; child's feelings about, 474

Pain: of illness, 44, 64–65, 212, 335–37; mechanism for, in hemophilia, 302; effect of clotting materials on, 303; in arthritis, 335–37; of diabetic neuropathy, 354; in leukemia, 390; in muscular dystrophy, 404, 414; in sickle cell anemia, 435ff
—of treatment: abortion, 150; peritoneal dialysis, 206, 209; in hemophilia, 317; by parents, in arthritis, 325; physical therapy, 332–33; in leukemia, 370–73; in muscular dystrophy, 407

Paraplegia, 243, 455, 481, 491, 496–97

Parents: substitutes for, 67, 285, 318, 383, 400–401; relationships, 96–98, 191–92; and satisfaction in adoption, 99f; education of, 159–60, 362, 366, 439; competence of, and foster care, 183; and school, 186; attitudes of, in asthma, 188f; use of asthma to affect, 189–90; role in asthma treatment, 192–93; hospital experience of, 214, 293; need for respite of, 279; groups, 286, 294, 366, 468; and brain-injured behavior, 295–96, 297; diabetic, as model, 363; participation in hospital care, 375–76; behavior of, at diagnosis, 377–81; as support to other parents, 399; reaction to spina bifida, 466, 468; and decisions in spina bifida, 467, 469. *See also* Employment; Father; Marriage; Mother

Parity as risk factor, 121f, 125, 131

Passivity: vs. autonomy, 211, 214; in sickle cell anemia, 450f

Patent ductus arteriosus, 235, 237f, 244, 245–47, 266f

Peer relationship: during hospitalization, 74; in asthma, 184; during dialysis, 227; in cystic fibrosis, 283–84; in hemophilia, 312, 315; in arthritis, 338; in diabetic adolescent, 359; in leukemia, 392; in muscular dystrophy, 421–23; in cord injury, 493, 495–96. *See also* Alienation; Socialization

Perception: and intellectual development, 27–28; emotional filters for, 28; social, after head injury, 291

Percussion, 272f

Permissiveness: excessive, in mother, 184; in physician in asthma, 188

Personality, 14; and stress, 19; and tasks of childhood, 57–64; in asthma, 170–71, 185, 187–89; in kidney disease, 195–96; before and after head injury, 291f; in hemophilia, 311, 319; in arthritis, 335, 341–42; in muscular dystrophy, 420–21; in sickle cell anemia, 449–51

Petechiae, 369, 390

Pets: and the asthmatic child, 181–83, 184; and the leukemic child, 391, 399

Physical education, 61; and asthma, 186; and sickle cell anemia, 449

Physical therapy: in hemophilia, 306; in arthritis, 325–34 *passim*; pain of, 332–33; in muscular dystrophy, 406ff, 425; in spina bifida, 474

Physicians: working with, 114–16, 213; requirements for and role of, 172–77 *passim*, 188, 194, 280, 303, 357, 360, 374–75, 419; communication with, 213, 439; barrier to use of, 256; as model, 318, 469

Placement, *see* Adoption; Institutionalization; Out-of-home care

Plasma transfusion, 303

Platelets, 368f, 372; donors, 371; transfusions of, 371, 385

Play: and development, 27ff; "playing" out experience, 214

Pneumoencephalogram, 290

Postural drainage, 272f, 276, 408

Potassium restriction, 206, 208

Poverty, 30, 122f. *See also* Socioeconomic status

Pregnancy: impact of experience during, 37–38; as proof of normalcy, 54, 145, 316, 365, 447, 453; risk factors in, 120–44; tasks of adolescence and, 129; and kidney disease, 137; and diabetes, 138–39, 365–66; in heart disease, 139–40, 141; prevention of, 144–47, 151–52; needs of, 157–63; in sickle cell trait, 451–52; in sickle cell anemia, 453; in cord-injured, 491
—illegitimate: as risk factor, 122, 130–33; and age, 128, 130, 131–32, 133f, 140; and race, 128, 131; and outcome, 131; and socioeconomic status, 131; and future reproductive behavior, 131–32, 133; needs of, 132–33; and physical handi-

cap in adolescent mother, 140; and availability of abortion, 150; and diabetes, 365
—unwanted: as risk factor, 122; vulnerability to, 147–48; and outcome, 162–63. See also Reproduction
Prematurity: factors associated with, 122–31 *passim*; as risk factor, 123–24
Prenatal care, 158–63; barriers to, 123, 131f; and toxemia, 137; and diabetes, 138; and rubella, 141; and Rh, 141, 143f
Preschool child: and importance of experience, 37; developmental needs of, and illness, 58–59, 211–12, 213f; and asthma, 164, 175f; urine collection in, 197; kidney disease in, 200, 211–15; dialysis and transplant in, 207, 210–11; interpretation of illness, 212; activity limitation in, 241; head injury in, 287f, 295; hemophilia in, 301; arthritis in, 338; as a diabetic, 358; effect of illness on, 389; fears of mutilation in, 389; sickle cell anemia in, 436, 440; screening for sickle cell trait in, 451; paraplegia in, 455
Pressure sores, 291, 354, 407, 408–9, 458, 485; to gain admission to hospital, 475–76; seriousness of, 486
Prevalence, 4; of chronic illness, 5; of chronic disabling conditions, 6; of congenital heart defects, 6; of asthma, 164, 171, 186; of allergy, 165; of emotional disorder in asthma, 187; of kidney-related disease, 195; of renal failure, 203; of rheumatic fever, 233; of congenital heart disease in schoolchildren, 234; of atrial septal defect in adults, 245; of cystic fibrosis, 269; of two or more siblings with cystic fibrosis, 270; of hemophilia, 300; of arthritis, 320; of diabetes, 343; of leukemia, 367; of muscular dystrophy, 403; of emotional problems in muscular dystrophy, 420–21; of sickle cell anemia, 433; of spina bifida, 456. See also Incidence
Prevention: of chronic conditions, and age, 4–5; and socioeconomic status, 122; of illegitimate pregnancy, 133; of high-risk infants, 135; of pregnancy in heart disease, 139; of rubella and Rh damage, 141–42, 142–43, 143–44; of pregnancy, 144–47; of genetic disease, 152–57; of asthma attack, 173; of bacterial endocarditis, 241; in cystic fibrosis, 274; in hemophilia, 302, 306; of hemophilia, 316; in arthritis, 320, 325–26; in diabetes, 352f; in leukemia, 371; in sickle cell anemia, 437, 439, 444; of paternal separation, 469; in cord injury, 485–86. See also Chap. 5
Prognosis, *see* Outlook
Psychosis: after transplant, 230; after cord injury, 492
Psychosomatic approach, 12–14
Public Health Nursing, 173, 179, 186, 252, 340, 416, 462, 464, 495; and the health team, 112–14; as support to foster mother, 279, 480; and death at home, 401
Publicity, effect of, on child and family, 274, 284, 381, 385, 392, 412, 428–29, 450
Public Social Services, 84–104
Pulmonary artery, 234; stenosis of, 235; banding of, 240, 244; in transposition of the great vessels, 243
Punishment: perception of illness as, 60, 192f, 212, 257, 382, 398; procedures viewed as, 336; immobilization viewed as, 337; methods of, in leukemia, 387
Pyelitis, 137
Pyelonephritis, 197f; progression of, 199; and renal failure, 203; in sickle cell anemia, 438; in cord injury, 485

Quadriplegia, 481, 497

Race: and death rate, 6; and one-parent families, 32; and birthrate, 121; and pregnancy in unwed adolescent, 140; and socioeconomic status, 445
Racial distribution: of poverty, 122; of illegitimacy in adolescence, 128; of illegitimacy, 131; of toxemia, 136; of legal abortion, 148; of spina bifida, 154–55, 455–56; of asthma, 164; of cystic fibrosis, 269, 432n; of diabetes, 343; of cancer, 368; of PKU, 432n; of Rh incompatibility, 432n; of sickle cell anemia, 432, 439, 445–46; and use of sickle cell trait screening, 452. See also Ethnicity
Radiation: as risk factor, 122, 149, 234, 368; in treating leukemia, 370, 371–72
Range of motion, 322, 325, 333
Rebellion: pregnancy as, 140; and diabetic diet, 359–60
Recreation and sports: in asthma, 186; in cystic fibrosis, 279, 283; in hemophilia, 303, 309, 315; in arthritis, 326; in diabetes, 364; in leukemia, 393; in muscular dystrophy, 409, 416–17, 427f; in sickle cell anemia, 449; in spina bifida, 477; in cord injury, 495–96
Regression: and stress, 26, 33, 66–67; and rejection, 168; in asthma, 168, 171, 192; in parents after head injury, 294
Rehabilitation: after head injury, 290–91;

INDEX

in cord injury, 483–84; cost of, 484–85; and bladder control, 487; work as, 497
Rejection: by parents, 55, 169, 184, 188–89, 191, 298, 319, 466–78 *passim*; of pregnancy, 162–63; of transplant, 210, 221, 228; by peers, 212–13, 284, 297, 422; by grandparents in hemophilia, 308; by teachers, 313
Religion: and prevention of pregnancy, 139; and prevalence of asthma, 171; and prolongation of life, 219; and treatment of heart defect, 253–54; in adolescent identity achievement, 283; and leukemia, 374, 380, 397–98, 399–400; reliance on prayer, 398; and muscular dystrophy, 418, 428; and hope for afterlife, 429ff; and sickle cell anemia, 447, 450–51. *See also* Clergy
Relinquishment of child, 40, 103, 453, 478
Remission, 322; in arthritis, 322f, 329; in leukemia, 367, 369, 372f, 382, 385–94; and muscular dystrophy, 404
Renal failure, *see under* Kidney
Reproduction: attitudes toward, 120; decisions about, 144, 145–46, 155, 316, 452; in diabetes, 344; attitudes of siblings toward, in muscular dystrophy, 424; in sickle cell anemia, 432, 446–47, 453; in sickle cell trait, 451–52; in cord-injured, 491. *See also* Pregnancy
Resentment: by parents, 176, 182, 192, 309, 311, 319, 413, 445–46, 470; by siblings, 181, 263, 276, 294, 310f, 387f, 493; by teachers, 185; by child, 226, 317, 413, 492f. *See also* Anger
Resistance to drugs in leukemia, 372
Respite, need for, 183, 279, 298, 358, 396, 413, 416, 426, 477, 479
Responsibility: vs. infantilization in asthma, 183–84; of parent vs. physician in asthma, 188; development of, in hemophilia, 302; mother vs. hospital staff in arthritis, 329. *See also* Burden; Decision making; Self-determination
Rheumatic fever, 233
Rh incompatibility: as risk in pregnancy, 143–44; testing for, 143, 158; racial distribution of, 432
Rho-Gam, 144
Rickets, renal, 204–5
Role intensification, 275, 309
Rubella: as risk in pregnancy, 141–43; tests for susceptibility to, 142f, 158; infectiousness of infant, 142; infectiousness of vaccinated children, 143; syndrome, 234, 245, 265–67

Salt loss, in cystic fibrosis, 270, 272
Salt restriction: in pregnancy, 129, 137f, 140; in kidney disease, 201f, 206, 208, 223–24
School: absence related to income, 6; in chronic illness, 45; junior high school, 61, 185, 215, 314, 450; and depression, 69–70; in teenage pregnancy, 130; and asthma, 164, 185–87; adjustment and the teacher, 185–86, 284, 312f, 364, 393f, 449; in kidney disease, 201, 211, 216; and dialysis, 226–27; in heart disease, 263–65; special schools or classes, 291, 296, 314–15, 340–41, 474, 479; after head injury, 292, 296; exclusion of handicapped from, 296; in hemophilia, 307, 312–15; as fun, 312; home teaching, 314–15, 394, 426, 448–49; in arthritis, 340–41; in diabetes, 363–64; in leukemia, 372, 391–94; in muscular dystrophy, 410, 416, 424–26; Life Experience Program, 425; in sickle cell anemia, 448–49, 450; in spina bifida, 458, 462, 474–75
School-age child, 60–61; and asthma, 183–87; heart disease in, 234, 241; and competition, 338; poverty as stress in, 338–39; as a diabetic, 345, 358–59; behavior of, in spina bifida, 473
Secondary gain, 169, 189–90, 314, 360
Self-care: in cystic fibrosis, 282; in hemophilia, 303–4; in diabetes, 348; in muscular dystrophy, 409; in spina bifida, 464–65, 476; in cord injury, 484–85, 486, 490
Self-control: need of child for, 193; effect of illness on, 211; eating as proof of, 214
Self-determination: and chronic illness, 59, 211–12; and decisions in kidney disease, 220; and postural drainage, 276; and bleeds, 317
Self-image: and chronically ill adolescents, 61f, 216, 282, 359; and limitation of competition, 62–63, 338; and dialysis, 224; and post-transplant obesity, 230; effect of school placement on, 296, 341; effect of poverty on, 338–39; effect of reproduction on, 453. *See also* Body image
Sensory information: in muscular dystrophy, 404; in spina bifida, 456f; in cord injury, 481, 483, 491
Separation: and age, 2, 59, 213, 389, 444; in chronic illness, 58; and outcome of adoption, 100; and unwanted pregnancy, 147; and asthma attacks, 169f, 189; in heart disease, 251; and surgery, 260; as reaction to illness, 377, 394–95, 418. *See also* Abdication of father

Septal defect, 235, 238–42 *passim*, 244–45
Sequentiality: of needs for development, 24; of growth, 28, 38–39, 57; of crises, 378
Seriousness: of status asthmaticus, 168; of asthma, 174–75, 191; of urinary infections, 198; of glomerulonephritis, 200f; of heart disease, 233; of cystic fibrosis early in life, 271; of concussion vs. skull fracture, 290; of head injury in hemophilia, 302; of diabetic coma, 353; of spina bifida, 455; of pressure sores, 486. *See also* Outlook
Severity as variable: in marriage of child, 62; in adoption, 100f, 318f; during pregnancy, 136f, 139; in asthma, 170, 175, 184, 187, 193–94; in kidney disease, 211; in heart defect, 247, 262; in cystic fibrosis, 283; in hemophilia, 302, 304, 307, 316, 318–19; in arthritis, 323, 328, 337; in muscular dystrophy, 407, 410; in sickle cell anemia, 432, 435f, 447; in hydrocephalus, 456; in spina bifida, 478
Sex, *see also* Development, sexual
—activity: and vasectomy, 151f; during dialysis, 207–8; of parents in cystic fibrosis, 276; brain control over, 289; in hemophilia, 316; in diabetic girl, 365–66; in cord injury, 483, 491
—difference: in hazard of prematurity, 124; in outgrowing asthma, 174; and dependency of mother in asthma, 192; and hazard of newborn urinary infection, 198; in kidney disease, 211; in effects of family impairment by illness, 218; in effect of growth retardation, 262; in separation of father, 301; in crippling of arthritis, 323; in effect of play restriction, 338; in problem of coma in diabetes, 353; in denial of diabetes, 360; in adjustment to diabetes, 365; in parents' experience of leukemia, 379; in meaning of baldness, 392; in employment in sickle cell anemia, 451; in bladder management after cord injury, 487–88
—distribution: of asthma, 164; and class in asthma, 171; of urinary infections, 198; of urinary anomalies, 200; of glomerulonephritis, 200; of nephrosis, 202; of cystic fibrosis, 283; of hemophilia, 301; of arthritis, 321; of cancer, 368; of muscular dystrophy, 403; of cord injury, 481
Sex-linkage, 154, 156–57, 301, 404–5
Shame, 62, 281–82, 284, 359, 412, 466
Shunts: for dialysis, 207f, 224–25; in heart defect, 246; in spina bifida, 458ff

Siblings: determinants of effect on, 56; deprivation of, 181f, 191, 263, 276, 294, 310, 363, 423; as social contact, 227; as kidney donors, 228; affected, 276, 311; female, and reproduction, 311, 424; as care providers, 339–40, 423; informing, of outlook, 387–88; discipline of, 387; and home death, 402. *See also under* Resentment
Sickle cell disease, *see also* Chap. 16
—anemia: and hospital admission, 6; and inheritance, 153; prenatal diagnosis of, 156; and urinary infection, 199
—trait: vs. sickle cell anemia, 432–33; significance of, 434–35; reproduction in, 451–52; adoption in, 453–54
Side effects: of oral contraception, 146; of hyposensitization, 173; of steroids, 173, 187, 196, 202, 210, 229f, 324; of aspirin, 324, 332; of anti-leukemic drugs, 370, 372; of radiation, 371; of screening for sickle cell trait, 439
Skin problems: in spina bifida, 457–65 *passim*; in cord injury, 485f, 488. *See also* Pressure sores
Sleep, 289; problems of family, 43, 176, 180, 276, 326, 334; and insulin dosage, 353
Smoking: as risk factor in pregnancy, 122, 127; in presence of asthmatic child, 168, 174
Social systems theory, 14–17
Socialization: and vulnerability of infant, 25; in asthma, 184–85, 187; in kidney disease, 212; in heart disease, 257, 263, 265; of family, 276, 308; in cystic fibrosis, 282, 283–84; in brain injury, 296–97; in hemophilia, 312; in diabetes, 359; in muscular dystrophy, 417, 425; in sickle cell anemia, 448; in spina bifida, 476f; in cord injury, 492. *See also* Peer relationships
Socioeconomic status: and treatment of chronic illness, 5; and health statistics, 6; and school absence, 6; and hospitalization, 6, 72; and health, 7; and life expectancy, 7; and stress, 19, 338–39; and employment of mother, 31–32; and marital status of mother, 32, 131; and adoption of handicapped, 100, 319; and birthrate, 121; and prevention of death, illness, handicaps, 122; and pregnancy, 122–23, 124ff, 136, 158–60; and race, 122, 440, 445; and family size, 123; and asthma, 171, 174, 180, 182f, 187; and allergy, 186; and kidney disease, 211, 218–19, 222, 227, 230; and heart disease, 249–50; and hemophilia, 301, 305, 309;

INDEX 555

and crippling in arthritis, 320; and diabetes, 343, 355–56, 361–62, 364, 366; and sickle cell anemia, 438, 440–42; and spina bifida, 455–56, 466–67, 472, 478
Sorrow, chronic, 52–53
Special needs: television, 180, 396, 399, 417, 477; vitamins, 204, 277; laundry equipment, 278, 417, 471; bathtub, 322, 325, 330, 437. *See also* Diet; Equipment; Housing; *and other major needs*
Speech retardation, 288; and maternal deprivation, 38; and head injury, 291
Spinal cord, 482–83; leukemia of, 371. *See also* Chap. 18
Spleen: in cystic fibrosis, 270; in sickle cell trait, 434; in sickle cell anemia, 436f
Squatting, 235f, 241, 246
Status asthmaticus, 167–68, 192
Sterilization, 139, 151–52
Steroids: in asthma, 173; in kidney disease, 202, 229–30; and virus infection, 210; in arthritis, 324f, 330; in leukemia, 369f. *See also under* Side effects
Stigma: and adolescent identity, 62; of sickle cell anemia, 438–39, 446
Still's disease, 321f
Stoma, 463, 465, 471–72
Stress: theory, 14–20; and regression, 26; and capacity to cope, 40f; determinants of degree, 64; number vs. quality of, 134; in asthma, 168ff, 176, 189; in kidney disease, 215, 224; in head injury, 293; effect of cryoprecipitate on, 308; in diabetes, 346, 353; in leukemia, 377, 380, 395–96; and sickle cell trait, 435; in sickle cell anemia, 436, 446; in spina bifida, 478
Stroke: and diagnostic procedures (heart), 237; in sickle cell anemia, 439, 441
Stunting, *see* Growth retardation
Suicide: in dialysis, 220; post-transplant, 230; in cord injury, 481, 491
Supplemental Security Income, 82–83, 277, 282, 337, 439, 467
Surgery: cardiovascular, 139, 141, 207, 235–36, 237–41, 248, 254–57, 266–68; urinary tract, 199f, 213, 463; intensive care after, 261–62; preparation for, 261f; in newborn with cystic fibrosis, 270; after head injury, 291; in hemophilia, 301, 303; in arthritis, 326–27, 329, 334–35, 339–40; in muscular dystrophy, 406, 408; and sickle cell trait, 434; in spina bifida, 455–65 *passim*, 471
Sweat, in cystic fibrosis, 269f
Swelling: in toxemia, 136f; in asthma, 165; in kidney disease, 201ff; in heart failure, 242

Syncope, 241
Synovectomy, 326–27

Tay-Sachs disease, 157
Teratogenic agents, 142, 149
Tetralogy of Fallot, 234f, 238–47 *passim*
Thalassemia, 434, 454
Thirst: in dialysis, 224; in diabetes, 345, 352
Time burden: of kidney disease, 211; of cystic fibrosis, 273, 276; in cord injury, 486; of bladder training, 488; for bowel management, in cord injury, 489–90
Timing: of need and resources, 24f; of experience, 37–38; of solicitude, related to illness, 67; of gestation and infection, 142; of abortion after amniocentesis, 150–51; of prenatal diagnosis and selective abortion, 156; of asthma attacks, 167, 175, 189, 192; in hyposensitization, 173; of dialysis and transplant, 227; of bleeds, 311f; in daily life in diabetes, 343; of sickle cell screening, 452; of foster home placement and special school entry, 479; of vocational counseling in cord injury, 496
Toilet training: and kidney tests, 197; in cystic fibrosis, 276, 281
Toxemia, 128f, 136–37, 138
Transplant, kidney, 118, 208–11, 218–23, 227–32; and paralysis, 204; use of dialysis, 206; and age, 206–7; source related to outcome, 209; removal of kidneys before, 227–28; donors, 228; adjustment to, 229–30; unsuccessful, 229, 232; and family reaction to, 230–32
Transportation: in asthma, 182f; in kidney disease, 215; in heart disease, 249–50; in cystic fibrosis, 278; in hemophilia, 306; in arthritis, 331; in leukemia, 396; in muscular dystrophy, 416–17; in sickle cell anemia, 439f, 442f, 449; in spina bifida, 470, 477; in cord injury, 486, 495
Transposition of the great vessels, 238, 242f
Trauma: in hemophilia, 304; of adoption and hemophilia, 319; in causation of arthritis, 321
Travel: effect of clotting materials on, 303; by air, 363–64, 436; in muscular dystrophy, 416
Tricuspid atresia, 238, 242
Triggering mechanisms, in asthma, 168–69, 189–94
Truncus arteriosus, 242
Trust: as a task of development, 57–58; ability to, and use of medical care, 135; and expression of fears, 429

Tubal ligation, 152

Unconsciousness: in asthma, 168; in heart disease, 235; in head injury, 290; in diabetes, 351
Unitary concept: of man, 12–13; of groups, 14–17; of family, 30
Unpredictability: in chronic illness, 45, 63; in hemophilia, 301–2, 308, 312, 316f, 319; in arthritis, 320f; in sickle cell anemia, 447
Uremia, 196f, 203; in chronic glomerulonephritis, 201; bone disease of, 204–5; during dialysis, 207, 224
Urinary tract, 196–97; infections of, 195–200 *passim*; anomalies, 199–200; surgery, 199f, 213, 463; complications in muscular dystrophy, 408f. *See also* Bladder; Kidney
Urination: difficulties in glomerulonephritis, 201; frequency of, in diabetes, 345, 347; Credé method of, 457, 462, 464, 488
Urine: analysis of, 197; collection of, 197; in kidney disease, 200f; testing in diabetes, 349–50, 352, 359f

Vasectomy, 139, 151–52
Ventricular septal defect, 239–42 *passim*
Ventriculitis, 460
Viruses: and fetal damage, 142; during steroid therapy, 210; in causation of leukemia, 392. *See also* Infection
Visiting Nurse Service, *see* Public Health Nursing

Vocational future: in fatal chronic illness, 69; in cystic fibrosis, 283; in head injury, 297; in hemophilia, 315–16; after arthritis, 320; in diabetes, 343, 354; in sickle cell anemia, 451; in sickle cell trait, 452; in spina bifida, 458, 474f; in cord injury, 496–97
Vulnerability, 11, 19f, 23–24, 25, 37–38; vulnerable-child syndrome, 55, 67, 447

Weakness: in kidney disease, 203; in arthritis, 322; in diabetes, 352; in muscular dystrophy, 403, 406; in spina bifida, 457
Weather as precipitant: in asthma, 166, 169, 187–88; in sickle cell anemia, 436, 440
Weight: low, at birth, 123ff, 127; in pregnancy, 125, 129, 137, 160; after transplant, 210, 229–30; in cystic fibrosis, 270f; in hemophilia, 315; in diabetes, 345; in muscular dystrophy, 406, 408, 415; in spina bifida, 457, 473
Wheezing, 167; causes of, 189–91; and depression, 190
Withdrawal: as normal response, 67; symptoms in infant, 127; in arthritis, 337; in muscular dystrophy, 422

X rays: in prenatal care, 158; in kidney testing, 197–98; in urinary abnormalities, 200; in heart defects, 236–37, 290; in cystic fibrosis, 271; in head injury, 290; as therapy, 371–72
X-linkage, *see* Sex-linkage

SAINT JOSEPH'S COLLEGE, INDIANA
RJ380 .T7   ISJA
Travis / Chronic illness in children : its impact on child a

3 2302 00081 8007